Tissue Engineering and Regenerative Medicine

Tissue Engineering and Regenerative Medicine

Edited by **Shay Fisher**

hayle
medical

New York

Published by Hayle Medical,
30 West, 37th Street, Suite 612,
New York, NY 10018, USA
www.haylemedical.com

Tissue Engineering and Regenerative Medicine
Edited by Shay Fisher

© 2016 Hayle Medical

International Standard Book Number: 978-1-63241-385-7 (Hardback)

Contents

Preface

This book aims to highlight the current researches and provides a platform to further the scope of innovations in this area. This book is a product of the combined efforts of many researchers and scientists from different parts of the world. The objective of this book is to provide the readers with the latest information in the field.

Tissue engineering is a branch of medicine that is majorly dependent on biomaterials. It combines material methods, cells, and biologically active molecules to form functionally active tissues. Regenerative medicine is a branch of tissue engineering which is based on the concept of self-healing with the help of some biological materials to rebuild and recreate tissues and organs. This book provides significant information of this discipline to help develop a good understanding of the core concepts and related aspects of these subjects. As these fields are emerging at a rapid pace, the contents of this book will help the readers get a better understanding of the modern concepts and applications of these subjects.

I would like to express my sincere thanks to the authors for their dedicated efforts in the completion of this book. I acknowledge the efforts of the publisher for providing constant support. Lastly, I would like to thank my family for their support in all academic endeavors.

Editor

Dual mode antibacterial activity of ion substituted calcium phosphate nanocarriers for bone infections

T. S. Sampath Kumar[1]*, K. Madhumathi*[1]*, Y. Rubaiya*[2] *and Mukesh Doble*[2]

[1] *Medical Materials Laboratory, Department of Metallurgical and Materials Engineering, Indian Institute of Technology Madras, Chennai, India,* [2] *Department of Biotechnology, Indian Institute of Technology Madras, Chennai, India*

Nanotechnology has tremendous potential for the management of infectious diseases caused by multi-drug resistant bacteria, through the development of newer antibacterial materials and efficient modes of antibiotic delivery. Calcium phosphate (CaP) bioceramics are commonly used as bone substitutes due to their similarity to bone mineral and are widely researched upon for the treatment of bone infections associated with bone loss. CaPs can be used as local antibiotic delivery agents for bone infections and can be substituted with antibacterial ions in their crystal structure to have a wide spectrum, sustained antibacterial activity even against drug resistant bacteria. In the present work, a dual mode antibiotic delivery system with antibacterial ion substituted calcium deficient hydroxyapatite (CDHA) nanoparticles has been developed. Antibacterial ions such as zinc, silver, and strontium have been incorporated into CDHA at concentrations of 6, 0.25–0.75, and 2.5–7.5 at. %, respectively. The samples were found to be phase pure, acicular nanoparticles of length 40–50 nm and width 5–6 nm approximately. The loading and release profile of doxycycline, a commonly used antibiotic, was studied from the nanocarriers. The drug release was studied for 5 days and the release profile was influenced by the ion concentrations. The release of antibacterial ions was studied over a period of 21 days. The ion substituted CDHA samples were tested for antibacterial efficacy on *Staphylococcus aureus* and *Escherichia coli* by MIC/MBC studies and time-kill assay. AgCDHA and ZnCDHA showed high antibacterial activity against both bacteria, while SrCDHA was weakly active against *S. aureus*. Present study shows that the antibiotic release can provide the initial high antibacterial activity, and the sustained ion release can provide a long-term antibacterial activity. Such dual mode antibiotic and antibacterial ion release offers an efficient and potent way to treat an incumbent drug resistant infection.

Keywords: doxycycline, calcium phosphate bioceramics, antibacterial ion substitutions, bone infections, silver, zinc, strontium, calcium deficient hydroxyapatite

Edited by:
Malcolm Xing,
University of Manitoba, Canada

Reviewed by:
Bingyun Li,
West Virginia University School of Medicine, USA
Wen Zhong,
University of Manitoba, Canada

*Correspondence:
T. S. Sampath Kumar,
Medical Materials Laboratory,
Department of Metallurgical and Materials Engineering, Indian Institute of Technology Madras, Chennai, Tamil Nadu 600036, India
tssk@iitm.ac.in

Introduction

Bone infections are becoming a frequent occurrence due to human longevity, increasing usage of prosthetic implants, and prevalence of drug resistant bacteria. These antibiotic resistant infections place immense burden on the health care system due to the medical complications, long duration of hospitalization, and associated costs. Bone and joint infections mostly fall into three types namely, osteomyelitis (infection of bones), septic arthritis (infection of joints), and prosthetic joint infections

(Bejon and Robinson, 2013). Gram-positive bacteria like *Staphylococcus aureus, β-hemolytic Streptococci, Enterococci, Coagulase-negative Staphylococci, Haemophilus influenza, Escherichia coli,* and *Enterobacteriaceae* are commonly implicated in these infections (Bejon and Robinson, 2013). Osteomyelitis is caused by bacteria introduced through trauma, surgery, direct colonization from a proximal infection, or through systemic circulation. Prosthetic joint infections are most often hospital acquired or nosocomial in origin. Contamination of implant site can occur from sources like the air of the operating room and resident bacteria on the patient's skin and body. Bacterial adhesion on the prosthesis results in biofilm formation, which renders bacteria resistant to most first-line antibiotics (Gristina, 1987). It is estimated that every year more than 2.2 million people are treated surgically for musculoskeletal disorders (Gentleman and Polak, 2006). Another study indicates the incidence of bone infections as approximately 5% of surgeries for fracture fixation devices, 2% of primary joint replacements, and 1.4–4% of total hip and knee replacements (Verron et al., 2012).

Treatment of bone infection involves systemic (intravenous) antibiotic administration in acute conditions and surgical excision of necrosed bone in chronic infections. Systemic administration of antibiotics suffers from side effects and is influenced by factors like the dosage interval and duration (Wu and Grainger, 2006). Bone infections associated with poorly vascularized or necrotic areas receive fluctuating and inadequate dose not capable of destroying the bacterial biofilm. Due to these problems, local drug delivery of antibiotics is favored. The advantages of local delivery include lowered dose, greater control over drug bioavailability and release profile, maintenance of therapeutic concentration at the infection site, avoidance of side effects, and lowered cost (Huh and Kwon, 2011). Currently, the gold standard in local delivery for bone infections is poly methyl methacrylate (PMMA) containing gentamycin available as beads and cement (McLaren, 2004). Various other biopolymers have been tried as drug carriers. However, most polymers are not bioactive, mostly non-biodegradable, and the degradation products produce inflammatory reactions at the local site (Madhumathi and Sampath Kumar, 2014). Bone destruction and defects commonly occur because of bone infections or post surgery. In such cases, osteoconductive or osteoinductive biomaterials promoting bone repair, and regeneration is preferable over polymers as delivery vehicles of antibiotics.

Bioactive ceramics such as calcium phosphate ceramics (CPCs) are attractive candidates for local drug delivery. Hydroxyapatite (HA), calcium deficient hydroxyapatite (CDHA), and tricalcium phosphate (TCP) are some of the CPCs of interest in bone therapeutics. Their degradation products are calcium and phosphate ions, which are commonly present in the human body (Bose and Tarafder, 2012). Human bone is considered as a composite of collagen biopolymer (~20%), reinforced with carbonated non-stoichiometric apatite (~70%) nanocrystals (Dorozhkin, 2010). These apatite nanocrystals have plate like morphology with width 15–30 nm and length 30–50 nm. Among the CPCs, CDHA [$Ca_{10-x}(HPO_4)_x(PO_4)_{6-x}(OH)_{2-x}$; Ca/P = 1.33–1.66] with tailorable Ca/P ratio and degradability is preferred for drug delivery applications (Victor and Kumar, 2008; Madhumathi and Sampath Kumar, 2014). CDHA is structurally similar to stoichiometric

HA (non-biodegradable) and compositionally can be varied even to that of TCP (rapidly biodegradable) (Victor and Kumar, 2008). The apatitic structure presents multiple functional groups to which many biomolecules can bind. Our earlier studies have shown that CDHA nanoparticles of Ca/P ratio 1.61 exhibit the maximum uptake and release of drugs like doxycycline and tetracycline (Victor and Kumar, 2008; Madhumathi and Sampath Kumar, 2014).

Although local drug delivery has more advantages compared to systemic delivery, the main challenge lies in treating drug resistant infections. Drug resistance results in reduced efficacy of antibacterial drugs, increasing the morbidity and mortality. The 2014 WHO global report on drug resistance projects an alarming scenario where common infections and minor injuries can kill humans in the near future (World Health Organization, 2014). Some alternate approaches explored include stimulation of the body's natural defense system by delivering biological molecules like cytokines that stimulate cell-mediated immunity (Li et al., 2009; Boyce et al., 2012), local delivery of antimicrobial peptides (Costa et al., 2011) etc., and developing antimicrobial materials such as antimicrobial polymers (Siedenbiedel and Tiller, 2012), antibacterial nanoparticles (Madhumathi et al., 2010), and a combination of these approaches (e.g., antibiotics with metallic nanoparticles) (Gu et al., 2003) to which drug resistant pathogens are susceptible. Ions such as silver, zinc, and strontium exhibit antibacterial activity against many bacteria. Their mode of action against bacteria is shown in **Figure 1**. Silver exerts its antibacterial activity by both deactivating the mitochondrial enzymes as well as denaturing the DNA of the bacterium (Rameshbabu et al., 2007). Strontium ions, in addition to being antibacterial, are known to up regulate osteoblast proliferation and down regulate osteoclast formation. The bacteriostatic activity of strontium substituted CDHA has been related to its highly negative zeta potential compared to pure CDHA (Ravi et al., 2012). Zinc is not only antibacterial, it also promotes the proliferation of osteoblasts while inhibiting osteoclastic bone resorption. In addition, it also exhibits anti-inflammatory properties. Zinc ions inhibit bacterial growth by binding to the bacterial membrane affecting calcium uptake and changing the membrane fluidity (Venkatasubbu et al., 2011). Some of the ions can also be toxic to mammalian cells. Hence, the above antimicrobial ions incorporated CPCs have been studied

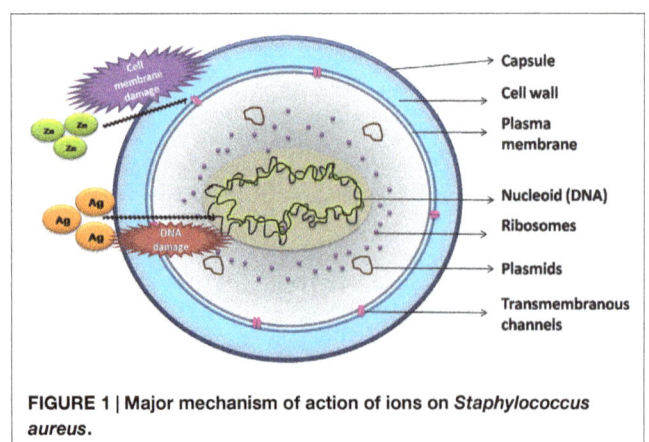

FIGURE 1 | Major mechanism of action of ions on *Staphylococcus aureus.*

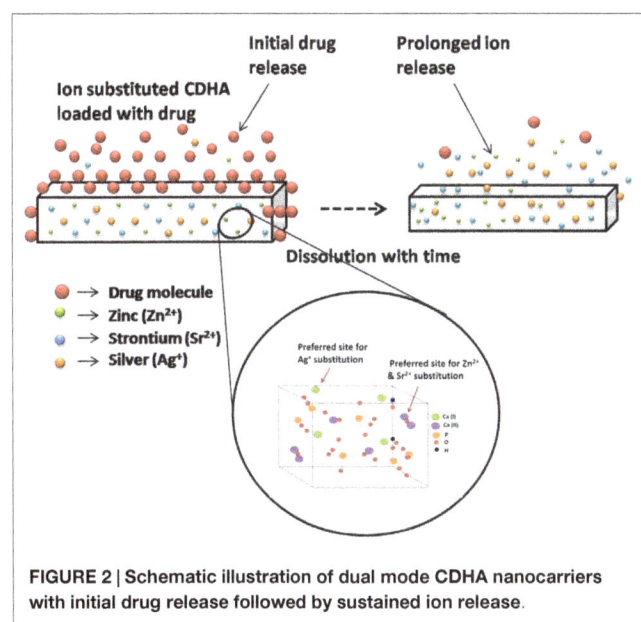

FIGURE 2 | Schematic illustration of dual mode CDHA nanocarriers with initial drug release followed by sustained ion release.

for their antibacterial activity and biocompatibility to establish the therapeutic limit of ion substitution (Rameshbabu et al., 2007; Venkatasubbu et al., 2011; Ravi et al., 2012). The ion substituted bioceramics present salient features such as cost effective preparation, long-term storage, and are amenable to sterilization (Huh and Kwon, 2011). Using the ion substituted bioceramics as carrier for antibiotics offers multiple advantages such as rapid and sustained antibacterial effect, broad-spectrum activity, and in some cases increased potency of drugs (Venkatasubbu et al., 2011).

In this work, an antibiotic delivery system based on antimicrobial ion substituted CDHA nanoparticles with dual mode activity as graphically represented in **Figure 2** was developed. The antibacterial activity was provided by the antibiotic released during the initial phase, which is followed by that of the sustained ion release to contain infections. Ion substituted CDHA of Ca/P 1.61 was prepared by incorporating zinc (Zn^{2+}), silver (Ag^+), and strontium (Sr^{2+}) ions separately at optimal concentrations for the antibacterial effect. All these ions are substituted at the calcium sites of apatite in exchange for calcium ions. While Ag^+ is substituted for Ca^{2+} at Ca(I) cation site, the Zn^{2+} and Sr^{2+} ions can be substituted at the Ca(II) site. The zinc substitution was fixed at 6 at. % since, zinc substituted HA was also shown to exhibit beneficial anti-inflammatory activity at 5% concentration (Velard et al., 2010). Concentrations more than 6% were avoided due to concerns of toxicity. Silver substitution in CDHA was fixed at 0.25–0.75 at. % substitution based on earlier studies, where silver substituted HAs exhibited both antibacterial activity and biocompatibility at 0.5% substitution while 1% substitution showed toxicity (Rameshbabu et al., 2007). Another study has shown that CDHA was both antibacterial and biocompatible at 5 at. % strontium substitution (Ravi et al., 2012). Hence, the strontium substitution was varied between 2.5 and 7.5 at. %. Pure as well as ion substituted CDHAs were synthesized by a microwave accelerated wet chemical synthesis method, which is a rapid method to produce highly pure nanoparticles of narrow size distribution (Siddharthan et al., 2004). Doxycycline is a potent

antibiotic, which also exhibits anti collagenase activity thereby preventing host mediated tissue destruction (Victor and Kumar, 2008). The effects of ion substitutions on the drug release, antibacterial activity, and biocompatibility of CDHA nanoparticles have been studied and analyzed.

Materials and Methods

Materials
Calcium nitrate [$Ca_3(NO_4)_2 \cdot 4H_2O$], diammonium hydrogen phosphate [$(NH_4)_2HPO_4$], zinc nitrate hexahydrate [$Zn(NO_3)_2 \cdot 6H_2O$], strontium nitrate [$Sr(NO_3)_2$], and ammonia (30% GR) were purchased from MERCK, India. Silver nitrate ($AgNO_3$) was purchased from SDFCL, India. All chemicals were pure and of analytical grade. Doxycycline hyclate was purchased from Sigma-Aldrich, India.

Synthesis
Pure and ion substituted CDHAs were prepared as reported earlier (Rameshbabu et al., 2007; Ravi et al., 2012). CDHA nanoparticles were synthesized using a microwave accelerated wet chemical synthesis method using $Ca_3(NO_4)_2 \cdot 4H_2O$ and $(NH_4)_2HPO_4$ as precursor solutions mixed at a Ca/P ratio of 1.61. The pH during the synthesis was maintained above 10 using ammonia. After complete mixing, the solution was subjected to irradiation in a microwave oven (BPL, India) of 800 W for about 30 min using 60% of the power. The precipitate was then washed thrice with distilled water to remove ions such as NH^{4+} and NO_3^{2-}, oven dried at 100°C, and ground to a fine powder using an agate mortar and pestle. The zinc, silver, and strontium substituted CDHAs were synthesized following the same procedure, with the addition of their respective solutions such as $Zn(NO_3)_2 \cdot 6H_2O$/$AgNO_3$/$Sr(NO_3)_2$ to the precursor solution of $Ca_3(NO_4)_2 \cdot 4H_2O$ and titrated with $(NH_4)_2HPO_4$ to obtain (Ca + X)/P ratio of 1.61 (where X = Zn or Ag or Sr). The ion substituted CDHAs with 6 at. % zinc, 0.25–0.75 at. % silver, and 2.5–7.5 at. % strontium were coded as listed in **Table 1**.

Material Characterization
The nanocarriers were characterized for phase purity and structural analysis by X-ray powder diffraction method (XRD, Bruker D8 DISCOVER, USA) using Cu Kα radiation ($\lambda = 1.54$ Å). The diffraction patterns were recorded with step size of 0.1°/step and at a scanning rate of 1 step/s. The functional groups present in pure CDHA and ion substituted CDHA nanocarriers were analyzed in the spectral range of 4000–510 cm^{-1} by Fourier transform infrared spectroscopy (Spectrum Two FT-IR spectrometer, Perkin-Elmer, USA) in the attenuated internal reflection (ATR) mode. Transmission electron microscopy was used to identify the morphology of the CDHA samples. The samples were dispersed in acetone and sonicated for 15 min using an ultrasonic bath (Citizen, India) at frequency of 45 kHz. The dispersions were dropped on carbon-coated copper grids, dried, and examined with a transmission electron microscope (Philips CM20 TEM, Netherlands) operated at 120 kV. The particle size analysis and zeta potential measurements of the pure and ion substituted CDHAs were carried out by dynamic light scattering (DLS) technique (Malvern

TABLE 1 | List of cell parameters, crystallite size, loading and release profiles for ion substituted CDHAs.

Sample code	% ionic substitution	Cell parameters (Å)		Cell volume (Å)³	Average crystallite size (nm)		Doxycycline loading percentage (%) (mean ± SD)	Doxycycline release percentage (%) (mean ± SD)
		a	c		XRD	TEM (mean ± SD)		
CDHA	–	9.110	6.80	519	25	(41 ± 0.6) × (5 ± 0.1)	68 ± 9	61 ± 1.0
ZnCDHA	6	9.014	6.72	509	19	(39 ± 0.7) × (4 ± 0.3)	47 ± 8	57 ± 1.2
0.25AgCDHA	0.25	9.190	6.82	524	27	(41 ± 0.5) × (6 ± 0.2)	37 ± 4	49 ± 1.6
0.5AgCDHA	0.5	9.195	6.81	527	28	(42 ± 0.9) × (6 ± 0.4)	30 ± 3	52 ± 0.8
0.75AgCDHA	0.75	9.198	6.83	529	29	(44 ± 0.5) × (6 ± 0.4)	27 ± 5	55 ± 0.8
2.5SrCDHA	2.5	9.410	6.80	541	34	(47 ± 0.5) × (6 ± 0.3)	31 ± 6	51 ± 1.1
5SrCDHA	5	9.440	6.82	547	38	(49 ± 0.4) × (6 ± 0.2)	26 ± 5	54 ± 0.7
7.5SrCDHA	7.5	9.460	6.83	549	38	(51 ± 0.2) × (6 ± 0.2)	21 ± 6	56 ± 0.9

Zetasizer Nano ZS-90, UK). One milligram of the samples were dispersed in 10 ml distilled water and sonicated for 15 min. One milliliter of the supernatant was then removed and used for DLS measurements.

In vitro Loading and Release Studies of Doxycycline
Loading and release studies of doxycycline from pure CDHA and ion substituted CDHA were performed as described earlier (Madhumathi and Sampath Kumar, 2014). About 10 mg of the drug was dispersed in 10 ml of phosphate buffer solution (PBS) of pH 7.4. To this, 10 mg of CDHA nanocarriers was added. The samples were placed in water bath at 37°C for 24 h. After 24 h, 2 ml of supernatant was removed for estimation of doxycycline concentration at 274 nm using UV-Vis spectrophotometer (Lambda 35, Perkin-Elmer, USA). The samples were centrifuged and dried at room temperature for 24 h. The amount of drug loaded onto the nanocarriers was determined by the following equation:

$$\%Drug\ loading = I_c - F_c/I_c \times 100 \qquad (1)$$

where I_c and F_c are initial and final concentration of doxycycline in PBS. The release study was performed by dispersing 10 mg of doxycycline loaded CDHA nanocarriers in PBS solution of pH 7.4 kept in a constant temperature water bath at 37°C. About 2 ml of supernatant was removed for doxycycline estimation and replaced by fresh PBS at periodic intervals over a period of 7 days. The drug release profile was determined by measuring the absorbance values at different time intervals (F_c) from the initial concentration (I_c). All the experiments were performed in triplicates.

In vitro Dissolution and Ion Release Studies
The in vitro dissolution studies were carried out in PBS of pH 7.4 kept in a constant temperature water bath and maintained at 37°C over a period of 21 days. Ten milligrams of the samples in powder form were dispersed in 10 ml of PBS at a concentration of 1 mg/ml. The weight loss of the samples, pH variations as well as the ionic concentration in the supernatant solution, was regularly monitored. At the end of each experiment, the samples were filtered, dried at 100°C, and weighed to calculate the percentage weight loss. The ion release studies were performed by removing 2 ml of the supernatant from each sample and diluting with 23 ml of distilled water to obtain a total volume of 25 ml.

The concentration of the released Zn^{2+}, Ag^+, and Sr^{2+} ions were determined using an inductively coupled plasma optical emission spectrometer (ICP-OES) (PerkinElmer Optima 5300 DV, USA). These studies were carried out in triplicates for 1st, 3rd, 7th, 14th, and 21st day.

In vitro Antibacterial Studies
Various antibacterial studies such as minimum inhibitory concentration (MIC), minimum bactericidal concentration (MBC), time-kill assays were performed on ion substituted CDHAs against the E. coli (NCIM 2931) and S. aureus (NCIM 5021), which were purchased from the National Chemical Laboratory, Pune, India. The bacteria were stored in glycerol stock at -20°C and used after revival as and when required. The stage of bacteria was determined by plotting a growth curve. They were found to be in stationary phase for MIC/MBC and bacterial growth inhibition studies. However, they were in log phase for time kill assay in view of the longer duration of the bacterial study. Pure CDHA was used as the control. All tests were performed in triplicates.

Minimum Inhibitory Concentration
Minimum inhibitory concentration is the lowest concentration of an antimicrobial agent that inhibited the visible growth of microorganism after incubation of 24 h. Ion substituted CDHA nanoparticles were suspended in nutrient broth at concentrations of 300, 200, 100, 75, 50, 25, 10, and 5 mg/ml and ultrasonicated to ensure optimal dispersion. After 24 h, 10 µl of the inoculum of each microorganism was added to the nanoparticulate suspension. The suspension was then incubated at 37°C for 24 h in a shaking incubator (180 rpm). Nanoparticle-free broths containing bacterial inoculum were used as negative controls. Resazurin dye was used to assess the viability of bacteria with presence of blue color indicating bacterial growth inhibition and a change to red color indicating viable bacteria. About 10 µl of 0.01% resazurin solution was added to the suspension and incubated for 2 h. The MIC of the ion substituted CDHAs was calculated as the lowest concentration of the nanoparticles that did not permit any visible growth of bacteria (blue color) during 24 h of incubation.

Minimum Bactericidal Concentration
Minimum bactericidal concentration refers to the lowest concentration of an antibacterial agent required to kill the bacteria. In

order to determine the MBC, the MIC samples prepared at various concentrations were plated in nutrient agar plates. The plates were incubated at 37°C for 24 h. The lowest concentration at which no bacterial colony was observed was taken as the MBC.

Time-Kill Curve

Pellets of pure and ion substituted CDHA samples were prepared by uniaxial compaction. About 300 mg of the nanoparticulate powder was weighed and compacted in a bench press at a force of 15 kN. The time-kill curve of these pellets was plotted by testing against *S. aureus* bacteria. The pellets were added to 2 ml of nutrient broth containing 1×10^8 CFU/ml in a 24-well plate and incubated at 37°C for 1, 3, 5, and 7 days. Pure CDHA was used as positive control while the bacteria containing broth without nanoparticles were used as negative control. After each incubation period, 100 µl of the broth solution was collected from the 24-well plate and was serially diluted to calculate the number of surviving colonies. About 50 µl of the aliquot of the latter was then added onto a nutrient agar and incubated at 37°C for 1 day for colony formation. The colonies formed were examined and counted. The time-kill curve was plotted as bacterial colony reduction (log CFU/ml) with time.

Bacterial Growth Inhibition Study on Drug Loaded Samples

Drug loaded ion substituted samples (1 mg) were added to 9 ml of the nutrient broth. The suspensions were then inoculated with 1 ml of *S. aureus* bacterial cultures and were incubated at 37°C for 24 h with shaking. The antibacterial efficacy of the drug loaded ion substituted samples was determined from the optical density (OD) of the cultures at 600 nm. The antimicrobial reduction percentage was calculated using the following equation

$$\text{Bacterial reduction}\% = \{1 - (\text{sample OD/control OD})\} \times 100\%. \quad (2)$$

In vitro Biocompatibility Studies

The biocompatibility of the drug loaded CDHA nanoparticles was tested against L6 myoblast cells (NCCS, Pune) by MTT [3-(4, 5-181dimethylthiazole-2-yl)-2, 5-diphenyl tetrazolium bromide] assay. MTT assay is a colorimetric test based on the selective ability of viable cells to reduce the tetrazolium component of MTT into purple colored formazan crystals. The L6 myoblast cells were grown to confluence with Dulbecco's modifed eagle's medium (DMEM), supplemented with 10% fetal bovine serum (FBS) and 1% 100× antibiotic-antimycotic liquid, and incubated at 37°C with 5% carbon dioxide in a CO_2 incubator (Astec, Japan). The cells were then trypsinized and the number of cells was counted with the help of a hemocytometer (Marienfeld, Germany). They were then diluted (10^4 cells per well) and seeded in 96-well plates and cultured for 24 h. One milligram of the CDHA samples was suspended in 1 ml of DMEM and incubated at 37°C for 24 h. The media in the 96-well plates were then replaced with 100 µl of the supernatant from the CDHA samples and again incubated for 24 h. About 20 µl of 5 mg/ml MTT was added to each well and incubated for 4 h. The formazan precipitates were solubilized in dimethyl sulfoxide (DMSO) and

the absorbance was measured at 570 nm using a multimode plate reader (EnSpire, Perkin-Elmer, Singapore). The percentage of viable cells was calculated as the percentage relative to the control (standard polystyrene tissue culture plates) using the following equation

$$\%\text{Cell viability} = (\text{mean OD/control OD}) \times 100. \quad (3)$$

Statistical Analysis

The values are expressed as mean ± SD. Statistical analysis was performed using one and two way ANOVA wherever applicable. The *p*-value <0.05 was considered statistically significant.

Results

Material Characterization

The XRD pattern of the CDHA and ion substituted CDHAs was compared with the standard HA pattern (JCPDS 09-432) as shown in **Figure 3A**. All the samples showed similar diffraction pattern corresponding to the characteristic peaks of HA. The absence of peaks other than HA confirms the formation of monophase CDHAs unaffected by ionic substitutions. The average crystallite size of the particles (*t*) was calculated from the broadening of the peak at 26° corresponding to (0 0 2) reflection using Scherrer's formula [$t = 0.9\lambda/B\cos\theta$], where λ = wavelength of CuKα radiation and B = full width at half maximum value (in radians) of the diffraction peak at 26°(2θ). The cell parameters and cell volume were calculated from the XRD data using the program "UnitCell" and are listed in **Table 1**, along with the crystallite size of the synthesized powders. It can be seen from **Table 1** that the cell parameters varied with the type and concentration of substituted ions. Compared to pure CDHAs, the cell parameters and cell volume for zinc substituted CDHA showed a decrease while there was an increase in the case of silver and strontium substitution. The average crystallite size of pure CDHA was 25 nm. The crystallite size showed variations on ion substitution with values ranging from 19 nm for zinc to 27–32 nm in case of silver and strontium substituted CDHAs. The functional groups present in the ion substituted CDHAs were identified using FT-IR spectroscopy. **Figure 3B** shows the typical FT-IR spectra of pure and ions substituted CDHAs. All the characteristic vibration bands of CDHA such as PO_4^{3-} (564, 603, 962, and 1032 cm^{-1}), structural OH^- (633 and 3570 cm^{-1}), and CO_3^{2-} (1403 and 1455 cm^{-1}) were present in all the samples (Siddharthan et al., 2004). The presence of HPO_4^{2-} at 876 cm^{-1} confirms that the samples were CDHAs in nature. The absence of any other new bands suggests that the ions have been substituted into the crystal structure without the formation of any other intermediate compounds.

The TEM images (**Figure 4**) show that the nanoparticles have a rod or acicular morphology. The particle sizes calculated from TEM micrographs using Image J software are listed in **Table 1**. Pure CDHA showed a size of $(41 \pm 0.6) \times (5 \pm 0.1)$ nm while the zinc substituted CDHA show a decrease in the size $(39 \pm 0.7) \times (4 \pm 0.3)$ nm. Both silver and strontium substituted CDHAs are larger compared to pure CDHA. In case of silver substitution, the size increases to a maximum of

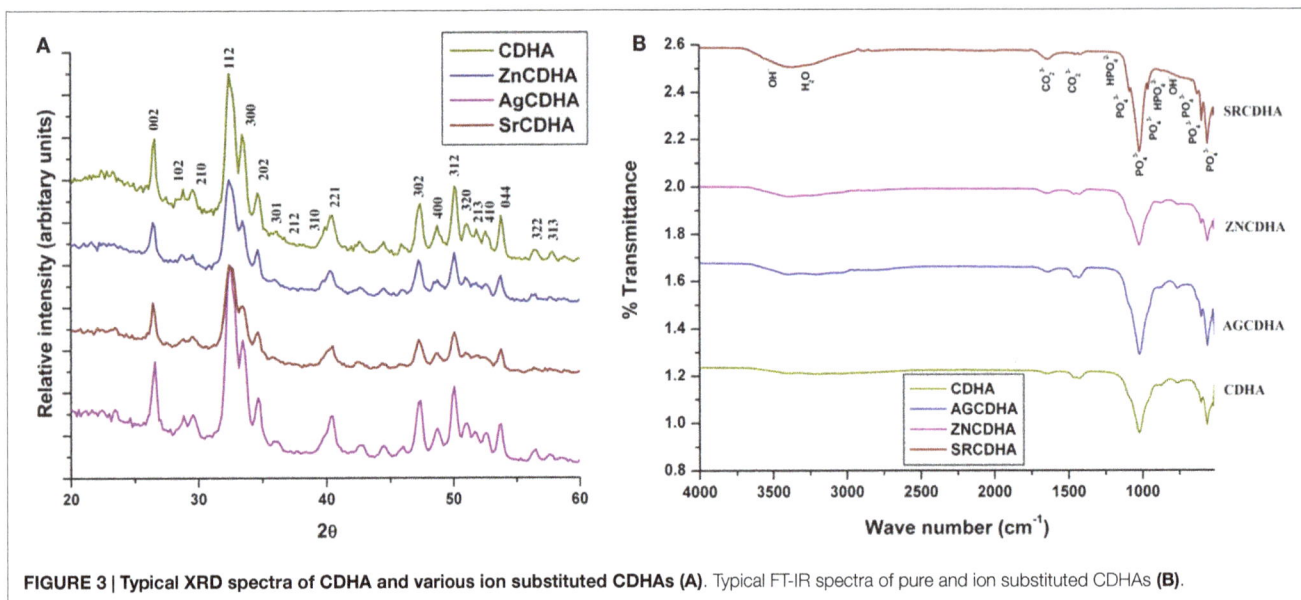

FIGURE 3 | Typical XRD spectra of CDHA and various ion substituted CDHAs (A). Typical FT-IR spectra of pure and ion substituted CDHAs (B).

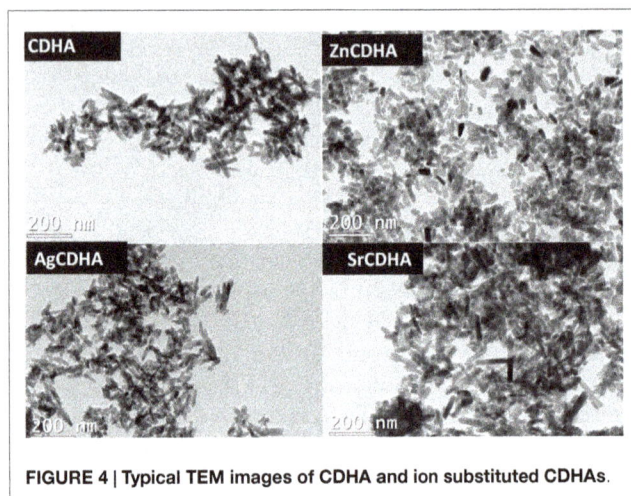

FIGURE 4 | Typical TEM images of CDHA and ion substituted CDHAs.

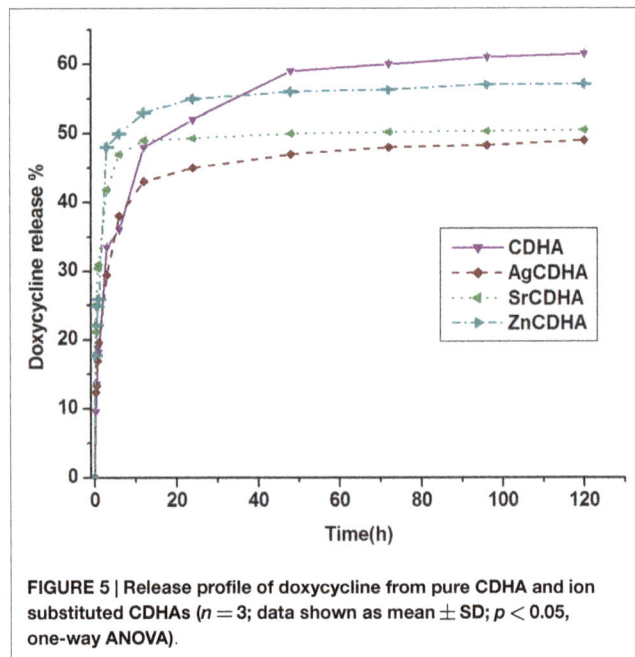

FIGURE 5 | Release profile of doxycycline from pure CDHA and ion substituted CDHAs ($n = 3$; data shown as mean $\pm$ SD; $p < 0.05$, one-way ANOVA).

$(44 \pm 0.5) \times (6 \pm 0.4)$ nm approximately while strontium substituted CDHAs show an even larger size of $(51 \pm 0.2) \times (6 \pm 0.2)$ nm approximately. The particle size obtained from TEM correlates with that of XRD crystallite results.

In vitro Drug Loading and Release Studies

The loading and release values of doxycycline from CDHA and ion substituted CDHAs are listed in **Table 1**. The loading and release percentage of doxycycline was found to be lower for all ion substituted samples compared to pure CDHA. In case of silver and strontium substituted samples, a decrease in loading of doxycycline with an increase in the amount of ion substitution was observed. Pure CDHA showed a doxycycline loading of $68 \pm 9\%$ and $69 \pm 5\%$ release. The zinc substituted CDHA showed a loading of $47 \pm 8\%$, while silver substituted CDHAs showed between (27 ± 5) and $(37 \pm 4)\%$, and strontium substituted CDHAs showed a loading of (21 ± 6)–$(31 \pm 6)\%$. One-way ANOVA test was used to statistically analyze the samples in triplicates and the results were statistically significant with $p < 0.05$.

The release percentage of doxycycline as listed in **Table 1** indicates a different trend. A classic two-stage release with an initial burst release in 6 h followed by sustained release was observed. The release percentage of doxycycline has been found to decrease for all the substituted CDHAs. However, an increase in release was observed with increased ion substitution. The 6% zinc substituted CDHA, 0.25% silver substituted CDHA, and 2.5% strontium substituted CDHA samples with maximum loading and higher amount of total drug release were selected as the best samples for further particle size analysis, in vitro dissolution, and biological studies. The samples were coded as ZnCDHA, AgCDHA, and SrCDHA, respectively. The doxycycline loading percentage and release profile of these nanocarriers are shown in **Table 1** and **Figure 5**.

TABLE 2 | List of particle size and zeta potential of CDHA samples.

Samples	Hydrodynamic diameter (d.nm) (mean ± SD)	Zeta potential (mV) (mean ± SD)
CDHA	1413 ± 16	−20.7 ± 0.4
AgCDHA	2181 ± 12	−14.9 ± 0.3
SrCDHA	1313 ± 07	−14.3 ± 1.0
ZnCDHA	2068 ± 21	−13.7 ± 0.3

Particle Size Analysis and Zeta Potential Measurements

The particle size analysis and zeta potential measurements of CDHA samples by DLS studies are listed in **Table 2**.

The hydrodynamic diameter obtained is more than 1000 nm for all samples. The hydrodynamic diameter of AgCDHA and ZnCDHA was significantly higher than pure CDHA, while that of SrCDHA was the lowest. The negative surface charge of CDHA is reflected in the zeta potential values as expected. The ion substituted samples exhibit highly negative zeta potential compared to pure CDHA (Ravi et al., 2012). The studies were conducted as triplicates. The one-way ANOVA test results were statistically significant with $p < 0.0001$.

In vitro Dissolution and Solubility Studies

The *in vitro* dissolution of CDHA and ion substituted CDHAs were measured by the weight loss and pH variation as shown in **Figures 6** and **7**, respectively. All the synthesized nanopowders showed weight loss from the first day onward (**Figure 6**). Compared to pure CDHA, silver substituted CDHAs show a reduced weight loss suggesting lower solubility and higher stability. Strontium substitution on the other hand appears to increase the solubility of the CDHAs with more than 90% weight loss in a 21 day period. Although, the ZnCDHA exhibited a greater initial solubility than CDHA for up to 3 days, they show lower solubility than CDHA from seventh day onward and the difference becomes statistically significant by 21st day. The dissolution studies were analyzed by a two-way ANOVA test. The difference between the samples was found to be statistically significant with $p < 0.0001$. The pH values of the PBS solution in which ion substituted CDHAs were dispersed have also been found to decrease during this duration as shown in **Figure 7A**. There was a slight decrease in the pH from initial 7.4 to 7.32 for AgCDHA and SrCDHA and reaches 7.15 for ZnCDHA at the end of 21 days. The ion release profiles obtained from dissolution studies of the samples are shown in **Figure 7B**. Zinc ions were found at higher concentration followed by strontium and silver ions.

In vitro Antibacterial Studies

The MIC and MBC values of the ion substituted samples are listed in **Table 3**. It can be seen that AgCDHA has the lowest MIC and MBC for both the bacteria even at low substitution. ZnCDHA showed a MIC of 200 µg/µl against both the bacteria. However, strontium substituted CDHAs showed very low antibacterial activity against *S. aureus* and no activity upto 300 µg/µl against *E. coli*. The MBC values also reflect a similar trend.

The time-kill studies on *S. aureus* showed a reduction in bacterial growth for ion substituted samples. AgCDHA and ZnCDHA

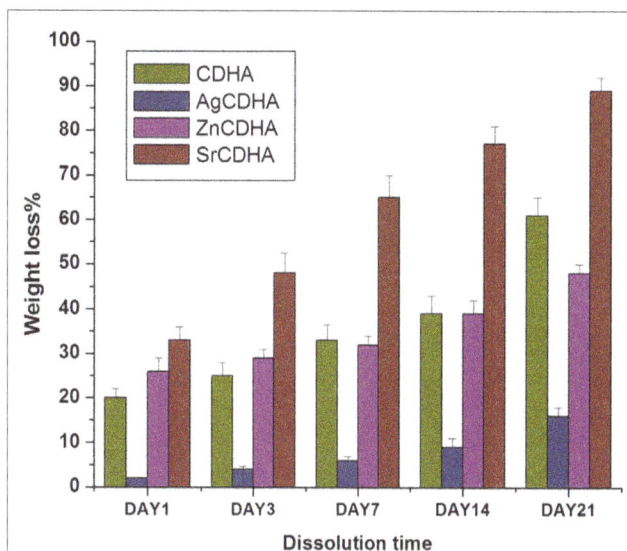

FIGURE 6 | *In vitro* solubility studies showing the weight loss of ion substituted CDHAs in PBS of pH 7.4 at 37°C ($n = 3$; data shown as mean ± SD; $p < 0.0001$, two-way ANOVA).

showed complete inhibition with absence of colonies on second day itself (**Figure 8A**). Two-way ANOVA was performed and a value of $p < 0.0001$ was obtained. The antibacterial activity of doxycycline loaded ion substituted CDHA nanoparticles were determined by incubating them with bacteria in a liquid broth. The results are shown in **Figure 8B**. It can be seen that there is a decrease in the antibacterial activity of the drug loaded substituted CDHAs compared to only drug loaded pure CDHA. Doxycycline loaded AgCDHA, especially, showed lower activity than other samples at the end of 24 h. The statistical analysis was calculated by one-way ANOVA with $p < 0.05$ considered significant.

In vitro Biocompatibility Studies

The biocompatibility of the samples before and after drug loading was tested by MTT assay and the results are shown in **Figure 9**. All samples were found to be biocompatible at a concentration of 1 mg/ml, with the cell viability above 80% at the end of 48 h. The biocompatibility of AgCDHA did not vary between 24 and 48 h of incubation while ZnCDHA and SrCDHA showed a decrease in cell viability after 24 h. Doxycycline loaded samples showed variations in biocompatibility in case of ZnCDHA and SrCDHA at the end of 24 h. Although, drug loaded AgCDHA did not show any statistical difference in cell viability, there was a reduction in cell viability for other drug loaded samples compared to pure samples at 24 h. At the end of 48 h, the cell viability of drug loaded samples showed no significant variation compared to that of 24 h incubation. The statistical analysis was conducted by two-way ANOVA test for triplicate samples with a significance of $p < 0.005$.

Discussion

Conventional treatment of bone infections suffer from problems like emergence of drug resistance and persistence of infections due to inadequate dose, leading to poor healing of bone that can be addressed with the help of nanotechnology. A dual strategy

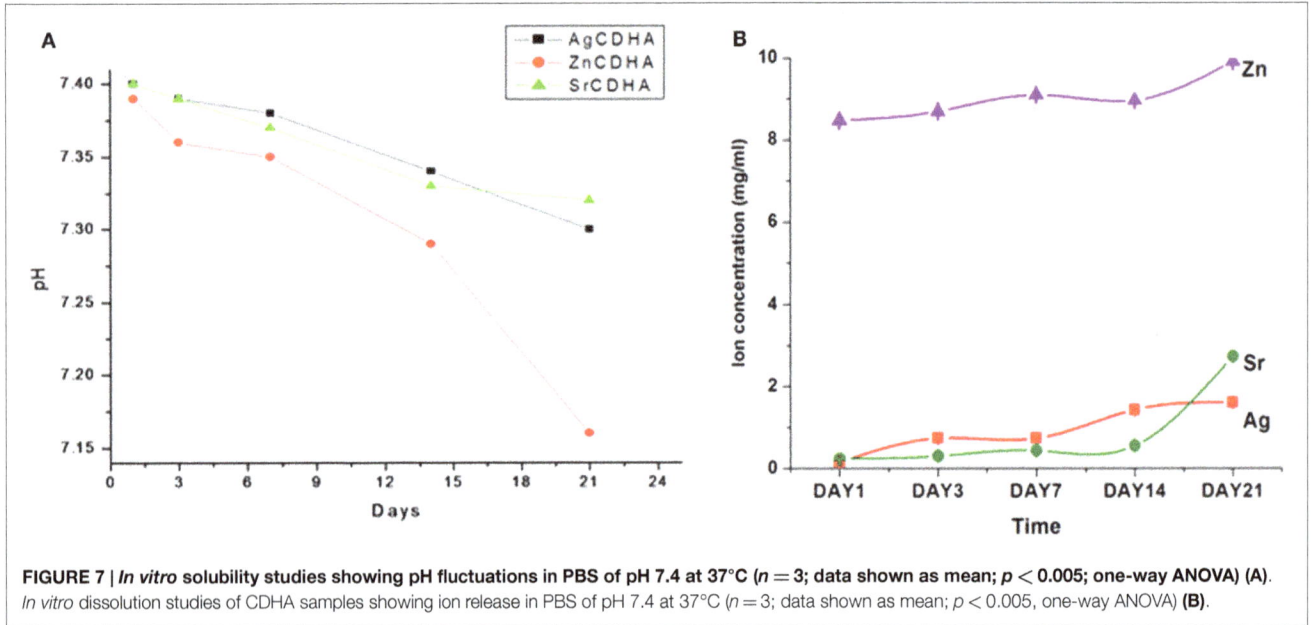

FIGURE 7 | *In vitro* solubility studies showing pH fluctuations in PBS of pH 7.4 at 37°C ($n = 3$; data shown as mean; $p < 0.005$; one-way ANOVA) **(A)**. *In vitro* dissolution studies of CDHA samples showing ion release in PBS of pH 7.4 at 37°C ($n = 3$; data shown as mean; $p < 0.005$, one-way ANOVA) **(B)**.

TABLE 3 | MIC and MBC values of various ion substituted CDHAs.

Samples	S. aureus		E. coli	
	MIC (µg/µl)	MBC (µg/µl)	MIC (µg/µl)	MBC (µg/µl)
ZnCDHA	200	200	200	300
AgCDHA	20	25	10	20
SrCDHA	200	300	–	–

of combining antibiotic release with antibacterial ion release can act effectively against persistent biofilms and can even prevent emergence of drug resistance. In this regard, CDHA nanoparticles offers a good platform for both ion substitution and drug release. The apatitic structure of CDHA provides multiple sites for ion substitution as well as drug/protein binding. CDHA also has higher bioactivity, higher specific surface area, and high efficient precipitation of bone like apatites compared to other calcium phosphates (Dorozhkin, 2010).

Highly pure ion substituted CDHA nanoparticles were obtained by microwave accelerated wet chemical method as evidenced from XRD, FT-IR, and TEM results. The ion substitutions have been found to influence structural parameters, drug loading and release capacity, particle stability, antibacterial activity, and biocompatibility. The cell volume, lattice parameters, and crystallite size vary with difference in the ionic radii of the substituting ions compared to calcium ions. ZnCDHA show a reduction in the cell parameters and size since Zn^{2+} ions have a smaller ionic radii of 0.74 Å compared to Ca^{2+} (0.99 Å). The above parameters have been found to increase in AgCDHAs and SrCDHAs, since Ag^+ (1.28 Å) and Sr^{2+} (1.18 Å) ions have higher ionic radii than Ca^{2+}.

The loading and release of doxycycline is also affected by the ion substitutions. Doxycycline binds to the Ca^{2+} site of CDHA (Victor and Kumar, 2008). A partial substitution of Ca^{2+} by other ions has reduced the binding sites for doxycycline as seen from the lower loading percentage. The loading decreases with increasing ion substitutions. It can be seen that even small amounts of silver substitution (<1at. %) show a high impact on doxycycline loading. The drug release percentage and profile was also affected by ion substitutions. The release profile shows the burst release of the drug from AgCDHA and SrCDHA, suggesting surface adsorption is the main mechanism of drug binding. It is surprising to observe that the biphasic release from ZnCDHA is closer to that of CDHA despite the relatively higher substitution. Since an optimal drug binding capacity is expected from the CDHA system, samples were selected based on the loading and release studies. Thus, 0.25% Ag^+ substituted CDHA and 2.5% Sr^{2+} substituted CDHA was selected for further studies along with 6% Zn substituted CDHA.

In vitro dissolution and stability studies are essential to understand the behavior of ion substituted CDHA in physiological system. Since, the antibacterial activity is not only dependant on drug release but also on ion release, these studies assume significance. A 21 day study showed that silver substitution lowered the solubility while strontium increased the solubility of CDHA. Substitutions with zinc showed a lower solubility than pure CDHA at 21st day. At the end of 21 day period, SrCDHA sample showed the maximum solubility with more than 90% weight loss. Strontium substitutions are known to decrease the crystallinity of CDHA, which can be a factor for the high solubility (Aina et al., 2012; Ravi et al., 2012). The order of weight loss was SrCDHA > CDHA > ZnCDHA > AgCDHA. This also correlates well with the ion release, since zinc and strontium ion concentration in PBS was higher than silver ions during this period. The pH study was done in a buffer solution where immediate variation may not be visible, while ICP analysis indicates the actual ion concentrations at a higher resolution. Hence, the trend of pH values may not correlate with Zn ion concentrations at day 1. The stability of the nanoparticles in a liquid medium was also investigated. The particle size obtained by TEM and the hydrodynamic

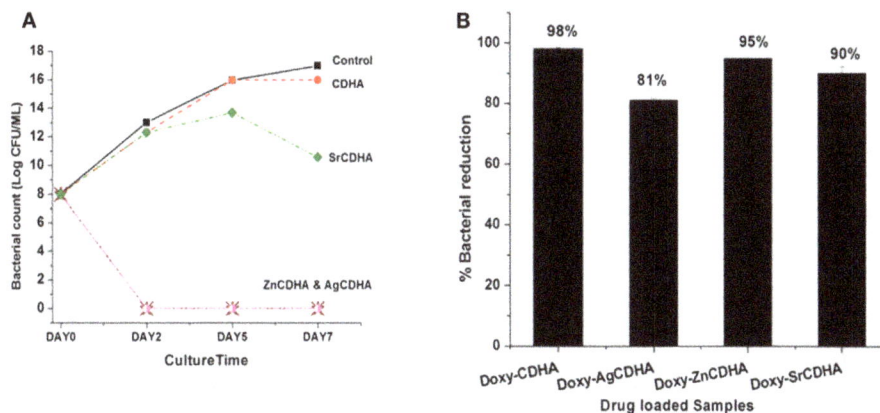

FIGURE 8 | Time-kill curve showing log reduction against *S. aureus* for ion substituted CDHA samples (A) (*n* = 3; data shown as mean; *p* < 0.0001, one-way ANOVA). Antibacterial activity of CDHA and ion substituted CDHA nanoparticles loaded with doxycycline (doxy – doxycycline) against *S. aureus* (B) (*n* = 3; data shown as mean ± SD; *p* < 0.005, one-way ANOVA).

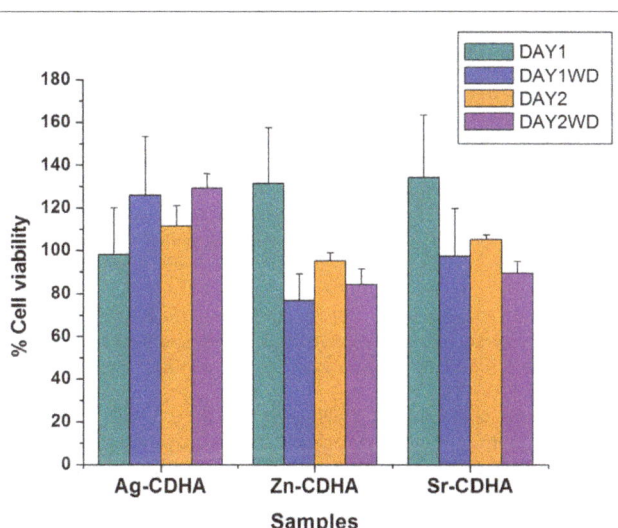

FIGURE 9 | Biocompatibility studies of pure and doxycycline loaded ion substituted CDHA samples (1 mg/ml) by MTT assay for 24 and 48 h (WD – with doxycycline) (*n* = 3; data shown as mean ± SD; *p* < 0.005, two-way ANOVA).

diameter obtained by DLS measurements do not correlate because of both anisotropic non-spherical nature as well as aggregation of the nanoparticles. Since, the particles are intended for local drug delivery, the aggregation of nanoparticles in aqueous medium should not pose any problem. The zeta potential values also reflect the unstable nature of the nanoparticles with values between -13.7 and -20.7 mV.

Antibacterial activity of ion substituted CDHAs before and after drug loading was evaluated by multiple studies including MIC/MBC determination and time-kill assay. The MIC and MBC studies test the bacteriostatic (growth inhibitory) and bactericidal (killing of bacteria) effects of the samples respectively. Of the three ions, silver is the most potent antibacterial agent, which is bactericidal in nature. AgCDHA is highly effective against both *S. aureus* and *E. coli*, as can be seen from the MIC and MBC values.

ZnCDHA shows moderate antibacterial activity against both bacteria with similar MIC values. However, the MBC of zinc is higher for *E. coli*. This is because gram-positive bacteria like *S. aureus* are more susceptible to zinc ions than gram-negative *E. coli* due to the difference in the protein constituents of their cell walls (Jain et al., 2013). SrCDHA showed a weak antibacterial activity against *S. aureus*. However, no antimicrobial activity was observed against *E. coli* at upto 300 µg/µl. The time-kill assay was used to evaluate the time dependant antibacterial effect of ion substituted CDHAs on *S. aureus* bacterial growth. This assay was found to be ideal to evaluate the antibacterial action of ions released from substituted CDHAs in a time dependant manner. Similar studies for zinc substituted HA have been reported earlier (Thian et al., 2013). The trend observed in the MIC/MBC studies was also reflected in time-kill studies, with both AgCDHA and ZnCDHA inhibiting the bacterial growth, as their concentration (300 µg/µl) was more than their MBC. SrCDHA showed an incomplete growth reduction since its MBC was more than 300 µg/µl. The antibacterial activity of doxycycline loaded ion substituted samples against *S. aureus* present interesting results. There is an overall marginal reduction in the antibacterial activity of doxycycline loaded ion substituted CDHAs compared to pure CDHA at the end of 24 h. This can be explained in conjunction with the drug loading. The initial antibacterial activity is provided by the doxycycline drug, which is loaded at lower amounts in ion substituted samples. Silver shows the lowest loading (~31%) and hence its antibacterial activity is also lower than other samples at 24 h. Thus, though silver ion is highly antibacterial, it is released only by the time dependant dissolution of the CDHA nanoparticles during which the drug released provides the antibacterial activity.

Biocompatibility of ion substituted CDHAs is an important criteria for its clinical applications. Though the ions were substituted at concentrations deemed biocompatible, the biocompatibility of drug loaded substituted CDHAs had to be evaluated using MTT assay. The doxycycline concentration was approximately 0.18 µg/µl for CDHA, 0.26 µg/µl for ZnCDHA, 0.12 µg/µl for AgCDHA, and 0.15 µg/µl for SrCDHA samples as calculated from drug release studies at the end of 24 h.

The doxycycline release reduces the cell viability during first 24 h for ZnCDHA and SrCDHA while no appreciable difference was observed for AgCDHA samples with and without drug loading. However, a statistically significant decrease in cell viability was observed for ZnCDHA and SrCDHA at the end of 48 h compared to 24 h. However, all the samples were found to be biocompatible at the given concentration. The results clearly demonstrate the advantage of ion substituted CDHAs, as the controlled release of ions incorporated into CDHAs plays an important role in improving the biocompatibility.

Among various ion substituted CDHAs, AgCDHA with 0.25% substitution shows the lowest doxycycline loading. However, it exhibits the highest antibacterial activity and is also biocompatible. The SrCDHA sample shows low loading of doxycycline and lowest antibacterial activity but exhibits higher biocompatibility. Although, the ZnCDHA sample exhibits reasonable drug loading and satisfactory antibacterial activity, it shows lower cell viability compared to pure CDHA and other ion substituted samples. The CDHA and AgCDHA samples exhibit drug release up to 5 days while there was no change in the drug release profile after first day for SrCDHA and ZnCDHA samples. But both ZnCDHA and AgCDHA show high antibacterial activity at day 2 in spite of their different drug release profiles. Although, SrCDHA show maximum drug release by first day, it exhibits antibacterial activity from day 2 onward. A long-term antibacterial and cytotoxic study may clearly bring out the combined role of ion substitution and drug release in combating antimicrobial resistance.

Thus, the present work demonstrates that by combining antibiotics and antimicrobial ions, a biocompatible, sustained, highly efficient antibacterial bioceramic system with additional beneficial properties such as anti-inflammatory activity or bone remodeling activity can be developed to efficiently contain and treat bone infections.

References

Aina, V., Lusvardi, G., Annaz, B., Gibson, I. R., Flora, E., and Malavasi, I. G. (2012). Magnesium- and strontium-co-substituted hydroxyapatite: the effects of doped ions on the structure and chemico-physical properties. *J. Mater. Sci. Mater. Med.* 23, 2867–2879. doi:10.1007/s10856-012-4767-3

Bejon, P., and Robinson, E. (2013). Bone and joint infection. *Medicine* 41, 719–722. doi:10.1016/j.mpmed.2013.09.008

Bose, S., and Tarafder, S. (2012). Calcium phosphate ceramic systems in growth factor and drug delivery. *Acta Biomater.* 8, 1401–1421. doi:10.1016/j.actbio.2011.11.017

Boyce, B. M., Lindsey, B. A., Clovis, N. B., Smith, S., Hobbs, G. R., Hubbard, D. F., et al. (2012). Additive effects of exogenous IL-12 supplementation and antibiotic treatment in infection prophylaxis. *J. Orthop. Res.* 30, 196–202. doi:10.1002/jor.21520

Costa, F., Carvalho, I. F., Montelaro, R. C., Gomes, P., and Martins, M. C. L. (2011). Covalent immobilization of antimicrobial peptides (AMPs) onto biomaterial surfaces. *Acta Biomater.* 7, 1431–1440. doi:10.1016/j.actbio.2010.11.005

Dorozhkin, S. V. (2010). Nanosized and nanocrystalline calcium orthophosphates. *Acta Biomater.* 6, 715–734. doi:10.1016/j.actbio.2009.10.031

Gentleman, E., and Polak, J. (2006). Historic and current strategies in bone tissue engineering: do we have a hope in hench? *J. Mater. Sci. Mater. Med.* 17, 1029–1035. doi:10.1007/s10856-006-0440-z

Gristina, A. G. (1987). Biomaterial-centered infection: microbial adhesion versus tissue integration. *Science* 237, 1588–1595. doi:10.1126/science.3629258

Gu, H., Ho, P. L., Tong, E., Wang, L., and Xu, B. (2003). Presenting vancomycin on nanoparticles to enhance antimicrobial activities. *Nano Lett.* 3, 1261–1263. doi:10.1021/nl034396z

Huh, A. J., and Kwon, Y. J. (2011). Nanoantibiotics: a new paradigm for treating infectious diseases using nanomaterials in the antibiotics resistant era. *J. Control. Release* 156, 128–145. doi:10.1016/j.jconrel.2011.07.002

Jain, A., Bhargava, R., and Poddar, P. (2013). Probing interaction of Gram-positive and Gram-negative bacterial cells with ZnO nanorods. *Mater. Sci. Eng. C* 33, 1247–1253. doi:10.1016/j.msec.2012.12.019

Li, B., Jiang, B., Boyce, B. M., and Lindsey, B. A. (2009). Multilayer polypeptide nanoscale coatings incorporating IL-12 for the prevention of biomedical device-associated infections. *Biomaterials* 30, 2552–2558. doi:10.1016/j.biomaterials.2009.01.042

Madhumathi, K., and Sampath Kumar, T. S. (2014). Regenerative potential and antibacterial activity of tetracycline loaded apatitic nanocarriers for the treatment of periodontitis. *Biomed. Mater.* 9, 035002. doi:10.1088/1748-6041/9/3/035002

Madhumathi, K., Sudeesh Kumar, P. T., Abhilash, S., Sreeja, V., Tamura, H., Manzoor, K., et al. (2010). Development of novel chitin/nanosilver composite scaffolds for wound dressing applications. *J. Mater. Sci. Mater. Med.* 21, 807–813. doi:10.1007/s10856-009-3877-z

McLaren, A. (2004). Alternative materials to acrylic bone cement for delivery of depot antibiotics in orthopaedic infections. *Clin. Orthop. Relat. Res.* 427, 101–106. doi:10.1097/01.blo.0000143554.56897.26

Rameshbabu, N., Kumar, T. S., Prabhakar, T., Sastry, V., Murty, K., and Rao, K. P. (2007). Antibacterial nanosized silver substituted hydroxyapatite: synthesis and characterization. *J. Biomed. Mater. Res. A* 80, 581–591. doi:10.1002/jbm.a.30958

Ravi, N. D., Balu, R., and Sampath Kumar, T. S. (2012). Strontium-substituted calcium deficient hydroxyapatite nanoparticles: synthesis, characterization, and antibacterial properties. *J. Am. Ceram. Soc.* 95, 2700–2708. doi:10.1111/j.1551-2916.2012.05262

Siddharthan, A., Seshadri, S. K., and Sampath Kumar, T. S. (2004). Microwave accelerated synthesis of nanosized calcium deficient hydroxyapatite. *J. Mater. Sci. Mater. Med.* 15, 1279–1284. doi:10.1007/s10856-004-5735-3

Siedenbiedel, F., and Tiller, J. C. (2012). Antimicrobial polymers in solution and on surfaces: overview and functional principles. *Polymers* 4, 46–71. doi:10.3390/polym4010046

Thian, E. S., Konishi, T., Kawanobe, Y., Lim, P. N., Choong, C., Ho, B., et al. (2013). Zinc-substituted hydroxyapatite: a biomaterial with enhanced bioactivity and antibacterial properties. *J. Mater. Sci. Mater. Med.* 24, 437–445. doi:10.1007/s10856-012-4817-x

Velard, F., Laurent-Maquin, D., Braux, J., Guillaume, C., Bouthors, S., Jallot, E., et al. (2010). The effect of zinc on hydroxyapatite-mediated activation of human polymorphonuclear neutrophils and bone implant-associated acute inflammation. *Biomaterials* 31, 2001–2009. doi:10.1016/j.biomaterials.2009.11.066

Venkatasubbu, G. D., Ramasamy, S., Ramakrishnan, V., and Kumar, J. (2011). Nanocrystalline hydroxyapatite and zinc-doped hydroxyapatite as carrier material for controlled delivery of ciprofloxacin. *3 Biotech* 1, 173–186. doi:10.1007/s13205-011-0021-9

Verron, E., Bouler, J. M., and Guicheux, J. (2012). Controlling the biological function of calcium phosphate bone substitutes with drugs. *Acta Biomater.* 8, 3541–3551. doi:10.1016/j.actbio.2012.06.022

Victor, S. P., and Kumar, T. S. (2008). Tailoring calcium-deficient hydroxyapatite nanocarriers for enhanced release of antibiotics. *J. Biomed. Nanotechnol.* 4, 1–7. doi:10.1166/jbn.2008.019

World Health Organization. (2014). *Antimicrobial Resistance Global Report on Surveillance*. Geneva: World Health Organization.

Wu, P., and Grainger, D. W. (2006). Drug/device combinations for local drug therapies and infection prophylaxis. *Biomaterials* 27, 2450–2467. doi:10.1016/j.biomaterials.2005.11.031

Conflict of Interest Statement: The authors declare that the research was conducted in the absence of any commercial or financial relationships that could be construed as a potential conflict of interest.

2

Strategies to stimulate mobilization and homing of endogenous stem and progenitor cells for bone tissue repair

Marietta Herrmann, Sophie Verrier and Mauro Alini*

AO Research Institute Davos, Davos, Switzerland

Edited by:
Bruno Peault,
University of California Los Angeles,
USA

Reviewed by:
Vasif Nejat Hasirci,
Middle East Technical University,
Turkey
Mikaël M. Martino,
Osaka University, Japan

*Correspondence:
Mauro Alini,
AO Research Institute Davos,
Clavadelerstrasse 8, Davos Platz,
7270, Switzerland
mauro.alini@aofoundation.org

The gold standard for the treatment of critical-size bone defects is autologous or allogenic bone graft. This has several limitations including donor site morbidity and the restricted supply of graft material. Cell-based tissue engineering strategies represent an alternative approach. Mesenchymal stem cells (MSCs) have been considered as a source of osteo-progenitor cells. More recently, focus has been placed on the use of endothelial progenitor cells (EPCs), since vascularization is a critical step in bone healing. Although many of these approaches have demonstrated effectiveness for bone regeneration, cell-based therapies require time consuming and cost-expensive *in vitro* cell expansion procedures. Accordingly, research is becoming increasingly focused on the homing and stimulation of native cells. The stromal cell-derived factor-1 (SDF-1) – CXCR4 axis has been shown to be critical for the recruitment of MSCs and EPCs. Vascular endothelial growth factor (VEGF) is a key factor in angiogenesis and has been targeted in many studies. Here, we present an overview of the different approaches for delivering homing factors to the defect site by absorption or incorporation to biomaterials, gene therapy, or via genetically manipulated cells. We further review strategies focusing on the stimulation of endogenous cells to support bone repair. Finally, we discuss the major challenges in the treatment of critical-size bone defects and fracture non-unions.

Keywords: bone repair, homing, stem cells, endothelial progenitor cells

Introduction

Bone fracture healing is a tightly regulated process involving different cell types. The first hours after trauma are characterized by hematoma formation and an acute inflammatory response. Blood and bone marrow-derived leukocytes express pro-inflammatory cytokines and initiate the healing process. Eventually, mesenchymal stem cells (MSC) are attracted from the surrounding tissue, bone marrow, and/or the circulation (Shirley et al., 2005) to serve as osteoprogenitor cells. Different mechanisms have been described for the homing of MSCs to the fracture site.

Mesenchymal stem cells express the chemokine receptor CXCR4, and MSC migration toward stromal cell-derived factor-1 (SDF-1) has been confirmed *in vitro* and *in vivo* (Abbott et al., 2004; Ji et al., 2004; Wynn et al., 2004). At injury sites, tissue ischemia induces expression of hypoxia-inducible factor-1 (HIF-1), which in turn triggers SDF-1 expression (Ceradini et al., 2004). Accordingly, upregulation of SDF-1 expression was shown during fracture healing in mice (Kitaori et al., 2009). Further, it has been shown that osteoblast progenitor cells express CXRC4 prompting their migration to regions of new bone formation (Otsuru et al., 2008). Inhibition of SDF-1 or blocking of its receptor, CXCR4, prevents MSC recruitment and results in impaired bone healing (Kitaori et al., 2009). It has also been shown that long-term administration of the CXCR4 antagonist AMD3000 specifically decreases hyaline cartilage volume at early time points, as well as the volume of callus and mineralized bone at later stages of the healing cascade (Toupadakis et al., 2013).

Along with other pro-inflammatory cytokines, tumor necrosis factor alpha (TNFα) accumulation peaks in the first 24 h after fracture and again during the remodeling phase (Kon et al., 2001). Transgenic mice lacking the TNFα receptor suffer from impaired intra-membranous bone formation suggesting a critical role of TNFα in fracture healing (Gerstenfeld et al., 2001). It has been further suggested that TNFα is specifically involved in the attraction of osteoprogenitor cells from surrounding soft tissues (Glass et al., 2011). However, depending on the concentration, TNFα may also have an anti-regenerative effect. In a murine model of subcutaneous bone formation, it has been demonstrated that T-lymphocyte secreted TNFα-induced apoptosis of transplanted MSCs, which resulted in inhibition of new bone formation (Liu et al., 2013).

Revascularization is a critical step in the process of fracture healing (Laroche, 2002). Vascularization ensures an adequate nutrient supply, the removal of metabolic waste products, and supports the influx of immune and progenitor cells from the circulation. Revascularization is mediated by two different mechanisms: (i) angiogenesis: involving sprouting and ingrowth from pre-existing blood vessels, i.e., from the periosteum and (ii) the *de novo* formation of blood vessels by endothelial progenitor cells (EPCs) referred to as neovascularization. The importance of neovascularization in bone healing is evident from the fact that mobilization of EPCs has been observed after musculoskeletal trauma (Laing et al., 2007), fracture (Matsumoto et al., 2008), and during fracture healing (Ma et al., 2012).

Endothelial progenitor cell mobilization and homing mechanisms have been studied in great detail in the context of ischemic diseases; for review, see Verloop et al. (2009); vascular endothelial growth factor (VEGF) and SDF-1 have been identified as key mediators of EPC mobilization (Asahara et al., 1999; Kawakami et al., 2015). Besides SDF-1, VEGF is also expressed in bone, and VEGF serum levels have been shown to increase after polytrauma (Grad et al., 1998). Thus, both factors contribute to the recruitment of EPCs to the fracture site. Furthermore, VEGF is expressed by hypertrophic chondrocytes and plays a crucial role in endochondral ossification (Gerber et al., 1999). Interestingly, it has been proposed that VEGF does not only stimulate angiogenesis during fracture repair but also has a direct effect on osteoblast attraction and differentiation as well as bone turnover (Mayr-Wohlfart et al., 2002; Street et al., 2002; Orlandini et al., 2006).

Stem cell recruitment is a critical step in bone regeneration, and failed healing has been correlated with a decreased MSC pool in patients suffering from atrophic non-union fractures (Mathieu et al., 2013). Similarly, a lack in vascularization leads to delayed or failed tissue regeneration. In this review, we first summarize tissue engineering strategies focusing on the local delivery of homing factors. We then present an overview of the approaches to mobilize stem cells from their niche in order to increase the pool of circulating stem cells. Finally, the clinical challenges of critical-size bone defects and fracture non-union repair are discussed in context to the development of future cell-based therapies.

Strategies to Promote Homing

Different approaches have been used to deliver homing factors to the fracture site (**Table 1, Figure 1B**).

In scaffold-based tissue engineering strategies, homing factors can be covalently bound or absorbed to the scaffold. Drug delivery systems such as hydrogels, microspheres, and nanoparticles have been used on their own or in combination with scaffolds and/or biomaterials (see Local delivery of Homing Factors). Of note, the carrier material has a significant impact on the release profile of the homing factor in question. Alternatively, protein may be delivered via plasmid- or virus-based induction of homing factors (see Delivery of Genes). A recent study incorporated angiogenic and osteogenic small interfering RNAs into a tissue-engineered construct for bone regeneration (Jia et al., 2014). Finally, co-transplanted cells have been targeted to promote expression of homing factors by genetic manipulation (see Genetically Manipulated Cells). In the case of MSCs, the natural secretome itself might be a source of chemoattractants (Caplan et al., 1998; Kinnaird et al., 2004; Stoddart et al., 2014), which in turn mediate recruitment of endothelial cells (Seebach et al., 2014).

Local Delivery of Homing Factors

For the local administration of growth factors, different delivery strategies have been investigated as reviewed by Chen et al. (2010). The delivery system determines the release profile of the growth factor and has to be carefully chosen based on the requirements of the targeted tissue. Most systems display a continuous release of the growth factor. Here, the direct adsorption of growth factors results in a burst release, while a sustained and delayed release can be achieved by encapsulation of growth factors in microspheres (Chen et al., 2010). A responsive system can be created, whereby growth factors are entrapped, ionically or covalently bonded to the carrier material. Growth factor release is then indirectly modulated by physical and chemical microenvironmental changes.

Vascular endothelial growth factor is a key mediator in angiogenesis, but has also been suggested to directly support bone formation. This dual function has made VEGF an attractive target for bone tissue engineering in the past decade. Recombinant VEGF has been delivered with various biomaterials and tested in different preclinical bone fracture models. VEGF delivery with poly(lactide-co-glycolide) (PLGA) scaffolds has been shown to increase vascular density as well as bone mineral formation in a critical-size cranium defect (Murphy et al., 2004) and calvarial defects (Kaigler et al., 2006) in rats. A similar positive outcome was reported when VEGF was administered on a (i) collagen sponge into mandibular (Kleinheinz et al., 2005) or calvarial defects (Behr et al., 2012; Jin and Giannobile, 2014); (ii) polymeric scaffolds with a bioactive glass coating (Leach et al., 2006) in a rat critical-size defect; and (iii) β-tricalcium phosphate scaffold in a rabbit ulna defect (Clarke et al., 2007). By contrast, other studies failed to

TABLE 1 | Homing factors for bone regeneration.

Agent	Delivery system	Animal model	Reference
Protein delivery			
FGF-2	Collagen sponge	Mouse, calvarial defect	Behr et al. (2012)
PDGF-BB	Fibrin gel	Rat, femur delayed union	Kaipel et al. (2012)
PDGF-BB + BMP-2	Fibrin gel (functionalized)	Rat, calvarial defect	Martino et al. (2011)
PDGF-BB/PlGF-2$_{123-144}$ + BMP-2 PlGF-2$_{123-144}$	Saline or fibrin gel	Rat, calvarial defect	Martino et al. (2014)
SDF-1	Collagen gel matrix	Mouse, DO model	Fujio et al. (2011)
	Fibrin gel	Mouse, tibial defect	Li et al. (2011)
	PCL/gelatin electrospun membranes	Rat, calvarial defect	Ji et al. (2013)
	Collagen sponge	Mouse, calvarial defect	Jin and Giannobile (2014)
	PLGA scaffold	Mouse, calvarial defect	Liu et al. (2014)
SDF-1 + BMP-2	Collagen sponge	Mouse, calvarial defect	Jin and Giannobile (2014)
SDF-1 + PDGF	Collagen sponge	Mouse, calvarial defect	Jin and Giannobile (2014)
SDF-1 + VEGF	Collagen sponge	Mouse, calvarial defect	Jin and Giannobile (2014)
Simvastatin	α-TCP	Rat, calvarial defect	Nyan et al. (2009)
	PLA scaffold	Rat, rabbit, calvarial defect	Yueyi et al. (2013)
	PLGA scaffold	Mouse, calvarial defect	Liu et al. (2014)
TNF	Saline	Mouse, tibial defect	Glass et al. (2011)
VEGF	β-TCP	Mouse, calvarial defect	Wernike et al. (2010)
		Rabbit, ulna defect	Clarke et al. (2007)
	CaP coated titanium	Pig, calvarial defect	Ramazanoglu et al. (2013)
	Chitosan sponge	Rabbit, intercondylar defect	De la Riva et al. (2010)
	Collagen	Rabbit, mandibular defect	Kleinheinz et al. (2005)
	Collagen sponge	Mouse, calvarial defect	Behr et al. (2012), Jin and Giannobile (2014)
	Fibrin	Rat, femur delayed union	Kaipel et al. (2012)
	Gelatin spheres, PPF scaffold	Rat, calvarial defect	Patel et al. (2008a)
		Rat, femoral defect	Kempen et al. (2009)
	Hyaluronic acid	Rabbit, tibial defect	Eckardt et al. (2005)
	PLGA scaffold	Rat, calvarial defect	Murphy et al. (2004), Kaigler et al. (2006)
	PLGA scaffold BG coated	Rat, calvarial defect	Leach et al. (2006)
	PLGA spheres, fibrin	Dog, femoral neck defect	Zhang et al. (2014a)
	Silk fibroin/CaP/PLGA	Rabbit, calvarial defect	Farokhi et al. (2014)
VEGF + BMP-2	Allograft, PLGA	Rat, femoral defect	Mattar et al. (2013)
	CaP coated titanium	Pig, calvarial defect	Ramazanoglu et al. (2013)
	Gelatin spheres in PPF scaffold	Rat, calvarial defect	Patel et al. (2008a)
		Rat, femoral defect	Kempen et al. (2009)
	PLGA, alginate	Mouse, femoral defect	Kanczler et al. (2010)
	Silk fibroin	Rabbit, maxillary sinus	Zhang et al. (2011)
		Rabbit, calvarial defect	Zhang et al. (2014b)
		Rat, calvarial defect	Zhang et al. (2014c)
VEGF + PDGF-BB	Silk fibroin/CaP/PLGA	Rabbit, calvarial defect	Farokhi et al. (2013)
Plasmid/virus delivery			
VEGF	AV, intramuscular injection	Rat, femur drill hole	Tarkka et al. (2003)
	plasmid-DNA	Rabbit, radius defect	Geiger et al. (2005)
	Corraline scaffold coated with plasmid-DNA	Rabbit, radius defect	Geiger et al. (2007)
Genetically manipulated cells			
MCP-3	LV-transduced MSC, bone graft	Mouse, fibular osteotomy	Shinohara et al. (2011)
SDF-1	AV-transduced MSC, collagen sponge	Rat, femoral defect	Ho et al. (2014)
	LV-transduced MSC, bone graft	Mouse, fibular osteotomy	Shinohara et al. (2011)
SDF-1 + BMP-2	AV-transduced fat tissue graft	Mouse, femoral defect	Zwingenberger et al. (2014)
VEGF	Plasmid-transfected MSC, corraline scaffold	Rabbit, radius defect	Geiger et al. (2007)
		Rabbit, orbital defect	Xiao et al. (2011)
	Plasmid-transfected fibroblasts, gelfoam	Rabbit, tibial defect	Li et al. (2009)
VEGF + BMP-2	AV-transduced MSC, corraline scaffold	Rabbit, orbital defect	Xiao et al. (2011)
	BV-transduced ASC, PLGA scaffold	Rabbit femoral defect	Lin et al. (2014)
VEGF + BMP-4	RV-transduced MDSC, gelfoam	Mouse, skull defect	Peng et al. (2002)

The table lists chemoattractants, which have been delivered as protein or on the gene level to the bone defect site. Alternatively, genetic manipulation has been applied to overexpress homing factors in transplanted cells. Of note, the table includes only factors, which have been tested in orthotopic models of bone regeneration in vivo. ASC, adipose-derived stem cells; AV, adenovirus; BV, hybrid baculovirus; DO, distraction osteogenesis; LV, lentivirus; MDSC, muscle-derived stem cells; PCL, poly(epsilon-caprolactone); PPF, poly(propylene fumarate); RV, retrovirus.

show a beneficial effect of VEGF delivery on bone regeneration in different models including a rabbit non-union model (Geiger et al., 2005), a rat model of delayed union (Kaipel et al., 2012), and an ectopic bone formation model using cancellous bone scaffolds (Lenze et al., 2014).

It has been shown that adsorbed VEGF is released within few days (Leach et al., 2006; Kempen et al., 2009). A too high local concentration of VEGF might, however, cause malformation and malfunction of blood vessels (Neufeld et al., 1999; Ozawa et al., 2004). In addition, a more sustained release of VEGF might be desirable to efficiently support vascularization and bone formation. Therefore, several studies attempted a more controlled release of VEGF aiming to sustain a low dose of VEGF during the first weeks after trauma. Mostly, these approaches follow the route of encapsulation of VEGF in microspheres or nanoparticles. Pre-encapsulation of VEGF in PLGA microspheres before scaffold fabrication has been shown to delay the growth factor release compared to direct incorporation into PLGA scaffolds (Ennett et al., 2006). Encapsulation of VEGF in alginate microspheres delivered with a chitosan/poly(lactide) scaffold has also been promising, showing only a 13% release within the first 24 h followed by a sustained release throughout 5 weeks (De la Riva et al., 2009, 2010). Similarly, encapsulation of VEGF in gelatin microparticles, which have been included in a composite scaffold, could maintain VEGF bioactivity above 90% over 14 days (Patel et al., 2008a). In orthotopic bone formation models, VEGF delivery via a PLGA-composite scaffold has shown a sustained VEGF release over 28 days, resulting in new bone formation observed 10 weeks after implantation in a rabbit cranial defect (Farokhi et al., 2013, 2014). Similarly, the combined administration of PLGA-encapsulated VEGF with fibrin resulted in a sustained VEGF release for up to 42 days, with improved vascularization and accelerated healing of a femoral head fracture model in dogs (Zhang et al., 2014a). Burst release of VEGF was also prevented by co-precipitating VEGF onto basic calcium phosphate (BCP), resulting in vascularization and osseointegration of the biomaterial, and finally to new bone formation in a critical-size cranial defect in Balb/c mice (Wernike et al., 2010).

Ehrbar and colleagues introduced an innovative approach to control the release of VEGF by cell-mediated enzyme activity (Ehrbar et al., 2004). Here, authors engineered a recombinant form of VEGF containing an $alpha_2$-plasmin inhibitor ($alpha_2$-PI_{1-8}) sequence, which is a substrate for factor XIIIa. Covalently linked to the fibrin matrix, $alpha_2$-PI_{1-8}-VEGF is released upon remodeling of the fibrin by cell-associated enzymatic activity, such as plasmin or matrix metalloproteinases. Authors demonstrated that cell-controlled release of the VEGF from the fibrin gel carrier led to an increase in formation of new arterial and venous branches in an embryonic chicken chorioallantoic membrane model (Ehrbar et al., 2004). Recently, it was shown that the system was therapeutically effective both in ischemic hind limb and wound-healing models (Sacchi et al., 2014).

Several studies have combined VEGF with other chemoattractive or osteoinductive factors. For example, VEGF has been applied in combination with BMP-2. Most of these studies showed the expected strong osteoinductive effect of BMP-2. However, further addition of VEGF, while leading to slightly increased vascular density, did not exhibit enhanced bone formation (Patel et al., 2008b;

Kempen et al., 2009; Young et al., 2009; Kanczler et al., 2010; Zhang et al., 2011, 2014b; Mattar et al., 2013; Ramazanoglu et al., 2013; Cai et al., 2014). Interestingly, Kempen and colleagues presented a delivery system allowing for a sequential release of the two growth factors. Here, BMP-2 was encapsulated in PLGA microspheres, which were delivered in a poly(propylene) scaffold surrounded by a gelatin hydrogel loaded with VEGF (Kempen et al., 2009).

Platelet-derived growth factor (PDGF) is involved in angiogenesis, in particular, it mediates migration of pericytes from the vessel wall toward sites of new vessel formation, which is thought to be critical for the stabilization of newly formed blood vessels (Armulik et al., 2005). In addition, a chemoattractive effect of PDGF-BB on MSCs has been reported (Fiedler et al., 2004). This was confirmed in a study testing the release of PDGF-BB from a poly(ϵ-caprolactone) (PCL) – collagen – hydroxyapatite scaffolds, showing a sustained release of bioactive PDGF-BB, which was able to stimulate MSC migration (Phipps et al., 2012). Interestingly, PDGF-BB has been FDA approved for periodontal repair (Pellegrini et al., 2009). Recently, PDGF delivery has been tested in orthotopic bone formation models. Here, administration of PDGF on a collagen sponge in a critical-size calvarial defect has been shown to increase bone mineral content to a similar extent than VEGF, but significantly less than BMP-2 (Jin and Giannobile, 2014). In line with this, in a rat model of delayed union, PDGF-BB delivery alone did not support bone formation (Kaipel et al., 2012). Farokhi et al. (2013) studied the controlled release of VEGF and PDGF from a silk/calcium phosphate/PLGA scaffolds and found that the combination of the two homing factors supported new bone formation and neovascularization in a rabbit drill hole model. Martino and co-workers reported that the delivery of PDGF-BB and BMP-2 in a fibrin gel functionalized with an integrin binding domain and allowing for sequestration of the growth factors greatly enhanced bone regeneration in a rat calvarial defect compared to growth factors encapsulated in unmodified fibrin (Martino et al., 2011). Recently, the same group reported on an interesting approach to fuse extracellular matrix super-affinity binding sites to growth factors. Applying such engineered variants of PDGF-BB and BMP-2 for the treatment of a calvarial defect in rats resulted in greater bone regeneration compared to wild type growth factors (Martino et al., 2014).

The recruitment of MSCs to the fracture site is predominantly regulated via the SDF-1 – CXCR4 axis (Kitaori et al., 2009). Interestingly, homing of EPCs may be triggered by the same pathway. Accordingly, several tissue engineering strategies have been using SDF-1 to stimulate MSC and EPC homing. Indeed, local administration of SDF-1 in a distraction osteogenesis mouse model has been shown to increase the recruitment of MSCs and EPCs, to induce callus formation and blood flow (Fujio et al., 2011). Li and colleagues reported that SDF-1 administered in fibrin glue enhanced the healing process in a mouse tibia fracture model with intramedullary fixation (Li et al., 2011).

Absorption of SDF-1 to an electrospun gelatin/PCL membrane was shown to efficiently recruit MSCs to a cranial defect and resulted in a sixfold increase in bone formation compared to membrane alone (Ji et al., 2013). A positive effect on MSC recruitment and bone formation was also shown for PLGA loaded with SDF-1 in a critical-size calvarial defect in mice (Liu et al., 2014). A comparative study evaluating the effect of different chemoattractants applied on a collagen sponge in a critical-size calvarial defect is presented by Jin and Giannobile (2014). The authors report on a moderate effect on bone formation by SDF-1 alone or in combination with PDGF or VEGF. By contrast, significant more bone volume was seen when SDF-1 was administered in combination with BMP-2. In a model of ectopic bone formation, Chim et al. (2012) used a customized microdelivery apparatus to maintain constant cytokine release over a period of 4 weeks within the subcutaneous implanted PLGA scaffolds. The experiment revealed that a higher cellular infiltration was seen when SDF-1 was administered in addition to BMP-2 or TGFβ.

It has been reported that statins, such as simvastatin, have the potential to induce bone formation (Mundy et al., 1999). Recent work suggested that this effect is driven by the stimulation of MSC and EPC homing. Accordingly, simvastatin-based tissue engineering strategies showed increased recruitment of osteoprogenitor cells and EPCs (Nyan et al., 2009; Yueyi et al., 2013). Furthermore, it has been suggested that the outcome of such approaches may be improved by combining simvastatin and SDF-1 (Liu et al., 2014). On the other hand, an *in vitro* study suggested that high doses of statins may have a cytotoxic effect on MSCs (Kupcsik et al., 2009).

Besides SDF-1, it has been suggested that TNFα plays a role in the recruitment of osteoprogenitor cells to the fracture site and local injection of TNFα upon initiation of trauma and the day after accelerated fracture healing (Glass et al., 2011).

An alternative approach to the use of defined amounts of recombinant growth factors are platelet-released growth factors. Platelet-rich plasma (PRP) refers to a concentrate of blood platelets, which upon activation releases various growth factors, including VEGF, CCL5, PDGF-AB, and PDGF-BB (Fekete et al., 2012). Although standard protocols for the preparation of PRP are missing and its efficacy is under debate, PRP in combination with scaffolds or bone graft has been variously used in preclinical and clinical approaches. These studies have been reviewed elsewhere and are not described in this article (Malhotra et al., 2013).

Another method is to use the secretome of MSCs. Wang et al. (2012) demonstrated that a galantine sponge soaked in MSC-conditioned medium supported angiogenesis and bone healing in a model of fracture non-union in diabetic rats.

Delivery of Genes

Gene therapies have been developed aiming to deliver the genetic information of homing factors into the defect site, with VEGF being the main target gene. Gene delivery methods have the main advantage to promote sustained and regulated expression of proteins at the defect site (Evans, 2012). Some approaches incorporate plasmids in tissue-engineered constructs; however, low efficacy prompted researchers to develop alternative approaches, such as adenoviral delivery of the genetic information. While dramatically increasing gene transfer efficiency, there are also drawbacks to the use of viral vectors. Lentiviral and retroviral vectors permanently modify the cells genome, with the risk of insertional mutagenesis. Adenoviral transduction has the advantage that the absence of vector genome integration minimizes the risk of germ-line transmission and insertional mutagenesis. It does, however, trigger an immunological response at higher doses. Adeno-associated virus

(AAV) is increasing in popularity due to its low immunogenicity and lack of integration. AAV vectors are currently difficult to produce to a high titer.

Geiger et al. (2005) report on a VEGF-gene-activated matrix promoting vascularization and bone formation in a critical-size radius defect in rabbits. A positive effect of VEGF on vascularization was also reported in an ectopic bone formation model in mice, while the most efficient bone formation was detected in constructs containing MSCs along with VEGF and BMP-4 plasmids (Huang et al., 2005). It has been shown that local administration of a VEGF adenovirus in the distal femur of rabbits was able to transduce endogenous bone marrow cells and in turn to enhance osteoblast number, osteoid volume, and bone volume (Hiltunen et al., 2003). In a rat femoral defect, injection of a VEGF adenovirus in the adjacent muscle has shown to promote endochondral bone healing (Tarkka et al., 2003). Similarly, it has been shown that a VEGF adenoviral vector containing chitosan/hydroxyapatite scaffold promoted recruitment of endogenous endothelial cells and supported ectopic bone formation (Koc et al., 2014).

Genetically Manipulated Cells

Transplantation of autologous stem cells is widely used in bone tissue engineering strategies. Several studies have used genetically modified cells to induce expression of homing factors, which in turn promotes the recruitment of host osteogenic and EPCs. Here, most studies have applied viral transduction strategies (for details, see **Table 1**) to introduce the specific gene sequence prior to transplantation of cells into the bone defect. Again, the main interest has been in overexpression of VEGF.

Promising results were reported for adipose-derived stem cells (ASCs) transduced with an adenovirus to release VEGF that led to vascular ingrowth into PLGA scaffolds (Jabbarzadeh et al., 2008). An approach using VEGF-plasmid-transfected fibroblasts showed improved vascularization and bridging of a segmental bone defect in rabbits, while unmodified fibroblasts did not support bone regeneration (Li et al., 2009). By contrast, a study comparing the healing of a critical-size radius defect in rabbits revealed that substantial bone formation was only seen in groups with MSCs transfected with control plasmid, while VEGF transfected MSCs prompted a higher vascular density (Geiger et al., 2007). In line with this, Helmrich and colleagues demonstrated that subcutaneously implanted osteogenic constructs containing MSCs, transduced with a retroviral vector to overexpress VEGF, led to an increase in vascular density but caused a global decrease in bone quality by increasing the recruitment of osteoclasts (Helmrich et al., 2013).

In order to also address osteoinduction, several groups followed a combined approach with overexpression of VEGF and BMP-2. Cell transplantation of human periosteum-derived cells transfected with VEGF and BMP-2 plasmids resulted in improved osteogenesis and vascularization in an ectopic bone formation model and a critical-size orbital defect (Samee et al., 2008). A similar finding was reported with adenoviral-transduced MSCs (Xiao et al., 2011). Long time evaluation of the healing of a rabbit femoral defect treated with baculovirus-engineered ASCs overexpressing VEGF/BMP-2 further revealed a positive effect on endochondral ossification and bone remodeling (Lin et al., 2014). A similar observation was made in a study applying retroviral-transduced muscle-derived stem cells overexpressing BMP-4 and VEGF in a skull defect in mice (Peng et al., 2002). Adenoviral delivery of the angiogenic factor angiopoitin-1 (ANG-1) along with BMP-2 and VEGF led to enhanced osteogenesis and angiogenesis in a rabbit radial defect treated with MSCs overexpressing all three factors compared to the other study groups (Hou et al., 2009).

A study from Shinohara et al. (2011) suggested that lentiviral-overexpression of SDF-1 or monocyte chemotactic protein-3 (MCP-3) may be used to attract MSCs to the fracture site. The authors performed a parabiosis of a GFP and a wild-type mouse and studied the homing of GFP-positive stem cells into an osteotomy gap in the wildtype mouse; this experiment revealed significantly enhanced cell recruitment when the defect was treated with MSCs overexpressing MCP-3 or SDF-1 (Shinohara et al., 2011). The stimulatory effect of SDF-1 on cell homing was confirmed in a study applying SDF-1- and/or BMP-2-lentivirus-transduced fat grafts in a femoral defect in mice (Zwingenberger et al., 2014), a significant increase in bone volume compared to untreated fat grafts was, however, only observed in groups with combined expression of both factors. A rat study testing the effect of SDF-1-adenovirus-transduced MSCs implanted on a collagen sponge in a femoral defect showed a significant increase in new bone formation compared to cell-free or untransduced control groups (Ho et al., 2014).

Stem Cell Stimulation

Local or systemic transplantation of stem- and progenitor cells has been used for bone tissue engineering and bone regeneration (**Figure 1A**). For example, transplantation of EPCs has shown promising results with regards to the regeneration of vascularized bone tissue (Matsumoto et al., 2006; Kuroda et al., 2011, 2014). These strategies have several limitations. Harvesting of cells is associated with donor site morbidity, pain, and additional hospitalization of the patient. Cell purification and expansion is expensive and time consuming and associated with safety concerns such as mutagenesis or contaminations. Therefore, there has been an interest to circumvent cell harvesting and amplification steps and to develop strategies to stimulate the mobilization of native endogenous stem cells (**Figure 1C**).

Granulocyte colony-stimulating factor (G-CSF) induces the mobilization of CD34-positive, hematopoietic cells representing a source of EPCs (Peichev et al., 2000). Subsequently, G-CSF has been used to enrich CD34-positive cells prior cell harvest and local or systemic transplantation (Mifune et al., 2008; Kuroda et al., 2011). In addition, G-CSF has been applied as a homing factor at the defect site in a segmental bone defect (Ishida et al., 2010). Finally, some studies evaluated the effect of G-CSF stimulation in bone defect models hypothesizing that the enhanced accumulation of CD34-positive progenitor cells may promote revascularization and thus bone healing (Bozlar et al., 2005; Kaygusuz et al., 2006; Marmotti et al., 2013). Indeed subcutaneous injection of G-CSF on seven consecutive days after creation of a tibia defect in rats accelerated bone healing (Bozlar et al., 2005); in line with this another study reported improved fracture healing scores in a tibia defect model in rats after administration of G-CSF

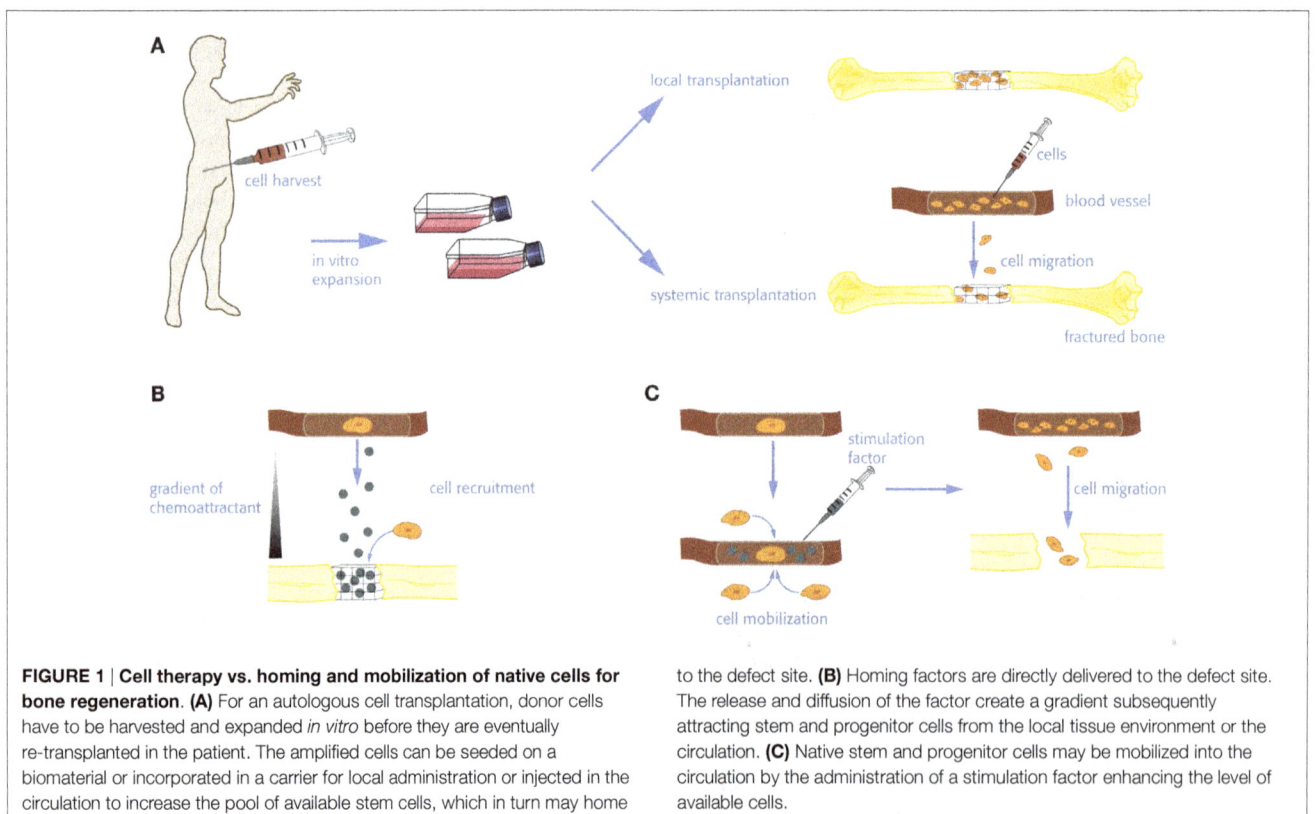

FIGURE 1 | Cell therapy vs. homing and mobilization of native cells for bone regeneration. (A) For an autologous cell transplantation, donor cells have to be harvested and expanded *in vitro* before they are eventually re-transplanted in the patient. The amplified cells can be seeded on a biomaterial or incorporated in a carrier for local administration or injected in the circulation to increase the pool of available stem cells, which in turn may home to the defect site. **(B)** Homing factors are directly delivered to the defect site. The release and diffusion of the factor create a gradient subsequently attracting stem and progenitor cells from the local tissue environment or the circulation. **(C)** Native stem and progenitor cells may be mobilized into the circulation by the administration of a stimulation factor enhancing the level of available cells.

(Kaygusuz et al., 2006). A recent phase II clinical trial evaluated the preoperative administration (three consecutive days) of G-CSF in patients undergoing opening-wedge high tibial valgus osteotomy (Marmotti et al., 2013). The study including 12 patients in both the G-CSF treated- and the control group, reported on a successful mobilization of CD34-positive cells upon surgery, which in turn resulted in an improved osseointegration of grafts (Marmotti et al., 2013).

The SDF-1/CXCR4 axis is involved in the retention of hematopoietic progenitor cells in the bone marrow (Levesque et al., 2003). Accordingly, it has been shown that AMD3100, a CXCR4 antagonist promotes stem cell mobilization into the circulation, with the most efficient cell mobilization seen in combination with G-CSF (Broxmeyer et al., 2005). Conversely, the biological function of AMD3100-mobilized cells has been questioned in an *in vitro* study (Yin et al., 2007). In addition, interference with the SDF-1/CXCR4 axis can also impair homing of stem cells toward the defect site (Toupadakis et al., 2013). Nonetheless, a positive effect of AMD3100 administration on the healing of a segmental defect in mice was reported (Kumar and Ponnazhagan, 2012). The authors show that a combined treatment with insulin-like growth factor-1 (IGF-1) and AMD3100 resulted expectably in an increased accumulation of colony-forming cells and finally augmented bone growth (Kumar and Ponnazhagan, 2012).

It has been suggested that low-intensity pulsed ultrasound (LIPUS) might be used to promote fracture healing (Duarte, 1983; Leung et al., 2004; Khan and Laurencin, 2008). Interestingly, a recent study investigating the underlying mechanisms revealed that LIPUS stimulates MSC homing to the fracture site by upregulating local and serum SDF-1 levels (Wei et al., 2014).

Sildenafil, a potent vasodilator and stimulator of angiogenesis, has been proposed to increase circulating EPCs (Foresta et al., 2009) and sildenafil has been used for the treatment of ischemic diseases (Hart et al., 2006; Koneru et al., 2008). Histing et al. (2011) investigated the effect of sildenafil during the process of fracture healing in a drill hole model in mice. The study revealed that daily oral administration of sildenafil accelerated bone healing indicated by increased osseous fracture bridging, biomechanical stiffness, and a smaller callus area after 2 weeks (Histing et al., 2011).

Challenges and Future Perspectives

Bone has a high natural regeneration capacity. Tissue engineering strategies and cell therapies for bone repair are focusing on critical-size defects and fracture non-unions, which fail to heal spontaneously. A main challenge is the treatment of atrophic non-unions, which are defined as bone defects showing no healing progress within 6 months after fracture. This has been associated with risk factors including smoking and chronic diseases like diabetes (Gaston and Simpson, 2007) but may also be idiopathic. In both cases, the underlying mechanisms still remain elusive. A better understanding of the pathology of non-unions will certainly help to find new treatment strategies. A major limitation preventing the development of efficient therapies so far is the lack of appropriate animal models. While various non-union models in rodents, rabbits, and sheep have been established (Garcia et al., 2013), most of these models only simulate the situation of a non-healing

critical-size defect in a healthy environment and those parameters resulting in non-unions in humans are not addressed. Accordingly, therapies proven successful in preclinical models might thus be ineffective upon clinical application.

The availability of stem and progenitor cells might be a crucial factor for bone healing. A low number of bone marrow progenitor cells were found in patients suffering from pseudoarthrosis (Hernigou and Beaujean, 1997). Similarly, it has been reported that the number of circulating progenitor cells was significantly lower in patients with non-union fractures compared to healthy individuals (Seebach et al., 2007). Interestingly, the authors further report on an elevated stem cell accumulation in polytrauma patients; at the same time polytrauma is also associated with increased serum accumulation of VEGF (Grad et al., 1998). Recent work evaluated the abundance of EPCs in patients with atrophic non-unions (Mathieu et al., 2013). In line with the previous studies, a decreased pool of MSCs was detected; but the EPC level was not affected. Future studies will be required to verify these results and to assess stem and progenitor cell availability, mobilization, and recruitment in non-union fractures in detail. However, assuming that fracture non-unions are indeed correlated with a decreased pool of circulating and bone marrow MSCs, this would be a major limitation for cell-based therapies in those patients. Besides preventing the mobilization and recruitment of endogenous cells, the cell harvest for transplantation is limited by a low frequency of MSCs. Recent work suggested a perivascular origin of MSCs suggesting that multipotent cells are available in virtually all vascularized tissues (Crisan et al., 2008). The function of these cells in (local) tissue regeneration has, however, not been explored to date. It has still not been determined to which extent the abundance and regeneration potential of these perivascular MSCs (pericytes) are affected by certain disease states, i.e., the situation of fracture non-union. The investigation of the endogenous regeneration potential of these cells might help to develop new strategies for MSC recruitment to the defect site.

Fracture non-union often occurs in elderly patients. Patient age might have an important influence on the bone regeneration capacities, representing another challenge for both the development of suitable models to test therapeutic strategies and finally the treatment of the patients. Preclinical studies are normally performed in young animals, which are in some cases not even skeletally mature and are not representative for bone healing in elderly patients. The age of patients is also an important consideration with regards to MSC functionality as it has been suggested that proliferation and differentiation abilities are altered in MSCs from donors above 50 years (Mendes et al., 2002; Zhou et al., 2008; Siegel et al., 2013).

Although atrophic non-unions are not always avascular (Reed et al., 2002) and EPC mobilization appears not to be affected (Mathieu et al., 2013), revascularization is an important event in bone regeneration and endochondral bone formation (Gerber et al., 1999; Keramaris et al., 2008). The molecular mechanisms and timing of the revascularization process are still poorly understood. Most importantly, little is known about how these processes are altered in non-union patients. For the development of strategies to improve the vascularization in bone defects, it might be of interest to adapt methods, which have been well established for the treatment of ischemic diseases.

Conclusion

Cell-bases therapies have shown promising results for the repair of bone tissue; for review, see Ma et al. (2014), Romagnoli and Brandi (2014), and Asatrian et al. (2015). Most of these approaches require, however, time- and cost-extensive *in vitro* expansion procedures and finally regulatory issues have to be considered. This has prompted the development of strategies to stimulate native cells. Homing factors supporting the migration of osteoprogenitor and EPCs toward the fracture site have been administered as microspheres, hydrogels, adsorbed to biomaterials, or delivered as

plasmid or viral vector. Here, the combination of a pro-angiogenic stimulus (e.g., VEGF) and an osteoinductive signal, such as BMP-2 has shown most promising results. Besides, mobilization of stem- and progenitor cells from their niche has been shown to facilitate bone healing. Although some of the approaches have shown a promising outcome in preclinical studies, the main challenge remains their translation to the clinical situation. In addition, the lack of a good understanding of the pathological mechanisms, in particularly of fracture non-unions, prevents the development of effective therapies.

Acknowledgments

The authors wish to thank Dr. Martin Stoddard and Dr. Jennifer Bara for proofreading this manuscript.

References

Abbott, J. D., Huang, Y., Liu, D., Hickey, R., Krause, D. S., and Giordano, F. J. (2004). Stromal cell-derived factor-1alpha plays a critical role in stem cell recruitment to the heart after myocardial infarction but is not sufficient to induce homing in the absence of injury. *Circulation* **110**, 3300–3305. doi:10.1161/01.CIR.0000147780.30124.CF

Armulik, A., Abramsson, A., and Betsholtz, C. (2005). Endothelial/pericyte interactions. *Circ. Res.* **97**, 512–523. doi:10.1161/01.RES.0000182903.16652.d7

Asahara, T., Takahashi, T., Masuda, H., Kalka, C., Chen, D., Iwaguro, H., et al. (1999). VEGF contributes to postnatal neovascularization by mobilizing bone marrow-derived endothelial progenitor cells. *EMBO J.* **18**, 3964–3972. doi:10.1093/emboj/18.14.3964

Asatrian, G., Pham, D., Hardy, W. R., James, A. W., and Peault, B. (2015). Stem cell technology for bone regeneration: current status and potential applications. *Stem Cells Cloning* **8**, 39–48. doi:10.2147/SCCAA.S48423

Behr, B., Sorkin, M., Lehnhardt, M., Renda, A., Longaker, M. T., and Quarto, N. (2012). A comparative analysis of the osteogenic effects of BMP-2, FGF-2, and VEGFA in a calvarial defect model. *Tissue Eng. Part A* **18**, 1079–1086. doi:10.1089/ten.TEA.2011.0537

Bozlar, M., Aslan, B., Kalaci, A., Baktiroglu, L., Yanat, A. N., and Tasci, A. (2005). Effects of human granulocyte-colony stimulating factor on fracture healing in rats. *Saudi Med. J.* **26**, 1250–1254.

Broxmeyer, H. E., Orschell, C. M., Clapp, D. W., Hangoc, G., Cooper, S., Plett, P. A., et al. (2005). Rapid mobilization of murine and human hematopoietic stem and progenitor cells with AMD3100, a CXCR4 antagonist. *J. Exp. Med.* **201**, 1307–1318. doi:10.1084/jem.20041385

Cai, W. X., Zheng, L. W., Li, C. L., Ma, L., Ehrbar, M., Weber, F. E., et al. (2014). Effect of different rhBMP-2 and TG-VEGF ratios on the formation of heterotopic bone and neovessels. *Biomed Res. Int.* **2014**, 571510. doi:10.1155/2014/571510

Caplan, A. I., Reuben, D., and Haynesworth, S. E. (1998). Cell-based tissue engineering therapies: the influence of whole body physiology. *Adv. Drug Deliv. Rev.* **33**, 3–14. doi:10.1016/S0169-409X(98)00016-7

Ceradini, D. J., Kulkarni, A. R., Callaghan, M. J., Tepper, O. M., Bastidas, N., Kleinman, M. E., et al. (2004). Progenitor cell trafficking is regulated by hypoxic gradients through HIF-1 induction of SDF-1. *Nat. Med.* **10**, 858–864. doi:10.1038/nm1075

Chen, F. M., Zhang, M., and Wu, Z. F. (2010). Toward delivery of multiple growth factors in tissue engineering. *Biomaterials* **31**, 6279–6308. doi:10.1016/j.biomaterials.2010.04.053

Chim, H., Miller, E., Gliniak, C., and Alsberg, E. (2012). Stromal-cell-derived factor (SDF) 1-alpha in combination with BMP-2 and TGF-beta1 induces site-directed cell homing and osteogenic and chondrogenic differentiation for tissue engineering without the requirement for cell seeding. *Cell Tissue Res.* **350**, 89–94. doi:10.1007/s00441-012-1449-x

Clarke, S. A., Hoskins, N. L., Jordan, G. R., and Marsh, D. R. (2007). Healing of an ulnar defect using a proprietary TCP bone graft substitute, JAX, in association with autologous osteogenic cells and growth factors. *Bone* **40**, 939–947. doi:10.1016/j.bone.2006.11.004

Crisan, M., Yap, S., Casteilla, L., Chen, C. W., Corselli, M., Park, T. S., et al. (2008). A perivascular origin for mesenchymal stem cells in multiple human organs. *Cell Stem Cell* **3**, 301–313. doi:10.1016/j.stem.2008.07.003

De la Riva, B., Nowak, C., Sanchez, E., Hernandez, A., Schulz-Siegmund, M., Pec, M. K., et al. (2009). VEGF-controlled release within a bone defect from alginate/chitosan/PLA-H scaffolds. *Eur. J. Pharm. Biopharm.* **73**, 50–58. doi:10.1016/j.ejpb.2009.04.014

De la Riva, B., Sanchez, E., Hernandez, A., Reyes, R., Tamimi, F., Lopez-Cabarcos, E., et al. (2010). Local controlled release of VEGF and PDGF from a combined brushite-chitosan system enhances bone regeneration. *J. Control Release* **143**, 45–52. doi:10.1016/j.jconrel.2009.11.026

Duarte, L. R. (1983). The stimulation of bone growth by ultrasound. *Arch. Orthop. Trauma Surg.* **101**, 153–159. doi:10.1007/BF00436764

Eckardt, H., Ding, M., Lind, M., Hansen, E. S., Christensen, K. S., and Hvid, I. (2005). Recombinant human vascular endothelial growth factor enhances bone healing in an experimental nonunion model. *J. Bone Joint Surg. Br.* **87**, 1434–1438. doi:10.1302/0301-620X.87B10.16226

Ehrbar, M., Djonov, V. G., Schnell, C., Tschanz, S. A., Martiny-Baron, G., Schenk, U., et al. (2004). Cell-demanded liberation of VEGF121 from fibrin implants induces local and controlled blood vessel growth. *Circ. Res.* **94**, 1124–1132. doi:10.1161/01.RES.0000126411.29641.08

Ennett, A. B., Kaigler, D., and Mooney, D. J. (2006). Temporally regulated delivery of VEGF in vitro and in vivo. *J. Biomed. Mater. Res. A* **79**, 176–184. doi:10.1002/jbm.a.30771

Evans, C. H. (2012). Gene delivery to bone. *Adv. Drug Deliv. Rev.* **64**, 1331–1340. doi:10.1016/j.addr.2012.03.013

Farokhi, M., Mottaghitalab, F., Ai, J., and Shokrgozar, M. A. (2013). Sustained release of platelet-derived growth factor and vascular endothelial growth factor from silk/calcium phosphate/PLGA based nanocomposite scaffold. *Int. J. Pharm.* **454**, 216–225. doi:10.1016/j.ijpharm.2013.06.080

Farokhi, M., Mottaghitalab, F., Shokrgozar, M. A., Ai, J., Hadjati, J., and Azami, M. (2014). Bio-hybrid silk fibroin/calcium phosphate/PLGA nanocomposite scaffold to control the delivery of vascular endothelial growth factor. *Mater. Sci. Eng. C Mater. Biol. Appl.* **35**, 401–410. doi:10.1016/j.msec.2013.11.023

Fekete, N., Gadelorge, M., Furst, D., Maurer, C., Dausend, J., Fleury-Cappellesso, S., et al. (2012). Platelet lysate from whole blood-derived pooled platelet concentrates and apheresis-derived platelet concentrates for the isolation and expansion of human bone marrow mesenchymal stromal cells: production process, content and identification of active components. *Cytotherapy* **14**, 540–554. doi:10.3109/14653249.2012.655420

Fiedler, J., Etzel, N., and Brenner, R. E. (2004). To go or not to go: migration of human mesenchymal progenitor cells stimulated by isoforms of PDGF. *J. Cell. Biochem.* **93**, 990–998. doi:10.1002/jcb.20219

Foresta, C., De Toni, L., Di Mambro, A., Garolla, A., Ferlin, A., and Zuccarello, D. (2009). The PDE5 inhibitor sildenafil increases circulating endothelial progenitor cells and CXCR4 expression. *J. Sex. Med.* **6**, 369–372. doi:10.1111/j.1743-6109.2008.01014.x

Fujio, M., Yamamoto, A., Ando, Y., Shohara, R., Kinoshita, K., Kaneko, T., et al. (2011). Stromal cell-derived factor-1 enhances distraction osteogenesis-mediated skeletal tissue regeneration through the recruitment of endothelial precursors. *Bone* **49**, 693–700. doi:10.1016/j.bone.2011.06.024

Garcia, P., Histing, T., Holstein, J. H., Klein, M., Laschke, M. W., Matthys, R., et al. (2013). Rodent animal models of delayed bone healing and non-union formation: a comprehensive review. *Eur. Cell. Mater.* **26**, 1–12.

Gaston, M. S., and Simpson, A. H. (2007). Inhibition of fracture healing. *J. Bone Joint Surg. Br.* **89**, 1553–1560. doi:10.1302/0301-620X.89B12.19671

Geiger, F., Bertram, H., Berger, I., Lorenz, H., Wall, O., Eckhardt, C., et al. (2005). Vascular endothelial growth factor gene-activated matrix (VEGF165-GAM) enhances osteogenesis and angiogenesis in large segmental bone defects. *J. Bone Miner. Res.* **20**, 2028–2035. doi:10.1359/JBMR.050701

Geiger, F., Lorenz, H., Xu, W., Szalay, K., Kasten, P., Claes, L., et al. (2007). VEGF producing bone marrow stromal cells (BMSC) enhance vascularization and resorption of a natural coral bone substitute. *Bone* **41**, 516–522. doi:10.1016/j.bone.2007.06.018

Gerber, H. P., Vu, T. H., Ryan, A. M., Kowalski, J., Werb, Z., and Ferrara, N. (1999). VEGF couples hypertrophic cartilage remodeling, ossification and angiogenesis during endochondral bone formation. *Nat. Med.* **5**, 623–628. doi:10.1038/9467

Gerstenfeld, L. C., Cho, T. J., Kon, T., Aizawa, T., Cruceta, J., Graves, B. D., et al. (2001). Impaired intramembranous bone formation during bone repair in the absence of tumor necrosis factor-alpha signaling. *Cells Tissues Organs* **169**, 285–294. doi:10.1159/000047893

Glass, G. E., Chan, J. K., Freidin, A., Feldmann, M., Horwood, N. J., and Nanchahal, J. (2011). TNF-alpha promotes fracture repair by augmenting the recruitment and differentiation of muscle-derived stromal cells. *Proc. Natl. Acad. Sci. U.S.A.* **108**, 1585–1590. doi:10.1073/pnas.1018501108

Grad, S., Ertel, W., Keel, M., Infanger, M., Vonderschmitt, D. J., and Maly, F. E. (1998). Strongly enhanced serum levels of vascular endothelial growth factor (VEGF) after polytrauma and burn. *Clin. Chem. Lab. Med.* **36**, 379–383. doi:10.1515/CCLM.1998.064

Hart, K., Baur, D., Hodam, J., Lesoon-Wood, L., Parham, M., Keith, K., et al. (2006). Short- and long-term effects of sildenafil on skin flap survival in rats. *Laryngoscope* **116**, 522–528. doi:10.1097/01.mlg.0000200792.67802.3b

Helmrich, U., Di Maggio, N., Guven, S., Groppa, E., Melly, L., Largo, R. D., et al. (2013). Osteogenic graft vascularization and bone resorption by VEGF-expressing human mesenchymal progenitors. *Biomaterials* **34**, 5025–5035. doi:10.1016/j.biomaterials.2013.03.040

Hernigou, P., and Beaujean, F. (1997). [Bone marrow in patients with pseudarthrosis. A study of progenitor cells by in vitro cloning]. *Rev. Chir. Orthop. Reparatrice. Appar. Mot.* **83**, 33–40.

Hiltunen, M. O., Ruuskanen, M., Huuskonen, J., Mahonen, A. J., Ahonen, M., Rutanen, J., et al. (2003). Adenovirus-mediated VEGF-A gene transfer induces bone formation in vivo. *FASEB J.* **17**, 1147–1149. doi:10.1096/fj.02-0514fje

Histing, T., Marciniak, K., Scheuer, C., Garcia, P., Holstein, J. H., Klein, M., et al. (2011). Sildenafil accelerates fracture healing in mice. *J. Orthop. Res.* **29**, 867–873. doi:10.1002/jor.21324

Ho, C. Y., Sanghani, A., Hua, J., Coathup, M., Kalia, P., and Blunn, G. (2014). Mesenchymal stem cells with increased stromal cell-derived factor 1 expression enhanced fracture healing. *Tissue Eng. Part A.* **21**, 594–602. doi:10.1089/ten.TEA.2013.0762

Hou, H., Zhang, X., Tang, T., Dai, K., and Ge, R. (2009). Enhancement of bone formation by genetically-engineered bone marrow stromal cells expressing BMP-2, VEGF and angiopoietin-1. *Biotechnol. Lett.* **31**, 1183–1189. doi:10.1007/s10529-009-0007-4

Huang, Y. C., Simmons, C., Kaigler, D., Rice, K. G., and Mooney, D. J. (2005). Bone regeneration in a rat cranial defect with delivery of PEI-condensed plasmid DNA encoding for bone morphogenetic protein-4 (BMP-4). *Gene Ther.* **12**, 418–426. doi:10.1038/sj.gt.3302439

Ishida, K., Matsumoto, T., Sasaki, K., Mifune, Y., Tei, K., Kubo, S., et al. (2010). Bone regeneration properties of granulocyte colony-stimulating factor via neovascularization and osteogenesis. *Tissue Eng. Part A* **16**, 3271–3284. doi:10.1089/ten.tea.2009.0268

Jabbarzadeh, E., Starnes, T., Khan, Y. M., Jiang, T., Wirtel, A. J., Deng, M., et al. (2008). Induction of angiogenesis in tissue-engineered scaffolds designed for bone repair: a combined gene therapy-cell transplantation approach. *Proc. Natl. Acad. Sci. U.S.A.* **105**, 11099–11104. doi:10.1073/pnas.0800069105

Ji, J. F., He, B. P., Dheen, S. T., and Tay, S. S. (2004). Interactions of chemokines and chemokine receptors mediate the migration of mesenchymal stem cells to the impaired site in the brain after hypoglossal nerve injury. *Stem Cells* **22**, 415–427. doi:10.1634/stemcells.22-3-415

Ji, W., Yang, F., Ma, J., Bouma, M. J., Boerman, O. C., Chen, Z., et al. (2013). Incorporation of stromal cell-derived factor-1alpha in PCL/gelatin electrospun membranes for guided bone regeneration. *Biomaterials* **34**, 735–745. doi:10.1016/j.biomaterials.2012.10.016

Jia, S., Yang, X., Song, W., Wang, L., Fang, K., Hu, Z., et al. (2014). Incorporation of osteogenic and angiogenic small interfering RNAs into chitosan sponge for bone tissue engineering. *Int. J. Nanomedicine* **9**, 5307–5316. doi:10.2147/IJN.S70457

Jin, Q., and Giannobile, W. V. (2014). SDF-1 enhances wound healing of critical-sized calvarial defects beyond self-repair capacity. *PLoS ONE* **9**:e97035. doi:10.1371/journal.pone.0097035

Kaigler, D., Wang, Z., Horger, K., Mooney, D. J., and Krebsbach, P. H. (2006). VEGF scaffolds enhance angiogenesis and bone regeneration in irradiated osseous defects. *J. Bone Miner. Res.* **21**, 735–744. doi:10.1359/jbmr.060120

Kaipel, M., Schutzenberger, S., Schultz, A., Ferguson, J., Slezak, P., Morton, T. J., et al. (2012). BMP-2 but not VEGF or PDGF in fibrin matrix supports bone healing in a delayed-union rat model. *J. Orthop. Res.* **30**, 1563–1569. doi:10.1002/jor.22132

Kanczler, J. M., Ginty, P. J., White, L., Clarke, N. M., Howdle, S. M., Shakesheff, K. M., et al. (2010). The effect of the delivery of vascular endothelial growth factor and bone morphogenic protein-2 to osteoprogenitor cell populations on bone formation. *Biomaterials* **31**, 1242–1250. doi:10.1016/j.biomaterials.2009.10.059

Kawakami, Y., Ii, M., Matsumoto, T., Kuroda, R., Kuroda, T., Kwon, S. M., et al. (2015). SDF-1/CXCR4 axis in Tie2-lineage cells including endothelial progenitor cells contributes to bone fracture healing. *J. Bone Miner. Res.* **30**, 95–105. doi:10.1002/jbmr.2318

Kaygusuz, M. A., Turan, C. C., Aydin, N. E., Temel, I., Firat, S., Bulut, T., et al. (2006). The effects of G-CSF and naproxen sodium on the serum TGF-beta1 level and fracture healing in rat tibias. *Life Sci.* **80**, 67–73. doi:10.1016/j.lfs.2006.08.023

Kempen, D. H., Lu, L., Heijink, A., Hefferan, T. E., Creemers, L. B., Maran, A., et al. (2009). Effect of local sequential VEGF and BMP-2 delivery on ectopic and orthotopic bone regeneration. *Biomaterials* **30**, 2816–2825. doi:10.1016/j.biomaterials.2009.01.031

Keramaris, N. C., Calori, G. M., Nikolaou, V. S., Schemitsch, E. H., and Giannoudis, P. V. (2008). Fracture vascularity and bone healing: a systematic review of the role of VEGF. *Injury* **39**(Suppl. 2), S45–S57. doi:10.1016/S0020-1383(08)70015-9

Khan, Y., and Laurencin, C. T. (2008). Fracture repair with ultrasound: clinical and cell-based evaluation. *J. Bone Joint Surg. Am.* **90**(Suppl. 1), 138–144. doi:10.2106/JBJS.G.01218

Kinnaird, T., Stabile, E., Burnett, M. S., and Epstein, S. E. (2004). Bone-marrow-derived cells for enhancing collateral development: mechanisms, animal data, and initial clinical experiences. *Circ. Res.* **95**, 354–363. doi:10.1161/01.RES.0000137878.26174.66

Kitaori, T., Ito, H., Schwarz, E. M., Tsutsumi, R., Yoshitomi, H., Oishi, S., et al. (2009). Stromal cell-derived factor 1/CXCR4 signaling is critical for the recruitment of mesenchymal stem cells to the fracture site during skeletal repair in a mouse model. *Arthritis Rheum.* **60**, 813–823. doi:10.1002/art.24330

Kleinheinz, J., Stratmann, U., Joos, U., and Wiesmann, H. P. (2005). VEGF-activated angiogenesis during bone regeneration. *J. Oral Maxillofac. Surg.* **63**, 1310–1316. doi:10.1016/j.joms.2005.05.303

Koc, A., Finkenzeller, G., Elcin, A. E., Stark, G. B., and Elcin, Y. M. (2014). Evaluation of adenoviral vascular endothelial growth factor-activated chitosan/hydroxyapatite scaffold for engineering vascularized bone tissue using human osteoblasts: in vitro and in vivo studies. *J. Biomater. Appl.* **29**, 748–760. doi:10.1177/0885328214544769

Kon, T., Cho, T. J., Aizawa, T., Yamazaki, M., Nooh, N., Graves, D., et al. (2001). Expression of osteoprotegerin, receptor activator of NF-kappaB ligand (osteoprotegerin ligand) and related proinflammatory cytokines during fracture healing. *J. Bone Miner. Res.* **16**, 1004–1014. doi:10.1359/jbmr.2001.16.6.1004

Koneru, S., Varma Penumathsa, S., Thirunavukkarasu, M., Vidavalur, R., Zhan, L., Singal, P. K., et al. (2008). Sildenafil-mediated neovascularization and protection against myocardial ischaemia reperfusion injury in rats: role of VEGF/angiopoietin-1. *J. Cell. Mol. Med.* **12**, 2651–2664. doi:10.1111/j.1582-4934.2008.00319.x

Kumar, S., and Ponnazhagan, S. (2012). Mobilization of bone marrow mesenchymal stem cells in vivo augments bone healing in a mouse model of segmental bone defect. *Bone* **50**, 1012–1018. doi:10.1016/j.bone.2012.01.027

Kupcsik, L., Meurya, T., Flury, M., Stoddart, M., and Alini, M. (2009). Statin-induced calcification in human mesenchymal stem cells is cell death related. *J. Cell. Mol. Med.* **13**, 4465–4473. doi:10.1111/j.1582-4934.2008.00545.x

Kuroda, R., Matsumoto, T., Miwa, M., Kawamoto, A., Mifune, Y., Fukui, T., et al. (2011). Local transplantation of G-CSF-mobilized CD34(+) cells in a patient with tibial nonunion: a case report. *Cell Transplant.* **20**, 1491–1496. doi:10.3727/096368910X550189

Kuroda, R., Matsumoto, T., Niikura, T., Kawakami, Y., Fukui, T., Lee, S. Y., et al. (2014). Local transplantation of granulocyte colony stimulating factor-mobilized CD34+

cells for patients with femoral and tibial nonunion: pilot clinical trial. *Stem Cells Transl. Med.* **3**, 128–134. doi:10.5966/sctm.2013-0106

Laing, A. J., Dillon, J. P., Condon, E. T., Street, J. T., Wang, J. H., Mcguinness, A. J., et al. (2007). Mobilization of endothelial precursor cells: systemic vascular response to musculoskeletal trauma. *J. Orthop. Res.* **25**, 44–50. doi:10.1002/jor.20228

Laroche, M. (2002). Intraosseous circulation from physiology to disease. *Joint Bone Spine* **69**, 262–269. doi:10.1016/S1297-319X(02)00391-3

Leach, J. K., Kaigler, D., Wang, Z., Krebsbach, P. H., and Mooney, D. J. (2006). Coating of VEGF-releasing scaffolds with bioactive glass for angiogenesis and bone regeneration. *Biomaterials* **27**, 3249–3255. doi:10.1016/j.biomaterials.2006.01.033

Lenze, U., Pohlig, F., Seitz, S., Ern, C., Milz, S., Docheva, D., et al. (2014). Influence of osteogenic stimulation and VEGF treatment on in vivo bone formation in hMSC-seeded cancellous bone scaffolds. *BMC Musculoskelet. Disord.* **15**:350. doi:10.1186/1471-2474-15-350

Leung, K. S., Lee, W. S., Tsui, H. F., Liu, P. P., and Cheung, W. H. (2004). Complex tibial fracture outcomes following treatment with low-intensity pulsed ultrasound. *Ultrasound Med. Biol.* **30**, 389–395. doi:10.1016/j.ultrasmedbio.2003.11.008

Levesque, J. P., Hendy, J., Takamatsu, Y., Simmons, P. J., and Bendall, L. J. (2003). Disruption of the CXCR4/CXCL12 chemotactic interaction during hematopoietic stem cell mobilization induced by GCSF or cyclophosphamide. *J. Clin. Invest.* **111**, 187–196. doi:10.1172/JCI15994

Li, R., Stewart, D. J., Von Schroeder, H. P., Mackinnon, E. S., and Schemitsch, E. H. (2009). Effect of cell-based VEGF gene therapy on healing of a segmental bone defect. *J. Orthop. Res.* **27**, 8–14. doi:10.1002/jor.20658

Li, X., Gao, Z., and Wang, J. (2011). Single percutaneous injection of stromal cell-derived factor-1 induces bone repair in mouse closed tibial fracture model. *Orthopedics* **34**, 450. doi:10.3928/01477447-20110427-19

Lin, C. Y., Chang, Y. H., Sung, L. Y., Chen, C. L., Lin, S. Y., Li, K. C., et al. (2014). Long-term tracking of segmental bone healing mediated by genetically engineered adipose-derived stem cells: focuses on bone remodeling and potential side effects. *Tissue Eng. Part A* **20**, 1392–1402. doi:10.1089/ten.TEA.2013.0314

Liu, J., Wang, J., Jiang, W., and Tang, Y. (2013). Effect of cytotoxic T-lymphocyte antigen-4, TNF-alpha polymorphisms on osteosarcoma: evidences from a meta-analysis. *Chin. J. Cancer Res.* **25**, 671–678. doi:10.3978/j.issn.1000-9604.2013.11.06

Liu, Y. S., Ou, M. E., Liu, H., Gu, M., Lv, L. W., Fan, C., et al. (2014). The effect of simvastatin on chemotactic capability of SDF-1alpha and the promotion of bone regeneration. *Biomaterials* **35**, 4489–4498. doi:10.1016/j.biomaterials.2014.02.025

Ma, J., Both, S. K., Yang, F., Cui, F. Z., Pan, J., Meijer, G. J., et al. (2014). Concise review: cell-based strategies in bone tissue engineering and regenerative medicine. *Stem Cells Transl. Med.* **3**, 98–107. doi:10.5966/sctm.2013-0126

Ma, X. L., Sun, X. L., Wan, C. Y., Ma, J. X., and Tian, P. (2012). Significance of circulating endothelial progenitor cells in patients with fracture healing process. *J. Orthop. Res.* **30**, 1860–1866. doi:10.1002/jor.22134

Malhotra, A., Pelletier, M. H., Yu, Y., and Walsh, W. R. (2013). Can platelet-rich plasma (PRP) improve bone healing? A comparison between the theory and experimental outcomes. *Arch. Orthop. Trauma Surg.* **133**, 153–165. doi:10.1007/s00402-012-1641-1

Marmotti, A., Castoldi, F., Rossi, R., Marenco, S., Risso, A., Ruella, M., et al. (2013). Bone marrow-derived cell mobilization by G-CSF to enhance osseointegration of bone substitute in high tibial osteotomy. *Knee Surg. Sports Traumatol. Arthrosc.* **21**, 237–248. doi:10.1007/s00167-012-2150-z

Martino, M. M., Briquez, P. S., Guc, E., Tortelli, F., Kilarski, W. W., Metzger, S., et al. (2014). Growth factors engineered for super-affinity to the extracellular matrix enhance tissue healing. *Science* **343**, 885–888. doi:10.1126/science.1247663

Martino, M. M., Tortelli, F., Mochizuki, M., Traub, S., Ben-David, D., Kuhn, G. A., et al. (2011). Engineering the growth factor microenvironment with fibronectin domains to promote wound and bone tissue healing. *Sci. Transl. Med.* **3**, 100ra189. doi:10.1126/scitranslmed.3002614

Mathieu, M., Rigutto, S., Ingels, A., Spruyt, D., Stricwant, N., Kharroubi, I., et al. (2013). Decreased pool of mesenchymal stem cells is associated with altered chemokines serum levels in atrophic nonunion fractures. *Bone* **53**, 391–398. doi:10.1016/j.bone.2013.01.005

Matsumoto, T., Kawamoto, A., Kuroda, R., Ishikawa, M., Mifune, Y., Iwasaki, H., et al. (2006). Therapeutic potential of vasculogenesis and osteogenesis promoted by peripheral blood CD34-positive cells for functional bone healing. *Am. J. Pathol.* **169**, 1440–1457. doi:10.2353/ajpath.2006.060064

Matsumoto, T., Mifune, Y., Kawamoto, A., Kuroda, R., Shoji, T., Iwasaki, H., et al. (2008). Fracture induced mobilization and incorporation of bone marrow-derived

endothelial progenitor cells for bone healing. *J. Cell. Physiol.* **215**, 234–242. doi:10.1002/jcp.21309

Mattar, T., Friedrich, P. F., and Bishop, A. T. (2013). Effect of rhBMP-2 and VEGF in a vascularized bone allotransplant experimental model based on surgical neoangiogenesis. *J. Orthop. Res.* **31**, 561–566. doi:10.1002/jor.22277

Mayr-Wohlfart, U., Waltenberger, J., Hausser, H., Kessler, S., Gunther, K. P., Dehio, C., et al. (2002). Vascular endothelial growth factor stimulates chemotactic migration of primary human osteoblasts. *Bone* **30**, 472–477. doi:10.1016/S8756-3282(01)00690-1

Mendes, S. C., Tibbe, J. M., Veenhof, M., Bakker, K., Both, S., Platenburg, P. P., et al. (2002). Bone tissue-engineered implants using human bone marrow stromal cells: effect of culture conditions and donor age. *Tissue Eng.* **8**, 911–920. doi:10.1089/107632702320934010

Mifune, Y., Matsumoto, T., Kawamoto, A., Kuroda, R., Shoji, T., Iwasaki, H., et al. (2008). Local delivery of granulocyte colony stimulating factor-mobilized CD34-positive progenitor cells using bioscaffold for modality of unhealing bone fracture. *Stem Cells* **26**, 1395–1405. doi:10.1634/stemcells.2007-0820

Mundy, G., Garrett, R., Harris, S., Chan, J., Chen, D., Rossini, G., et al. (1999). Stimulation of bone formation in vitro and in rodents by statins. *Science* **286**, 1946–1949. doi:10.1126/science.286.5446.1946

Murphy, W. L., Simmons, C. A., Kaigler, D., and Mooney, D. J. (2004). Bone regeneration via a mineral substrate and induced angiogenesis. *J. Dent. Res.* **83**, 204–210. doi:10.1177/154405910408300304

Neufeld, G., Cohen, T., Gengrinovitch, S., and Poltorak, Z. (1999). Vascular endothelial growth factor (VEGF) and its receptors. *FASEB J.* **13**, 9–22.

Nyan, M., Sato, D., Kihara, H., Machida, T., Ohya, K., and Kasugai, S. (2009). Effects of the combination with alpha-tricalcium phosphate and simvastatin on bone regeneration. *Clin. Oral Implants Res.* **20**, 280–287. doi:10.1111/j.1600-0501.2008.01639.x

Orlandini, M., Spreafico, A., Bardelli, M., Rocchigiani, M., Salameh, A., Nucciotti, S., et al. (2006). Vascular endothelial growth factor-D activates VEGFR-3 expressed in osteoblasts inducing their differentiation. *J. Biol. Chem.* **281**, 17961–17967. doi:10.1074/jbc.M600413200

Otsuru, S., Tamai, K., Yamazaki, T., Yoshikawa, H., and Kaneda, Y. (2008). Circulating bone marrow-derived osteoblast progenitor cells are recruited to the bone-forming site by the CXCR4/stromal cell-derived factor-1 pathway. *Stem Cells* **26**, 223–234. doi:10.1634/stemcells.2007-0515

Ozawa, C. R., Banfi, A., Glazer, N. L., Thurston, G., Springer, M. L., Kraft, P. E., et al. (2004). Microenvironmental VEGF concentration, not total dose, determines a threshold between normal and aberrant angiogenesis. *J. Clin. Invest.* **113**, 516–527. doi:10.1172/JCI18420

Patel, Z. S., Ueda, H., Yamamoto, M., Tabata, Y., and Mikos, A. G. (2008a). In vitro and in vivo release of vascular endothelial growth factor from gelatin microparticles and biodegradable composite scaffolds. *Pharm. Res.* **25**, 2370–2378. doi:10.1007/s11095-008-9685-1

Patel, Z. S., Young, S., Tabata, Y., Jansen, J. A., Wong, M. E., and Mikos, A. G. (2008b). Dual delivery of an angiogenic and an osteogenic growth factor for bone regeneration in a critical size defect model. *Bone* **43**, 931–940. doi:10.1016/j.bone.2008.06.019

Peichev, M., Naiyer, A. J., Pereira, D., Zhu, Z., Lane, W. J., Williams, M., et al. (2000). Expression of VEGFR-2 and AC133 by circulating human CD34(+) cells identifies a population of functional endothelial precursors. *Blood* **95**, 952–958.

Pellegrini, G., Seol, Y. J., Gruber, R., and Giannobile, W. V. (2009). Pre-clinical models for oral and periodontal reconstructive therapies. *J. Dent. Res.* **88**, 1065–1076. doi:10.1177/0022034509349748

Peng, H., Wright, V., Usas, A., Gearhart, B., Shen, H. C., Cummins, J., et al. (2002). Synergistic enhancement of bone formation and healing by stem cell-expressed VEGF and bone morphogenetic protein-4. *J. Clin. Invest.* **110**, 751–759. doi:10.1172/JCI15153

Phipps, M. C., Xu, Y., and Bellis, S. L. (2012). Delivery of platelet-derived growth factor as a chemotactic factor for mesenchymal stem cells by bone-mimetic electrospun scaffolds. *PLoS ONE* **7**:e40831. doi:10.1371/journal.pone.0040831

Ramazanoglu, M., Lutz, R., Rusche, P., Trabzon, L., Kose, G. T., Prechtl, C., et al. (2013). Bone response to biomimetic implants delivering BMP-2 and VEGF: an immunohistochemical study. *J. Craniomaxillofac. Surg.* **41**, 826–835. doi:10.1016/j.jcms.2013.01.037

Reed, A. A., Joyner, C. J., Brownlow, H. C., and Simpson, A. H. (2002). Human atrophic fracture non-unions are not avascular. *J. Orthop. Res.* **20**, 593–599. doi:10.1016/S0736-0266(01)00142-5

Romagnoli, C., and Brandi, M. L. (2014). Adipose mesenchymal stem cells in the field of bone tissue engineering. *World J. Stem Cells* **6**, 144–152. doi:10.4252/wjsc.v6.i2.144

Sacchi, V., Mittermayr, R., Hartinger, J., Martino, M. M., Lorentz, K. M., Wolbank, S., et al. (2014). Long-lasting fibrin matrices ensure stable and functional angiogenesis by highly tunable, sustained delivery of recombinant VEGF164. *Proc. Natl. Acad. Sci. U.S.A.* **111**, 6952–6957. doi:10.1073/pnas.1404605111

Samee, M., Kasugai, S., Kondo, H., Ohya, K., Shimokawa, H., and Kuroda, S. (2008). Bone morphogenetic protein-2 (BMP-2) and vascular endothelial growth factor (VEGF) transfection to human periosteal cells enhances osteoblast differentiation and bone formation. *J. Pharmacol. Sci.* **108**, 18–31. doi:10.1254/jphs.08036FP

Seebach, C., Henrich, D., Tewksbury, R., Wilhelm, K., and Marzi, I. (2007). Number and proliferative capacity of human mesenchymal stem cells are modulated positively in multiple trauma patients and negatively in atrophic nonunions. *Calcif. Tissue Int.* **80**, 294–300. doi:10.1007/s00223-007-9020-6

Seebach, E., Freischmidt, H., Holschbach, J., Fellenberg, J., and Richter, W. (2014). Mesenchymal stroma cells trigger early attraction of M1 macrophages and endothelial cells into fibrin hydrogels, stimulating long bone healing without long-term engraftment. *Acta Biomater.* **10**, 4730–4741. doi:10.1016/j.actbio.2014.07.017

Shinohara, K., Greenfield, S., Pan, H., Vasanji, A., Kumagai, K., Midura, R. J., et al. (2011). Stromal cell-derived factor-1 and monocyte chemotactic protein-3 improve recruitment of osteogenic cells into sites of musculoskeletal repair. *J. Orthop. Res.* **29**, 1064–1069. doi:10.1002/jor.21374

Shirley, D., Marsh, D., Jordan, G., Mcquaid, S., and Li, G. (2005). Systemic recruitment of osteoblastic cells in fracture healing. *J. Orthop. Res.* **23**, 1013–1021. doi:10.1016/j.orthres.2005.01.013

Siegel, G., Kluba, T., Hermanutz-Klein, U., Bieback, K., Northoff, H., and Schafer, R. (2013). Phenotype, donor age and gender affect function of human bone marrow-derived mesenchymal stromal cells. *BMC Med.* **11**:146. doi:10.1186/1741-7015-11-146

Stoddart, M. J., Bara, J., and Alini, M. (2014). Cells and secretome – towards endogenous cell re-activation for cartilage repair. *Adv. Drug Deliv. Rev.* **84**, 135–145. doi:10.1016/j.addr.2014.08.007

Street, J., Bao, M., Deguzman, L., Bunting, S., Peale, F. V. Jr., Ferrara, N., et al. (2002). Vascular endothelial growth factor stimulates bone repair by promoting angiogenesis and bone turnover. *Proc. Natl. Acad. Sci. U.S.A.* **99**, 9656–9661. doi:10.1073/pnas.152324099

Tarkka, T., Sipola, A., Jamsa, T., Soini, Y., Yla-Herttuala, S., Tuukkanen, J., et al. (2003). Adenoviral VEGF-A gene transfer induces angiogenesis and promotes bone formation in healing osseous tissues. *J. Gene Med.* **5**, 560–566. doi:10.1002/jgm.392

Toupadakis, C. A., Granick, J. L., Sagy, M., Wong, A., Ghassemi, E., Chung, D. J., et al. (2013). Mobilization of endogenous stem cell populations enhances fracture healing in a murine femoral fracture model. *Cytotherapy* **15**, 1136–1147. doi:10.1016/j.jcyt.2013.05.004

Verloop, R. E., Koolwijk, P., Van Zonneveld, A. J., and Van Hinsbergh, V. W. (2009). Proteases and receptors in the recruitment of endothelial progenitor cells in neovascularization. *Eur. Cytokine Netw.* **20**, 207–219. doi:10.1684/ecn.2009.0174

Wang, C. Y., Yang, H. B., Hsu, H. S., Chen, L. L., Tsai, C. C., Tsai, K. S., et al. (2012). Mesenchymal stem cell-conditioned medium facilitates angiogenesis and fracture healing in diabetic rats. *J. Tissue Eng. Regen. Med.* **6**, 559–569. doi:10.1002/term.461

Wei, F. Y., Leung, K. S., Li, G., Qin, J., Chow, S. K., Huang, S., et al. (2014). Low intensity pulsed ultrasound enhanced mesenchymal stem cell recruitment through stromal derived factor-1 signaling in fracture healing. *PLoS ONE* **9**:e106722. doi:10.1371/journal.pone.0106722

Wernike, E., Montjovent, M. O., Liu, Y., Wismeijer, D., Hunziker, E. B., Siebenrock, K. A., et al. (2010). VEGF incorporated into calcium phosphate ceramics promotes vascularisation and bone formation in vivo. *Eur. Cell. Mater.* **19**, 30–40.

Wynn, R. F., Hart, C. A., Corradi-Perini, C., O'Neill, L., Evans, C. A., Wraith, J. E., et al. (2004). A small proportion of mesenchymal stem cells strongly expresses functionally active CXCR4 receptor capable of promoting migration to bone marrow. *Blood* **104**, 2643–2645. doi:10.1182/blood-2004-02-0526

Xiao, C., Zhou, H., Liu, G., Zhang, P., Fu, Y., Gu, P., et al. (2011). Bone marrow stromal cells with a combined expression of BMP-2 and VEGF-165 enhanced bone regeneration. *Biomed. Mater.* **6**, 015013. doi:10.1088/1748-6041/6/1/015013

Yin, Y., Huang, L., Zhao, X., Fang, Y., Yu, S., Zhao, J., et al. (2007). AMD3100 mobilizes endothelial progenitor cells in mice, but inhibits its biological functions by blocking an autocrine/paracrine regulatory loop of stromal cell derived factor-1 in vitro. *J. Cardiovasc. Pharmacol.* **50**, 61–67. doi:10.1097/FJC.0b013e3180587e4d

Young, S., Patel, Z. S., Kretlow, J. D., Murphy, M. B., Mountziaris, P. M., Baggett, L. S., et al. (2009). Dose effect of dual delivery of vascular endothelial growth factor and bone morphogenetic protein-2 on bone regeneration in a rat critical-size defect model. *Tissue Eng. Part A* **15**, 2347–2362. doi:10.1089/ten.tea.2008.0510

Yueyi, C., Xiaoguang, H., Jingying, W., Quansheng, S., Jie, T., Xin, F., et al. (2013). Calvarial defect healing by recruitment of autogenous osteogenic stem cells using locally applied simvastatin. *Biomaterials* **34**, 9373–9380. doi:10.1016/j.biomaterials.2013.08.060

Zhang, L., Zhang, L., Lan, X., Xu, M., Mao, Z., Lv, H., et al. (2014a). Improvement in angiogenesis and osteogenesis with modified cannulated screws combined with VEGF/PLGA/fibrin glue in femoral neck fractures. *J. Mater. Sci. Mater. Med.* **25**, 1165–1172. doi:10.1007/s10856-013-5138-4

Zhang, W., Zhu, C., Wu, Y., Ye, D., Wang, S., Zou, D., et al. (2014b). VEGF and BMP-2 promote bone regeneration by facilitating bone marrow stem cell homing and differentiation. *Eur. Cell. Mater.* **27**, 1–11. doi:10.1016/j.eurpolymj.2014.08.007

Zhang, W., Zhu, C., Ye, D., Xu, L., Zhang, X., Wu, Q., et al. (2014c). Porous silk scaffolds for delivery of growth factors and stem cells to enhance bone regeneration. *PLoS One* **9**:e102371. doi:10.1371/journal.pone.0102371

Zhang, W., Wang, X., Wang, S., Zhao, J., Xu, L., Zhu, C., et al. (2011). The use of injectable sonication-induced silk hydrogel for VEGF(165) and BMP-2 delivery for elevation of the maxillary sinus floor. *Biomaterials* **32**, 9415–9424. doi:10.1016/j.biomaterials.2011.08.047

Zhou, S., Greenberger, J. S., Epperly, M. W., Goff, J. P., Adler, C., Leboff, M. S., et al. (2008). Age-related intrinsic changes in human bone-marrow-derived mesenchymal stem cells and their differentiation to osteoblasts. *Aging Cell* **7**, 335–343. doi:10.1111/j.1474-9726.2008.00377.x

Zwingenberger, S., Yao, Z., Jacobi, A., Vater, C., Valladares, R. D., Li, C., et al. (2014). Enhancement of BMP-2 induced bone regeneration by SDF-1alpha mediated stem cell recruitment. *Tissue Eng. Part A* **20**, 810–818. doi:10.1089/ten.TEA.2013.0222

Conflict of Interest Statement: The authors declare that the research was conducted in the absence of any commercial or financial relationships that could be construed as a potential conflict of interest.

3

Depot-based delivery systems for pro-angiogenic peptides: a review

Amy H. Van Hove[1] and Danielle S. W. Benoit[1,2,3,4]*

[1]Department of Biomedical Engineering, University of Rochester, Rochester, NY, USA, [2]Department of Chemical Engineering, University of Rochester, Rochester, NY, USA, [3]Department of Biomedical Genetics, University of Rochester Medical Center, Rochester, NY, USA, [4]Department of Orthopaedics, Center for Musculoskeletal Research, University of Rochester Medical Center, Rochester, NY, USA

Edited by:
Jian Yang,
The Pennsylvania State University,
USA

Reviewed by:
Heike Boehm,
Max Planck Institute for Intelligent
Systems, Germany
Lauren Flynn,
The University of Western Ontario,
Canada

*Correspondence:
Danielle S. W. Benoit,
Department of Biomedical
Engineering, University of Rochester,
207 Robert B. Goergen Hall,
Rochester, NY 14627, USA
benoit@bme.rochester.edu

Insufficient vascularization currently limits the size and complexity for all tissue engineering approaches. Additionally, increasing or re-initiating blood flow is the first step toward restoration of ischemic tissue homeostasis. However, no FDA-approved pro-angiogenic treatments exist, despite the many pre-clinical approaches that have been developed. The relatively small size of peptides gives advantages over protein-based treatments, specifically with respect to synthesis and stability. While many pro-angiogenic peptides have been identified and shown promising results in vitro and in vivo, the majority of biomaterials developed for pro-angiogenic drug delivery focus on protein delivery. This narrow focus limits pro-angiogenic therapeutics as peptides, similar to proteins, suffer from poor pharmacokinetics in vivo, necessitating the development of controlled release systems. This review discusses pro-angiogenic peptides and the biomaterials delivery systems that have been developed, or that could easily be adapted for peptide delivery, with a particular focus on depot-based delivery systems.

Keywords: angiogenesis, controlled release, biomaterials, drug delivery, hydrogels, depot-based, review

Introduction

Therapeutic angiogenesis holds great potential for supporting developing engineered tissues, where insufficient vascularization limits size and complexity. Additionally, a number of ischemic tissue disorders would benefit from pro-angiogenic therapies by restoring blood flow to the tissue. However, no FDA-approved treatments exist to reproducibly enhance vascularization (Muir, 2009; Zachary and Morgan, 2011; Chu and Wang, 2012).

The field of tissue engineering has made remarkable progress in developing tissues to restore, augment, or replace the function of damaged tissues within the body. For example, engineered urethras remained functional for 6 years (Raya-Rivera et al., 2011). Similarly, tissue-engineered bladders (Atala et al., 2006) and trachea (Macchiarini et al., 2008) have been successfully implanted in humans, and remained functional at 46- and 4-month follow up exams, respectively. However, the success of engineered tissues has been limited to thin tissues, with engineering larger, more complex structures slowed by challenges associated with development of necessary vascularization to sustain growing/remodeling tissues (Atala, 2004).

$500 billion is spent each year in the United States to treat cardiovascular diseases, such as peripheral arterial and coronary heart disease (Go et al., 2014). Peripheral arterial disease affects 8.5 million Americans, and coronary heart disease is the leading cause of death in the United States, responsible for ~1 in every 6 deaths in 2010 (Go et al., 2014). Currently, treatment of peripheral arterial and coronary heart disease focuses on maximizing function of existing vasculature using vasodilators and anti-clotting agents, or through surgical interventions, such as angioplasty, stent placement, or bypass grafts, rather than encouraging development of new vasculature to support the tissue (Muir, 2009; Lloyd-Jones et al., 2010).

Diabetes affects 20.8 million people in the United States, with 15% of this population also affected by diabetic foot ulcers. Diabetic ulcers precede 84% of diabetes-related lower limb amputations and are a cause significant morbidity, making them a significant public health burden (Brem and Tomic-Canic, 2007). These wounds are resistant to healing due in part to decreased angiogenic response (Galiano et al., 2004), and improvements in ulcer healing have been obtained with repeated topical treatment with pro-angiogenic growth factors. However, becaplermin (recombinant platelet-derived growth factor, PDGF) is currently the only FDA-approved pro-angiogenic treatment for diabetic ulcers, and even with daily application, only 48% of patients exhibit complete wound closure over 20 weeks (Steed, 1995).

This review focuses on pro-angiogenic peptides and biomaterials exploited for their delivery. First, the process of angiogenesis including the critical factors and cell types involved in this process is briefly reviewed. The relative merits of pro-angiogenic peptides as compared to proteins are discussed, as are particular challenges associated with the use of peptide drugs. While many of the biomaterials that have been developed for the delivery of pro-angiogenic factors focus on delivery of large proteins, this review focuses on identifying materials that can be adapted for delivery of the many promising pro-angiogenic peptides that have been identified, as well as materials designed specifically for peptide delivery. Both natural and synthetic biomaterials are discussed, with a focus on depot-based (rather than injectable or orally delivered) biomaterials as they present advantages for pro-angiogenic applications.

Angiogenesis

Vascularization is involved in tissue homeostasis, wound repair, tissue healing, and during the female reproductive cycle. In healthy tissue, development of new vasculature is a carefully orchestrated process controlled by growth factor signals. New vasculature within the body is formed by three processes: vasculogenesis, angiogenesis, and arteriogenesis (Heil et al., 2006). Vasculogenesis occurs early in development and gives rise to the primitive circulatory system, but does not occur during adulthood. Angiogenesis and arteriogenesis, however, frequently occur in adult tissue (Chu and Wang, 2012). Angiogenesis is the sprouting and growth of new, small vessels from existing vasculature, followed by the subsequent remodeling and maturation of the newly developed vasculature. Arteriogenesis typically occurs when larger arteries are occluded, and involves the remodeling of pre-existing vasculature into fully developed, functional arteries (Heil et al., 2006; Chu and Wang, 2012).

While arteriogenesis occurs in response to changes in shear stress within a vessel, angiogenesis responds to tissue hypoxia or insufficient tissue oxygen tension (Adams and Alitalo, 2007). This initiates growth factor signaling cascades that drive the formation of new vasculature toward the ischemic tissue. A schematic representation of this process is shown in **Figure 1**, which includes a summary of key growth factors involved in the process. First, low

oxygen tension inhibits the intracellular degradation of hypoxia inducible factor-1α (HIF-1α), causing HIF-1α accumulation and allowing it to bind with HIF-1β and activate hypoxia-responsive elements within target genes (Hirota and Semenza, 2006). This causes production of a number of angiogenic growth factors, such as vascular endothelial growth factor (VEGF) (Forsythe et al., 1996), which then diffuse into the nearby tissue (**Figure 1A**) (Hirota and

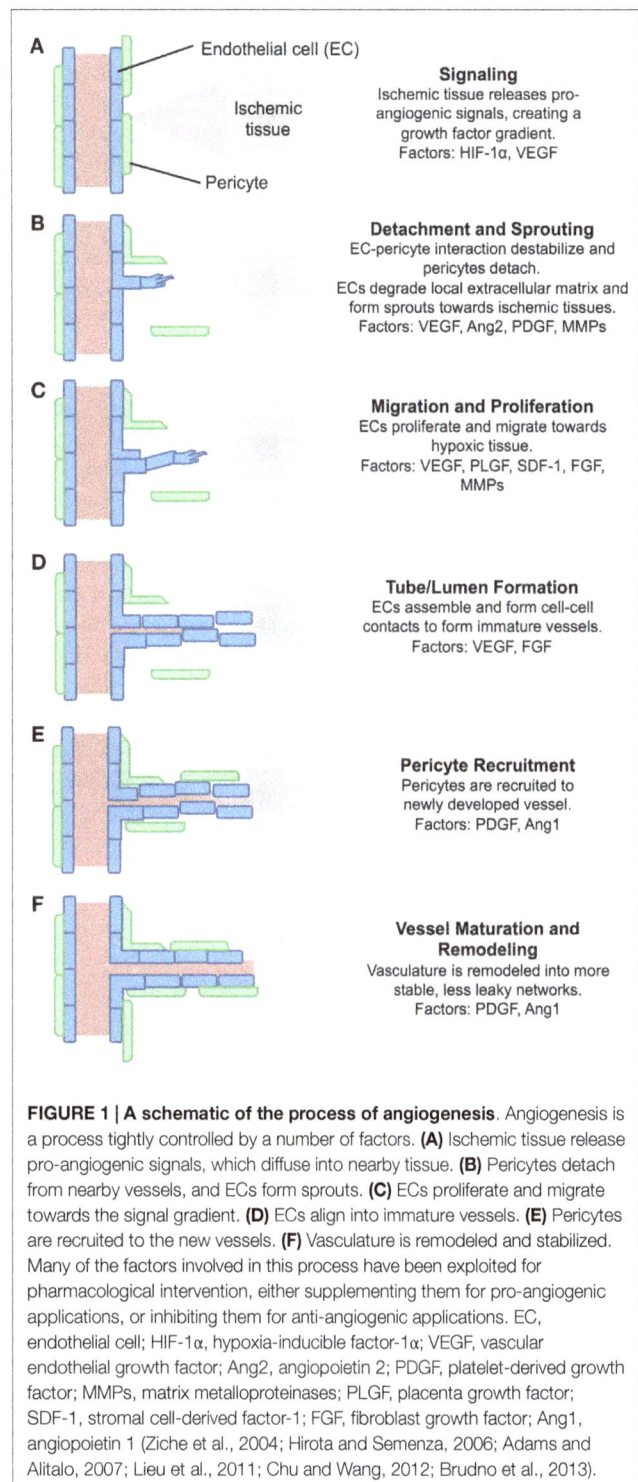

FIGURE 1 | A schematic of the process of angiogenesis. Angiogenesis is a process tightly controlled by a number of factors. **(A)** Ischemic tissue release pro-angiogenic signals, which diffuse into nearby tissue. **(B)** Pericytes detach from nearby vessels, and ECs form sprouts. **(C)** ECs proliferate and migrate towards the signal gradient. **(D)** ECs align into immature vessels. **(E)** Pericytes are recruited to the new vessels. **(F)** Vasculature is remodeled and stabilized. Many of the factors involved in this process have been exploited for pharmacological intervention, either supplementing them for pro-angiogenic applications, or inhibiting them for anti-angiogenic applications. EC, endothelial cell; HIF-1α, hypoxia-inducible factor-1α; VEGF, vascular endothelial growth factor; Ang2, angiopoietin 2; PDGF, platelet-derived growth factor; MMPs, matrix metalloproteinases; PLGF, placenta growth factor; SDF-1, stromal cell-derived factor-1; FGF, fibroblast growth factor; Ang1, angiopoietin 1 (Ziche et al., 2004; Hirota and Semenza, 2006; Adams and Alitalo, 2007; Lieu et al., 2011; Chu and Wang, 2012; Brudno et al., 2013).

Semenza, 2006). These factors signal nearby vasculature, causing detachment of pericytes and sprouting of endothelial cells (ECs) toward the VEGF gradient (**Figure 1B**) (Hirota and Semenza, 2006; Adams and Alitalo, 2007). ECs then migrate in the direction of the gradient, degrading the local extracellular matrix and proliferating in response to factors, such as VEGF, fibroblast growth factor (FGF), and stromal cell-derived factor-1 (SDF-1), producing the required number of cells for vessel formation (**Figure 1C**) (Kuhlmann et al., 2005; Adams and Alitalo, 2007; Lieu et al., 2011). ECs align in tube-like lumen structures, forming an immature vascular network (**Figure 1D**). Pericytes are then recruited to the newly formed vasculature (**Figure 1E**) and the pericyte–EC interaction is stabilized by factors, such as PDGF and Angiopoietin 1 (**Figure 1F**) (Ang1) (Hirota and Semenza, 2006). A variety of growth factors are involved in this process as indicated in **Figure 1**, with some produced by the ischemic tissue itself and others by ECs and pericytes, often in response to previously expressed factors (Forsythe et al., 1996; Ziche et al., 2004; Kuhlmann et al., 2005; Hirota and Semenza, 2006; Adams and Alitalo, 2007; Lieu et al., 2011; Chu and Wang, 2012; Brudno et al., 2013).

Dysfunctions in angiogenesis can lead to serious pathological conditions. Excessive angiogenesis occur in diseases such as cancer, rheumatoid arthritis, age-related macular degeneration, and diabetic retinopathy, while insufficient angiogenesis is associated with diseases like coronary arterial diseases, stroke, and impaired wound healing (Ziche et al., 2004). The development and delivery of anti-angiogenic drugs are a large, exciting area of current research that has been reviewed elsewhere (Nishida et al., 2006; Folkman, 2007; Segal and Satchi-Fainaro, 2009; Welti et al., 2013; Vasudev and Reynolds, 2014). Restoring vascular homeostasis holds great potential for the treatment of ischemic tissue diseases, and as a result, has become an area of great interest in the fields of drug discovery, drug delivery, and tissue engineering (Atala, 2004; Ziche et al., 2004; Vinoth Prabhu et al., 2011; Chu and Wang, 2012). In this review, we focus on biomaterials for the delivery of pro-angiogenic drugs, with a particular focus on delivery of pro-angiogenic peptides.

Pro-Angiogenic Therapies

Pro-angiogenic approaches include delivery of angiogenic proteins (Losordo and Dimmeler, 2004; Silva and Mooney, 2010) or gene therapy resulting in the expression of these proteins (Henry et al., 2007; Gupta et al., 2009), peptide drugs (Lane et al., 1994; Finetti et al., 2012), a limited number of small molecule drugs (Wieghaus et al., 2008), as well as cell-based approaches (Rustad et al., 2012). However, all pro-angiogenic therapeutic strategies reaching clinical trials have had disappointing results (Chu and Wang, 2012). While the reason for failure is specific for each therapeutic approach, many can be attributed to the classic challenges of drug delivery: failure to deliver the therapeutic to the target tissue at the necessary doses and for the required duration, while avoiding degradation and delivery to off-target tissues (Bader and Putnam, 2014).

Protein Therapeutics
Pro-angiogenic approaches have largely focused on delivery of angiogenic proteins including but not limited to vascular

endothelial-, fibroblast-, or platelet-derived growth factor (Losordo and Dimmeler, 2004; Papanas and Maltezos, 2007). Delivery of these factors is considered one of the more straightforward pro-angiogenic approaches; it is simpler and more controllable than cell- and gene-based therapies, and many pro-angiogenic proteins are commercially available (Chu and Wang, 2012). However, simple injection is an inefficient and ineffectual delivery method, as proteins suffer from poor localization and rapid clearance (Laham et al., 1999). These drawbacks present significant challenges, as tight spatio-temporal control over pro-angiogenic proteins, such as VEGF, is required to induce formation of stable and functional vessels (Ozawa et al., 2004; Silva and Mooney, 2007). Additionally, as angiogenesis is a highly regulated process controlled by a number of growth factors, some work suggests that delivery of multiple pro-angiogenic proteins that more closely recapitulate the pro-angiogenic signaling cascade may be required to produce therapeutically relevant and long-lasting vascularization (Mooney et al., 2007; Sylven et al., 2007; Layman et al., 2009; Brudno et al., 2013). While many recombinant human proteins do not elicit a notable immune response in clinical trials, some have induced an immune reaction substantial enough to prevent their use, underlying the importance of addressing this possibility in translational studies (Porter, 2001).

Peptide Therapeutics
As peptides have smaller sequences than proteins (generally <50 amino acids), peptides can be produced either synthetically or grown biologically in *Escherichia coli* or yeast, giving them more versatile production schemes than proteins (Lehninger et al., 2000). Their smaller size allows peptides to be delivered at higher concentrations to target tissue. Additionally, peptides often do not require complex tertiary structures for bioactivity (Finetti et al., 2012). While some pro-angiogenic peptides consist of entirely novel sequences (Hardy et al., 2008), many mimic the bioactive region of pro-angiogenic growth factors (Lane et al., 1994; Finetti et al., 2012) or the extracellular matrix (Demidova-Rice et al., 2011, 2012), facilitating rationally designed therapeutic sequences. There are many modifications to peptides that can be made to increase their thermal and protease stability, such as cyclization, substitution of amino acids not critical for biological effects, and use of non-natural amino acids (Rozek et al., 2003; Diana et al., 2008; Gentilucci et al., 2010). Peptide sequences have been identified that are sensitive to protease cleavage (West and Hubbell, 1999; Patterson and Hubbell, 2010), and that enhance cell penetration and uptake (Lindgren et al., 2000; Copolovici et al., 2014), which are attractive for use in drug delivery applications. Together, these many advantages make peptides an attractive drug class for any number of therapeutic applications.

However, there are drawbacks to the use of peptide drugs. In some situations, peptides do not fully retain the bioactivity of the parent protein and must be delivered at higher doses than protein counterparts to achieve similar effects (Ben-Sasson et al., 2003). This is not always the case, and some peptides afford comparable bioactivities to the parent protein (Santulli et al., 2009). Peptides are still susceptible to protease degradation (Frackenpohl et al., 2001), and similar to proteins, peptides suffer from rapid clearance by the liver and kidneys, leading to poor pharmacokinetics when delivered systemically (Vlieghe et al., 2010; Craik et al., 2013). Peptides that act intracellularly may have difficulty penetrating the hydrophobic cell membrane, reducing their efficacy (Copolovici et al., 2014). Similar to proteins, peptides may elicit an immune response (Niman et al., 1983), and flexible peptide conformations can result in off-target receptor interactions (Vlieghe et al., 2010). These drawbacks have likely contributed to the delayed development and approval of peptides as compared to small molecule and antibody-based therapeutics (Kaspar and Reichert, 2013). However, new synthetic strategies, increased interest in drugs delivered via routes beyond oral and parenteral routes, and the development of improved delivery systems have recently increased their popularity (Vlieghe et al., 2010).

This renewed interest in therapeutic peptides has resulted in the identification and use of peptides as pro-angiogenic therapies, as well as a number of other applications. In 2011, over 500 peptides were in pre-clinical studies, and as of 2013, there were 128 therapeutic peptides in the FDA-approval pipeline: 40 in phase I, 74 in Phase I/II or Phase II, and 14 in Phase II/III or Phase III trials. The peptides currently in clinical trials are designed to treat a variety of diseases, including cancers, acute bacterial infections, type 2 diabetes, osteoporosis, and chronic foot ulcers (Kaspar and Reichert, 2013; Thomas et al., 2014). The number of therapeutic peptides that have been identified but are still in pre-clinical trials is even greater, and they too encompass a variety of therapeutic actions, including chemotherapeutic (Selivanova et al., 1997; Yang et al., 2003) and anti-inflammatory (Akeson et al., 1996; Schultz et al., 2005) peptides, as well as the pro-angiogenic peptides, which are of primary interest here (Lane et al., 1994; Demidova-Rice et al., 2012; Finetti et al., 2012). Select therapeutic peptides, their sources, and current phases of development are listed in **Table 1**, and a number of pro-angiogenic peptides that have shown promising results are summarized in **Table 2**, with specific interesting examples further discussed here.

Qk

The potent pro-angiogenic peptide Qk was designed to mimic the receptor binding α-helix region of VEGF, a key factor in the early stages of angiogenesis (**Figure 1**). Based on the 17–25 amino acid region

of VEGF, Qk was strategically modified such that it would maintain the α-helix secondary structure of the corresponding segment of the full-length protein and the three-dimensional presentation of amino acids critical for VEGF receptor interactions. Qk is able to induce ERK1/2 and Akt phosphorylation similar to full-length VEGF, and results in similar cell proliferation and migration *in vitro* (D'Andrea et al., 2005; Diana et al., 2008; Finetti et al., 2012). While more stable than VEGF$_{17-25}$, Qk still has a serum half-life of only ~4 h, making simple injection an inefficient method to maintain therapeutic levels of bioactive peptide (Finetti et al., 2012). As spatial and temporal control over VEGF concentration is critical for vessel formation (Mooney et al., 2007), it is reasonable that Qk would require similar control. This need for controlled delivery of this peptide is emphasized by the controlled release systems exploited in the *in vivo* studies performed with Qk. An infusion pump was used to deliver Qk to ischemic hind limbs, increasing vessel density; Matrigel and Pluronic gels have been used to sustain the delivery of Qk subcutaneously and to cutaneous wounds, increasing vessel density and the rate of wound closure, respectively (Santulli et al., 2009).

PAB2-1c

PAB2-1c was designed to mimic PDGF, a protein involved in vessel detachment and sprouting, pericyte recruitment, and vessel maturation and remodeling (**Figure 1**) (Lin et al., 2007). PAB2-1c was shown to bind PDGF receptors α and β and induce Akt and ERK1/2 phosphorylation, albeit to a lesser extent than full-length PDGF. Additionally, while PAB2-1c induced similar cell proliferation and migration, higher doses of the peptide were required to match the full-length protein (Lin et al., 2007). While no *in vivo* data have been published exploiting this peptide, it holds great potential for future applications attempting to more mimic the pro-angiogenic signaling cascade shown in **Figure 1**. For example, materials could be developed by delivering peptides that first stimulate the early phases of vessel development (i.e., the VEGF mimic Qk) followed by peptides that stimulate pericyte recruitment and vessel remodeling (i.e., the PDGF

TABLE 1 | Examples of therapeutic peptides.

Therapeutic application	Name	Source	Phase of development	Reference
Wound healing	DSC127	Angiotensin (1–7)	Phase III	Rodgers and Dizerega (2013), Derma Sciences (2015)
	GHK	Cu^{2+} binding region of SPARC	Failed phase III trials for venous stasis ulcers	Pickart (2008)
Cosmetic	GHK (and analogues)	Cu^{2+} binding region of SPARC	FDA-approved for both wrinkle treatment and hair regrowth	Pickart (2008)
Anti-inflammatory	AF12198	Phage display	Pre-clinical	Akeson et al. (1996), Mandrup-Poulsen (2012)
	CBX129801	Cleavage product of proinsulin	Phase IIb	Henriksson et al. (2005), Cebix (2013)
Chemotherapeutic	Endostatin peptide fragment I (180–199)	Collagen XVIII	Pre-clinical	Olsson et al. (2004)
	VEGF-derived peptide	Exon 6a of VEGF gene	Pre-clinical	Lee et al. (2010)
	ATN-161	Fibronectin	Phase II	Plunkett et al. (2002), Cianfrocca et al. (2006)
Osteoporosis	BA058	Parathyroid hormone receptor (PTHR) agonist	Phase III	Radius Health (2015)
Anti-bacterial	Oritavancin (LY333328)	Semisynthetic lipoglycopeptide analogue of vancomycin	FDA approved	Zhanel et al. (2012), FDA (2014)

A selection of bioactive peptides and intended therapeutic applications.

TABLE 2 | Pro-angiogenic peptides.

Pro-angiogenic peptide	Sequence	Source	Demonstrated effects	Reference
Qk	KLTWQELYQLKYKGI	α-helix region of VEGF	Causes similar signaling and *in vitro* effects to full-length VEGF. *In vivo*, Qk increased vessel density in ischemic hind limbs and Matrigel plugs, as well as the rate of cutaneous wound closure	Santulli et al. (2009), Finetti et al. (2012)
PAB2-1c	(C*VRKIEIVRKK)$_2$–Ahx–Ahx–Ahx–RKRKLERIAR–NH$_2$	Mimic of PDGF	Stimulates cell proliferation, migration, and collagen gel contraction similar to full-length PDGF *in vitro*	Lin et al. (2007)
T7 vasculotide	(PEG-CHHHRHSF) tetramer	Tie-2-binding region of Ang1	Increases serum-free cell survival and cell migration as compared to controls *in vitro*. Increases vessel number and size when delivered from Matrigel, and increase the rate of diabetic wound closure when delivered using Intrasite Topical Gel *in vivo*	Van Slyke et al. (2009), Slyke (2011)
GHK, GHK-Cu, or SPARC$_{120-122}$	GHK	Cu^{2+}-binding region of SPARC	Induces a wide range of cellular effects, including reducing inflammatory while increasing anti-inflammatory factors, increasing extracellular matrix protein production, and matrix metalloproteinase expression. *In vivo* effects have been shown ranging from increasing vascularization in the rabbit eye, increasing the rate of uncomplicated and diabetic wound healing, and inhibiting gastric ulcer formation	Pickart (2008)
Comb1	DINECEIGAPAGEETEVTVEGLEPG	Combination of the epidermal growth factor -like domains of fibrillin 1 and tenascin X	Increases cell proliferation, tube formation, and sprouting compared to controls *in vitro*. Increased chemically impaired cutaneous wound healing when co-delivered daily with UN3	Demidova-Rice et al. (2011, 2012)
UN3	NH$_2$-ELLESYIDGRPTATSEYQTFFNPR-amide	Previously unknown peptide fragment from platelet lysate	Significantly increased cell migration, proliferation, and tube formation *in vitro*. Significantly increased vessel density in impaired cutaneous wounds. Increased chemically impaired cutaneous wound healing when co-delivered daily with Comb1	Demidova-Rice et al. (2012)
KRX-725	MRPYDANKR	Second intercellular loop of sphingosine 1-phosphate (S1P) 3	Increases aortic ring sprouting as compared to controls with greater smooth muscle cell co-localization to endothelial cells than VEGF. Increases in vascularization of the rabbit cornea were obtained by co-treatment with KRX-725 and VEGF or bFGF as compared to factors alone	Ben-Sasson et al. (2003)
Pep-12	NYLTHRQ	Ig-like domain II of VEGF receptor 1	Facilitates integrin-mediated cell adhesion and cause tube formation *in vitro*. Significantly increases angiogenesis in the rabbit cornea as compared to controls, albeit to a lesser extent than VEGF	Soro et al. (2008)
LL-37	LLGDFFRKSKEKIGKEFKRIVQR IKDFLRNLVPRTES	The 134–170 amino acid region of the human cationic anti-microbial protein 18	Originally identified as an anti-microbial peptide produced in response to inflammation or infection, it was shown to have pro-angiogenic effects in addition to anti-microbial action. LL-37 caused dose-dependent increases in cell proliferation and increased collateral blood flow, capillary density, and blood velocity in a rabbit hind-limb ischemia model	Koczulla et al. (2003)
YR or RoY	YPHIDSLGHWRR	Identified by phage display for binding to endothelial cells	Increased cell proliferation and migration *in vitro*. Increases vessel density when injected into a mouse ear and hindlimb reperfusion when delivered intramuscularly	Hardy et al. (2007, 2008)
AcSDKP	AcSDKP	A naturally expressed regulator of hematopoiesis found in bone marrow	AcSDKP increases cell migration and tube formation, with increasing then decreasing responses as the concentration is increased beyond the optimal dose. Similar results were seen *in vivo* using the Matrigel plug assay, with greater vascularization induced with 10^{-9} M than 10^{-5} M of peptide	Liu et al. (2003)

A selection of pro-angiogenic peptides, all which are in pre-clinical testing. Standard amino acid abbreviations are used. C, disulfide bridge; Ahx, aminohexanoic acid; Ac, acetyl.*

mimic PAB2-1c). Additionally, PAB2-1c is a multi-domain peptide, containing two copies of PDGF-BB$_{153-162}$ as well as a heparin-binding domain RKRKLERIAR (Verrecchio et al., 2000), which could be exploited for controlled release purposes (further discussed below).

GHK

The secreted protein acidic and rich in cysteine (SPARC) (also known as osteonectin) is an extracellular matrix protein expressed during embryogenesis and tissue repair/remodeling. *In vivo*, SPARC is cleaved by proteases into distinct fragments, with fragments from each domain producing drastically different cellular responses (Motamed, 1999). Fragments from the cysteine-rich follistatin-like region that contain the copper-binding sequence GHK have been shown to have numerous pro-angiogenic and healing effects, increasing fibroblast production of VEGF and FGF, increasing extracellular matrix production and remodeling, increasing vessel formation in the rabbit cornea, accelerating dermal wound healing, increasing hair follicle growth, and acting as a chemoattractant for macrophages, capillary cells, and mast cells, to name a few (Pickart, 2008). While the delivery system, dose, and model varies widely across the many studies exploiting GHK and its analogues, the peptide is generally delivered using a controlled release system or by repeated administration (Pickart, 2008). Interestingly, when coupled to alginate hydrogels, GHK increased VEGF and FGF production by mesenchymal stem cells (Jose et al., 2014), potentially increasing their pro-angiogenic efficacy and capacity for tissue repair (Rustad et al., 2012; Hoffman et al., 2013). Together, the numerous and diverse effects of this peptide make it an intriguing drug for use in pro-angiogenic, wound repair, and tissue engineering applications.

Synergistic Effects Upon Delivery of Multiple Factors

Numerous peptides have improved efficacy upon co-delivery with other peptides or factors. Qk caused synergistic increases in cell migration when delivered with VEGF or FGF-2 (Finetti et al., 2012). While UN3 (a peptide fragment identified from platelet lysate) alone was able to increase vascularization of cutaneous wounds, increased wound quality was only observed when UN3 was co-delivered with Comb1 (a combination of the fibrillin 1 and tenascin X) (Demidova-Rice et al., 2012). KRX-725 showed similar additive effects when co-delivered with bFGF, significantly increasing vascularization of the rabbit cornea as compared to delivery of the peptide or protein alone (Ben-Sasson et al., 2003). This suggests that pro-angiogenic peptides, similar to their protein counterparts, could benefit from controlled release strategies that deliver multiple factors, either all peptides, or a combination of peptides and proteins.

Delivery of multiple proteins from a material that more closely replicating their temporal expression in the pro-angiogenic signaling cascade has been shown to improve pro-angiogenic effects as compared to singular protein delivery, or delivery of multiple proteins without this temporal control (Mooney et al., 2007; Brudno et al., 2013). For example, delivery of VEGF followed by PDGF, which more closely recapitulates the native pro-angiogenic healing cascade (**Figure 1**), improves vessel density, size, and maturity as compared to delivery of either factor alone (Richardson et al., 2001; Sylven et al., 2007). Similarly, delivery of multiple pro-angiogenic (VEGF and Ang2) followed by pro-maturation (PDGF and Ang1) factors with temporal delivery motivated by healthy angiogenic signaling-induced formation of more mature, larger vessels than controls (Brudno et al., 2013). As previously discussed, one could envision exploiting peptide mimics of these two factors (Qk and PAB2-1c) similarly. Additionally, the Ang1 mimic T7 could be employed as a pro-maturation peptide delivered in conjunction with a pro-angiogenic peptide, such as Qk, as Ang1 is important for pericyte recruitment and vessel maturation/remodeling (**Figure 1**).

Drug Delivery Systems for Pro-Angiogenic Peptides

Drug delivery systems are often used to address delivery challenges associated with therapeutic efficacy. While the specific goal of each delivery system depends on the drug being delivered and its target tissue/disease state, the over-arching goal is to maintain or increase the efficacy of the therapeutic while minimizing or eliminating toxicity and side effects (Bader and Putnam, 2014). To achieve these goals, drug delivery systems can be designed to improve the solubility of the drug, protect it from degradation, increase its circulation/retention time, improve preferential tissue accumulation, and/or prolong its retention at the target site (Bader and Putnam, 2014). Of particular concern when delivering pro-angiogenic drugs is off-target delivery, which could potentially encourage the development of tumors (Carmeliet and Jain, 2000), or increasing the severity of diseases associated with excessive angiogenesis, such as macular degeneration (Kent, 2014).

The most commonly exploited drug delivery systems can be broadly classified into three categories: orally delivered, soluble (or injectable), and depot-based implantable systems. Delivery of proteins and peptides using alternate entry routes (e.g., nasal, pulmonary, and transdermal) are not commonly exploited for pro-angiogenic applications, and are reviewed elsewhere (Agu et al., 2001; Shoyele and Cawthorne, 2006; Antosova et al., 2009). Methods to improve oral delivery of protein and peptide drugs have been recently reviewed (Al-Hilal et al., 2013; Renukuntla et al., 2013). Du and Stenzel have published a thorough review that focuses on chemical conjugation methods for peptide drug delivery using soluble polymeric delivery systems (liposomes, nanoparticles, etc.) (Du and Stenzel, 2014). These soluble and oral delivery systems are less desirable for pro-angiogenic applications, such as cardiac ischemia and diabetic wounds, due to difficulty achieving preferential accumulation at target tissues, and previously mentioned concerns over systemic delivery of pro-angiogenic factors encouraging tumor development (Carmeliet and Jain, 2000).

Depot-Based Drug Delivery Systems

Depot-based delivery systems are associated with improved patient compliance and have been successfully used for decades for longitudinal delivery of drugs, such as contraceptives (Graesslin and Korver, 2008). This delivery route avoids the need for the drug to pass through the harsh conditions of the digestive system, and through the intestinal epithelium. Placing the drug delivery depot directly at the target tissue site allows preferential delivery to the target tissue, achieving higher doses and reducing unwanted off-target tissue side effects. Additionally, by designing the depot to contain a high dose of drug and slowly release it over time, a single treatment can maintain drug dose within the therapeutic window for extended durations (Bader and Putnam, 2014).

Osmotic pumps are commonly used to achieve prolonged drug delivery (Santulli et al., 2009; Bader and Putnam, 2014). However, pumps must be removed after payload delivery, necessitating additional surgeries. Biomaterial-based peptide delivery systems that provide longitudinal release are an alternate method to locally deliver proteins and peptides, and the use of degradable biomaterials avoids the need for surgical recovery. While many depot-based delivery systems are formed externally and then implanted, some biomaterials allow for *in situ* formation, where precursor material can be injected and then polymerized in place, allowing for minimally invasive implantation (Anseth et al., 2002), particularly attractive for cardiac applications.

Depot-based methods present many specific advantages for pro-angiogenic therapies, including providing localized drug delivery

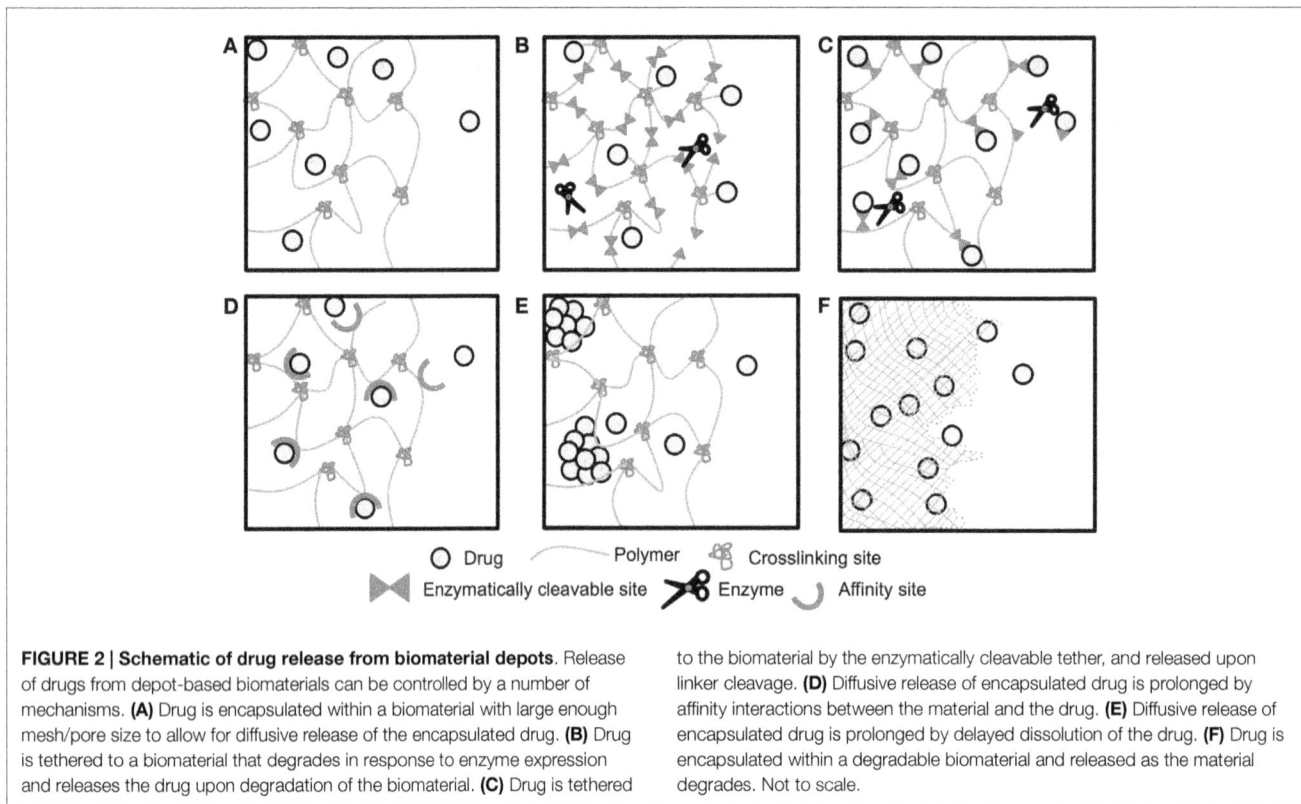

FIGURE 2 | Schematic of drug release from biomaterial depots. Release of drugs from depot-based biomaterials can be controlled by a number of mechanisms. (A) Drug is encapsulated within a biomaterial with large enough mesh/pore size to allow for diffusive release of the encapsulated drug. (B) Drug is tethered to a biomaterial that degrades in response to enzyme expression and releases the drug upon degradation of the biomaterial. (C) Drug is tethered to the biomaterial by the enzymatically cleavable tether, and released upon linker cleavage. (D) Diffusive release of encapsulated drug is prolonged by affinity interactions between the material and the drug. (E) Diffusive release of encapsulated drug is prolonged by delayed dissolution of the drug. (F) Drug is encapsulated within a degradable biomaterial and released as the material degrades. Not to scale.

thereby reducing concerns over off-target effects (Chu and Wang, 2012). Depot methods can also provide the spatial and temporal delivery of factors necessary for the development of stable, functional vessels (Mooney et al., 2007; Brudno et al., 2013). A schematic depicting select modes drugs have been released from biomaterial depots is shown in **Figure 2**. To date, the pro-angiogenic biomaterials field has largely focused on delivery of full-length proteins, and few depot-based methods for peptides have been developed (Du and Stenzel, 2014). This is likely due to the previously discussed historical difficulties associated with the use of peptide drugs. However, the recent identification of numerous pro-angiogenic peptides (**Table 2**) combined with new and improved peptide synthesis strategies have opened up an entirely new class of pro-angiogenic drugs for delivery. Herein, we focus on those biomaterials that have been developed for delivery of pro-angiogenic peptides, and those that could be easily adapted for peptide delivery, laying the foundation for a whole host of potential pro-angiogenic therapies.

Hydrogels

Hydrogels are highly hydrated crosslinked polymeric networks often used to provide sustained, localized drug delivery. The highly hydrated nature of hydrogels is similar to native tissues, and the aqueous network can stabilize peptide and protein drugs. Depending on the polymer used to form the gel, hydrogels can have highly tunable physical and chemical properties, to provide a wide degree of control over hydrogel properties and drug release behavior (Lin and Anseth, 2009b; Liechty et al., 2010).

Hydrogels can be formed using a variety of approaches. These include physical crosslinks (entanglements, hydrogen bonding,

or hydrophobic forces), covalent bonds, ionic crosslinks, or a combination of these approaches (Peppas et al., 2006). These gels may be physically stable, or may degrade or dissolve, either due to the nature of the polymer used, or as a result of specific chemical functionalities introduced for degradability. While a wide range of polymers have been used to form hydrogels, they can be broadly classified as either natural or synthetic polymers, although "hybrid hydrogels" can be formed that use both natural and synthetic polymers (Slaughter et al., 2009). Select examples of hydrogels used for controlled drug delivery are listed in **Table 3**.

Generally speaking, the rate of drug release from hydrogels is controlled by the diffusion of drug out of the crosslinked gel network (**Figure 2A**) (Slaughter et al., 2009). However, diffusion alone often does not facilitate long-term delivery of small drugs, such as peptides and small molecule drugs, as hydrodynamic radius is proportional to release rate, resulting in faster release relative to larger molecules, such as proteins (Lustig and Peppas, 1988). Therefore, to deliver these small drugs from hydrogels, more advanced modifications are often required to control the release (**Figures 2B–E**).

Naturally derived polymers

Polymers from natural sources, such as alginate, agarose, chitosan, collagen, digested extracellular matrix, fibrin, gelatin, and hyaluronic acid (HA) can be used to form hydrogels. As they are derived from plant or animal sources, natural polymers generally have low toxicity and good biocompatibility. However, the physical and chemical properties of naturally derived hydrogels can be difficult to control. Additionally, due to their biological sources, these materials often present signals that can be recognized by cells

TABLE 3 | Hydrogel-based biomaterials for controlled drug delivery.

Type	Polymer	Drug delivered	Drug type	Mode of release	Reference
Natural hydrogels	Alginate	VEGF	Protein	Diffusive	Silva and Mooney (2007, 2010)
	Alginate	VEGF and PDGF	Dual proteins	Diffusive	Sylven et al. (2007)
	Fibrin	VEGF	Protein	Proteolytic degradation	Ehrbar et al. (2004)
	Extracellular matrix	bFGF	Protein	sGAG-binding affinity	Seif-Naraghi et al. (2012)
	Extracellular matrix	HGF-f	Protein fragment	sGAG-binding affinity	Sonnenberg et al. (2015)
	Gelatin	FGF-2 and G-CSF	Dual proteins	Diffusive and ionic interactions	Layman et al. (2009)
	Hyaluronic acid	TGF-β1	Protein	Heparin-binding affinity	Jha et al. (2015)
	Matrigel	T7 Vasculotide	PEG-peptide tetramer	Diffusive	Van Slyke et al. (2009)
	Matrigel	Qk	Peptide	Diffusive	Santulli et al. (2009)
Synthetic hydrogels	Poly(ethylene glycol) multiacrylate and dithiolthreitol	hGH	Protein	Dissolution and diffusion	van de Wetering et al. (2005)
	Poly(ethylene glycol) vinyl sulfone and proteolytically cleavable peptide	VEGF	Protein	Enzymatically responsive	Zisch et al. (2003)
	Poly(ethylene glycol) diacrylate and proteolytically cleavable peptide	VEGF	Protein	Enzymatically responsive	Phelps et al. (2010)
	Poly(ethylene glycol) norbornene and enzymatically cleavable peptide	Qk, SPARC$_{113}$, SPARC$_{118}$, and model peptides	Peptide	Enzymatically responsive	Van Hove et al. (2014)
	Poly(N-isopropylacrylamide-co-propylacrylic acid-co-butyl acrylate)	bFGF	Protein	pH-responsive and diffusive	Garbern et al. (2010), Murry et al. (2011)
Combinatory/ hybrid hydrogels	Poly(ethylene glycol)-bis-butanoic acid and hydrazide-functionalized heparin	VEGF	Protein	Heparin-binding affinity	Tae et al. (2006)
	Multi-arm poly(ethylene glycol) thiol and dextran vinyl sulfone	IgG, BSA, Lysozyme, and bFGF	Protein	Diffusive	Hiemstra et al. (2007)
	Poly(ether)urethane–polydimethylsiloxane + fibrin	VEGF and bFGF	Dual proteins	Diffusive	Losi et al. (2010)
	Hyaluronic acid + PEG	VEGF and bFGF	Protein	Heparin-binding affinity	Pike et al. (2006)

Select examples of hydrogel-based biomaterials used for controlled drug delivery.

within the body, which can be advantageous or disadvantageous depending upon the application (Peppas et al., 2006).

Alginate

Alginate is a naturally occurring linear polysaccharide that is soluble in water, but due to negatively charged side groups can be ionically crosslinked by the addition of divalent cations, such as Ca^{2+}. While they are generally biocompatible, without additional modification alginate hydrogels undergo slow and uncontrolled degradation *in vivo* (Bouhadir et al., 2001; Silva and Mooney, 2007). Alginate hydrogels have been used for the controlled delivery of growth factors in a number of studies, and have shown the importance of extended delivery of VEGF to ischemic tissue (Silva and Mooney, 2007, 2010). Additionally, alginate hydrogels delivering VEGF followed by PDGF resulted in the same capillary density within infarcted tissues versus gels delivering VEGF, but significantly improved the number of mature vessels over gels delivering either PDGF or VEGF alone (Sylven et al., 2007), demonstrating the improvement in angiogenesis that can be obtained by more closely recapitulating the natural pro-angiogenic signaling cascade reviewed in **Figure 1**. While able to controllably deliver large proteins, unmodified alginate hydrogels are not well suited for delivery of peptide drugs. The mesh size of alginate hydrogels varies depending on the percentage of alginate used,

but is generally on the order of magnitude of 10 nm (Turco et al., 2011). This facilitates hindered diffusion of larger proteins, such as VEGF and PDGF, but would likely be less successful delivering small peptides.

Extracellular matrix

Hydrogels derived from decellularized, digested extracellular matrix (ECM) have also been exploited for delivery of pro-angiogenic factors. These materials provide a physical structure that supports cell infiltration and vascularization and provides structural support to the tissue, which has been shown beneficial in limiting post-myocardial infarction damage to cardiac tissue (Okada et al., 2010; Singelyn et al., 2012). These materials are highly heterogeneous, and some ECM-based materials have caused inflammatory responses *in vivo* (Seif-Naraghi et al., 2012), while others reduce the extent of chronic inflammation (Faulk et al., 2014). Decellularized, digested porcine pericardiac tissue has been exploited for the sustained delivery of bFGF. Release of bFGF from the ECM material occurred at approximately half the rate as from collagen gels, likely due to affinity interactions between bFGF and sulfated glycosaminoglycans (GAGs) within the ECM (**Figure 2D**). Upon injection into cardiac tissue, approximately three times more bFGF was retained after 5 days when the protein was delivered in the ECM material compared to direct injection. Additionally, the bFGF-releasing ECM significantly increased the number of small (10–50 µm) vessels within the tissue. However, the bFGF-releasing ECM caused a significant increase in inflammation, undesirable in many tissue repair applications (Seif-Naraghi et al., 2012).

Similar porcine pericardial ECM hydrogels were used for sustained delivery of a hepatocyte growth factor (HGF) fragment (HGF-f), which shows similar bioactivity to full-length HGF while being less than half the size of the full-length protein (Liu et al., 2014). The ECM-based hydrogel provided sustained release of HGF-f, releasing ~30% over 5 days and significantly increased arteriole density in infarcted cardiac tissue. However, it only caused trending improvements in function as assessed by ejection fraction (Sonnenberg et al., 2015). The HGF-f released from these gels is still substantial larger than a peptide (~40 kDa), and sustained delivery of smaller peptides from these hydrogels would likely not occur without similarly exploiting GAG affinity interactions. This would require modification of the peptide with a heparin-binding sequence, such as RKRKLERIAR (Lin et al., 2007), $(XBBXBX)_n$, or $(XBBXXBX)_n$, where X is uncharged or hydrophobic, and B is a basic amino acid (Verrecchio et al., 2000). Additionally, any inflammatory reaction to these ECM materials would need to be addressed, as this is a significant concern for translation.

Fibrin

Fibrin hydrogels have been used for a number of biomaterial and drug delivery applications. Similar to fibrin clots formed after vascular injury, fibrin hydrogels are formed by reacting fibrinogen and thrombin (Ehrbar et al., 2004; Schmoekel et al., 2005). They are highly biocompatible, and can be degraded by plasmin and other enzymes in the body (Ye et al., 2000; Ahmed et al., 2007). In an attempt to improve the efficacy of VEGF by providing long-term delivery of the growth factor, Ehrbar et al. conjugated VEGF to a fibrin matrix such that the VEGF molecule could only be released when the fibrin matrix was proteolytically degraded (**Figure 2B**). This greatly extended the duration of VEGF release, and the fibrin-released VEGF increased the formation of new arterial and venous structures within the chick chorioallantoic membrane, while passively released VEGF (**Figure 2A**) primarily resulted in chaotic changes to the vasculature (Ehrbar et al., 2004). This enzymatically responsive gel could easily be adapted for delivery of pro-angiogenic peptides. By including the factor XIIIa substrate NQEQVSPL onto either the C- or N-termini of the peptide, peptides could similarly be covalently integrated into the fibrin network via factor XIIIa activation (Zisch et al., 2001). However, proteins/peptides released from these gels contain residual fragments of the fibrin gel, which could affect bioactivity. Testing of released VEGF showed comparable bioactivity to non-tethered, encapsulated protein (Ehrbar et al., 2004), but this would not necessarily be the case for all drugs.

One disadvantage to the use of fibrin gels is that they do not afford control over the rate of gel degradation and associated drug release. Some degree of control over the time course of VEGF release was achieved by introducing a plasmin-sensitive substrate between the growth factor and the Factor XIIIa substrate (NQEQVSPL-LIK↓MKP-VEGF, ↓ indicates cleavage site) (Ehrbar et al., 2005). However, this modification to the system only accelerated growth factor release by ~25%, and does not provide a means to easily tune protein/peptide release kinetics.

Gelatin

Gelatin is a natural hydrogel derived from collagen used in drug delivery applications because of its biocompatibility and controllable degradation (Tabata and Ikada, 1998; Young et al., 2005). Covalently crosslinked gelatin hydrogels were exploited for the controlled delivery of FGF-2 and granulocyte-colony stimulating factor (G-CSF). While release of both FGF-2 and G-CSF were diffusion mediated, FGF-2 release was delayed as compared to G-CSF, likely due to ionic interactions between the anionic gelatin and cationic FGF-2 (**Figures 2A,D**). Hydrogels releasing both growth factors improved ischemic hind limb reperfusion assessed via increased capillary density and maturity as compared to PBS or singularly delivered growth factor controls (Layman et al., 2009). By processing collagen in either acidic or alkaline conditions, its isoelectric point can be modified. This allows oppositely charged molecules to interact with the gelatin and form a polyion complex, extending release by affinity interactions (Tabata and Ikada, 1998; Young et al., 2005). Yamamoto et al. showed this when they demonstrated that encapsulation of bFGF and transforming growth factor-β1 (TGF-β1) in acidic gelatin hydrogels prolonged *in vivo* delivery as compared to direct injection. However, despite similar isoelectric points, prolonged delivery of bone morphogenetic protein-2 (BMP-2) and VEGF was not achieved possibly due to differences in 3D structure and charge exposure (Yamamoto et al., 2001). In addition to being unable to deliver the potent pro-angiogenic protein VEGF, these gelatin hydrogels are not ideal for the delivery of smaller peptides. The strength of the interaction between the drug and the gelatin decreases as the size of and number of charges on the drug being delivered decreases (Tabata and Ikada, 1998), making it likely that gelatin would not prolong the delivery of smaller peptides. This was illustrated by Saramento et al., who attempted to use polyion interactions to deliver insulin, which at 51 amino acids is on the cusp of what is considered a peptide versus a protein (Sarmento et al., 2007). By combining this negatively charged peptide with negatively charged fibrin and positively charged chitosan, nanoparticles were formed crosslinked by electrostatic forces. However, release of the peptide was rapid, with ~60% released in 2 h, demonstrating the limitations of using ionic interactions to control the release of small peptides (Sarmento et al., 2007).

Hyaluronic acid

Hyaluronan or HA is a naturally occurring component of the extracellular matrix. HA degradation *in vivo* is mediated by hyaluronidases, six enzymes that hydrolyze HA (Stern, 2004). The released HA fragments have been shown to have pro-angiogenic effects *in vivo* (Montesano et al., 1996), making it a promising material for delivery of pro-angiogenic factors, as both the material and drug being delivered could contribute to the desired pro-angiogenic response. However, this convolutes drug-specific effects, and excessive pro-angiogenic signaling can sometimes lead to the development of leaky vasculature (Yancopoulos et al., 2000). HA hydrogels with mesh sizes and degradation controllable based upon the degree of HA methacrylation can be formed by

UV polymerization. These hydrogels exhibit good biocompatibility upon subcutaneous implantation (Leach et al., 2003) but their mesh sizes are very large (~600 nm), causing rapid release of encapsulated proteins (Leach and Schmidt, 2005) and making this an unattractive approach for delivery of small pro-angiogenic peptides. Enzymatically degradable HA hydrogels were formed by functionalizing HA with acrylate groups and reacting with di-thiol containing matrix metalloproteinase (MMP)-degradable crosslinking peptides and thiolated heparin for affinity-controlled protein release (**Figure 2D**). Release of encapsulated TGF-β1 was prolonged over >3 weeks, with the release rate affected by the molecular weight of heparin used, as well as the amounts of heparin and TGF-β1 used in hydrogel formation (Jha et al., 2015). While this study did not investigate *in vivo* degradation or the pro-angiogenic/wound healing effects of the material, it did demonstrate the highly tunable protein release that can be achieved using heparin-functionalized HA hydrogels. However, due to the number of growth factors that have affinity for heparin (Peysselon and Ricard-Blum, 2014), it is possible that host proteins with greater affinity for heparin may displace drug molecules when introduced *in vivo*.

Supramolecular interactions of adamantine and cyclodextrin have also been exploited to form shear-thinning, self-healing HA hydrogels, by combining adamantane- and cyclodextrin-functionalized HA. The physical properties of these HA gels, such as stiffness and degradation rate, can be modified by varying the weight percentage of HA, as well as the extent of functionalization (Rodell et al., 2013). These hydrogels can be rendered enzymatically degradable by tethering the adamantane to the HA by an MMP-degradable peptide sequence (Rodell et al., 2015). This material holds great promise for the delivery of pro-angiogenic peptides due to the affinity interactions of cyclodextrin with peptides (Tiwari et al., 2010), particularly those containing hydrophobic and aromatic amino acids (Castronuovo et al., 1995; Aachmann et al., 2012). However, due to these fairly non-specific interactions, these materials have the same potential concern as heparin gels whereby host molecules may displace drug molecules, drastically affecting drug release. Many HA hydrogels are formed using poly(ethylene glycol) (PEG) crosslinkers, and are further discussed in the Section "Hybrid materials" below.

Matrigel

Matrigel is a mixture of extracellular matrix molecules produced by Engelbreth–Holm–Swarm (EHS) mouse sarcoma cells that is soluble at 4°C but polymerizes when incubated at 37°C. Due to the gentle polymerization conditions required to form gels, and ability of a variety of cells to interact with the gel during vascularization, Matrigel is commonly used *in vivo* to provide diffusive release (**Figure 2A**) and evaluate the efficacy of pro- and anti-angiogenic proteins and peptides (Kleinman and Martin, 2005; Santulli et al., 2009; Van Slyke et al., 2009). However, Matrigel has inherent biological activity that varies between production lots based on residual-growth factors left in the matrix (Kleinman and Martin, 2005). Concerns over its tumor source prevents Matrigel from being used for translational drug delivery purposes, and many studies using Matrigel to deliver therapeutic factors *in vivo* do not characterize the release of the factor from the gel (Santulli et al., 2009; Van Slyke et al., 2009).

Synthetic polymers

Many synthetic polymers have also been exploited for controlled drug delivery. As compared to natural polymers, synthetic polymers afford a greater degree of control over resulting hydrogel networks. Hydrogel properties, such as crosslinking density, mechanical strength, degradation, drug release profile, and even stimuli-responsive behavior can be controlled by altering the composition of the polymer network. While many synthetic polymers are bio-inert, they are frequently engineered to incorporate functional groups that allow cells to bind to and interact with the hydrogel (Peppas et al., 2006).

Poly(ethylene glycol)

Poly(ethylene glycol) hydrogels are a commonly used synthetic biomaterial for drug delivery (Peppas et al., 2006; Lin and Anseth, 2009b; Slaughter et al., 2009). PEG hydrogels are highly hydrophilic, inert, and biocompatible, and PEG has been approved by the FDA for a number of clinical uses (Peppas et al., 2006). Additionally, PEG hydrogels have been shown to have highly tunable degradation profiles and mechanical properties (Lin and Anseth, 2009b). While PEG hydrogels are inherently bio-inert, they can be functionalized with cell adhesion molecules, such as the RGD peptide to facilitate cellular interactions (Hern and Hubbell, 1998).

To facilitate hydrogel formation, PEG can be crosslinked by two mechanisms: step-growth and chain-growth, or a combination of the two, termed mixed-mode. Chain-growth polymerization occurs when PEG macromers contain self-reactive terminal groups (predominantly acrylates and methacrylates). These gels do not require the use of an additional crosslinking agent, but produce heterogeneous networks structures that contain dense crosslinking regions (Lin and Anseth, 2009b; Van Hove et al., 2013). Step-growth polymerization occurs when PEG macromers preferentially react with a second functionality on a crosslinker (thiol-acrylate, thiol-norbornene, alkyne-azide, tetrazine-azide, etc.). Step-growth polymerization provides an easy method to incorporate peptides into hydrogel networks; by exploiting thiol groups on cysteine amino acids and unsaturated carbon bonds of functionalities introduced to PEG (norbornene, acrylate, etc.), peptides can be incorporated into hydrogels as crosslinking agents or tethered pendant groups (Fairbanks et al., 2009; Shih and Lin, 2012; Van Hove et al., 2014).

PEG hydrogels for pro-angiogenic drug delivery

Poly(ethylene glycol) hydrogels have been used to deliver a number of therapeutic molecules. This specific topic was previously reviewed by Lin and Anseth (2009b). Herein, we will focus on recent developments and their specific utility in pro-angiogenic applications. Controlled delivery of human growth hormone (hGH) from step-growth polymerized PEG hydrogel networks formed by reacting multi-arm PEG acrylate (PEGA) with dithiothreitol (DTT) has been demonstrated. Precipitation of hGH with Zn^{2+} prior to encapsulation protected the protein during polymerization and delayed release from the gels via delayed dissolution (**Figure 2E**). Varying the PEG macromers used to form hydrogels controlled hydrogel swelling ratios, which subsequently extended protein release beyond 25 days (van de Wetering et al., 2005).

While all gels studied were hydrolytically degradable, only one macromer configuration produced gels that degraded and release drug over similar time frames (21 days). The other gels developed persisted long after releasing their payload: gels releasing hGH over 1 day took 21 days to degrade, and gels releasing hGH over ~8 weeks (extrapolated based on first-order release data) were still intact after 15 weeks (van de Wetering et al., 2005). hGH has been shown to have both pro- and anti-angiogenic effects depending if it is presented in full-length protein or as the 16 kDa N-terminal fragment (Struman et al., 1999). Therefore, while these hydrogels were intended for treatment of growth hormone deficiency, Turner's syndrome, and chronic renal failure, they could also present a promising pro-angiogenic strategy. While to the best of our knowledge, this delayed dissolution approach has not yet been exploited for delivery of peptide drugs, it could theoretically be used for delivery of hydrophobic peptides, such as Qk, which has 53% hydrophobic amino acids (Lehninger et al., 2000) and a Hopp–Woods average value of −0.2 (Hopp and Woods, 1981). Additionally, Qk forms an α-helix, which has been shown to increase peptide self-assembly in aqueous solution (Kisiday et al., 2002), making it an attractive candidate for delivery using this delayed dissolution approach.

poly(ethylene glycol) hydrogels designed by West and Hubbell to degrade in response to local enzyme levels have recently been adapted for drug delivery applications. In their seminal work, enzymatically responsive PEG macromers were formed by reacting a degradable peptide with PEG, forming an peptide-PEG-peptide block copolymer which was then functionalized with terminal acrylate groups, allowing for hydrogel formation (West and Hubbell, 1999). Building upon this foundation, additional enzymatically responsive PEG hydrogels have been developed, with the specific degradable peptide used controlling enzyme specific and hydrogel degradation kinetics (Hubbell et al., 2003; Patterson and Hubbell, 2010).

As a pro-angiogenic approach, Zisch et al. used Michael-type addition reactions to form PEG hydrogels that degrade and release VEGF in response to local enzymes. Multi-arm PEG vinyl sulfone was reacted with cysteine flanked MMP-degradable peptides, as well as VEGF engineered with a plasmin-sensitive tether and terminal cysteine. This formed hydrogels that released VEGF both upon MMP-mediated hydrogel degradation and plasmin-mediated tether cleavage (**Figures 2B,C**). When used in the chick chorioallantoic membrane assay, VEGF-conjugated hydrogels resulted in the formation of new vessels highly localized to the hydrogel, and improved vessel infiltration upon subcutaneous implantation as compared to controls (Zisch et al., 2003). These hydrogels simultaneously degrade and release the pro-angiogenic protein, attractive behavior for an implantable or injectable drug delivery system as the gel will not persist after delivering its payload. This system could be easily adapted for delivery of pro-angiogenic peptides like those shown in **Table 2**. However, some of the drug is release tethered to a PEG molecule. While testing showed that VEGF remained bioactive with the PEG "tail" (Zisch et al., 2003), this would not necessarily be the case for all proteins or peptides.

Phelps et al. also exploited PEG hydrogels to provide enzymatically responsive protein release. By reacting proteolytically cleavable peptide linkers with acrylate-PEG-N-hydroxysuccinimide (NHS), an acrylate–PEG-peptide–PEG-acrylate macromer was formed. These macromers were then polymerized to form enzymatically degradable PEG hydrogels, with VEGF tethered via a non-degradable PEG linker, resulting in protein release only when the gel is degraded (**Figure 2B**). Similar to the system developed by Zisch et al., the VEGF is released from the gel tethered to residual PEG macromers. While enzymatically responsive hydrogel degradation was shown, protein release was not quantified in parallel. Nevertheless, there was significantly greater vascular ingrowth into VEGF-releasing hydrogel as compared to the enzymatically responsive hydrogels alone. Additionally, treatment with the enzymatically responsive, VEGF-releasing hydrogels caused greater reperfusion of ischemic hindlimb tissue than bolus VEGF delivery (Phelps et al., 2010).

Our group recently developed hydrogels providing sustained, enzymatically responsive peptide release (**Figure 2B**). Peptide drugs were synthesized flanked by enzymatically degradable sequences with terminal cysteine amino acids (C-degradable linker-drug-degradable linker-C). This allowed for step-growth thiolene reactions with multi-arm norbornene-functionalized PEG (PEGN). These hydrogels demonstrated enzymatically responsive degradation and peptide release, and were confirmed to release bioactive components able to induce tube network formation *in vitro*. Similar to the previously discussed systems, simultaneous hydrogel degradation and peptide release occurs. However, in this system, the peptide drugs are released with only four amino acids residues on either side of the drug, rather than entire PEG macromers. These residual amino acids still had a substantial effect of peptide bioactivity, with only three of the six pro-angiogenic peptides screened retaining bioactivity *in vitro*. While this work generated a novel biomaterial to provide enzymatically responsive delivery of peptide drugs and identified key drug properties that affect gel behavior, it did not investigate hydrogel pro-angiogenic efficacy *in vivo* (Van Hove et al., 2014).

pH and temperature-responsive materials have also been exploited for controlled delivery of pro-angiogenic factors. Temperature and pH-responsive copolymers were formed from N-isopropylacrylamide (NIPAAM), propylacrylic acid (PAA), and butyl acrylate (BA) monomers [p(NIPAAm-co-PAA-co-BA)]. These copolymers form physical hydrogels (undergoing solution-to-gel, or sol-to-gel, transition) as temperature is increased and pH decreased, with the transition point affected by the relative amounts of each monomer used. p(NIPAAm-co-PAA) (83 mol% NIPAAm, 17 mol% PAA, 37 kDa) copolymers produced hydrogels that released encapsulated VEGF via diffusion over ~7 days at pH 7.4 and over ~3 weeks when pH was lowered to 5 or 6, pH levels consistent with ischemic tissue microenvironments (Garbern et al., 2010). Similar p(NIPAAm-co-PAA-co-BA) copolymers (67 mol% NIPAAm, 18 mol% PAA, 15 mol% BA, 28 kDa) delivered encapsulated bFGF *in vivo* to infarcted myocardium over ~7 days, and improved fractional shortening of and blood flow to the heart, as well as capillary and arteriolar densities as compared to controls (Murry et al., 2011). pH-responsive nanospheres formed from p(pAA-PEG) have been used to provide stimuli-responsive release of insulin (Foss et al., 2004), demonstrating the potential of these similar pH-responsive hydrogels for the delivery of pro-angiogenic peptide drugs.

Hybrid materials

Combinations of natural and synthetic polymers have also been used to form hybrid hydrogels for controlled drug delivery. Heparin is often exploited as a natural polymer, as many pro-angiogenic proteins contain heparin-binding domains. Via heparin-protein affinity interactions, protein release can be sustained for days to weeks, depending upon the protein, amount of heparin included, and the tissue microenvironment. For example, covalently crosslinked heparin-PEG gels were formed by step-growth reactions between hydrazide-functionalized heparin (Hep-ADH) and poly(ethylene glycol)-bis-butanoic acid (SBA-PEG-SBA). After gel formation, gels were partially dried and injected with a high concentration of VEGF before being incubated overnight to allow the protein to equilibrate within the gel. Release of VEGF from these hydrogels was nearly linear and occurred over >3 weeks, with the extended release attributed to affinity interactions between VEGF and heparin (**Figure 2D**). Subcutaneous implantation of the hydrogels showed increased CD31-staining as compared to control gels, indicating increased vessel formation (Tae et al., 2006).

Numerous proteins beyond VEGF contain heparin-binding domains (Peysselon and Ricard-Blum, 2014), and as a result, heparin affinity has been exploited for controlled delivery of a variety of proteins from a number of materials. This includes delivery of bFGF and BMP-2 from PEG hydrogels (Benoit and Anseth, 2005; Benoit et al., 2007; Nie et al., 2007), bFGF and β-nerve growth factor (β-NGF) from fibrin hydrogels (Sakiyama-Elbert and Hubbell, 2000a,b), and transforming growth factor β1 (TGF-β1), FGF-2, VEGF, and BMP-2 from alginate hydrogels (Jeon et al., 2011), all which incorporated heparin functionalities to prolong growth factor delivery. These materials are well suited for delivery of pro-angiogenic peptides, such as PAB2-1c, which contains the heparin-binding region RKRKLERIAR (Lin et al., 2007). Additional pro-angiogenic peptides could be delivered from heparin-functionalized hydrogels by including this or another heparin-binding sequence (Verrecchio et al., 2000) on either the C- or N-termini of the drug sequence, provided the addition of the heparin-binding region did not inhibit peptide bioactivity. However, as previously discussed, materials exploiting heparin affinity have the potential to sequester a variety of host proteins with affinity for heparin (Peysselon and Ricard-Blum, 2014).

Similarly, short peptides have been identified that mimic the heparin-binding capacity of VEGF (Maynard and Hubbell, 2005) and NGF (Willerth et al., 2007). By conjugating these peptides to hydrogels, affinity-controlled release of NGF from fibrin hydrogels (Willerth et al., 2007) and bFGF from PEG hydrogels (Lin and Anseth, 2009a) was demonstrated. While not explicitly used for pro-angiogenic applications, the potential for these approaches to deliver a number of pro-angiogenic proteins make them promising materials that could be further exploited for pro-angiogenic applications. However, these binding peptides would not necessarily have the same ability to bind and control the release of peptides mimics, as these mimics do not necessarily contain the region responsible for the drug-binding peptide interaction.

Other hybrid materials approaches for pro-angiogenic factor release include step-growth PEG-dextran hydrogels. These networks were formed by Michael Addition reactions between dextran vinyl sulfone (dex-VS) and multi-arm PEG thiol. Controlling

the molecular weight of the dextran molecule and the degree of substitution was shown to control hydrogel degradation kinetics and delivery of encapsulated proteins, such as immunoglobulin G (IgG) and bovine serum albumin (BSA). Lysozyme and bFGF release was achieved over 2 weeks to 1 month, with release rates affected by hydrogel composition. While the ability of the bFGF-releasing hydrogels to induce angiogenesis was not studied *in vivo*, this material successfully delivered the pro-angiogenic factor over 28 days with first-order release kinetics, with hydrogel degradation occurring over a similar time scale (Hiemstra et al., 2007). These dextran-PEG hydrogels release encapsulated protein by hindered diffusion (**Figure 2A**), and would likely release peptides at an accelerated rate due to the smaller size of the peptide drugs. However, it is possible that extended release could be achieved by further increasing the degree of substitution on the dextran or decreasing the molecular weight, both of which prolonged the protein delivery (Hiemstra et al., 2007).

Hybrid scaffolds have been formed using semi-interpenetrating polymeric network (semi-IPN) of poly(ether)urethane-polydimethylsiloxane (PEtU-PDMS) networks coated with protein-laden fibrin gels. These materials combined the mechanical strength of the PEtU-PDMS scaffold with controlled release provided by fibrin gels. This combination material provided simultaneous release of bFGF and VEGF, and significantly improved capillary density and perfusion of ischemic murine hind limbs as compared to controls (Losi et al., 2010). However, these materials must be formed *ex vivo*, and the PEtU-PDMS scaffold persists over a longer time scale (~6–24 months) (Soldani et al., 2010) than they deliver the drug (~1–2 weeks) (Losi et al., 2010). These scaffolds relied on diffusional release of the protein from the fibrin gels, rather than covalently linking the protein to the gel as discussed in the Section "Fibrin." This makes them an unattractive approach for delivery of pro-angiogenic peptides, as the release of the drug is governed by diffusion (**Figure 2A**) rather than degradation, and would likely result in accelerated release of pro-angiogenic peptides. Alternately, one could envision combining the enzymatically responsive fibrin material used by Zisch et al. and Ehrbar et al. with the PDMS scaffold exploited here to combine the benefits of prolonged, enzymatically responsive drug delivery with the strength of the PDMS scaffold (Zisch et al., 2001; Ehrbar et al., 2004, 2005).

Many HA-based hydrogels are crosslinked by functionalizing HA and PEG with mutually reactive groups (Peattie et al., 2004; Cai et al., 2005; Pike et al., 2006; Riley et al., 2006; Hosack et al., 2008). Hydrogels have been formed by reacting thiol-functionalized HA with PEG diacrylate (Peattie et al., 2006; Pike et al., 2006; Riley et al., 2006; Hosack et al., 2008), hydrazide-functionalized HA with PEG propiondialdehyde (Peattie et al., 2004), and methacrylate-functionalized HA with PEGA (Leach and Schmidt, 2005). HA hydrogels containing tethered gelatin and heparin were formed containing encapsulated VEGF or bFGF, and showed extended release of encapsulated protein, with tunable release varying from 19 to 96% after 42 days. Inclusion of thiol-functionalized gelatin increased the rate of protein release, while increasing amounts of heparin decreased the rate of drug delivery, with similar trends observed for both VEGF and bFGF. Heparin-functionalized HA gels releasing VEGF and bFGF both increased vascularization index

28 days after implantation in the mouse ear, but vessel density was unaffected (Pike et al., 2006). Excitingly, HA hydrogels crosslinked with PEG releasing encapsulated VEGF and/or keratinocyte growth factor (KGF) showed an additive increase in vessel number after implantation in the mouse ear when compared to HA gels, VEGF, or KGF alone. However, this study did not report the rate of drug release or degradation of the material (Peattie et al., 2006). These hydrogels could potentially be adapted for peptide delivery, but would require similar modification of peptides with a heparin-binding region as discussed above, to facilitate extended release.

Scaffold-Based Systems

Many studies have exploited poly(lactide-co-glycolide) (PLG) scaffolds for drug delivery applications. PLG materials are bio-degradable, biocompatible, and have received FDA approval for drug delivery applications (Jain, 2000; Makadia and Siegel, 2011). By altering the relative amounts of poly(lactic acid) (PLA) and poly(glycolic acid) (PGA) in the copolymer, the rate of degradation and subsequent release of encapsulated drug can be controlled. While commonly used to form nano- and microparticles for systemic drug delivery, PLG can also be fabricated into scaffolds for depot-based drug delivery. One important considerations for use of PLG scaffolds is that the rate of degradation and associated drug release is dependent on many factors (lactide/glycolide ratio, polymer molecular weight, degree of crystallinity, glass transition temperature, etc.) and can be difficult to predict (Makadia and Siegel, 2011). Additionally, degradation of PLG scaffolds releases lactic and glycolic acid, which can accelerate the rate of degradation and affect local tissue pH, potentially damaging nearby tissue (Liu et al., 2006). Select examples of scaffolds used for controlled drug delivery are listed in **Table 4**.

For pro-angiogenic applications, PLG scaffolds have been developed using a high-pressure carbon dioxide/salt leaching method where the delivery of VEGF is controlled by the rate of scaffold degradation (**Figure 2F**). Sustained VEGF delivery over ~1 month was achieved, with the PLG–VEGF scaffold significantly increasing reperfusion of, and capillary density within, ischemic murine hindlimb as compared to empty scaffolds (Sun et al., 2005). In an attempt to mimic the temporal growth factor expression occurring in healthy tissue (**Figure 1**), PLG scaffolds were formed releasing VEGF followed by PDGF. In layer 1, PDGF was pre-encapsulated in PLG microspheres and mixed with VEGF prior

to scaffold formation, while layer 2 only contained VEGF. This resulted in spatially patterned scaffolds that provided delayed release of PDGF compared to VEGF. These dual-delivery scaffolds induced the formation of more, larger vessels than empty PLG scaffolds. However, due to the spatial patterning of the two layers, local protein delivery to the tissue was dependent on scaffold orientation during implantation (Mooney et al., 2007).

Alternately, by forming PLG scaffolds with microspheres already containing PDGF, which are subsequently mixed with VEGF, sustained release of both factors was achieved, with VEGF being released more rapidly than PDGF. Similar to the system just discussed, this biomaterial attempts to mimic the native pro-angiogenic signaling cascade (**Figure 1**); however, this system has the advantage of spatial uniformity, causing temporal protein delivery to be independent of scaffold orientation. This dual-growth factor delivery system increased vessel density within the scaffold after subcutaneous implantation compared to scaffolds delivering either factor alone. Dual factor delivery also increased vessel size and maturity as compared to blank scaffolds or scaffolds releasing VEGF or PDGF alone (Richardson et al., 2001). This biomaterials strategy has also been used to temporally control the delivery of multiple pro-angiogenic (VEGF and Ang2) and pro-maturation (PDGF and Ang1) factors from a single scaffold. Scaffolds delivering all four growth factors over time courses motivated by healthy angiogenic signaling (**Figure 1**) and *in vitro* testing resulted in the formation of more mature vessels than controls and the formation of the largest vessels of any group investigated (Brudno et al., 2013). These PLG scaffold systems could easily be adapted for controlled delivery of peptide drugs, as the drugs (protein or peptide) are released upon degradation of the biomaterial and do not rely on size-hindered diffusion through the material (**Figure 2F**). Similar to the results showing improved vascularization upon co-delivery of VEGF and PDGF, PLG scaffolds could be developed that deliver Qk (the VEGF mimic) followed by PAB2-1c (the PDGF mimic) or T7 (Ang1 mimic).

Engineering Successful Pro-Angiogenic Biomaterials

While a number of pro-angiogenic biomaterials have been discussed here, they are not equally well-suited to all pro-angiogenic therapeutic applications. All materials meet the over-arching requirement of biocompatibility, but the different environments and demands of ischemic peripheral tissue, ischemic cardiac tissue, diabetic ulcers, and tissue engineering applications result in vastly different material requirements. Ischemic cardiac tissue, for example, is most likely to be successfully treated by injectable materials that can be delivered laparoscopically, to provide initial structural support to the damaged heart, produce extended growth factor release, and eventually degrade (Chen et al., 2008). These design requirements makes the alginate, fibrin, ECM-based, enzymatically degradable PEG, and PEG-dextran gels discussed here very promising for cardiac applications, as they can be crosslinked *in situ,* either using a dual barrel syringe or UV-initiated photopolymerizations. For all materials, testing would be required to ensure *in situ* polymerization produces gels that provide similar drug

TABLE 4 | Scaffold-based biomaterials for controlled drug delivery.

Polymer	Drug Delivered	Drug Type	Mode of release	Reference
Poly(lactide-co-glycolide) (PLG)	VEGF	Protein	Scaffold degradation	Sun et al. (2005)
PLG	VEGF and PDGF	Dual proteins	Diffusion and scaffold degradation	Mooney et al. (2007)
PLG	VEGF and PDGF	Dual proteins	Diffusion and scaffold degradation	Richardson et al. (2001)
PLG	VEGF/Ang2 and PDGF/Ang1	Multiple proteins	Diffusive and scaffold degradation	Brudno et al. (2013)

Select examples of scaffold-based biomaterials used for controlled drug delivery.

release and vascularization as *ex situ* polymerization, to address potential differences in crosslinking efficiency and drug encapsulation that could occur. The pH and temperature-responsive p(NIPAAm-co-PAA-co-BA) hydrogels have the added benefit of being crosslinked by the native tissue environment, thus avoiding the need for external stimuli for gelation (Garbern et al., 2010; Murry et al., 2011). Ischemic peripheral tissue has similar design requirements as cardiac applications and would likely be best treated by the same types of materials as cardiac tissue. While the use of biomaterials for cardiac regeneration has largely focused on delivery of pro-angiogenic proteins, multiple pro-angiogenic peptides could instead be delivered to ischemic cardiac tissue, such as Qk, AcSDKP, and T7, all of which have shown promising results in other *in vivo* models (Liu et al., 2003; Santulli et al., 2009; Slyke, 2011).

Diabetic wounds are readily accessible, and therefore do not require *in situ* gel formation or degradation, as the biomaterial can simply be placed on the wound and removed after delivering its payload. Therefore, these ulcers could be treated by a wider range of materials, including the gelatin and PEtU-PDMS materials discussed here. Diabetic ulcers are associated with myriad deficiencies beyond insufficient angiogenesis (Lobmann et al., 2002; Lerman et al., 2003; Galiano et al., 2004), and as such, would likely benefit from delivery of multiple protein or peptide drugs, or drugs that have more broad effects, such as GHK-containing peptides (Pickart, 2008). Additionally, some of the pro-angiogenic peptides discussed here have already been shown efficacious in treating diabetic wounds, such as T7 and GHK, making them even more attractive candidates for incorporation into biomaterials for treatment of these wounds (Pickart, 2008; Van Slyke et al., 2009). As PLG scaffolds must be formed externally and then implanted, they could also be used for diabetic ulcer treatment, but are not ideal for cardiac applications. However, these scaffolds present a unique material compared to the other gels discussed here, in that they have significantly greater structural integrity (Makadia and Siegel, 2011). This makes them the most attractive biomaterial discussed here for engineering tissues, such as bone, while softer gels are better suited for engineering more compliant tissues, such as kidney and liver. However, as previously discussed, the acidic environment caused by degradation of the PLG scaffolds can negatively affect tissue, and must be considered when using these biomaterials (Liu et al., 2006).

Concluding Remarks

From natural to synthetic, diffusion controlled to stimuli-responsive, a number of biomaterials delivery systems have been developed to deliver pro-angiogenic factors, each presenting unique advantages and disadvantages. Building off seminal research, current research is producing more complex and intricate materials delivering pro-angiogenic drugs, inducing robust pro-angiogenic effects *in vivo*. Delivery of multiple factors, with tight temporal control over factor release has been shown to induce formation of more mature vasculature than delivery of a single factor. Similarly, materials delivering pro-angiogenic factors in response to enzyme expression present a promising means to deliver drugs based on local tissue demands. While current research focuses largely on delivery of pro-angiogenic proteins, we feel that delivery of peptide drugs that mimic the bioactivity of these proteins presents a unique opportunity to develop novel, potent pro-angiogenic therapies. Additionally, materials combining many of the promising techniques already developed could present even more potent methods to induce therapeutic angiogenesis, such as temporally controlling stimuli-responsive release, or delivery of multiple factors in a stimuli-responsive manner.

Author Contributions

Literature review was performed by AVH with assistance by DB. AVH generated all figures and tables, and wrote the article. AVH and DB critically revised the work and approved the final version to be published.

Acknowledgments

The authors would like to thank the Howard Hughes Medical Institute Med-into-Grade fellowship in Cardiovascular Sciences (AVH), the National Institute of Health (R01 AR064200), and the National Science Foundation (CAREER 1450987) for funding.

References

Aachmann, F. L., Larsen, K. L., and Wimmer, R. (2012). Interactions of cyclodextrins with aromatic amino acids: a basis for protein interactions. *J. Incl. Phenom. Macrocycl. Chem.* 73, 349–357. doi:10.1007/s10847-011-0071-y

Adams, R. H., and Alitalo, K. (2007). Molecular regulation of angiogenesis and lymphangiogenesis. *Nat. Rev. Mol. Cell Biol.* 8, 464–478. doi:10.1038/nrm2183

Agu, R. U., Ugwoke, M. I., Armand, M., Kinget, R., and Verbeke, N. (2001). The lung as a route for systemic delivery of therapeutic proteins and peptides. *Respir. Res.* 2, 198–209. doi:10.1186/rr58

Ahmed, T. A. E., Griffith, M., and Hincke, M. (2007). Characterization and inhibition of fibrin hydrogel-degrading enzymes during development of tissue engineering scaffolds. *Tissue Eng.* 13, 1469–1477. doi:10.1089/ten.2006.0354

Akeson, A. L., Woods, C. W., Hsieh, L. C., Bohnke, R. A., Ackermann, B. L., Chan, K. Y., et al. (1996). AF12198, a novel low molecular weight antagonist, selectively binds the human type I interleukin (IL)-1 receptor and blocks in vivo responses to IL-1. *J. Biol. Chem.* 271, 30517–30523. doi:10.1074/jbc.271.48.30517

Al-Hilal, T. A., Alam, F., and Byun, Y. (2013). Oral drug delivery systems using chemical conjugates or physical complexes. *Adv. Drug Deliv. Rev.* 65, 845–864. doi:10.1016/j.addr.2012.11.002

Anseth, K. S., Metters, A. T., Bryant, S. J., Martens, P. J., Elisseeff, J. H., and Bowman, C. N. (2002). In situ forming degradable networks and their application in tissue engineering and drug delivery. *J. Control. Release* 78, 199–209. doi:10.1016/S0168-3659(01)00500-4

Antosova, Z., Mackova, M., Kral, V., and Macek, T. (2009). Therapeutic application of peptides and proteins: parenteral forever? *Trends Biotechnol.* 27, 628–635. doi:10.1016/j.tibtech.2009.07.009

Atala, A. (2004). Tissue engineering and regenerative medicine: concepts for clinical application. *Rejuvenation Res.* 7, 15–31. doi:10.1089/154916804323105053

Atala, A., Bauer, S. B., Soker, S., Yoo, J. J., and Retik, A. B. (2006). Tissue-engineered autologous bladders for patients needing cystoplasty. *Lancet* 367, 1241–1246. doi:10.1016/S0140-6736(06)68438-9

Bader, R. A., and Putnam, D. A. (2014). *Engineering Polymer Systems for Improved Drug Delivery*. Hoboken, NJ: John Wiley & Sons, Inc.

Benoit, D. S. W., and Anseth, K. S. (2005). Heparin functionalized PEG gels that modulate protein adsorption for hMSC adhesion and differentiation. *Acta Biomater.* 1, 461–470. doi:10.1016/j.actbio.2005.03.002

Benoit, D. S. W., Durney, A. R., and Anseth, K. S. (2007). The effect of heparin-functionalized PEG hydrogels on three-dimensional human mesenchymal stem cell osteogenic differentiation. *Biomaterials* 28, 66–77. doi:10.1016/j.biomaterials.2006.08.033

Ben-Sasson, S. A., Licht, T., Tsirulnikov, L., Reuveni, H., and Yarnitzky, T. (2003). Induction of pro-angiogenic signaling by a synthetic peptide derived from the second intracellular loop of S1P(3) (EDG3). *Blood* 102, 2099–2107. doi:10.1182/blood-2002-12-3634

Bouhadir, K. H., Lee, K. Y., Alsberg, E., Damm, K. L., Anderson, K. W., and Mooney, D. J. (2001). Degradation of partially oxidized alginate and its potential application for tissue engineering. *Biotechnol. Prog.* 17, 945–950. doi:10.1021/bp010070p

Brem, H., and Tomic-Canic, M. (2007). Cellular and molecular basis of wound healing in diabetes. *J. Clin. Invest.* 117, 1219–1222. doi:10.1172/JCI32169

Brudno, Y., Ennett-Shepard, A. B., Chen, R. R., Aizenberg, M., and Mooney, D. J. (2013). Enhancing microvascular formation and vessel maturation through temporal control over multiple pro-angiogenic and pro-maturation factors. *Biomaterials* 34, 9201–9209. doi:10.1016/j.biomaterials.2013.08.007

Cai, S. S., Liu, Y. C., Shu, X. Z., and Prestwich, G. D. (2005). Injectable glycosaminoglycan hydrogels for controlled release of human basic fibroblast growth factor. *Biomaterials* 26, 6054–6067. doi:10.1016/j.biomaterials.2005.03.012

Carmeliet, P., and Jain, R. K. (2000). Angiogenesis in cancer and other diseases. *Nature* 407, 249–257. doi:10.1038/35025220

Castronuovo, G., Elia, V., Fessas, D., Giordano, A., and Velleca, F. (1995). Thermodynamics of the interaction of cyclodextrins with aromatic and alpha, omega-amino acids in aqueous-solutions – a calorimetric study at 25-degrees-C. *Carbohydr. Res.* 272, 31–39. doi:10.1016/0008-6215(95)00000-J

Cebix. (2013). *A Phase 2b, Randomized, Double-Blind, Placebo Controlled Study to Evaluate the Safety and Efficacy of CBX129801 (Ersatta™), Long-Acting Synthetic C-Peptide, in Type 1 Diabetes Mellitus Subjects*. ClinicalTrials.gov Identifier: NCT01681290.

Chen, Q. Z., Harding, S. E., Ali, N. N., Lyon, A. R., and Boccaccini, A. R. (2008). Biomaterials in cardiac tissue engineering: ten years of research survey. *Mater. Sci. Eng. R Rep.* 59, 1–37. doi:10.1016/j.mser.2007.08.001

Chu, H., and Wang, Y. (2012). Therapeutic angiogenesis: controlled delivery of angiogenic factors. *Ther. Deliv.* 3, 693–714. doi:10.4155/tde.12.50

Cianfrocca, M. E., Kimmel, K. A., Gallo, J., Cardoso, T., Brown, M. M., Hudes, G., et al. (2006). Phase 1 trial of the antiangiogenic peptide ATN-161 (Ac-PHSCN-NH2), a beta integrin antagonist, in patients with solid tumours. *Br. J. Cancer* 94, 1621–1626. doi:10.1038/sj.bjc.6603171

Copolovici, D. M., Langel, K., Eriste, E., and Langel, U. (2014). Cell-penetrating peptides: design, synthesis, and applications. *ACS Nano* 8, 1972–1994. doi:10.1021/nn4057269

Craik, D. J., Fairlie, D. P., Liras, S., and Price, D. (2013). The future of peptide-based drugs. *Chem. Biol. Drug Des.* 81, 136–147. doi:10.1111/cbdd.12055

D'Andrea, L. D., Iaccarino, G., Fattorusso, R., Sorriento, D., Carannante, C., Capasso, D., et al. (2005). Targeting angiogenesis: structural characterization and biological properties of a de novo engineered VEGF mimicking peptide. *Proc. Natl. Acad. Sci. U.S.A.* 102, 14215–14220. doi:10.1073/pnas.0505047102

Demidova-Rice, T. N., Geevarghese, A., and Herman, I. M. (2011). Bioactive peptides derived from vascular endothelial cell extracellular matrices promote microvascular morphogenesis and wound healing in vitro. *Wound Repair Regen.* 19, 59–70. doi:10.1111/j.1524-475X.2010.00642.x

Demidova-Rice, T. N., Wolf, L., Deckenback, J., Hamblin, M. R., and Herman, I. M. (2012). Human platelet-rich plasma- and extracellular matrix-derived peptides promote impaired cutaneous wound healing in vivo. *PLoS ONE* 7:e32146. doi:10.1371/journal.pone.0032146

Derma Sciences, I. (2015). *Phase III Study to Evaluate Efficacy and Safety of DSC127 in Diabetic Foot Ulcers (STRIDE 1)*. ClinicalTrials.gov Identifier: NCT01830348.

Diana, D., Ziaco, B., Colombo, G., Scarabelli, G., Romanelli, A., Fedone, C., et al. (2008). Structural determinants of the unusual helix stability of a de novo engineered vascular endothelial growth factor (VEGF) mimicking peptide. *Chemistry* 14, 4164–4166. doi:10.1002/chem.200800180

Du, A. W., and Stenzel, M. H. (2014). Drug carriers for the delivery of therapeutic peptides. *Biomacromolecules* 15, 1097–1114. doi:10.1021/bm500169p

Ehrbar, M., Djonov, V. G., Schnell, C., Tschanz, S. A., Martiny-Baron, G., Schenk, U., et al. (2004). Cell-demanded liberation of VEGF121 from fibrin implants induces local and controlled blood vessel growth. *Circ. Res.* 94, 1124–1132. doi:10.1161/01.RES.0000126411.29641.08

Ehrbar, M., Metters, A., Zammaretti, P., Hubbell, J. A., and Zisch, A. H. (2005). Endothelial cell proliferation and progenitor maturation by fibrin-bound VEGF variants with differential susceptibilities to local cellular activity. *J. Control. Release* 101, 93–109. doi:10.1016/j.jconrel.2004.07.018

Fairbanks, B. D., Schwartz, M. P., Halevi, A. E., Nuttelman, C. R., Bowman, C. N., and Anseth, K. S. (2009). A versatile synthetic extracellular matrix mimic via thiol-norbornene photopolymerization. *Adv. Mater. Weinheim* 21, 5005–5010. doi:10.1002/adma.200901808

Faulk, D. M., Londono, R., Wolf, M. T., Ranallo, C. A., Carruthers, C. A., Wildemann, J. D., et al. (2014). ECM hydrogel coating mitigates the chronic inflammatory response to polypropylene mesh. *Biomaterials* 35, 8585–8595. doi:10.1016/j.biomaterials.2014.06.057

FDA. (2014). *FDA Approves Orbactiv to Treat Skin Infections*. Silver Spring, MD: U.S. Food and Drug Administration.

Finetti, F., Basile, A., Capasso, D., Di Gaetano, S., Di Stasi, R., Pascale, M., et al. (2012). Functional and pharmacological characterization of a VEGF mimetic peptide on reparative angiogenesis. *Biochem. Pharmacol.* 84, 303–311. doi:10.1016/j.bcp.2012.04.011

Folkman, J. (2007). Angiogenesis: an organizing principle for drug discovery? *Nat. Rev. Drug Discov.* 6, 273–286. doi:10.1038/nrd2115

Forsythe, J. A., Jiang, B. H., Iyer, N. V., Agani, F., Leung, S. W., Koos, R. D., et al. (1996). Activation of vascular endothelial growth factor gene transcription by hypoxia-inducible factor 1. *Mol. Cell. Biol.* 16, 4604–4613.

Foss, A. C., Goto, T., Morishita, M., and Peppas, N. A. (2004). Development of acrylic-based copolymers for oral insulin delivery. *Eur. J. Pharm. Biopharm.* 57, 163–169. doi:10.1016/S0939-6411(03)00145-0

Frackenpohl, J., Arvidsson, P. I., Schreiber, J. V., and Seebach, D. (2001). The outstanding biological stability of beta- and gamma-peptides toward proteolytic enzymes: an in vitro investigation with fifteen peptidases. *Chembiochem* 2, 445–455. doi:10.1002/1439-7633(20010601)2:6<445::AID-CBIC445>3.3.CO;2-I

Galiano, R. D., Tepper, O. M., Pelo, C. R., Bhatt, K. A., Callaghan, M., Bastidas, N., et al. (2004). Topical vascular endothelial growth factor accelerates diabetic wound healing through increased angiogenesis and by mobilizing and recruiting bone marrow-derived cells. *Am. J. Pathol.* 164, 1935–1947. doi:10.1016/S0002-9440(10)63754-6

Garbern, J. C., Hoffman, A. S., and Stayton, P. S. (2010). Injectable pH- and temperature-responsive poly(N-isopropylacrylamide-co-propylacrylic acid) copolymers for delivery of angiogenic growth factors. *Biomacromolecules* 11, 1833–1839. doi:10.1021/bm100318z

Gentilucci, L., De Marco, R., and Cerisoli, L. (2010). Chemical modifications designed to improve peptide stability: incorporation of non-natural amino acids, pseudo-peptide bonds, and cyclization. *Curr. Pharm. Des.* 16, 3185–3203. doi:10.2174/138161210793292555

Go, A. S., Mozaffarian, D., Roger, V. L., Benjamin, E. J., Berry, J. D., Blaha, M. J., et al. (2014). Heart disease and stroke statistics-2014 update a report from the American heart association. *Circulation* 129, E28–E292. doi:10.1161/01.cir.0000442015.53336.12

Graesslin, O., and Korver, T. (2008). The contraceptive efficacy of implanon: a review of clinical trials and marketing experience. *Eur. J. Contracept. Reprod. Health Care* 13(Suppl. 1), 4–12. doi:10.1080/13625180801942754

Gupta, R., Tongers, J., and Losordo, D. W. (2009). Human studies of angiogenic gene therapy. *Circ. Res.* 105, 724–736. doi:10.1161/CIRCRESAHA.109.200386

Hardy, B., Battler, A., Weiss, C., Kudasi, O., and Raiter, A. (2008). Therapeutic angiogenesis of mouse hind limb ischemia by novel peptide activating GRP78 receptor on endothelial cells. *Biochem. Pharmacol.* 75, 891–899. doi:10.1016/j.bcp.2007.10.008

Hardy, B., Raiter, A., Weiss, C., Kaplan, B., Tenenbaum, A., and Battler, A. (2007). Angiogenesis induced by novel peptides selected from a phage display library by screening human vascular endothelial cells under different physiological conditions. *Peptides* 28, 691–701. doi:10.1016/j.peptides.2006.11.008

Heil, M., Eitenmuller, I., Schmitz-Rixen, T., and Schaper, W. (2006). Arteriogenesis versus angiogenesis: similarities and differences. *J. Cell. Mol. Med.* 10, 45–55. doi:10.1111/j.1582-4934.2006.tb00290.x

Henriksson, M., Nordling, E., Melles, E., Shafqat, J., Stahlberg, M., Ekberg, K., et al. (2005). Separate functional features of proinsulin C-peptide. *Cell. Mol. Life Sci.* 62, 1772–1778. doi:10.1007/s00018-005-5180-6

Henry, T. D., Grines, C. L., Watkins, M. W., Dib, N., Barbeau, G., Moreadith, R., et al. (2007). Effect of Ad5FGF-4 in patients with angina – an analysis of pooled data from the AGENT-3 and AGENT-4 trials. *J. Am. Coll. Cardiol.* 50, 1038–1046. doi:10.1016/j.jacc.2007.06.010

Hern, D. L., and Hubbell, J. A. (1998). Incorporation of adhesion peptides into nonadhesive hydrogels useful for tissue resurfacing. *J. Biomed. Mater. Res.* 39, 266–276. doi:10.1002/(SICI)1097-4636(199802)39:2<266::AID-JBM14>3.0.CO;2-B

Hiemstra, C., Zhong, Z. Y., Van Steenbergen, M. J., Hennink, W. E., and Feijen, J. (2007). Release of model proteins and basic fibroblast growth factor from in situ forming degradable dextran hydrogels. *J. Control. Release* 122, 71–78. doi:10.1016/j.jconrel.2007.06.011

Hirota, K., and Semenza, G. L. (2006). Regulation of angiogenesis by hypoxia-inducible factor 1. *Crit. Rev. Oncol. Hematol.* 59, 15–26. doi:10.1016/j.critrevonc.2005.12.003

Hoffman, M. D., Xie, C., Zhang, X., and Benoit, D. S. (2013). The effect of mesenchymal stem cells delivered via hydrogel-based tissue engineered periosteum on bone allograft healing. *Biomaterials* 34, 8887–8898. doi:10.1016/j.biomaterials.2013.08.005

Hopp, T. P., and Woods, K. R. (1981). Prediction of protein antigenic determinants from amino-acid-sequences. *Proc. Natl. Acad. Sci. U.S.A.* 78, 3824–3828. doi:10.1073/pnas.78.6.3824

Hosack, L. W., Firpo, M. A., Scott, J. A., Prestwich, G. D., and Peattie, R. A. (2008). Microvascular maturity elicited in tissue treated with cytokine-loaded hyaluronan-based hydrogels. *Biomaterials* 29, 2336–2347. doi:10.1016/j.biomaterials.2008.01.033

Hubbell, J. A., Lutolf, M. P., Raeber, G. P., Zisch, A. H., and Tirelli, N. (2003). Cell-responsive synthetic hydrogels. *Adv. Mater. Weinheim* 15, 888–892. doi:10.1002/adma.200304621

Jain, R. A. (2000). The manufacturing techniques of various drug loaded biodegradable poly(lactide-co-glycolide) (PLGA) devices. *Biomaterials* 21, 2475–2490. doi:10.1016/S0142-9612(00)00115-0

Jeon, O., Powell, C., Solorio, L. D., Krebs, M. D., and Alsberg, E. (2011). Affinity-based growth factor delivery using biodegradable, photocrosslinked heparin-alginate hydrogels. *J. Control. Release* 154, 258–266. doi:10.1016/j.jconrel.2011.06.027

Jha, A. K., Mathur, A., Svedlund, F. L., Ye, J., Yeghiazarians, Y., and Healy, K. E. (2015). Molecular weight and concentration of heparin in hyaluronic acid-based matrices modulates growth factor retention kinetics and stem cell fate. *J. Control. Release* 209, 308–316. doi:10.1016/j.jconrel.2015.04.034

Jose, S., Hughbanks, M. L., Binder, B. Y., Ingavle, G. C., and Leach, J. K. (2014). Enhanced trophic factor secretion by mesenchymal stem/stromal cells with glycine-histidine-lysine (GHK)-modified alginate hydrogels. *Acta Biomater.* 10, 1955–1964. doi:10.1016/j.actbio.2014.01.020

Kaspar, A. A., and Reichert, J. M. (2013). Future directions for peptide therapeutics development. *Drug Discov. Today* 18, 807–817. doi:10.1016/j.drudis.2013.05.011

Rodgers, K. E., and Dizerega, G. S. *Methods for Treating Diabetic Foot Ulcers.* USA Patent Application US 13/467,253 (2013).

Kent, D. L. (2014). Age-related macular degeneration: beyond anti-angiogenesis. *Mol. Vis.* 20, 46–55.

Kisiday, J., Jin, M., Kurz, B., Hung, H., Semino, C., Zhang, S., et al. (2002). Self-assembling peptide hydrogel fosters chondrocyte extracellular matrix production and cell division: implications for cartilage tissue repair. *Proc. Natl. Acad. Sci. U.S.A.* 99, 9996–10001. doi:10.1073/pnas.142309999

Kleinman, H. K., and Martin, G. R. (2005). Matrigel: basement membrane matrix with biological activity. *Semin. Cancer Biol.* 15, 378–386. doi:10.1016/j.semcancer.2005.05.004

Koczulla, R., Von Degenfeld, G., Kupatt, C., Krotz, F., Zahler, S., Gloe, T., et al. (2003). An angiogenic role for the human peptide antibiotic LL-37/hCAP-18. *J. Clin. Invest.* 111, 1665–1672. doi:10.1172/JCI17545

Kuhlmann, C. R., Schaefer, C. A., Reinhold, L., Tillmanns, H., and Erdogan, A. (2005). Signalling mechanisms of SDF-induced endothelial cell proliferation and migration. *Biochem. Biophys. Res. Commun.* 335, 1107–1114. doi:10.1016/j.bbrc.2005.08.006

Laham, R. J., Rezaee, M., Post, M., Sellke, F. W., Braeckman, R. A., Hung, D., et al. (1999). Intracoronary and intravenous administration of basic fibroblast growth factor: myocardial and tissue distribution. *Drug Metab. Dispos.* 27, 821–826.

Lane, T. F., Iruelaarispe, M. L., Johnson, R. S., and Sage, E. H. (1994). Sparc is a source of copper-binding peptides that stimulate angiogenesis. *J. Cell Biol.* 125, 929–943. doi:10.1083/jcb.125.4.929

Layman, H., Sacasa, M., Murphy, A. E., Murphy, A. M., Pham, S. M., and Andreopoulos, F. M. (2009). Co-delivery of FGF-2 and G-CSF from gelatin-based hydrogels as angiogenic therapy in a murine critical limb ischemic model. *Acta Biomater.* 5, 230–239. doi:10.1016/j.actbio.2008.07.024

Leach, J. B., Bivens, K. A., Patrick, C. W., and Schmidt, C. E. (2003). Photocrosslinked hyaluronic acid hydrogels: natural, biodegradable tissue engineering scaffolds. *Biotechnol. Bioeng.* 82, 578–589. doi:10.1002/bit.10605

Leach, J. B., and Schmidt, C. E. (2005). Characterization of protein release from photocrosslinkable hyaluronic acid-polyethylene glycol hydrogel tissue engineering scaffolds. *Biomaterials* 26, 125–135. doi:10.1016/j.biomaterials.2004.02.018

Lee, T. Y., Folkman, J., and Javaherian, K. (2010). HSPG-binding peptide corresponding to the exon 6a-encoded domain of VEGF inhibits tumor growth by blocking angiogenesis in murine model. *PLoS ONE* 5:e9945. doi:10.1371/journal.pone.0009945

Lehninger, A. L., Nelson, D. L., and Cox, M. M. (2000). *Lehninger Principles of Biochemistry.* New York, NY: Worth Publishers.

Lerman, O. Z., Galiano, R. D., Armour, M., Levine, J. P., and Gurtner, G. C. (2003). Cellular dysfunction in the diabetic fibroblast – impairment in migration, vascular endothelial growth factor production, and response to hypoxia. *Am. J. Pathol.* 162, 303–312. doi:10.1016/S0002-9440(10)63821-7

Liechty, W. B., Kryscio, D. R., Slaughter, B. V., and Peppas, N. A. (2010). Polymers for drug delivery systems. *Annu. Rev. Chem. Biomol. Eng.* 1, 149–173. doi:10.1146/annurev-chembioeng-073009-100847

Lieu, C., Heymach, J., Overman, M., Tran, H., and Kopetz, S. (2011). Beyond VEGF: inhibition of the fibroblast growth factor pathway and antiangiogenesis. *Clin. Cancer Res.* 17, 6130–6139. doi:10.1158/1078-0432.CCR-11-0659

Lin, C. C., and Anseth, K. S. (2009a). Controlling affinity binding with peptide-functionalized poly(ethylene glycol) hydrogels. *Adv. Funct. Mater.* 19, 2325–2331. doi:10.1002/adfm.200900107

Lin, C. C., and Anseth, K. S. (2009b). PEG hydrogels for the controlled release of biomolecules in regenerative medicine. *Pharm. Res.* 26, 631–643. doi:10.1007/s11095-008-9801-2

Lin, X. H., Takahashi, K., Liu, Y., Derrien, A., and Zamora, P. O. (2007). A synthetic, bioactive PDGF mimetic with binding to both alpha-PDGF and beta-PDGF receptors. *Growth Factors* 25, 87–93. doi:10.1080/08977190701553449

Lindgren, M., Hallbrink, M., Prochiantz, A., and Langel, U. (2000). Cell-penetrating peptides. *Trends Pharmacol. Sci.* 21, 99–103. doi:10.1016/S0165-6147(00)01447-4

Liu, C. J., Jones, D. S., Tsai, P. C., Venkataramana, A., and Cochran, J. R. (2014). An engineered dimeric fragment of hepatocyte growth factor is a potent c-MET agonist. *FEBS Lett.* 588, 4831–4837. doi:10.1016/j.febslet.2014.11.018

Liu, H., Slamovich, E. B., and Webster, T. J. (2006). Less harmful acidic degradation of poly(lactic-co-glycolic acid) bone tissue engineering scaffolds through titania nanoparticle addition. *Int. J. Nanomedicine* 1, 541–545. doi:10.2147/nano.2006.1.4.541

Liu, J. M., Lawrence, F., Kovacevic, M., Bignon, J., Papadimitriou, E., Lallemand, J. Y., et al. (2003). The tetrapeptide AcSDKP, an inhibitor of primitive hematopoietic cell proliferation, induces angiogenesis in vitro and in vivo. *Blood* 101, 3014–3020. doi:10.1182/blood-2002-07-2315

Lloyd-Jones, D., Adams, R. J., Brown, T. M., Carnethon, M., Dai, S., De Simone, G., et al. (2010). Heart disease and stroke statistics – 2010 update: a report from the American heart association. *Circulation* 121, e46–e215. doi:10.1161/CIRCULATIONAHA.109.192667

Lobmann, R., Ambrosch, A., Schultz, G., Waldmann, K., Schiweck, S., and Lehnert, H. (2002). Expression of matrix-metalloproteinases and their inhibitors in the wounds of diabetic and non-diabetic patients. *Diabetologia* 45, 1011–1016. doi:10.1007/s00125-002-0868-8

Losi, P., Briganti, E., Magera, A., Spiller, D., Ristori, C., Battolla, B., et al. (2010). Tissue response to poly(ether)urethane-polydimethylsiloxane-fibrin composite scaffolds for controlled delivery of pro-angiogenic growth factors. *Biomaterials* 31, 5336–5344. doi:10.1016/j.biomaterials.2010.03.033

Losordo, D. W., and Dimmeler, S. (2004). Therapeutic angiogenesis and vasculogenesis for ischemic disease. Part I: angiogenic cytokines. *Circulation* 109, 2487–2491. doi:10.1161/01.CIR.0000128595.79378.FA

Lustig, S. R., and Peppas, N. A. (1988). Solute diffusion in swollen membranes.9. Scaling laws for solute diffusion in gels. *J. Appl. Polym. Sci.* 36, 735–747. doi:10.1002/app.1988.070360401

Macchiarini, P., Jungebluth, P., Go, T., Asnaghi, M. A., Rees, L. E., Cogan, T. A., et al. (2008). Clinical transplantation of a tissue-engineered airway. *Lancet* 372, 2023–2030. doi:10.1016/S0140-6736(08)61598-6

Makadia, H. K., and Siegel, S. J. (2011). Poly lactic-co-glycolic acid (PLGA) as biodegradable controlled drug delivery carrier. *Polymers* 3, 1377–1397. doi:10.3390/polym3031377

Mandrup-Poulsen, T. (2012). Interleukin-1 antagonists and other cytokine blockade strategies for type 1 diabetes. *Rev. Diabet. Stud.* 9, 338–347. doi:10.1900/RDS.2012.9.338

Maynard, H. D., and Hubbell, J. A. (2005). Discovery of a sulfated tetrapeptide that binds to vascular endothelial growth factor. *Acta Biomater.* 1, 451–459. doi:10.1016/j.actbio.2005.04.004

Montesano, R., Kumar, S., Orci, L., and Pepper, M. S. (1996). Synergistic effect of hyaluronan oligosaccharides and vascular endothelial growth factor on angiogenesis in vitro. *Lab. Invest.* 75, 249–262.

Mooney, D. J., Chen, R. R., Silva, E. A., and Yuen, W. W. (2007). Spatio-temporal VEGF and PDGF delivery patterns blood vessel formation and maturation. *Pharm. Res.* 24, 258–264. doi:10.1007/s11095-006-9173-4

Motamed, K. (1999). SPARC (osteonectin/BM-40). *Int. J. Biochem. Cell Biol.* 31, 1363–1366. doi:10.1016/S1357-2725(99)00090-4

Muir, R. L. (2009). Peripheral arterial disease: pathophysiology, risk factors, diagnosis, treatment, and prevention. *J. Vasc. Nurs.* 27, 26–30. doi:10.1016/j.jvn.2009.03.001

Murry, C. E., Garbern, J. C., Minami, E., and Stayton, P. S. (2011). Delivery of basic fibroblast growth factor with a pH-responsive, injectable hydrogel to improve angiogenesis in infarcted myocardium. *Biomaterials* 32, 2407–2416. doi:10.1016/j.biomaterials.2010.11.075

Nie, T., Baldwin, A., Yamaguchi, N., and Kiick, K. L. (2007). Production of heparin-functionalized hydrogels for the development of responsive and controlled growth factor delivery systems. *J. Control. Release* 122, 287–296. doi:10.1016/j.jconrel.2007.04.019

Niman, H. L., Houghten, R. A., Walker, L. E., Reisfeld, R. A., Wilson, I. A., Hogle, J. M., et al. (1983). Generation of protein-reactive antibodies by short peptides is an event of high-frequency – implications for the structural basis of immune recognition. *Proc. Natl. Acad. Sci. U.S.A.* 80, 4949–4953. doi:10.1073/pnas.80.16.4949

Nishida, N., Yano, H., Nishida, T., Kamura, T., and Kojiro, M. (2006). Angiogenesis in cancer. *Vasc. Health Risk Manag.* 2, 213–219. doi:10.2147/vhrm.2006.2.3.213

Okada, M., Payne, T. R., Oshima, H., Momoi, N., Tobita, K., and Huard, J. (2010). Differential efficacy of gels derived from small intestinal submucosa as an injectable biomaterial for myocardial infarct repair. *Biomaterials* 31, 7678–7683. doi:10.1016/j.biomaterials.2010.06.056

Olsson, A. K., Johansson, I., Akerud, H., Einarsson, B., Christofferson, R., Sasaki, T., et al. (2004). The minimal active domain of endostatin is a heparin-binding motif that mediates inhibition of tumor vascularization. *Cancer Res.* 64, 9012–9017. doi:10.1158/0008-5472.CAN-04-2172

Ozawa, C. R., Banfi, A., Glazer, N. L., Thurston, G., Springer, M. L., Kraft, P. E., et al. (2004). Microenvironmental VEGF concentration, not total dose, determines a threshold between normal and aberrant angiogenesis. *J. Clin. Invest.* 113, 516–527. doi:10.1172/JCI18420

Papanas, N., and Maltezos, E. (2007). Growth factors in the treatment of diabetic foot ulcers: new technologies, any promises? *Int. J. Low. Extrem. Wounds* 6, 37–53. doi:10.1177/1534734606298416

Patterson, J., and Hubbell, J. A. (2010). Enhanced proteolytic degradation of molecularly engineered PEG hydrogels in response to MMP-1 and MMP-2. *Biomaterials* 31, 7836–7845. doi:10.1016/j.biomaterials.2010.06.061

Peattie, R. A., Nayate, A. P., Firpo, M. A., Shelby, J., Fisher, R. J., and Prestwich, G. D. (2004). Stimulation of in vivo angiogenesis by cytokine-loaded hyaluronic acid hydrogel implants. *Biomaterials* 25, 2789–2798. doi:10.1016/j.biomaterials.2003.09.054

Peattie, R. A., Rieke, E. R., Hewett, E. M., Fisher, R. J., Shu, X. Z., and Prestwich, G. D. (2006). Dual growth factor-induced angiogenesis in vivo using hyaluronan hydrogel implants. *Biomaterials* 27, 1868–1875. doi:10.1016/j.biomaterials.2005.09.035

Peppas, N. A., Hilt, J. Z., Khademhosseini, A., and Langer, R. (2006). Hydrogels in biology and medicine: from molecular principles to bionanotechnology. *Adv. Mater. Weinheim* 18, 1345–1360. doi:10.1002/adma.200501612

Peysselon, F., and Ricard-Blum, S. (2014). Heparin-protein interactions: from affinity and kinetics to biological roles. Application to an interaction network regulating angiogenesis. *Matrix Biol.* 35, 73–81. doi:10.1016/j.matbio.2013.11.001

Phelps, E. A., Landazuri, N., Thule, P. M., Taylor, W. R., and Garcia, A. J. (2010). Bioartificial matrices for therapeutic vascularization. *Proc. Natl. Acad. Sci. U.S.A.* 107, 3323–3328. doi:10.1073/pnas.0905447107

Pickart, L. (2008). The human tri-peptide GHK and tissue remodeling. *J. Biomater. Sci. Polym. Ed.* 19, 969–988. doi:10.1163/156856208784909435

Pike, D. B., Cai, S. S., Pomraning, K. R., Firpo, M. A., Fisher, R. J., Shu, X. Z., et al. (2006). Heparin-regulated release of growth factors in vitro and angiogenic response in vivo to implanted hyaluronan hydrogels containing VEGF and bFGF. *Biomaterials* 27, 5242–5251. doi:10.1016/j.biomaterials.2006.05.018

Plunkett, M. L., Tel-Tsur, Z., Bera, M., Beck, I., Avery, J., Livant, D. L., et al. (2002). A novel anti-angiogenic/anti-metastatic peptide, ATN-161 (Ac-PHSCN-NH2), which targets multiple fully activated integrins including alpha-5 beta-1 and alpha-v beta-3, leads to increased anti-tumor activity and increased survival in multiple tumor models when combined with chemotherapy. *Eur. J. Cancer* 38, S79. doi:10.1016/S0959-8049(02)80901-7

Porter, S. (2001). Human immune response to recombinant human proteins. *J. Pharm. Sci.* 90, 1–11. doi:10.1002/1520-6017(200101)90:1<1::AID-JPS1>3.0.CO;2-K

Radius Health, I. (2015). *Study to Evaluate the Safety and Efficacy of BA058 (Abaloparatide) for Prevention of Fracture in Postmenopausal Women (ACTIVE)*. Available from: ClinicalTrials.gov.

Raya-Rivera, A., Esquiliano, D. R., Yoo, J. J., Lopez-Bayghen, E., Soker, S., and Atala, A. (2011). Tissue-engineered autologous urethras for patients who need reconstruction: an observational study. *Lancet* 377, 1175–1182. doi:10.1016/S0140-6736(10)62354-9

Renukuntla, J., Vadlapudi, A. D., Patel, A., Boddu, S. H. S., and Mitra, A. K. (2013). Approaches for enhancing oral bioavailability of peptides and proteins. *Int. J. Pharm.* 447, 75–93. doi:10.1016/j.ijpharm.2013.02.030

Richardson, T. P., Peters, M. C., Ennett, A. B., and Mooney, D. J. (2001). Polymeric system for dual growth factor delivery. *Nat. Biotechnol.* 19, 1029–1034. doi:10.1038/nbt1101-1029

Riley, C. M., Fuegy, P. W., Firpo, M. A., Shu, X. Z., Prestwich, G. D., and Peattie, R. A. (2006). Stimulation of in vivo angiogenesis using dual growth factor-loaded cross-linked glycosaminoglycan hydrogels. *Biomaterials* 27, 5935–5943. doi:10.1016/j.biomaterials.2006.08.029

Rodell, C. B., Kaminski, A. L., and Burdick, J. A. (2013). Rational design of network properties in guest-host assembled and shear-thinning hyaluronic acid hydrogels. *Biomacromolecules* 14, 4125–4134. doi:10.1021/bm401280z

Rodell, C. B., Wade, R. J., Purcell, B. P., Dusaj, N. N., and Burdick, J. A. (2015). Selective proteolytic degradation of guest−host assembled, injectable hyaluronic acid hydrogels. *ACS Biomater. Sci. Eng.* 1, 277–286. doi:10.1021/ab5001673

Rozek, A., Powers, J. P. S., Friedrich, C. L., and Hancock, R. E. W. (2003). Structure-based design of an indolicidin peptide analogue with increased protease stability. *Biochemistry* 42, 14130–14138. doi:10.1021/bi035643g

Rustad, K. C., Wong, V. W., Sorkin, M., Glotzbach, J. P., Major, M. R., Rajadas, J., et al. (2012). Enhancement of mesenchymal stem cell angiogenic capacity and stemness by a biomimetic hydrogel scaffold. *Biomaterials* 33, 80–90. doi:10.1016/j.biomaterials.2011.09.041

Sakiyama-Elbert, S. E., and Hubbell, J. A. (2000a). Controlled release of nerve growth factor from a heparin-containing fibrin-based cell ingrowth matrix. *J. Control. Release* 69, 149–158. doi:10.1016/S0168-3659(00)00296-0

Sakiyama-Elbert, S. E., and Hubbell, J. A. (2000b). Development of fibrin derivatives for controlled release of heparin-binding growth factors. *J. Control. Release* 65, 389–402. doi:10.1016/S0168-3659(99)00221-7

Santulli, G., Ciccarelli, M., Palumbo, G., Campanile, A., Galasso, G., Ziaco, B., et al. (2009). In vivo properties of the proangiogenic peptide QK. *J. Transl. Med.* 7, 41. doi:10.1186/1479-5876-7-41

Sarmento, B., Ferreira, D. C., Jorgensen, L., and Van De Weert, M. (2007). Probing insulin's secondary structure after entrapment into alginate/chitosan nanoparticles. *Eur. J. Pharm. Biopharm.* 65, 10–17. doi:10.1016/j.ejpb.2006.09.005

Schmoekel, H. G., Weber, F. E., Schense, J. C., Gratz, K. W., Schawalder, P., and Hubbell, J. A. (2005). Bone repair with a form of BMP-2 engineered for incorporation into fibrin cell ingrowth matrices. *Biotechnol. Bioeng.* 89, 253–262. doi:10.1002/bit.20168

Schultz, P., Vautier, D., Richert, L., Jessel, N., Haikel, Y., Schaaf, P., et al. (2005). Polyelectrolyte multilayers functionalized by a synthetic analogue of an anti-inflammatory peptide, alpha-MSH, for coating a tracheal prosthesis. *Biomaterials* 26, 2621–2630. doi:10.1016/j.biomaterials.2004.06.049

Segal, E., and Satchi-Fainaro, R. (2009). Design and development of polymer conjugates as anti-angiogenic agents. *Adv. Drug Deliv. Rev.* 61, 1159–1176. doi:10.1016/j.addr.2009.06.005

Seif-Naraghi, S. B., Horn, D., Schup-Magoffin, P. J., and Christman, K. L. (2012). Injectable extracellular matrix derived hydrogel provides a platform for enhanced retention and delivery of a heparin-binding growth factor. *Acta Biomater.* 8, 3695–3703. doi:10.1016/j.actbio.2012.06.030

Selivanova, G., Iotsova, V., Okan, I., Fritsche, M., Strom, M., Groner, B., et al. (1997). Restoration of the growth suppression function of mutant p53 by a synthetic peptide derived from the p53 C-terminal domain. *Nat. Med.* 3, 632–638. doi:10.1038/nm0697-632

Shih, H., and Lin, C. C. (2012). Cross-linking and degradation of step-growth hydrogels formed by thiol-ene photoclick chemistry. *Biomacromolecules* 13, 2003–2012. doi:10.1021/bm300752j

Shoyele, S. A., and Cawthorne, S. (2006). Particle engineering techniques for inhaled biopharmaceuticals. *Adv. Drug Deliv. Rev.* 58, 1009–1029. doi:10.1016/j.addr.2006.07.010

Silva, E. A., and Mooney, D. J. (2007). Spatiotemporal control of vascular endothelial growth factor delivery from injectable hydrogels enhances angiogenesis. *J. Thromb. Haemost.* 5, 590–598. doi:10.1111/j.1538-7836.2007.02386.x

Silva, E. A., and Mooney, D. J. (2010). Effects of VEGF temporal and spatial presentation on angiogenesis. *Biomaterials* 31, 1235–1241. doi:10.1016/j.biomaterials.2009.10.052

Singelyn, J. M., Sundaramurthy, P., Johnson, T. D., Schup-Magoffin, P. J., Hu, D. P., Faulk, D. M., et al. (2012). Catheter-deliverable hydrogel derived from decellularized ventricular extracellular matrix increases endogenous cardiomyocytes and preserves cardiac function post-myocardial infarction. *J. Am. Coll. Cardiol.* 59, 751–763. doi:10.1016/j.jacc.2011.10.888

Slaughter, B. V., Khurshid, S. S., Fisher, O. Z., Khademhosseini, A., and Peppas, N. A. (2009). Hydrogels in regenerative medicine. *Adv. Mater. Weinheim* 21, 3307–3329. doi:10.1002/adma.200802106

Slyke, P. V. *Multimeric TIE 2 Agonists and Uses Thereof in Stimulating Angiogenesis.* USA Patent Application 12/446,511 (2011).

Soldani, G., Losi, P., Bernabei, M., Burchielli, S., Chiappino, D., Kull, S., et al. (2010). Long term performance of small-diameter vascular grafts made of a poly(ether) urethane-polydimethylsiloxane semi-interpenetrating polymeric network. *Biomaterials* 31, 2592–2605. doi:10.1016/j.biomaterials.2009.12.017

Sonnenberg, S. B., Rane, A. A., Liu, C. J., Rao, N., Agmon, G., Suarez, S., et al. (2015). Delivery of an engineered HGF fragment in an extracellular matrix-derived hydrogel prevents negative LV remodeling post-myocardial infarction. *Biomaterials* 45, 56–63. doi:10.1016/j.biomaterials.2014.12.021

Soro, S., Orecchia, A., Morbidelli, L., Lacal, P. M., Morea, V., Ballmer-Hofer, K., et al. (2008). A proangiogenic peptide derived from vascular endothelial growth factor receptor-1 acts through alpha 5 beta 1 integrin. *Blood* 111, 3479–3488. doi:10.1182/blood-2007-03-077537

Steed, D. L. (1995). Clinical evaluation of recombinant human platelet-derived growth factor for the treatment of lower extremity diabetic ulcers. Diabetic ulcer study group. *J. Vasc. Surg.* 21, 71–78. doi:10.1016/S0741-5214(95)70245-8

Stern, R. (2004). Hyaluronan catabolism: a new metabolic pathway. *Eur. J. Cell Biol.* 83, 317–325. doi:10.1078/0171-9335-00392

Struman, I., Bentzien, F., Lee, H. Y., Mainfroid, V., D'Angelo, G., Goffin, V., et al. (1999). Opposing actions of intact and N-terminal fragments of the human prolactin growth hormone family members on angiogenesis: an efficient mechanism for the regulation of angiogenesis. *Proc. Natl. Acad. Sci. U.S.A.* 96, 1246–1251. doi:10.1073/pnas.96.4.1246

Sun, Q. H., Chen, R. R., Shen, Y. C., Mooney, D. J., Rajagopalan, S., and Grossman, P. M. (2005). Sustained vascular endothelial growth factor delivery enhances angiogenesis and perfusion in ischemic hind limb. *Pharm. Res.* 22, 1110–1116. doi:10.1007/s11095-005-5644-2

Sylven, C., Hao, X. J., Silva, E. A., Mansson-Broberg, A., Grinnemo, K. H., Siddiqui, A. J., et al. (2007). Angiogenic effects of sequential release of VEGF-A(165) and PDGF-BB with alginate hydrogels after myocardial infarction. *Cardiovasc. Res.* 75, 178–185. doi:10.1016/j.cardiores.2007.03.028

Tabata, Y., and Ikada, Y. (1998). Protein release from gelatin matrices. *Adv. Drug Deliv. Rev.* 31, 287–301. doi:10.1016/S0169-409X(97)00125-7

Tae, G., Scatena, M., Stayton, P. S., and Hoffman, A. S. (2006). PEG-cross-linked heparin is an affinity hydrogel for sustained release of vascular endothelial growth factor. *J. Biomater. Sci. Polym. Ed.* 17, 187–197. doi:10.1163/156856206774879090

Thomas, U., Themis, K., Filippo, G. M., Carlo Alberto, O., Dave, H., Diederik, H., et al. (2014). The emergence of peptides in the pharmaceutical business: from exploration to exploitation. *EuPA Open Proteom.* 4, 58–69. doi:10.1016/j.euprot.2014.05.003

Tiwari, G., Tiwari, R., and Rai, A. K. (2010). Cyclodextrins in delivery systems: applications. *J. Pharm. Bioallied Sci.* 2, 72–79. doi:10.4103/0975-7406.67003

Turco, G., Donati, I., Grassi, M., Marchioli, G., Lapasin, R., and Paoletti, S. (2011). Mechanical spectroscopy and relaxometry on alginate hydrogels: a comparative analysis for structural characterization and network mesh size determination. *Biomacromolecules* 12, 1272–1282. doi:10.1021/bm101556m

van de Wetering, P., Metters, A. T., Schoenmakers, R. G., and Hubbell, J. A. (2005). Poly(ethylene glycol) hydrogels formed by conjugate addition with controllable swelling, degradation, and release of pharmaceutically active proteins. *J. Control. Release* 102, 619–627. doi:10.1016/j.jconrel.2004.10.029

Van Hove, A. H., Beltejar, M. J., and Benoit, D. S. (2014). Development and in vitro assessment of enzymatically responsive poly(ethylene glycol) hydrogels for the delivery of therapeutic peptides. *Biomaterials* 35, 9719–9730. doi:10.1016/j.biomaterials.2014.08.019

Van Hove, A. H., Willson, B., and Benoit, D. S. (2013). Microwave-assisted functionalization of poly(ethylene glycol) and on-resin peptides for use in chain polymerizations and hydrogel formation. *J. Vis. Exp.* 80, e50890. doi:10.3791/50890

Van Slyke, P., Alami, J., Martin, D., Kuliszewski, M., Leong-Poi, H., Sefton, M. V., et al. (2009). Acceleration of diabetic wound healing by an angiopoietin peptide mimetic. *Tissue Eng. Part A* 15, 1269–1280. doi:10.1089/ten.tea.2007.0400

Vasudev, N. S., and Reynolds, A. R. (2014). Anti-angiogenic therapy for cancer: current progress, unresolved questions and future directions. *Angiogenesis* 17, 471–494. doi:10.1007/s10456-014-9420-y

Verrecchio, A., Germann, M. W., Schick, B. P., Kung, B., Twardowski, T., and San Antonio, J. D. (2000). Design of peptides with high affinities for heparin and endothelial cell proteoglycans. *J. Biol. Chem.* 275, 7701–7707. doi:10.1074/jbc.275.11.7701

Vinoth Prabhu, V., Chidambaranathan, N., and Gopal, V. (2011). A historical review on current medication and therapies for inducing and inhibiting angiogenesis. *J. Chem. Pharm. Res.* 3, 526–533.

Vlieghe, P., Lisowski, V., Martinez, J., and Khrestchatisky, M. (2010). Synthetic therapeutic peptides: science and market. *Drug Discov. Today* 15, 40–56. doi:10.1016/j.drudis.2009.10.009

Welti, J., Loges, S., Dimmeler, S., and Carmeliet, P. (2013). Recent molecular discoveries in angiogenesis and antiangiogenic therapies in cancer. *J. Clin. Invest.* 123, 3190–3200. doi:10.1172/JCI70212

West, J. L., and Hubbell, J. A. (1999). Polymeric biomaterials with degradation sites for proteases involved in cell migration. *Macromolecules* 32, 241–244. doi:10.1021/ma981296k

Wieghaus, K. A., Nickerson, M. M., Petrie Aronin, C. E., Sefcik, L. S., Price, R. J., Paige, M. A., et al. (2008). Expansion of microvascular networks in vivo by phthalimide neovascular factor 1 (PNF1). *Biomaterials* 29, 4698–4708. doi:10.1016/j.biomaterials.2008.08.029

Willerth, S. M., Johnson, P. J., Maxwell, D. J., Parsons, S. R., Doukas, M. E., and Sakiyama-Elbert, S. E. (2007). Rationally designed peptides for controlled release of nerve growth factor from fibrin matrices. *J. Biomed. Mater. Res. A.* 80A, 13–23. doi:10.1002/jbm.a.30844

Yamamoto, M., Ikada, Y., and Tabata, Y. (2001). Controlled release of growth factors based on biodegradation of gelatin hydrogel. *J. Biomater. Sci. Polym. Ed.* 12, 77–88. doi:10.1163/156856201744461

Yancopoulos, G. D., Davis, S., Gale, N. W., Rudge, J. S., Wiegand, S. J., and Holash, J. (2000). Vascular-specific growth factors and blood vessel formation. *Nature* 407, 242–248. doi:10.1038/35025215

Yang, L. L., Mashima, T., Sato, S., Mochizuki, M., Sakamoto, H., Yamori, T., et al. (2003). Predominant suppression of apoptosome by inhibitor of apoptosis protein in non-small cell lung cancer H460 cells: therapeutic effect of a novel polyarginine-conjugated Smac peptide. *Cancer Res.* 63, 831–837.

Ye, Q., Zund, G., Benedikt, P., Jockenhoevel, S., Hoerstrup, S. P., Sakyama, S., et al. (2000). Fibrin gel as a three dimensional matrix in cardiovascular tissue engineering. *Eur. J. Cardiothorac. Surg.* 17, 587–591. doi:10.1016/S1010-7940(00)00373-0

Young, S., Wong, M., Tabata, Y., and Mikos, A. G. (2005). Gelatin as a delivery vehicle for the controlled release of bioactive molecules. *J. Control. Release* 109, 256–274. doi:10.1016/j.jconrel.2005.09.023

Zachary, I., and Morgan, R. D. (2011). Therapeutic angiogenesis for cardiovascular disease: biological context, challenges, prospects. *Heart* 97, 181–189. doi:10.1136/hrt.2009.180414

Zhanel, G. G., Schweizer, F., and Karlowsky, J. A. (2012). Oritavancin: mechanism of action. *Clin. Infect. Dis.* 54(Suppl. 3), S214–S219. doi:10.1093/cid/cir920

Ziche, M., Donnini, S., and Morbidelli, L. (2004). Development of new drugs in angiogenesis. *Curr. Drug Targets* 5, 485–493. doi:10.2174/1389450043345371

Zisch, A. H., Lutolf, M. P., Ehrbar, M., Raeber, G. P., Rizzi, S. C., Davies, N., et al. (2003). Cell-demanded release of VEGF from synthetic, biointeractive cell-ingrowth matrices for vascularized tissue growth. *FASEB J.* 17, 2260–2262. doi:10.1096/fj.02-1041fje

Zisch, A. H., Schenk, U., Schense, J. C., Sakiyama-Elbert, S. E., and Hubbell, J. A. (2001). Covalently conjugated VEGF – fibrin matrices for endothelialization. *J. Control. Release* 72, 101–113. doi:10.1016/S0168-3659(01)00266-8

Conflict of Interest Statement: The authors declare that they have no financial conflicts of interest related to the submitted work. They have a patent pending on one of the pro-angiogenic biomaterial discussed (Amy H. Van Hove and Danielle S. W. Benoit. Compositions and Methods for Stimuli-Responsive Release of a Therapeutic Agent. PCT/US14/49774 (filed). Assignee: University of Rochester. 5 August 2014.)

4

Biomaterial-mediated modification of the local inflammatory environment

Shane Browne and Abhay Pandit*

Network of Excellence for Functional Biomaterials (NFB), National University of Ireland, Galway, Ireland

Inflammation plays a major role in the rejection of biomaterial implants. In addition, despite playing an important role in the early stages of wound healing, dysregulated inflammation has a negative impact on the wound healing processes. Thus, strategies to modulate excessive inflammation are needed. Through the use of biomaterials to control the release of anti-inflammatory therapeutics, increased control over inflammation is possible in a range of pathological conditions. However, the choice of biomaterial (natural or synthetic), and the form it takes (solid, hydrogel, or micro/nanoparticle) is dependent on both the cause and tissue location of inflammation. These considerations also influence the nature of the anti-inflammatory therapeutic that is incorporated into the biomaterial to be delivered. In this report, the range of biomaterials and anti-inflammatory therapeutics that have been combined will be discussed, as well as the functional benefit observed. Furthermore, we point toward future strategies in the field that will bring more efficacious anti-inflammatory therapeutics closer to realization.

Keywords: biomaterials, foreign body response, inflammation, drug delivery, controlled release

Edited by:
Gilson Khang,
Chonbuk National University,
South Korea

Reviewed by:
Mikaël M. Martino,
Osaka University, Japan
Elizabeth R. Balmayor,
Technical University Munich, Germany

*Correspondence:
Abhay Pandit,
Network of Excellence for Functional
Biomaterials (NFB), Biosciences,
National University of Ireland, Galway,
Ireland
abhay.pandit@nuigalway.ie

Introduction

The inflammatory response is an essential part of the healing process (Martin and Leibovich, 2005; Li et al., 2007). Inflammation is initiated by necrosis and tissue injury, through the recognition of damage associated molecular patterns (DAMPs). DAMPs that trigger inflammation include intracellular proteins and nucleic acids released by dying cells, and extracellular matrix (ECM) fragments such as low molecular weight hyaluronic acid (HA) (Kataoka et al., 2014). In addition, stores of inflammatory cytokines including IL-1α and IL-33 present in cells are released following necrotic cell death (Chen and Nunez, 2010). Inflammation is required to remove necrotic and apoptotic cells, cleaved ECM molecules, and to initiate subsequent angiogenesis and tissue repair (Jiang and Liao, 2010). In fact, inflammatory cells have been shown to play a role in regeneration (Kim et al., 2013). However, excessive and chronic inflammation leads to the formation of a hostile environment for regeneration and repair, resulting in further cell death. Excessive inflammation and ECM remodeling lead to the formation of a fibrotic scar through the upregulation of matrix metalloproteinases (MMPs) and increased deposition of collagen type I and III (Dobaczewski and Frangogiannis, 2008). This is typically characterized by increased neutrophils infiltration and pro-inflammatory macrophage retention. This amplifies the pro-inflammatory cytokine response, along with MMP activity and the presence of radical oxygen species (ROS). It has been shown that improved wound healing occurs following a lesser inflammatory response in fetal wound healing (Redd et al., 2004), with a reduced expression of pro-inflammatory cytokines, transforming growth factor-beta (TGF-β), and overexpression of interleukin-10 (IL-10) (Lo et al., 2012). A similar effect has been observed in fetal myocardium, with reduced inflammation allowing for complete functional restoration (Herdrich et al., 2010). Furthermore, reduction in inflammation has been shown to promote mesenchymal stem cell (MSC)-mediated bone tissue regeneration (Liu et al., 2011; Chang et al., 2013). While scarless healing cannot be completely attributed to the absence of inflammation, it does present evidence that a reduced inflammatory response can result in a more favorable outcome.

Thus, strategies to reduce inflammation can prove to be of benefit to treat conditions in which excessive inflammation causes damage to the tissue, or when inflammation becomes chronic.

Biomaterials to Modulate Inflammation

Implanted biomaterials can cause an inflammatory response, with the level of this response dependent on the material of choice along with the site in the body into which it is implanted (Luttikhuizen et al., 2006a,b; Anderson et al., 2008). This is known as the foreign body response (FBR) and is the response of the host to the implant. Following implantation, a biomaterial acquires a layer of host proteins that is associated with the surface chemistry of the material. This occurs before any interaction with host cells, and governs the type of cells that interact and their phenotypes. Material properties and, particularly, surface chemistry have an effect on protein deposition on the surface. The proteins that typically absorb on the surface include fibrinogen, albumin, and fibronectin. These proteins form a provisional matrix composed mostly of fibrin around the implant. This matrix acts like a thrombus and initiates a wound healing-like inflammatory response. Inflammatory cells such as neutrophils and macrophages are attracted by the build-up of chemokines and other chemoattractants in the provisional matrix. Therefore, the choice of biomaterial is of the utmost importance, with an obvious preference for materials that cause a minimal acute response. Typically, anti-inflammatory strategies using biomaterials have involved loading of therapeutics into biomaterial systems, with therapeutic release *in vivo* aiding to alleviate inflammation. These anti-inflammatory signals are composed of anti-inflammatory drugs, proteins, or nucleic acids, while the delivery of stem cells has also been shown to result in a reduced inflammatory response. In addition, a number of naturally occurring biomaterials have intrinsic anti-inflammatory signals. These include high molecular weight HA (Nakamura et al., 2004; Hirabara et al., 2013) and chitosan, which have ROS-scavenging properties (Je and Kim, 2006). However, in the case of most materials, loading of anti-inflammatory therapeutics is necessary to modulate the inflammatory microenvironment.

A wide variety of therapies to reduce inflammation exist, from gene therapy to receptor blocking antibodies, protein delivery, and cell therapy (see **Figure 1B**). However, as yet, no outstanding candidate has emerged that can convincingly reduce inflammation in all situations. Each therapy has associated advantages and disadvantages. However, the main drawback associated with most therapies is inadequate efficacy as a result of an insufficient local concentration. This may be due to minimal localization at the appropriate site of action when administered systemically, or as a result of clearance and destruction by inflammatory cells when administered locally. One route to address this concern is by the use of biomaterial systems as reservoirs of therapeutics to locally deliver and sustain effective concentrations for a prolonged period of time. Protein and gene delivery through scaffolds holds much promise to produce efficacious therapies (O'Rorke et al., 2010; Monaghan and Pandit, 2011; Censi et al., 2012). Natural biomaterials are capable of loading and releasing therapeutics through MMP-mediated biodegradation, with collagen in particular standing out for its usefulness (Browne et al., 2013). However, synthetic materials may allow for increased control over degradation and release kinetics of therapeutics, with the caveat that the material itself and its degradation products must cause a minimal response when implanted *in vivo*.

A further consideration that must be taken into account is the form the biomaterial system takes. Three typical structures that biomaterials can take are solid scaffolds, hydrogels, and particles, shown in **Figure 1A**. The choice of biomaterial structure is dependent on a number of factors, primarily the tissue being targeted and also the nature of the anti-inflammatory therapeutic incorporated. For example, solid scaffolds require surgery to implant, and thus are more suitable for wound healing applications

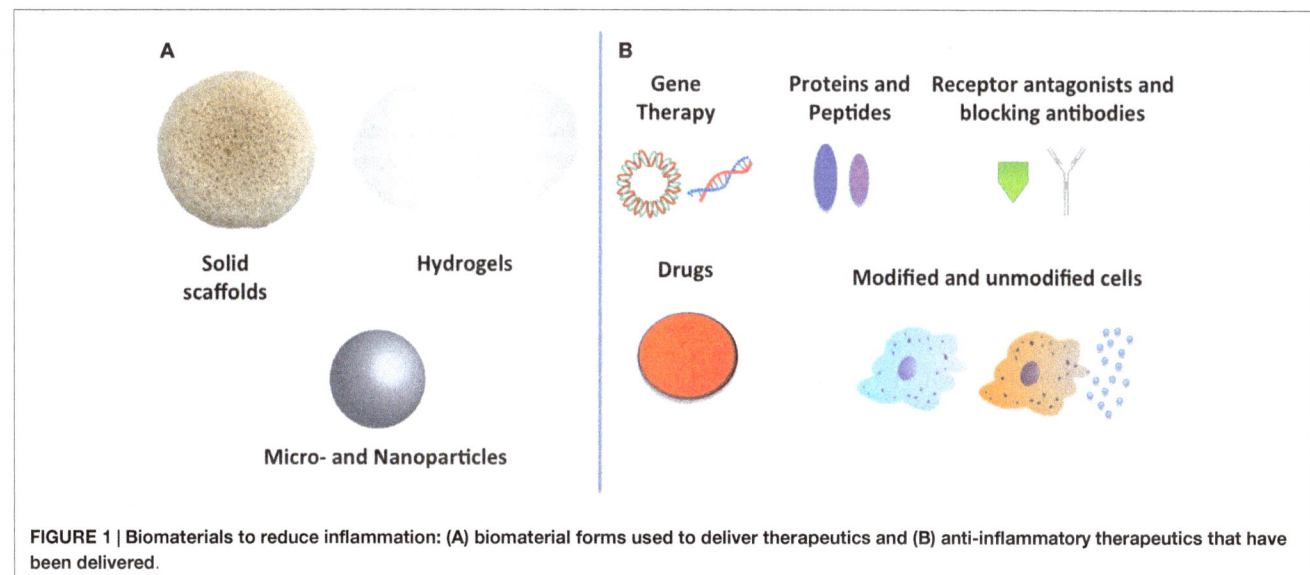

FIGURE 1 | Biomaterials to reduce inflammation: (A) biomaterial forms used to deliver therapeutics and (B) anti-inflammatory therapeutics that have been delivered.

in which they may be applied to an open wound. In contrast, *in situ* gelling hydrogels and particles can typically be delivered in a minimally invasive manner using a syringe without the need for open surgery. Thus, hydrogels and particles are suitable for delivery directly into tissues such as muscle and the myocardium. However, in terms of loading, they differ. Particles are most suited for protein, gene, and drug delivery (Sehgal and Srinivasan, 2009; Browne et al., 2012; Kraskiewicz et al., 2013). Hydrogels may not only be used for protein, gene, and drug delivery but also for cells. Hydrogels can be designed to provide a microenvironment that can be tuned to protect implanted cells, promoting cell survival, and improving function (Seliktar, 2012). Meanwhile, solid scaffolds have also been loaded with proteins, nucleic acids, and drugs, in addition to acting as matrices to enhance cell transplantation (Thevenot et al., 2010; Holladay et al., 2011; Hortensius et al., 2015). Thus, the choice of biomaterial form is dependent on the tissue into which it will be implanted, and the anti-inflammatory agent being delivered. The main biomaterial approaches to reducing inflammation will be discussed in terms of the type of biomaterial structure used.

Solid Scaffolds

The incorporation of stromal cell-derived factor-1 alpha (SDF-1α) into a poly (lactic-co-glycolic acid) PLGA scaffold reduced the inflammatory response when implanted into the subcutaneous space in mice (Thevenot et al., 2010). While SDF-1α is typically associated with increased angiogenesis, it can also exert anti-inflammatory effects through its mobilization and homing effect on stem cells (Ceradini et al., 2004; Ceradini and Gurtner, 2005). Thus, it was shown that incorporation of SDF-1α in PLGA scaffolds reduced the inflammatory tissue response through an increase in autologous stem recruitment to the implant site. Furthermore, a reduction in pro-inflammatory cytokines was detected, with reduced expression of a number of key mediators including interleukin-1 alpha (IL-1α), interleukin-6 (IL-6), and tumor necrosis factor alpha (TNF-α), while there was an increase in vascular endothelial growth factor (VEGF) expression.

Modification of the inflammatory response to a carbodiimide crosslinked collagen scaffold was achieved by codelivery of a plasmid encoding IL-10 (*p*IL-10). Treatment with the *p*IL-10 reduced the inflammatory response to the implanted collagen scaffolds in a subcutaneous model, with a reduction seen in infiltrating macrophages (ED1 positive cells). However, a subsequent reduction in vascularization was also observed (van Putten et al., 2009). A collagen scaffold with MSCs incorporated was further functionalized with *p*IL-10 polyplexes in an effort to reduce inflammation in an intramuscular model, and to promote the survival of the MSCs. It was observed that *p*IL-10 polyplex treatment reduced inflammation and increased MSC survival (Holladay et al., 2011). When this system was implanted in a rodent model of myocardial infarction (MI), reduced inflammation was detected along with functional recovery of the heart, in terms of improved ejection fraction (Holladay et al., 2012). Furthermore, a change in macrophage phenotype was detected. Macrophages were seen to change from a classically activated, pro-inflammatory phenotype in control groups to an alternatively activated, anti-inflammatory phenotype following treatment with *p*IL-10 polyplexes and MSCs.

Macrophage phenotype has been shown to be a key component of the inflammatory response to implanted biomaterials (van Putten et al., 2013; Spiller et al., 2014), and thus strategies to control the phenotype of macrophages may prove vital to modify inflammation. Incorporation of highly sulfated glycosaminoglycans (GAGs) into collagen scaffolds has enabled the control of monocyte differentiation and macrophage phenotype *in vitro* (Kajahn et al., 2012). A reduction of pro-inflammatory cytokine secretion and an increase in anti-inflammatory cytokines were observed when primary macrophages were cultured with a collagen scaffold containing highly sulfated GAGs, in comparison with a collagen scaffold with either no GAGs incorporated or a less sulfated GAG incorporated. However, the application of this system in pre-clinical models is crucial to determine its potential usefulness in controlling macrophage phenotype in disease states.

A silk-fibroin/HA scaffold was used to treat post-MI inflammation. In addition to providing a structural support to the damaged myocardium, it was found that treatment with the composite silk-fibroin/HA reduced macrophage infiltration (CD68 positive cells) in comparison with a non-treated infarct (Chi et al., 2012). In addition, there was an increase in macrophages when bone marrow mesenchymal stem cells (BMSCs) were incorporated within the scaffold. The authors attribute this to the fact that the cells were obtained from male rats and transplanted in female rats. However, incorporation of the BMSCs improved myocardial function (wall thickness and fractional shortening), primarily through an increase in angiogenic factors and a resultant increase in vascular area. This emphasizes that reducing inflammation is an important factor, but that a multi-faceted approach is typically necessary to ensure adequate healing. Conversely, it was found in a separate study that a HA-based scaffold did not reduce inflammation unless it was coupled with MSCs (Muscari et al., 2013). This could be related to possible differences in the molecular weight of HA used. An increase in the vascular density was observed with MSC delivery, as with the previous study.

Delivery of ibuprofen from an electrospun, acid responsive poly (L-lactide) (PLLA) scaffold improved regeneration in a muscle wound model. Incorporation of sodium bicarbonate induced acid responsiveness of the PLLA scaffold, as it was observed that ibuprofen release was increased when the pH was changed from 7.4 to 5, whereas this property was not observed without the incorporation of the sodium bicarbonate. It was found that the ibuprofen reduced the inflammatory response as measured by immunohistochemical staining and assessment of gene expression of IL-6 and TNF-α, which resulted in improved muscle regeneration (Yuan et al., 2014). In a similar study, tetrandrine, an anti-inflammatory agent, was incorporated into a PLLA scaffold. It was found that this system could reduce the production of pro-inflammatory cytokines both *in vitro* and *in vivo* (Wang et al., 2014a). A subcutaneous study revealed that the tetrandrine-loaded scaffold had a reduced inflammatory response compared with the unloaded scaffold at 1, 4, and 12 weeks.

Delivery of *p*IL-10 was proposed as a mechanism by which to reduce the inflammatory response to porous poly (lactide-co-glycolide) (PLG) scaffolds. It was found that a macrophage cell line, RAW 264.7 cells, markedly reduced TNF-α and increased IL-10 expression when cultured in the presence of the PLG scaffolds, the IL-10 gene, and lipopolysaccharide (LPS) (Gower et al., 2014). This indicates a more anti-inflammatory nature of the macrophages following treatment with the IL-10 gene-loaded scaffold. Increased expression of IL-10 *in vivo* resulted in a reduction in leukocyte infiltration in the PLG scaffolds after 7 days. A decrease was also observed in the expression of interferon gamma (IFN-), but no difference was observed in the expression of IL-1β or TNF-α when compared with the control scaffolds. A follow-on study revealed that the mechanism behind this anti-inflammatory nature was a change in the phenotype of macrophages following treatment with the *p*IL-10 gene. It was found that transduction of RAW 264.7 macrophages with *p*IL-10 resulted in a switch toward a more regulatory macrophage phenotype, as well as preventing a shift toward a more inflammatory phenotype when in a pro-inflammatory environment (IFN- and LPS) (Boehler et al., 2014). A reduction in NF-kB activation was also observed following *p*IL-10 delivery, which was consistent with the reduction observed in TNF-α expression.

A sphingosine 1-phosphate receptor-3 agonist (FTY720) was used to modify the inflammatory response to a PLGA film. It was found that following implantation of a PLGA film, FTY720 delivery increased the arteriole and length density (Awojoodu et al., 2013). This was found to be as a result of an increase in the infiltration of anti-inflammatory monocytes to the site of implantation. *In vitro* studies revealed that FTY720 treatment changed the profile of inflammatory and regenerative cytokine secretion in both pro- and anti-inflammatory macrophages as well as human umbilical vein endothelial cells (HUVECs).

The examples discussed above (summarized in **Table 1**) provide an overview of the range of therapeutics that have been incorporated into solid biomaterial scaffolds. Therapeutics can be added to the scaffold immediately prior to implantation, or conjugated via linker systems. The incorporated therapeutics can help to overcome inflammation associated with the FBR, as well as any pre-existing pathological inflammation. The choice of therapeutic is dependent on the biomaterial itself, as well as the site into which it will be implanted. Thus, it is imperative to consider each pathology individually, rather than a 'one size fits all' approach. Furthermore, depending on the context of the injury, as well as the selected material, solid scaffold may be capable of providing mechanical support, i.e., in the case of bone scaffolds, or functions as a barrier in the case of dermal wounds.

Hydrogels

One of the main reasons why anti-inflammatory therapy has become important in relation to biomaterials is to protect implanted cells and prevent rejection by the host. This can be elucidated with the example of islet cell delivery. Ideally, implanted islet cells will not be rejected by the body, and can produce insulin efficiently to correct diabetes. However, this is not the case in actuality, as the host often rejects the implanted cells and their function is compromised. Attempts to immuno-isolate cells using biomaterials have not proven successful, and thus anti-inflammatory signals are necessary to prevent rejection by the host immune system. Encapsulation in a biomaterial alone has not proved efficacious, and thus the incorporation of anti-inflammatory agent is the next logical step. Su et al. encapsulated islet cells in a

PEG-based hydrogel, and conjugated an inhibitory peptide to the IL-1 receptor (IL-R1) (Su et al., 2010). This increased the survival of encapsulated cells *in vitro* following exposure to IL-1β, IFN- , and TNF-α, while islet cells were also able to continue glucose-stimulated release of insulin when incubated with β-cell specific T-lymphocytes.

Hyaluronic acid hydrogels have been extensively studied as materials to deliver anti-inflammatory therapies due to their biodegradable nature, as well as their own potential anti-inflammatory nature, which is dependent on the molecular weight chosen (Nakamura et al., 2004). Conjugation of dexamethasone to the HA was performed to increase drug retention by reducing diffusion from the hydrogel (Ito et al., 2007). *In vitro* studies revealed that the released dexamethasone reduced the expression of TNF-α and IL-6 from LPS-treated macrophages in a dose-dependent manner. Furthermore, *in vivo* studies showed that dexamethasone conjugated hydrogels had a reduced inflammatory response after 2 days when implanted subcutaneously. In a similar study, an anti-TNF-α antibody was conjugated to a HA hydrogel and applied to a burn wound (Friedrich et al., 2014). This treatment appeared to reduce the thickness of non-viable tissue, as well as IL-1β concentration and macrophage infiltration compared with the control.

Chitosan is a polysaccharide derived from crustaceans. It has been used for many biomedical applications (Khor and Lim, 2003; Jayakumar et al., 2010, 2007; Prabaharan, 2008). Specifically, it is commercially available as a bandage due to its clotting ability and its anti-bacterial properties (Chirkov, 2002). The addition of adipose-derived mesenchymal stem cells (ADSCs) to a chitosan hydrogel was seen to improve their survival in the infarcted myocardium (Liu et al., 2012). *In vitro* studies demonstrated the ROS scavenging properties of chitosan and its degradation products. MI was induced by permanent ligation of the coronary artery, followed by injection of the chitosan/ADSCs system. Treatment with the chitosan/ADSCs system resulted in a reduction in ROS, as observed by a reduction in dihydroethidium (DHE) staining. An improvement was observed at 4 weeks in ejection fraction and fractional shortening, while there was a reduction in apoptosis seen at 1 week. Additionally, there was a reduction in infarct size as well as an increase in wall thickness and vessel density in the infarct site. This study demonstrates the anti-ROS properties of chitosan, as it is hypothesized that chitosan enhances stem cell retention and survival in the myocardium (which was confirmed by *in vivo* bioluminescence imaging), partly due to its ability to scavenge ROS. This system was also utilized to treat ischemic injury in the kidney (Gao et al., 2012). A similar effect was observed, with a reduction in ROS expression, increased cell retention, and increased number of blood vessels.

A large-scale study was performed to identify a suitable anti-inflammatory drug for local immunosuppression of islet cells. From a large range of anti-inflammatory drugs, curcumin was identified as being capable of reducing inflammation and ensuing fibrosis following implantation of PLGA particles (Dang et al., 2013). Subsequent encapsulation of islet cells in alginate microcapsules, along with the identified anti-inflammatory curcumin, improved survival of the islet cells *in vivo*, with reduced fibrosis

TABLE 1 | Examples of anti-inflammatory therapies delivered from solid scaffolds.

Biomaterial system	Therapeutic	Dose	*In vitro* characterization	*In vivo* model	*In vivo* outcome	Reference
PLGA	SDF-1α	50 μg SDF-1α	Stem cell migration assay	Mouse subcutaneous implantation	Increased vessel density Enhanced MSC engraftment Reduced inflammatory response (IL-1α, IL-6, TNF-α)	Thevenot et al. (2010)
Collagen	IL-10 pDNA	2.5 μg IL-10 pDNA	n/a	Rat subcutaneous model	Reduced cell infiltration Reduced EDI+ cells Reduced collagenase activity	van Putten et al. (2009)
Collagen	IL-10 pDNA polyplexes and MSCs	2 μg IL-10 pDNA	IL-10 secretion Metabolic activity	Rat intramuscular implantation model	Increased stem cell survival Increased ratio of regulatory to inflammatory macrophages	Holladay et al. (2011)
Collagen	IL-10 pDNA polyplexes and MSCs	2 μg IL-10 pDNA	n/a	Rat myocardial infarction model	Improved cardiac function and stem cell survival Increased ratio of regulatory to inflammatory macrophages Reduction in apoptosis	Holladay et al. (2012)
Silk-fibroin/ hyaluronic acid	n/a	n/a	n/a	Rat myocardial infarction model	Reduced CD68+ cells Improved wall thickness and fractional shortening Reduced apoptosis Increased vascular density, and VEGF, bFGF, and HGF expression	Chi et al. (2012)
Hyaluronic acid	MSCs	0.2–1 × 10^6	MSC proliferations VEGF expression	Porcine myocardial infarction model	Reduced CD3+ cells Reduced inflammatory score	Muscari et al. (2013)
Poly (L-lactide)	Ibuprofen	Not specified	Ibuprofen release prolife in neutral and acidic pH Fiber diameter	Rat muscle wound model	Improved muscle regeneration Reduced IL-6 and TNF-α and IL-6 (protein and gene expression) Increased VEGF and TGF-β (protein and gene expression)	Yuan et al. (2014)
Poly (L-lactic acid)	Tetrandrine	5–20 mg/g	Tetrandrine release Cell viability RAW 264.7 production of NO, TNF-α, and IL-6 on scaffold Reduction in gene expression of iNOS, TNF-α, IL-6, and Cox-II	Rat wound healing model	Reduction in inflammation in 20 mg/g tetrandrine group observed on H&E stained sections	Wang et al. (2014a,b)
Poly (lactide-co-Glycolide)	IL-10 viral vector	2 × 10^7 viral particles	Reduced RAW 264.7 production of TNF-α and increased IL-10 following LPS treatment	Implantation into intraperitoneal mouse fat pad	Reduced leukocyte infiltration Increased IL-10 expression and reduced IFN- expression	Gower et al. (2014)
Poly (lactic-co-Glycolic acid) film	FTY720	1:200 drug-to-polymer weight	Change in cytokine secretion of RAW 264.7 and HUVEC	Dorsal skinfold and muscle ischemia models	Increase in presence of anti-inflammatory macrophages Increased arteriole and length density	Awojoodu et al. (2013)

of the capsules and improved glycemic control in a chemically induced mouse type 1 diabetes model.

The anti-inflammatory drug resveratrol reduced inflammation in a cartilage defect model when delivered via a collagen hydrogel (Wang et al., 2014b). Resveratrol was grafted to poly (acrylic acid) and incorporated within a type I collagen hydrogel. Following delivery within a rabbit osteochondral defect model, treatment with resveratrol reduced inflammatory gene expression (IL-1β, MMP-13 and COX-2), with a resultant increase in bone and cartilage related genes (SOX-9, aggrecan, and collagen I and III). Gross

and histological examination revealed the formation of cartilage-like neotissue, which compared favorably with no treatment and a collagen hydrogel without resveratrol.

A gelatin hydrogel was loaded with an anti-inflammatory peptide (triptolide) and BMP-2 to increase bone regeneration (Ratanavaraporn et al., 2012). It was found that incorporation of the anti-inflammatory peptide reduced the infiltration of inflammatory cells, except at the highest dose (10 mg), which indicates the importance of dose-response studies. Expression of IL-6, TNF-α, and NF-kB mRNA was also reduced. Reduced infiltration of inflammatory cells resulted in an increase in bone formation and bone mineral density, when accompanied by BMP-2 delivery. This study highlights the possibility of combining anti-inflammatory therapies with complementary therapeutics for the treatment of complex pathologies. In this case, addition of an osteoinductive protein, BMP-2, was essential for the formation of bone, while reduced inflammation serves to enhance this function.

A peptide nanofiber gel was loaded with dexamethasone to modify the inflammatory response (Webber et al., 2012). *In vitro* studies revealed that delivery of the dexamethasone from the peptide nanofiber gel reduced NF-kB activation in LPS treated THP-1 monocytes. An *in vivo* subcutaneous study revealed that in comparison with an unloaded peptide nanofiber gel, dexamethasone loaded gels reduced the presence of ROS and inflammatory cells after 3 and 21 days.

A PEG-maleimide hydrogel was developed with on-demand protease sensitive release of IL-1RA, the naturally occurring antagonist to the IL-1R. This system was used as a coating to reduce inflammation associated with implantation of neural electrodes (Gutowski et al., 2015). Immunofluorescent staining of inflammatory cell infiltration showed no difference between samples, while RT-PCR analysis showed minimal differences, with increases in IL-6, MMP-13, and ciliary neurotrophic factor (CNTF) the only changes detected. However, the gene expression analysis does allow for the specific-targeting of genes to reduce the inflammatory response in future studies.

Hydrogels have been utilized for the delivery of a range of anti-inflammatory therapeutics (see **Table 2**). Hydrogels have proven particularly attractive as a matrix to assist cell transplantation. They provide an ideal substrate for cell encapsulation and protection from the host response. By engineering a suitable matrix to encourage cell adhesion and proliferation, along with the incorporation of an anti-inflammatory agent to be released in the microenvironment, the survival of implanted cells can be promoted.

Micro and Nanoparticles

Nanoparticles have been widely used to deliver anti-inflammatory therapies. Whitmire et al. fabricated a new block copolymer that assembles into sub-micron particles and contains a moiety for tethering proteins (Whitmire et al., 2012). To this moiety, IL-1RA was conjugated. These particles were injected into the intra-articular joint space, where it was shown that they significantly enhanced the retention time of IL-1RA. However, to further increase retention time, the authors hypothesized that increased particle size could prove beneficial. To achieve this, a new self-assembling polymer composed of a polyhydroxyethylmethacrylate (pHEMA) backbone with a functionalized hydrophobic side chain of pyridine was fabricated, which allowed for variation in particle sizes (Singh et al., 2014). Particles of size 500 and 900 nm were fabricated and a fibronectin targeting ligand attached. Retention of BSA-loaded particles in the intra-articular space in the rat stifle joint was assessed using fluorescence imaging. It was found that the 900 nm particles were retained in the joint to a greater extent that either the soluble protein or the 500 nm particles.

This emphasizes the importance of the design of appropriate and efficient systems to deliver therapeutics.

Polymer particles fabricated from poly (cyclohexane-1,4-diylacetone dimethylene ketal) (PCADK) were loaded with a p38 inhibitor to modulate the post-infarction inflammatory response in the myocardium (Sy et al., 2008). In an intramuscular model, the particles themselves were found to be non-inflammatory; while in an MI model, the particles significantly reduced superoxide and TNF-α production. This resulted in a reduction in fibrotic area as well as improved cardiac function. A similar study utilized the same particles to deliver superoxide dismutase (SOD) to the infarcted heart, which reduced superoxide expression and apoptosis (Seshadri et al., 2010). A subsequent improvement in cardiac function was also observed.

Encapsulating dexamethasone within PLGA particles reduced the *in vivo* inflammatory response to PLGA particles (Dang et al., 2011). It was found that encapsulation of dexamethasone within PLGA particles reduced both coverage of the PLGA particles with immune cells as well as cathepsin activity. Further investigation of the infiltration of inflammatory cells by examining histological sections revealed a reduction in the dexamethasone-loaded group compared with the unloaded control. Methylprednisolone (MP) was loaded within PLGA particles in an attempt to modify inflammation following injury of the spinal cord. The PLGA particles were suspended within an agarose gel to keep them in the local microenvironment of the injury (Chvatal et al., 2008). It was found that treatment with MP-loaded PLGA particles reduced the number of activated maicroglia, as well as the expression of the pro-inflammatory calpain and iNOS. This resulted in a reduction in lesion volume, indicating the potential of anti-inflammatory therapies in the spinal cord.

Delivery of siRNA targeting mitogen-activated protein kinase kinase kinase kinase 4 (MAP4K4) via β1,3-D-glucan particles suppressed systemic inflammation (Aouadi et al., 2009). Delivery of the siRNA orally resulted in a reduction in MAP4K4 gene expression in the lungs, liver, and spleen. In addition, when compared to a scrambled siRNA, MAP4K4 reduced the presence of LPS-induced TNF-α in both the serum and peritoneal fluid. The administration of MAP4K4 siRNA reduced LPS-induced lethality by inhibiting the expression of TNF-α and IL-1β. In a similar study using the same glucan particles, siRNA targeting TNF-α and osteopontin (OPN) was delivered systemically and localized to the macrophages present in the adipose tissue (Aouadi et al., 2013). It was found that silencing either TNF-α or OPN in the adipose tissue improved the glucose tolerance in ob/ob mice. Similarly, galactosylated trimethyl chitosanecysteine (GTC) nanoparticles were conjugated with MAP4K4 siRNA and delivered orally to treat ulcerative colitis (Zhang et al., 2013). It was found that this treatment reduced MAP4K4 and TNF-α mRNA, as well as TNF-α protein expression and MPO activity in the colon. Galactosylated particles showed increased efficacy compared with non-galactosylated nanoparticles, indicating the usefulness of targeting activated macrophages.

Utilization of PLGA particles to deliver PEI-conjugated Fc RIII-targeting siRNA to reduce inflammation proved efficacious in a rat model of temporomandibular joint (TMJ) inflammation (Mountziaris et al., 2012). Meal pattern analysis revealed

TABLE 2 | Examples of anti-inflammatory therapies delivered from hydrogels.

Biomaterial system	Therapeutic	Dose	*In vitro* characterization	*In vivo* model	*In vivo* outcome	Reference
PEG hydrogel (10,000 Mw)	IL-1R inhibitory peptide (IL-1RIP)	1% IL-1RIP	Cell viability and insulin secretion from MIN6 cells	n/a	n/a	Su et al. (2010)
Hyaluronic acid	Dexamethasone	$2.2-4.4 \times 10^{-5}$ M	Cell viability Hydrogel swelling ratio Dexamethasone release profile Reduced IL-6 and TNF-α production by RAW 264.7	Subcutaneous implantation model	Reduced infiltration of macrophages and neutrophils observed on H&E stained sections	Ito et al. (2007)
Hyaluronic acid	Anti TNF-α antibody	400 µg/ml	Binding affinity	Rat burn models	Reduced inflammatory cell infiltration observed on H&E stained sections Reduced non-viable tissue Reduced IL-1β protein expression	Friedrich et al. (2014)
Chitosan hydrogel	ADSCs	4×10^6 ADSCs	Cell adhesion and expression of adhesion genes in response to ROS	Rat myocardial infarction model	Increased ICAM-1, VCAM-1, and SDF-1 expression and ADSC retention Reduction in ROS, apoptosis, and infarct size Increased wall thickness and blood vessel density, improved cardiac function	Liu et al. (2012)
Chitosan hydrogel	ADSCs	2×10^6 ADSCs	n/a	Rat acute renal ischemia-reperfusion model	Reduction in apoptosis and ROS expression Increased stem cell retention and renal cell proliferation Reduction in serum levels of creatinine and blood urea nitrogen	Gao et al. (2012)
Alginate microcapsules containing islet cells	Curcumin	1 mg/ml	n/a	STZ-induced diabetic mouse model	Improved blood glucose level Reduced gene expression of CD68, CD19, CD74, CD8, TNF-α, TGF-β, and αSMA	Dang et al. (2013)
Collagen hydrogel	Resveratrol	0.5%	Compressive strength free radical scavenging Collagen degradation Cell viability	Rabbit osteochondral defect	Reduction in IL-1β, MMP-13, and Cox-II mRNA Increased SOX-9, aggrecan, collagen I and III mRNA Improved neotissue formation and integration Increased collagen II deposition	Wang et al. (2014a,b)
Gelatin	Triptolide [and BMP-2]	2.5, 5, or 10 mg	Release profile Relationship between degradation and release profile Reduction in IL-6 and IL-10 protein expression in J774.1 macrophage-like cells Proliferation and ALP activity in MC3T3-E1 cells	Rat critical-sized bone defect	Reduced lymphocytes, netrophils, and mast cells Reduced mRNA expression of IL-6, IL-10, TNF-α, NF-kB, and MMP-14 Increased bone mineral density	Ratanavaraporn et al. (2012)
Peptide amphiphile	Dexamethasone	Not specified	Dexamethasone release Reduced NF-kB activity in THP-1 cells following LPS activation Cell viability following treatment with Dex-PA	Mouse subcutaneous model	Reduced ROS formation Reduced inflammatory cell infiltration observed on H&E stained sections	Webber et al. (2012)
Poly (ethylene glycol)-maleimide (Coating on a neural electrode)	IL-1RA	150 pg	Coating thickness Cell adhesion Reduced expression of IL-1β and TNF-α in microglia/astrocytes treated with GMCSF IL-1RA release profile	Rat neural implantation model	Increased IL-6, MMP-2, and CNTF	Gutowski et al. (2015)

an improvement following Fc RIII siRNA treatment, while a reduction was observed in the levels of two key pro-inflammatory cytokines, IL-1β and IL-6. Similarly, PLGA particles were used to delivery anti-TNF-α siRNA to treat inflammation associated with rheumatoid arthritis (RA) (Présumey et al., 2012). *In vitro* studies revealed that delivery of anti-TNF-α siRNA via PLGA particles could reduce LPS-induced TNF-α production in mouse monocytic J774 cells. Translation to an *in vivo* model of RA resulted in a reduction in TNF-α production and inflammation in the joint. Loading of PLGA particles with COX-2 siRNA and dexamethasone has also been proposed as a means by which to modify RA associated inflammation (Park et al., 2012). PLGA particles were loaded with dexamethasone, and then these drug-loaded particles had PEI/siRNA complexes attached to them. Pretreatment of C28/I2 cells with TNF-α and IL-1β *in vitro* resulted in increased expression of COX-2 and iNOS. However, treatment with PLGA particles combined with dexamethasone and COX-2 siRNA reduced this induced expression. Interestingly, it was observed that dexamethasone had a minimal effect on inflammatory gene expression unless it was delivered via PLGA particles. This emphasizes the importance of the mode of delivery of an anti-inflammatory therapy, and suggests biomaterial systems as reservoirs of such therapeutics.

An annexin-A1 mimetic-peptide (Ac2-26) showed increased efficacy, when loaded within nanoparticles. Nanoparticles were fabricated from a biodegradable PLGA-b-PEG polymer using a nanoprecipitation method, with a collagen IV-targeting conjugate (Kamaly et al., 2013). These targeting nanoparticles loaded with Ac2-26 showed an increased ability to reduce the number of macrophages in an *in vivo* murine peritonitis model compared with non-targeting particles, srambled peptide-loaded particles, and also non-loaded particles. In an *in vivo* model of ischemia, targeted particles again compared favorably with scrambled-peptide loaded targeting particles and also non-targeting peptide loaded particles, with a reduction observed in myeloperoxidase activity. A similar formulation, but without the collagen IV-targeting conjugate, was used to form nanoparticles and deliver an anti-inflammatory synthetic liver X receptor agonist (GW3965) (Gadde et al., 2014). In peritoneal macrophages *in vitro*, it was shown that treatment with GW3965 in nanoparticle form reduced expression of monocyte chemoattractant protein 1 (MCP-1) and TNF-α. In an *in vivo* model of peritonitis, a reduction was observed in macrophage numbers, and MCP-1 and TNF-α gene and protein expression at a similar level to dexamethasone treatment.

A lipid nanoparticle was used to deliver a therapeutic siRNA that reduced the accumulation of pro-inflammatory monocytes to inflamed tissue (Leuschner et al., 2011). An siRNA targeting the chemokine receptor CCR2 was administered systemically, and shown to reduce the infarct size in an MI model, reduce inflammatory cells in atherosclerotic lesion, improve the survival of pancreatic islet allografts, and reduce tumor volume. This emphasizes the power of siRNA as a therapeutic modality capable of controlling cell phenotype, in this case pro-inflammatory macrophages.

Urethane acrylate non-ionomer (UAN) nanoparticles were functionalized with a targeting moiety to increase localization to tumors (Park et al., 2013). By conjugating an ICAM-1 targeting ligand to nanoparticles, localization to tumors and inflamed tissue was increased. UAN nanoparticles loaded with paclitaxel reduced the tumor volume compared without a targeting ligand. This shows the potential to target inflammation with nanoparticles and a targeting moiety. This system could be adapted to load various therapeutics, and also conjugated with different ligands for targeting of specific sights.

PLGA and chitosan were used to form bilayered nanoparticles for the delivery of two anti-inflammatory drugs, spantide II (SP) and ketoprofen (KP) (Shah et al., 2012). These nanoparticles were combined with a skin-permeating nanogel, and used in two models of allergic contact dermatitis (ACD) and psoriatic plaque. Ear thickness was reduced in the ACD model, while trans-epidermal water loss was reduced in the psoriatic model, the two primary endpoints in both models, indicating the power of anti-inflammatory delivery via nanoparticles.

Particulate systems, whether in the micro or nano range, are versatile delivery systems capable of delivering drugs, proteins, and nucleic acids, or combinations thereof (see **Table 3**). However, issues with retention at the inflamed site persist, amplified by the fact that activated macrophages clear particles in a size and shape-dependent manner (Champion and Mitragotri, 2006). Thus, choice of particle size/shape is imperative, as well as other strategies to avoid uptake and clearance. These may include tethering of "self" peptides to particles (Rodriguez et al., 2013), or combination with solid or hydrogel scaffolds to increase bulk retention in the target tissue.

Future Directions

Modulation of inflammation is a key component for the success of biomaterial and tissue engineering based strategies. This is the case both in terms of modulating the FBR to ensure the survival and functionality of implanted devices and also in delivering anti-inflammatory therapeutics to sites of pathological inflammation. Thus, strategies to improve the efficacy of anti-inflammatory therapies are vital.

The inflammatory response is often quantified in terms of the number of macrophages present, the phenotype of these macrophages, or both. Thus, the macrophage is and has been identified as a key component of inflammation (Wynn and Barron, 2010; Koh and DiPietro, 2011) and the FBR to biomaterials (Xia and Triffitt, 2006; Brown et al., 2012). Furthermore, where along the spectrum of macrophage activity, these macropahages are a key determinant in whether inflammation will become resolved in a satisfactory manner (Mosser and Edwards, 2009). Thus, control over macrophage can be key to modulating inflammation and resolving it. Cytokines such as IL-4, IL-10, and IL-13 (see **Figure 2**) have been identified as playing a role in shifting the balance from a pro-inflammatory macrophage to that of a macrophage more anti-inflammatory in nature, promoting tissue repair and remodeling (Mantovani et al., 2013). A number of biomaterial systems have been developed to deliver pDNA to macrophages (Helary et al., 2012; Mahor et al., 2012). Thus, specific delivery of molecules to direct macrophages toward an anti-inflammatory phenotype rather than a pro-inflammatory phenotype holds promise as a treatment for inflammation.

TABLE 3 | Micro and nanoparticles used to deliver anti-inflammatory therapies.

Biomaterial system	Therapeutic	Dose	*In vitro* characterization	*In vivo* model	*In vivo* outcome	Reference
Tetraethylene glycol and cyclohexyl methacrylate nanoparticles	IL-1RA	5 µg IL-1RA	Nanoparticle size Target specificity NF-κβ activity in NIH3T3 fibroblasts	Rat intra-articular model	Increased retention of IL-1RA compared with saline delivery	Whitmire et al. (2012)
Poly (hydroxy-ethyl-methacrylate) [p(HEMA)]	(BSA as a model protein)	500 µg Vivo-Tag-S750-BSA	Particle size Cell viability	Rat intra-articular injection	Increased retention compared with soluble protein	Singh et al. (2014)
Poly (cyclohexane-1,4-diylacetone dimethylene ketal) (PCADK)	P38 inhibitor	50 µg P38 inhibitor	Particle size Activation of RAW 264.7 macrophages	Rat myocardial infarction model	Reduced P38 activation, superoxide, and TNF-α production Reduced fibrotic area and improved cardiac function	Sy et al. (2008)
Poly (cyclohexane-1,4-diylacetone dimethylene ketal) (PCADK)	Superoxide dismutase (SOD)	80U SOD	Particle size Superoxide scavenging	Rat myocardial infarction model	Reduced superoxide production and apoptosis Improved cardiac function	Seshadri et al. (2010)
PLGA	Dexamethasone	1.3 and 26 wt%	Dexamthasone loading and release	Mouse subcutaneous injection	Reduced cathepsin activity up to 10 days Reduced inflammatory cell infiltration up to 30 days	Dang et al. (2011)
PLGA	Methylprednisolone	156 µg	Methylprednisolone release NO production by LPS-treated microglia	Rat spinal cord contusion model	Reduced ED1+ cells Reduced Calplain and iNOS Reduced lesion volume	Chvatal et al. (2008)
β1,3-d-glucan	MAP4K4 siRNA	20 µg/kg body weight	MAP4K4 and TNF-α knockdown	Mouse LPS-induced lethality	Reduced MAP4K4 mRNA in peritoneal macrophages, spleen, liver, and lung Reduced TNF-α and IL-1β mRNA Reduced serum and peritoneal TNF-α	Aouadi et al. (2009)
Galactosylated Trimethyl Chitosanecysteine	MAP4K4 siRNA	250 µg/kg body weight/day	Charge and cell uptake MAP4K4 and TNF-α mRNA knockdown Reduced TNF-α protein expression	Mouse ulcerative colitis	MAP4K4 and TNF-α mRNA knockdown Reduced colonic TNF-α protein and MPO activity Reduced infiltration of mononucleur cells observed on H&E sections	Zhang et al. (2013)
PLGA	Fc RIII-targeting siRNA	≈16–23 µg	siRNA release siRNA loading efficiency	Rat temporo-mandibular inflammation	Reduced IL-1β and IL-6 protein expression Reduced Fc RIII expression	Mountziaris et al. (2012)
PLGA	TNF-α siRNA	0.12 nM	Particle size siRNA release Reduced TNF-α mRNA and protein expression	Mouse collagen induced arthritis	Reduced synovial inflammatory score Reduced TNF-α protein expression	Présumey et al. (2012)
PLGA	Dexamethasone and COX-2 siRNA	n/a	Dexamethasone and siRNA loading Particle size, charge, cell viability, uptake, and transfection efficiency PGE$_2$ secretion COX-2 and iNOS knockdown in C28-I2 Reduced mPGES-1, COX-2, and iNOS protein expression Reduced caspase-3	n/a	n/a	Park et al. (2012)
PLGA-b-PEG	Ac2-26 (annexin-A1 mimetic peptide)	100 ng	Particle size Ac2-26 release	Murine peritonitis Muscle ischemia	Reduced number of PMNs Reduced MPO activity	Kamaly et al. (2013)

(Continued)

TABLE 3 | Continued

Biomaterial system	Therapeutic	Dose	*In vitro* characterization	*In vivo* model	*In vivo* outcome	Reference
PLGA-b-PEG	GW3965 (liver X receptor agonist)	8 mg/kg	Particle size GW3965 release profile Reduced TNF-α and MCP-1 gene and protein expression in peritoneal macrophages	Mouse zymosan-induced Peritonitis	Reduced PMN infiltration Reduced TNF-α and MCP-1 gene and protein expression in peritoneal exudates	Gadde et al. (2014)
C12-200 lipid, dis-teroylphosphatidyl choline, cholesterol, and PEG-DMG	CCR2 siRNA	1 mg/kg	n/a	Mouse ischemia/ reperfusion	Reduced CCR2 expression	Leuschner et al. (2011)
				Mouse permanent ligation	Reduced myocardial area-at-risk	
				Mouse streptozotocin-induced diabetes	Reduced Ly-6C^{high} macrophages, CD11b+ cells, and lesion volume in atheresclerotic plaque	
				Mouse islet transplantation	Increased survival of pancreatic islet allografts	
				Mouse tumor xenograft model	Reduced tumor volume, tumor associated macrophages, and CD11b+ cells	
Urethane acrylate non-ionomer (UAN)	Paclitaxel	200 µg UAN-Paclitaxel nanoparti-cles	Viability and dose response	Mouse tumor cytotoxicity assay	Reduced tumor volume	Park et al. (2013)
PLGA and chitosan	Spantide II and ketoprofen	Not specified	Particle loading efficiency Spantide II and ketoprofen release profile	Mouse allergic contact dermatitis	Increased drug retention Reduced ear Reduced IL-17 and IL-23 expression Reduced trans-epidermal water loss	Shah et al. (2012)

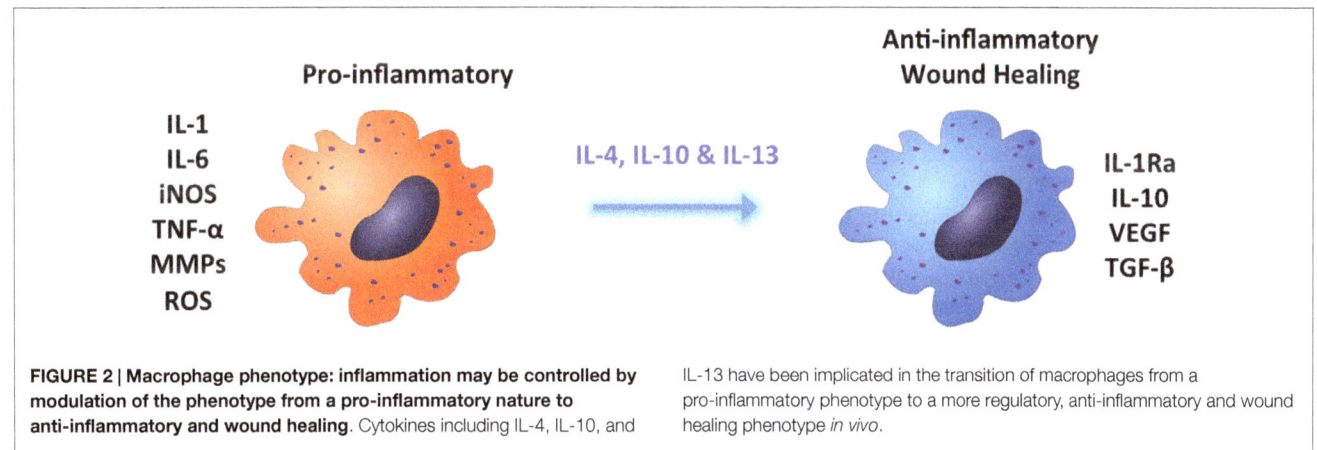

FIGURE 2 | Macrophage phenotype: inflammation may be controlled by modulation of the phenotype from a pro-inflammatory nature to anti-inflammatory and wound healing. Cytokines including IL-4, IL-10, and IL-13 have been implicated in the transition of macrophages from a pro-inflammatory phenotype to a more regulatory, anti-inflammatory and wound healing phenotype *in vivo*.

A number of natural biomaterials have intrinsic anti-inflammatory properties, including HA and chitosan. Thus, they are suitable as carriers for anti-inflammatory therapeutics. However, synthetic materials are also capable of acting in an anti-inflammatory way. Dead and dying cells release their contents, including nucleic acids, both RNA and DNA. These nucleic acids act as DAMPs and activate toll like receptors (TLRs), stimulating an inflammatory response. It was found that binding of nucleic acids produced by injury by cationic polymers reduces associated inflammation, both *in vitro* and *in vivo* (Lee et al.,

2011). This ability to act as a molecular scavenger for nucleic acids could be adapted for other molecules, with a biomaterial acting as a "sponge" to scavenge and absorb pro-inflammatory cytokines in an inflamed environment. However, a more specific approach, possibly involving conjugation of pro-inflammatory targeting antibodies, would be necessary to avoid the uptake of all cytokines and growth factors. In a similar way, materials may be protected from an inflammatory response by the conjugation of immunomodulatory "self" proteins. Attachment of CD200 protein to a biomaterial surface reduced the production of TNF-α and IL-6 *in vitro* in response to LPS and IFN- stimulation, by activating pathways that inhibit inflammation (Kim et al., 2014). This anti-inflammatory nature was confirmed *in vivo* using bioluminescence imaging to detect ROS activity. In comparison with unmodified materials, the CD200 modified material displayed a drastically reduced tissue response. Strategies such as this may reduce inflammation in the context of implantable devices, but may also be used as a means by which to reduce inflammation locally in a pathological condition.

Nanoparticles can be used to deliver multiple therapeutics. Codelivery of IL-10 siRNA and a pDNA vaccine using PLGA-PEI nanoparticles were used to modify the Th1 to Th2 balance during immunotherapy (Singh et al., 2008). Similarly, lipid-like nanoparticles were used to simultaneously deliver both pDNA and siRNA (Dong et al., 2014). *In vivo* studies showed the potential to upregulate luciferase activity and reduce Tie-2 expression using a luciferase pDNA, and a Tie-2 targeting siRNA. Selection of different nucleic acids creates an opportunity to upregulate an anti-inflammatory mediator while knocking down a pro-inflammatory mediator concurrently. This may prove key as inflammation is a complex phenomenon that requires multiple points of control.

Responsive systems are a well-utilized facet of biomaterial design. In order to design biodegradable systems, crosslinkers with MMP-cleavable sequences are incorporated into typically non-degradable sequences. In this way, MMP sensitivity is built into the system. Therapeutics may also be conjugated to biomaterials using sensitive linker systems. That is, the therapeutic will be released in response to a pre-determined stimulus. For example, previously therapeutics have been conjugated to a fibrin scaffold such that they would only be released by MMP activity, resulting in improved efficacy (Zisch et al., 2003; Ehrbar et al., 2004). ROS sensitivity has been identified as a key mediator for the release of therapeutics (Yoshitomi and Nagasaki, 2014). Nanoparticles composed of β-cyclodextrin were engineered with ROS sensitivity, and tested *in vitro* and *in vivo*. ROS responsive-release of docetaxal from nanoparticles *in vivo* was assessed as a means by which to reduce tumor volume (Zhang et al., 2015).

As stated, inflammation is a key determinant in the FBR and how it progresses. In addition, in plays a key role in the progression of a number of pathological conditions in which it is dysregulated. However, in most cases, dysregulation of and excessive inflammation is not the only process involved. For instance, in the case of diabetic wound healing, inflammation is excessive, but there are also issues with insufficient angiogenesis as well as ECM turnover. Thus, approaches that aim to reduce inflammation and also modulate other processes are needed. Biomaterial systems can be designed to load and release multiple, complementary therapeutics (Browne and Pandit, 2014). A multi-modal system composed of fibrin microspheres in a fibrin hydrogel was used to modify inflammation and angiogenesis, through the delivery of two pDNAs encoding Rab18 and endothelial nitric oxide synthase (eNOS) (Kulkarni et al., 2014). This improved healing in a diabetic rabbit wound model. A similar system composed of collagen spheres-in-hydrogel was used to deliver IL-10 and eNOS pDNA in a staggered manner *in vitro* (Alexander et al., 2013), while *in vivo* assessment of dual delivery of anti-inflammatory and pro-angiogenic peptides showed a combinatorial effect (Zachman et al., 2012).

Outlook

Control over inflammation is vital for the success of biomaterial and tissue engineered therapies. Modification of inflammation is key to reducing the impact of the FBR. In addition, biomaterials also offer the opportunity to control inflammation in pathological conditions, through increased localization and retention of therapies in the inflamed microenvironment. The form of biomaterial used (solid scaffold, hydrogel, or micro/nanoparticle) is dependent on the target site, with considerations such as ease of access and retention paramount. In addition, the choice of anti-inflammatory therapeutics is typically dependent on the cause of inflammation.

Future therapeutics will focus on control of macrophage phenotype, the use of anti-inflammatory materials, complementary combinations of anti-inflammatory therapeutics, and biomaterial systems that release anti-inflammatory therapeutics in response to inflammatory stimuli, such as ROS and MMPs.

Acknowledgments

The authors would like to acknowledge financial support from Science Foundation Ireland (Grant nos. 07/SRC/B1163, 13/RC/2073). The authors would like to thank Mr. Maciej Doczyk for assistance with graphics and Mr. Anthony Sloan for editorial assistance.

References

Alexander, J. C., Browne, S., Pandit, A., and Rochev, Y. (2013). Biomaterial constructs for delivery of multiple therapeutic genes: a spatiotemporal evaluation of efficacy using molecular beacons. *PLoS ONE* 8:e65749. doi:10.1371/journal.pone.0065749

Anderson, J. M., Rodriguez, A., and Chang, D. T. (2008). Foreign body reaction to biomaterials. *Semin. Immunol.* 20, 86–100. doi:10.1016/j.smim.2007.11.004

Aouadi, M., Tencerova, M., Vangala, P., Yawe, J. C., Nicoloro, S. M., Amano, S. U., et al. (2013). Gene silencing in adipose tissue macrophages regulates whole-body metabolism in obese mice. *Proc. Natl. Acad. Sci. U.S.A.* 110, 8278–8283. doi:10.1073/pnas.1300492110

Aouadi, M., Tesz, G. J., Nicoloro, S. M., Wang, M., Chouinard, M., Soto, E., et al. (2009). Orally delivered siRNA targeting macrophage Map4k4 suppresses systemic inflammation. *Nature* 458, 1180–1184. doi:10.1038/nature07774

Awojoodu, A. O., Ogle, M. E., Sefcik, L. S., Bowers, D. T., Martin, K., Brayman, K. L., et al. (2013). Sphingosine 1-phosphate receptor 3 regulates recruitment of anti-inflammatory monocytes to microvessels during implant arteriogenesis. *Proc. Natl. Acad. Sci. U.S.A.* 110, 13785–13790. doi:10.1073/pnas.1221309110

Boehler, R. M., Kuo, R., Shin, S., Goodman, A. G., Pilecki, M. A., Leonard, J. N., et al. (2014). Lentivirus delivery of IL-10 to promote and sustain macrophage polarization towards an anti-inflammatory phenotype. *Biotechnol. Bioeng.* 111, 1210–1221. doi:10.1002/bit.25175

Brown, B. N., Londono, R., Tottey, S., Zhang, L., Kukla, K. A., Wolf, M. T., et al. (2012). Macrophage phenotype as a predictor of constructive remodeling following the implantation of biologically derived surgical mesh materials. *Acta Biomater.* 8, 978–987. doi:10.1016/j.actbio.2011.11.031

Browne, S., Fontana, G., Rodriguez, B. J., and Pandit, A. (2012). A protective extracellular matrix-based gene delivery reservoir fabricated by electrostatic charge manipulation. *Mol. Pharm.* 9, 3099–3106. doi:10.1021/mp300231d

Browne, S., and Pandit, A. (2014). Multi-modal delivery of therapeutics using biomaterial scaffolds. *J. Mater. Chem. B Mater. Biol. Med.* 2, 6692–6707. doi:10. 1039/C4TB00863D

Browne, S., Zeugolis, D. I., and Pandit, A. (2013). Collagen: finding a solution for the source. *Tissue Eng. Part A* 19, 1491–1494. doi:10.1089/ten.TEA.2012.0721

Censi, R., Di Martino, P., Vermonden, T., and Hennink, W. E. (2012). Hydrogels for protein delivery in tissue engineering. *J. Control Release* 161, 680–692. doi:10. 1016/j.jconrel.2012.03.002

Ceradini, D. J., and Gurtner, G. C. (2005). Homing to hypoxia: HIF-1 as a mediator of progenitor cell recruitment to injured tissue. *Trends Cardiovasc. Med.* 15, 57–63. doi:10.1016/j.tcm.2005.02.002

Ceradini, D. J., Kulkarni, A. R., Callaghan, M. J., Tepper, O. M., Bastidas, N., Kleinman, M. E., et al. (2004). Progenitor cell trafficking is regulated by hypoxic gradients through HIF-1 induction of SDF-1. *Nat. Med.* 10, 858–864. doi:10. 1038/nm1075

Champion, J. A., and Mitragotri, S. (2006). Role of target geometry in phagocytosis. *Proc. Natl. Acad. Sci. U.S.A.* 103, 9430–9434. doi:10.1073/pnas.0600997103

Chang, J., Liu, F., Lee, M., Wu, B., Ting, K., Zara, J. N., et al. (2013). NF- B inhibits osteogenic differentiation of mesenchymal stem cells by promoting β-catenin degradation. *Proc. Natl. Acad. Sci. U.S.A.* 110, 9469–9474. doi:10.1073/pnas. 1300532110

Chen, G. Y., and Nunez, G. (2010). Sterile inflammation: sensing and reacting to damage. *Nat. Rev. Immun.* 10, 826–837. doi:10.1038/nri2873

Chi, N. H., Yang, M. C., Chung, T. W., Chen, J.-Y., Chou, N. K., and Wang, S. S. (2012). Cardiac repair achieved by bone marrow mesenchymal stem cells/silk fibroin/hyaluronic acid patches in a rat of myocardial infarction model. *Biomaterials* 33, 5541–5551. doi:10.1016/j.biomaterials.2012.04.030

Chirkov, S. N. (2002). The antiviral activity of chitosan. *Appl. Biochem. Microbiol.* 38, 5–13. doi:10.1023/A:1013206517442

Chvatal, S. A., Kim, Y. T., Bratt-Leal, A. M., Lee, H., and Bellamkonda, R. V. (2008). Spatial distribution and acute anti-inflammatory effects of methylprednisolone after sustained local delivery to the contused spinal cord. *Biomaterials* 29, 1967–1975. doi:10.1016/j.biomaterials.2008.01.002

Dang, T. T., Bratlie, K. M., Bogatyrev, S. R., Chen, X. Y., Langer, R., and Anderson, D. G. (2011). Spatiotemporal effects of a controlled-release anti-inflammatory drug on the cellular dynamics of host response. *Biomaterials* 32, 4464–4470. doi:10.1016/j.biomaterials.2011.02.048

Dang, T. T., Thai, A. V., Cohen, J., Slosberg, J. E., Siniakowicz, K., Doloff, J. C., et al. (2013). Enhanced function of immuno-isolated islets in diabetes therapy by co-encapsulation with an anti-inflammatory drug. *Biomaterials* 34, 5792–5801. doi:10.1016/j.biomaterials.2013.04.016

Dobaczewski, M., and Frangogiannis, N. G. (2008). Chemokines and cardiac fibrosis. *Front. Biosci. (Schol Ed)* 22:391–405. doi:10.1016/j.bbi.2008.05.010

Dong, Y., Eltoukhy, A. A., Alabi, C. A., Khan, O. F., Veiseh, O., Dorkin, J. R., et al. (2014). Lipid-like nanomaterials for simultaneous gene expression and silencing in vivo. *Adv. Healthc. Mater.* 3, 1392–1397. doi:10.1002/adhm.201400054

Ehrbar, M., Djonov, V. G., Schnell, C., Tschanz, S. A., Martiny-Baron, G., Schenk, U., et al. (2004). Cell-demanded liberation of VEGF$_{121}$ from fibrin implants induces local and controlled blood vessel growth. *Circ. Res.* 94, 1124–1132. doi:10.1161/01.RES.0000126411.29641.08

Friedrich, E. E., Sun, L. T., Natesan, S., Zamora, D. O., Christy, R. J., and Washburn, N. R. (2014). Effects of hyaluronic acid conjugation on anti-TNF-α inhibition of inflammation in burns. *J. Biomed. Mater. Res. A* 102, 1527–1536. doi:10.1002/ jbm.a.34829

Gadde, S., Even-Or, O., Kamaly, N., Hasija, A., Gagnon, P. G., Adusumilli, K. H., et al. (2014). Development of therapeutic polymeric nanoparticles for the resolution of inflammation. *Adv. Healthc. Mater.* 3, 1448–1456. doi:10.1002/ adhm.201300688

Gao, J., Liu, R., Wu, J., Liu, Z., Li, J., Zhou, J., et al. (2012). The use of chitosan based hydrogel for enhancing the therapeutic benefits of adipose-derived MSCs for acute kidney injury. *Biomaterials* 33, 3673–3681. doi:10.1016/j.biomaterials. 2012.01.061

Gower, R. M., Boehler, R. M., Azarin, S. M., Ricci, C. F., Leonard, J. N., and Shea, L. D. (2014). Modulation of leukocyte infiltration and phenotype in microporous tissue engineering scaffolds via vector induced IL-10 expression. *Biomaterials* 35, 2024–2031. doi:10.1016/j.biomaterials.2013.11.036

Gutowski, S. M., Shoemaker, J. T., Templeman, K. L., Wei, Y., Latour, R. A., Bellamkonda, R. V., et al. (2015). Protease-degradable PEG-maleimide coating with

on-demand release of IL-1Ra to improve tissue response to neural electrodes. *Biomaterials* 44, 55–70. doi:10.1016/j.biomaterials.2014.12.009

Helary, C., Browne, S., Mathew, A., Wang, W., and Pandit, A. (2012). Transfection of macrophages by collagen hollow spheres loaded with polyplexes: a step towards modulating inflammation. *Acta Biomater.* 8, 4208–4214. doi:10.1016/j.actbio. 2012.06.017

Herdrich, B. J., Danzer, E., Davey, M. G., Allukian, M., Englefield, V., Gorman, J. H., et al. (2010). Regenerative healing following foetal myocardial infarction. *Eur. J. Cardiothorac. Surg.* 38, 691–698. doi:10.1016/j.ejcts.2010.03.049

Hirabara, S., Kojima, T., Takahashi, N., Hanabayashi, M., and Ishiguro, N. (2013). Hyaluronan inhibits TLR-4 dependent cathepsin K and matrix metalloproteinase 1 expression in human fibroblasts. *Biochem. Biophys. Res. Commun.* 430, 519–522. doi:10.1016/j.bbrc.2012.12.003

Holladay, C., Power, K., Sefton, M., O'Brien, T., Gallagher, W. M., and Pandit, A. (2011). Functionalized scaffold-mediated interleukin 10 gene delivery significantly improves survival rates of stem cells in vivo. *Mol. Ther.* 19, 969–978. doi:10.1038/mt.2010.311

Holladay, C. A., Duffy, A. M., Chen, X., Sefton, M. V., O'Brien, T. D., and Pandit, A. S. (2012). Recovery of cardiac function mediated by MSC and interleukin-10 plasmid functionalised scaffold. *Biomaterials* 33, 1303–1314. doi:10.1016/j. biomaterials.2011.10.019

Hortensius, R. A., Becraft, J. R., Pack, D. W., and Harley, B. A. C. (2015). The effect of glycosaminoglycan content on polyethylenimine-based gene delivery within three-dimensional collagen-GAG scaffolds. *Biomater. Sci.* 3, 645–654. doi:10.1039/c5bm00033e

Ito, T., Fraser, I. P., Yeo, Y., Highley, C. B., Bellas, E., and Kohane, D. S. (2007). Anti-inflammatory function of an in situ cross-linkable conjugate hydrogel of hyaluronic acid and dexamethasone. *Biomaterials* 28, 1778–1786. doi:10.1016/j. biomaterials.2006.12.012

Jayakumar, R., Menon, D., Manzoor, K., Nair, S. V., and Tamura, H. (2010). Biomedical applications of chitin and chitosan based nanomaterials – a short review. *Carbohydr. Polym.* 82, 227–232. doi:10.1016/j.carbpol.2010.04.074

Jayakumar, R., Nwe, N., Tokura, S., and Tamura, H. (2007). Sulfated chitin and chitosan as novel biomaterials. *Int. J. Biol. Macromol.* 40, 175–181. doi:10.1016/ j.ijbiomac.2006.06.021

Je, J. Y., and Kim, S. K. (2006). Reactive oxygen species scavenging activity of aminoderivatized chitosan with different degree of deacetylation. *Bioorg. Med. Chem.* 14, 5989–5994. doi:10.1016/j.bmc.2006.05.016

Jiang, B., and Liao, R. (2010). The paradoxical role of inflammation in cardiac repair and regeneration. *J. Cardiovasc. Transl. Res.* 3, 410–416. doi:10.1007/ s12265-010-9193-7

Kajahn, J., Franz, S., Rueckert, E., Forstreuter, I., Hintze, V., Moeller, S., et al. (2012). Artificial extracellular matrices composed of collagen I and high sulfated hyaluronan modulate monocyte to macrophage differentiation under conditions of sterile inflammation. *Biomatter* 2, 226–236. doi:10.4161/biom.22855

Kamaly, N., Fredman, G., Subramanian, M., Gadde, S., Pesic, A., and Cheung, L. (2013). Development and in vivo efficacy of targeted polymeric inflammation-resolving nanoparticles. *Proc. Natl. Acad. Sci. U.S.A.* 110, 6506–6511. doi:10. 1073/pnas.1303377110

Kataoka, H., Kono, H., Patel, Z., and Rock, K. L. (2014). Evaluation of the contribution of multiple DAMPs and DAMP receptors in cell death-induced sterile inflammatory responses. *PLoS ONE* 9:e104741. doi:10.1371/journal.pone. 0104741

Khor, E., and Lim, L. Y. (2003). Implantable applications of chitin and chitosan. *Biomaterials* 24, 2339–2349. doi:10.1016/S0142-9612(03)00026-7

Kim, Y. H., Furuya, H., and Tabata, Y. (2013). Enhancement of bone regeneration by dual release of a macrophage recruitment agent and platelet-rich plasma from gelatin hydrogels. *Biomaterials* 35, 214–224. doi:10.1016/j.biomaterials. 2013.09.103

Kim, Y. K., Que, R., Wang, S. W., and Liu, W. F. (2014). Modification of biomaterials with a self-protein inhibits the macrophage response. *Adv. Healthc. Mater.* 3, 989–994. doi:10.1002/adhm.201300532

Koh, T. J., and DiPietro, L. A. (2011). Inflammation and wound healing: the role of the macrophage. *Expert Rev. Mol. Med.* 13, 1–12. doi:10.1017/ S1462399411001943

Kraskiewicz, H., Breen, B., Sargeant, T., Mcmahon, S., and Pandit, A. (2013). Assembly of protein-based hollow spheres encapsulating a therapeutic factor. *ACS Chem. Neurosci.* 4, 1297–1304. doi:10.1021/cn400080h

Kulkarni, M., Loughlin, A. O., Vazquez, R., Mashayekhi, K., Rooney, P., Greiser, U., et al. (2014). Use of a fibrin-based system for enhancing angiogenesis and modulating inflammation in the treatment of hyperglycemic wounds. *Biomaterials* 35, 2001–2010. doi:10.1016/j.biomaterials.2013.11.003

Lee, J., Sohn, J. W., Zhang, Y., Leong, K. W., Pisetsky, D., and Sullenger, B. A. (2011). Nucleic acid-binding polymers as anti-inflammatory agents. *Proc. Natl. Acad. Sci. U.S.A.* 108, 14055–14060. doi:10.1073/pnas.1105777108

Leuschner, F., Dutta, P., Gorbatov, R., Novobrantseva, T. I., Donahoe, J. S., Courties, G., et al. (2011). Therapeutic siRNA silencing in inflammatory monocytes in mice. *Nat. Biotechnol.* 29, 1005–1010. doi:10.1038/nbt.1989

Li, J., Chen, J., and Kirsner, R. (2007). Pathophysiology of acute wound healing. *Clin. Dermatol.* 25, 9–18. doi:10.1016/j.clindermatol.2006.09.007

Liu, Y., Wang, L., Kikuiri, T., Akiyama, K., Chen, C., Xu, X., et al. (2011). Mesenchymal stem cell–based tissue regeneration is governed by recipient T lymphocytes via IFN- and TNF-α. *Nat. Med.* 17, 1594–1602. doi:10.1038/nm.2542

Liu, Z., Wang, H., Wang, Y., Lin, Q., Yao, A., Cao, F., et al. (2012). The influence of chitosan hydrogel on stem cell engraftment, survival and homing in the ischemic myocardial microenvironment. *Biomaterials* 33, 3093–3106. doi:10.1016/j.biomaterials.2011.12.044

Lo, D. D., Zimmermann, A. S., Nauta, A., Longaker, M. T., and Lorenz, H. P. (2012). Scarless fetal skin wound healing update. *Birth Defects Res. C Embryo Today* 96, 237–247. doi:10.1002/bdrc.21018

Luttikhuizen, D. T., van Amerongen, M. J., de Feijter, P. C., Petersen, A. H., Harmsen, M. C., and van Luyn, M. J. A. (2006a). The correlation between difference in foreign body reaction between implant locations and cytokine and MMP expression. *Biomaterials* 27, 5763–5770. doi:10.1016/j.biomaterials.2006.07.004

Luttikhuizen, D. T., Harmsen, M. C., and Van Luyn, M. J. A. (2006b). Cellular and molecular dynamics in the foreign body reaction. *Tissue Eng.* 12, 1955–1971. doi:10.1243/EMED_JOUR_1983_012_027_02

Mahor, S., Dash, B. C., O'Connor, S., and Pandit, A. (2012). Mannosylated polyethyleneimine-hyaluronan nanohybrids for targeted gene delivery to macrophage-like cell lines. *Bioconjug. Chem.* 23, 1138–1148. doi:10.1021/bc200599k

Mantovani, A., Biswas, S. K., Galdiero, M. R., Sica, A., and Locati, M. (2013). Macrophage plasticity and polarization in tissue repair and remodelling. *J. Pathol.* 229, 176–185. doi:10.1002/path.4133

Martin, P., and Leibovich, S. J. (2005). Inflammatory cells during wound repair: the good, the bad and the ugly. *Trends Cell Biol.* 15, 599–607. doi:10.1016/j.tcb.2005.09.002

Monaghan, M., and Pandit, A. (2011). RNA interference therapy via functionalized scaffolds. *Adv. Drug Deliv. Rev.* 63, 197–208. doi:10.1016/j.addr.2011.01.006

Mosser, D. M., and Edwards, J. P. (2009). Exploring the full spectrum of macrophage activation. *Genetics* 8, 958–969. doi:10.1038/nri2448

Mountziaris, P. M., Tzouanas, S. N., Sing, D. C., Kramer, P. R., Kurtis Kasper, F., and Mikos, A. G. (2012). Intra-articular controlled release of anti-inflammatory siRNA with biodegradable polymer microparticles ameliorates temporomandibular joint inflammation. *Acta Biomater.* 8, 3552–3560. doi:10.1016/j.actbio.2012.06.031

Muscari, C., Bonafè, F., Martin-Suarez, S., Valgimigli, S., Valente, S., Fiumana, E., et al. (2013). Restored perfusion and reduced inflammation in the infarcted heart after grafting stem cells with a hyaluronan-based scaffold. *J. Cell. Mol. Med.* 17, 518–530. doi:10.1111/jcmm.12039

Nakamura, K., Yokohama, S., Yoneda, M., Okamoto, S., Tamaki, Y., Ito, T., et al. (2004). High, but not low, molecular weight hyaluronan prevents T-cell-mediated liver injury by reducing proinflammatory cytokines in mice. *J. Gastroenterol.* 39, 346–354. doi:10.1007/s00535-003-1301-x

O'Rorke, S., Keeney, M., and Pandit, A. (2010). Non-viral polyplexes: scaffold mediated delivery for gene therapy. *Prog. Polym. Sci.* 35, 441–458. doi:10.1016/j.progpolymsci.2010.01.005

Park, J. S., Yang, H. N., Jeon, S. Y., Woo, D. G., Kim, M. S., and Park, K. H. (2012). The use of anti-COX2 siRNA coated onto PLGA nanoparticles loading dexamethasone in the treatment of rheumatoid arthritis. *Biomaterials* 33, 8600–8612. doi:10.1016/j.biomaterials.2012.08.008

Park, S., Kang, S., Chen, X., Kim, E. J., Kim, J., Kim, N., et al. (2013). Tumor suppression via paclitaxel-loaded drug carriers that target inflammation marker upregulated in tumor vasculature and macrophages. *Biomaterials* 34, 598–605. doi:10.1016/j.biomaterials.2012.10.004

Prabaharan, M. (2008). Review paper: chitosan derivatives as promising materials for controlled drug delivery. *J. Biomater. Appl.* 23, 5–36. doi:10.1177/0885328208091562

Présumey, J., Salzano, G., Courties, G., Shires, M., Ponchel, F., Jorgensen, C., et al. (2012). PLGA microspheres encapsulating siRNA anti-TNFalpha: efficient RNAi-mediated treatment of arthritic joints. *Eur. J. Pharm. Biopharm.* 82, 457–464. doi:10.1016/j.ejpb.2012.07.021

Ratanavaraporn, J., Furuya, H., and Tabata, Y. (2012). Local suppression of pro-inflammatory cytokines and the effects in BMP-2-induced bone regeneration. *Biomaterials* 33, 304–316. doi:10.1016/j.biomaterials.2011.09.050

Redd, M. J., Cooper, L., Wood, W., Stramer, B., and Martin, P. (2004). Wound healing and inflammation: embryos reveal the way to perfect repair. *Philos. Trans. R Soc. Lond. B Biol. Sci.* 359, 777–784. doi:10.1098/rstb.2004.1466

Rodriguez, P. L., Harada, T., Christian, D. A., Pantano, D. A., Tsai, R. K., and Discher, D. A. (2013). Minimal "self" peptides that inhibit phagocytic clearance and enhance delivery of nanoparticles. *Science* 339, 971–975. doi:10.1126/science.122956

Sehgal, P. K., and Srinivasan, A. (2009). Collagen-coated microparticles in drug delivery. *Expert Opin. Drug Deliv.* 6, 687–695. doi:10.1517/17425240903025736

Seliktar, D. (2012). Designing cell-compatible hydrogels. *Science* 336, 1124–1129. doi:10.1126/science.1214804

Seshadri, G, Sy, J. C., Brown, M., Dikalov, S., Yang, S. C., Murthy, N., et al. (2010). The delivery of superoxide dismutase encapsulated in polyketal microparticles to rat myocardium and protection from myocardial ischemia-reperfusion injury. *Biomaterials* 31, 1372–1379. doi:10.1016/j.biomaterials.2009.10.045

Shah, P. P., Desai, P. R., Patel, A. R., and Singh, M. S. (2012). Skin permeating nanogel for the cutaneous co-delivery of two anti-inflammatory drugs. *Biomaterials* 33, 1607–1617. doi:10.1016/j.biomaterials.2011.11.011

Singh, A., Agarwal, R., Diaz-Ruiz, C. A., Willett, N. J., Wang, P., Lee, L. A., et al. (2014). Nanoengineered particles for enhanced intra-articular retention and delivery of proteins. *Adv. Healthc. Mater.* 3, 1562–1567. doi:10.1002/adhm.201400051

Singh, A., Nie, H., Ghosn, B., Qin, H., Kwak, L. W., and Roy, K. (2008). Efficient modulation of T-cell response by dual-mode, single-carrier delivery of cytokine-targeted siRNA and DNA vaccine to antigen-presenting cells. *Mol. Ther.* 16, 2011–2021. doi:10.1038/mt.2008.206

Spiller, K. L., Anfang, R. R., Spiller, K. J., Ng, J., Nakazawa, K. R., Daulton, J. W., et al. (2014). The role of macrophage phenotype in vascularization of tissue engineering scaffolds. *Biomaterials* 35, 4477–4488. doi:10.1016/j.biomaterials.2014.02.012

Su, J., Hu, B. H., Lowe, W. L., Kaufman, D. B., and Messersmith, P. B. (2010). Anti-inflammatory peptide-functionalized hydrogels for insulin-secreting cell encapsulation. *Biomaterials* 31, 308–314. doi:10.1016/j.biomaterials.2009.09.045

Sy, J. C., Seshadri, G., Yang, S. C., Brown, M., Oh, T., Dikalov, S., et al. (2008). Sustained release of a p38 inhibitor from non-inflammatory microspheres inhibits cardiac dysfunction. *Nat. Mater.* 7, 863–868. doi:10.1038/nmat2299

Thevenot, P. T., Nair, A. M., Shen, J., Lotfi, P., Ko, C. Y., and Tang, L. (2010). The effect of incorporation of SDF-1α into PLGA scaffolds on stem cell recruitment and the inflammatory response. *Biomaterials* 31, 3997–4008. doi:10.1016/j.biomaterials.2010.01.144

van Putten, S. M., Ploeger, D. T. A., Popa, E. R., and Bank, R. A. (2013). Macrophage phenotypes in the collagen-induced foreign body reaction in rats. *Acta Biomater.* 9, 6502–6510. doi:10.1016/j.actbio.2013.01.022

van Putten, S. M., Wübben, M., Hennink, W. E., van Luyn, M. J. A., and Harmsen, M. C. (2009). The downmodulation of the foreign body reaction by cytomegalovirus encoded interleukin-10. *Biomaterials* 30, 730–735. doi:10.1016/j.biomaterials.2008.10.043

Wang, Q. S., Cui, Y. L., Gao, L. N., Guo, Y., Li, R. X., and Zhang, X. Z. (2014a). Reduction of the pro-inflammatory response by tetrandrine-loading poly(l-lactic acid) films in vitro and in vivo. *J. Biomed. Mater. Res. A* 102A, 4098–4107. doi:10.1002/jbm.a.35083

Wang, W., Sun, L., Zhang, P., Song, J., and Liu, W. (2014b). An anti-inflammatory cell-free collagen/resveratrol scaffold for repairing osteochondral defects in rabbits. *Acta Biomater.* 10, 4983–4995. doi:10.1016/j.actbio.2014.08.022

Webber, M. J., Matson, J. B., Tamboli, V. K., and Stupp, S. I. (2012). Controlled release of dexamethasone from peptide nanofiber gels to modulate inflammatory response. *Biomaterials* 33, 6823–6832. doi:10.1016/j.biomaterials.2012.06.003

Whitmire, R. E., Wilson, D. S., Singh, A., Levenston, M. E., Murthy, N., and García, A. J. (2012). Self-assembling nanoparticles for intra-articular delivery of anti-inflammatory proteins. *Biomaterials* 33, 7665–7675. doi:10.1016/j.biomaterials.2012.06.101

Wynn, T. A., and Barron, L. (2010). Macrophages: master regulators of inflammation and fibrosis. *Semin. Liver Dis.* 30, 245–257. doi:10.1055/s-0030-1255354

Xia, Z., and Triffitt, J. T. (2006). A review on macrophage responses to biomaterials. *Biomed. Mater.* 1, R1–R9. doi:10.1088/1748-6041/1/1/R01

Yoshitomi, T., and Nagasaki, Y. (2014). Reactive oxygen species-scavenging nanomedicines for the treatment of oxidative stress injuries. *Adv. Healthc. Mater.* 3, 1149–1161. doi:10.1002/adhm.201300576

Yuan, Z., Zhao, J., Zhu, W., Yang, Z., Li, B., Yang, H., et al. (2014). Ibuprofen-loaded electrospun fibrous scaffold doped with sodium bicarbonate for responsively inhibiting inflammation and promoting muscle wound healing in vivo. *Biomater. Sci.* 2, 502–511. doi:10.1039/c3bm60198f

Zachman, A. L., Crowder, S. W., Ortiz, O., Zienkiewicz, K. J., Bronikowski, C. M., Yu, S. S., et al. (2012). Pro-angiogenic and anti-inflammatory regulation by functional peptides loaded in polymeric implants for soft tissue regeneration. *Tissue Eng. Part A* 19, 437. doi:10.1089/ten.tea.2012.0158

Zhang, D., Wei, Y., Chen, K., Zhang, X., Xu, X., and Shi, Q. (2015). Biocompatible reactive oxygen species (ROS)-responsive nanoparticles as superior drug delivery vehicles. *Adv. Healthc. Mater.* 4, 69–76. doi:10.1002/adhm.201400299

Zhang, J., Tang, C., and Yin, C. (2013). Galactosylated trimethyl chitosan-cysteine nanoparticles loaded with Map4k4 siRNA for targeting activated macrophages. *Biomaterials* 34, 3667–3677. doi:10.1016/j.biomaterials.2013.01.079

Zisch, A. H., Lutolf, M. P., Ehrbar, M., Raeber, G. P., Rizzi, S. C., Davies, N., et al. (2003). Cell-demanded release of VEGF from synthetic, biointeractive cell ingrowth matrices for vascularized tissue growth. *FASEB J.* 17, 2260–2262. doi:10.1096/fj.02-1041fje

Conflict of Interest Statement: The authors declare that the research was conducted in the absence of any commercial or financial relationships that could be construed as a potential conflict of interest.

5

Uniform surface modification of 3D Bioglass®-based scaffolds with mesoporous silica particles (MCM-41) for enhancing drug delivery capability

Elena Boccardi[1], Anahí Philippart[1], Judith A. Juhasz-Bortuzzo[1], Ana M. Beltrán[2†],
Giorgia Novajra[3], Chiara Vitale-Brovarone[3], Erdmann Spiecker[2] and Aldo R. Boccaccini[1]*

[1] Institute of Biomaterials, Department of Materials Science and Engineering, Friedrich-Alexander University Erlangen-Nürnberg, Erlangen, Germany, [2] Center for Nanoanalysis and Electron Microscopy (CENEM), Institute of Micro- and Nanostructure Research, Department of Materials Science and Engineering, Friedrich-Alexander University Erlangen-Nürnberg, Erlangen, Germany, [3] Institute of Materials Physics and Engineering, Applied Science and Technology Department, Politecnico di Torino, Turin, Italy

Edited by:
Malcolm Xing,
University of Manitoba, Canada

Reviewed by:
Hélder A. Santos,
University of Helsinki, Finland
Ahmed El-Fiqi,
Dankook University, South Korea

*Correspondence:
Aldo R. Boccaccini
aldo.boccaccini@ww.uni-erlangen.de

†Present address:
Ana M. Beltrán,
Instituto de Ciencia de Materiales de Sevilla (ICMS), CSIC-Universidad de Sevilla, Seville, Spain

The design and characterization of a new family of multifunctional scaffolds based on bioactive glass (BG) of 45S5 composition for bone tissue engineering and drug delivery applications are presented. These BG-based scaffolds are developed via a replication method of polyurethane packaging foam. In order to increase the therapeutic functionality, the scaffolds were coated with mesoporous silica particles (MCM-41), which act as an *in situ* drug delivery system. These sub-micron spheres are characterized by large surface area and pore volume with a narrow pore diameter distribution. The solution used for the synthesis of the silica mesoporous particles was designed to obtain a high-ordered mesoporous structure and spherical shape – both are key factors for achieving the desired controlled drug release. The MCM-41 particles were synthesized directly inside the BG-based scaffolds, and the drug-release capability of this combined system was evaluated. Moreover, the effect of MCM-41 particle coating on the bioactivity of the BG-based scaffolds was assessed. The results indicate that it is possible to obtain a multifunctional scaffold system characterized by high and interconnected porosity, high bioactivity, and sustained drug delivery capability.

Keywords: ordered mesoporosity, silica, MCM-41, bioactive glass, scaffolds, drug release, ibuprofen

INTRODUCTION

One of the most promising fields of tissue engineering is the development of porous 3D engineered scaffolds to enhance bone regeneration and neovascularization (Porter et al., 2009). The main challenge is the design of materials able to match at the same time the biological and the mechanical properties of the natural bone tissue (Mastrogiacomo et al., 2006; Stevens, 2008; Philippart et al., 2015). However, the design of the scaffolds is not the only challenge, in fact the first problem after implantation is the exposure to inflammatory and infection risks with further complications, e.g., septicemia and potential implant failure (Misch and Wang, 2008). To avoid these consequences, a large amount of antibiotics and anti-inflammatory drugs are administered to the patient, which can increase the healing time, the stay at the hospital, and costs (Neut et al., 2003). Nowadays, the most popular ways for drug intake are oral administration and injection. However, these methods may be affected by a lack of efficiency especially since the release of the drug is not targeted to the area that needs to be treated (Vallet-Regí et al., 2012a). For all these reasons, the development of local drug-release systems, which enable controlled release kinetics, has increased considerably during the past few years (Vallet-Regí, 2006a; Slowing et al., 2007; Cotí et al., 2009; Vitale-Brovarone et al., 2009; Wu et al., 2013). In this context, the combination of bioactive scaffolds with local drug delivery carriers is gaining increasing research efforts in the bone tissue engineering field (Philippart et al., 2015). Several matrices have been tested so far, such as organic polymers, organic–inorganic hybrid materials, bioactive glasses (BG), and ceramics (Wu and Chang, 2014). One approach gaining increasing interest involves obtaining drug carriers that are structured at the nanoscale. Since 1992, when silica-based MCM-41 was developed (Mobil Composition of Matter No. 41) (Beck et al., 1992), highly ordered mesoporous materials have attracted the attention of many scientists and in 2001 they were proposed as drug delivery system (Vallet-Regí et al., 2001). The most interesting features of these materials are the regular pore system, high specific surface area and high pore volume (Vallet-Regí et al., 2001, 2012a,b; Vallet-Regí, 2006b; Zhao et al., 2013). These silica-based mesoporous materials are able to incorporate relatively high content of drugs into the mesopores. Moreover, their silanol groups can be functionalized (**Figure 1**) and the pore diameter can be modulated, allowing a better control of the drug-release kinetic (Grün et al., 1997; Vallet-Regí et al., 2001, 2012b; Vallet-Regí, 2006b; Wu and Chang, 2014). Two mechanisms have been proposed to describe mesoporous silica material formation. The first model describes the addition of silicate to micelles formed using n-decyltrimethylammonium bromide. In this way, the silica precursor polymerizes around the already formed micelles (Zhao et al., 2013). The second proposed mechanism is that the addition of the silica precursor to an aqueous n-decyltrimethylammonium bromide solution induces the ordering of silica-encased surfactant micelles simultaneously. In this case, the micelle formation requires the silica precursor to be present (Vallet-Regí et al., 2012a; Zhao et al., 2013).

MCM-41 has become the most popular member of the mesoporous silicate materials family, and it has been considered also as drug carrier.(Vallet-Regí et al., 2012b) Nowadays, it is possible to find in literature different approaches for the synthesis of spherical MCM-41 (Grün et al., 1999; Cai et al., 2001; Zeleňák et al., 2008; Liu et al., 2009). Grün et al. (1997, 1999) proposed a novel pathway for the production of spherical MCM-41 applying a modification of the Stöber reaction (Stober and Fink, 1968) for the synthesis of spherical non-porous silica particles. The approach involves introducing a low-boiling alcohol, such as ethanol or isopropanol, as co-solvent for the silica source in order to get a more homogeneous solution (Grün et al., 1999). Starting from the work of Grün et al. (1999), it is possible to obtain well-shaped spherical particles; however, the mesoporosity is not homogeneously present. On the other hand, following a standard procedure reported by Zeleňák et al. (2008), it is possible to obtain well-ordered mesoporous structures; however, the particles are not spherical and the size distribution is usually broad. Combining these two synthesis pathways, a new solution for the synthesis of spherical mesoporous silica particles has been proposed in this study. Thus, the aim of the present work is the synthesis of spherical silica mesoporous particles (MCM-41) inside porous BG-based scaffolds [45S5 BG composition (Hench, 2015)] to combine in the same system the drug uptake and release capabilities of this mesoporous material with the bioactivity properties of the BG. The concept of incorporating a silica drug carrier into bioactive silicate scaffolds has been previously explored (Mortera et al., 2008); however, the main advantage of the approach introduced in this paper is the possibility to obtain a highly homogeneous coating of the BG scaffold struts with highly ordered mesoporous silica particles without affecting the BG bioactivity. Moreover, the total amount of produced particles obtained per single batch increases by ~60% combining the two standard procedures reported in literature (Grün et al., 1999; Zeleňák et al., 2008), which represents another advantage of the present approach.

MATERIALS AND METHODS

MCM-41 Particle Synthesis

The procedure adopted to prepare MCM-41 was a combination of the standard pathway for the production of mesoporous silica particles and a modification of the Stöber reaction (Stober and Fink, 1968) for the preparation of non-porous silica spheres proposed by Grün et al. (1999). In this way, the reaction took place in a more homogeneous environment, resulting in the formation of sub-micron sized spherical MCM-41 particles and the total amount of the cationic surfactant, which is extremely toxic, can be

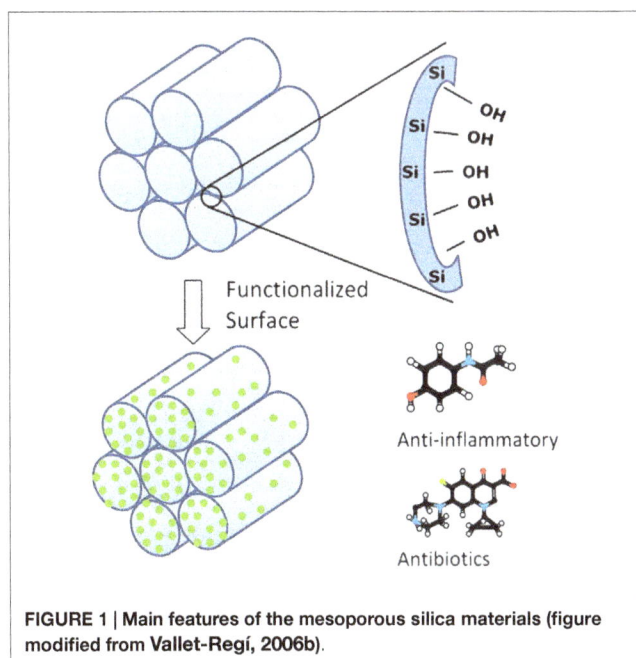

FIGURE 1 | Main features of the mesoporous silica materials (figure modified from Vallet-Regí, 2006b).

reduced (Grün et al., 1999). A low-boiling alcohol such as ethanol was added as co-solvent for the tetra-n-alkoxysilane to make it soluble. The reactants were ammonia (catalyst of the reaction), n-hexadecyltrimethylammonium bromide (CTAB, surfactant), pure ethanol (co-solvent of silica source), and tetraethyl orthosilicate (TEOS), all purchased from Sigma-Aldrich (Germany). Pure ethanol and ammonia (28–30 wt.%) solution were mixed with deionized water. The cationic surfactant was added to the solution under continuous stirring for 20 min. Once the solution was clear, TEOS was added (0.25 mL min^{-1}). All synthesis steps were carried out at room temperature (RT), which is the optimal temperature condition for the reaction with cationic surfactant in basic conditions as reported by Zhao et al. (2013). After 2 h of stirring, the resulting dispersion was centrifuged and washed once with deionized water and twice with ethanol in order to remove completely every trace of ammonia, collected in a ceramic crucible, dried, and calcined in air. The solutions used are reported in **Table 1**. For samples MCM-41_A (Zeleňák et al., 2008), MCM-41_B, and MCM-41_C, the thermal treatment was 60°C (2°C min^{-1}) for 12 h and 550°C (2°C min^{-1}) for 6 h; for sample MCM-41_D (Grün et al., 1999), the thermal treatment was 90°C (2°C min^{-1}) for 12 h and 550°C (1°C min^{-1}) for 5 h.

Scaffolds Preparation

The template used to prepare 3D porous scaffolds was polyurethane (PU) packaging foams (45 ppi) (Eurofoam Deutschland GmbH Schaumstoffe). BG powder (particle size 5 µm of 45S5 composition) was used. 45S5 BG-based scaffolds were produced by the replica technique, according to the method described by Chen et al. (2006). Briefly, the slurry for the scaffolds fabrication was prepared by dissolving polyvinyl alcohol (PVA) in deionized water at 80°C for 1 h, the concentration being 0.01 mol L^{-1}. Then, 45S5 BG powder was added to 25 mL PVA–water solution to obtain a concentration of 40 wt.%. Each procedure was carried out under vigorous stirring using a magnetic stirrer for 1 h. The sacrificial PU templates, cut to cylinders (7 mm in height and 5 mm in diameter), were immersed in the slurry for 10 min. The foams were retrieved and the extra slurry was completely squeezed out manually. The samples were then dried at RT for at least 12 h. The dip coating in the slurry was repeated three times to increase the coating thickness and consequently the mechanical properties. After the second and third coating, the extra slurry was completely removed using compressed air as explained elsewhere (Boccardi et al., 2015). Post-foaming heat treatment for the burning-out of the sacrificial template

and sintering of the BG structure was programed. The burning and sintering conditions were: 400°C for 1 h and 1050°C for 1 h, respectively. The heating and cooling rates were 2 and 5°C min^{-1}, respectively.

Composite System Preparation

MCM-41_A, MCM-41_B, and MCM-41_D samples were used for the preparation of BG_MCM-41 composite scaffolds. MCM-41_C solution was not used because it did not show any ordered mesoporosity. The coating procedure used here was similar to the one reported by Mortera et al. (2008). The procedure consisted of four steps, i.e., hydrolysis of TEOS in MCM-41-synthesis solution, dipping of scaffolds for particles impregnation, drying of the scaffolds, and calcination (heat treatment) for the removal of the surfactant. After TEOS addition, the solution was stirred for 10 min to promote the hydrolysis of the silica precursor. Scaffolds were then immersed in the silica synthesis batch for 10 min and meanwhile the solution was kept under vigorous stirring in order to enhance the coating of the inner core of the BG scaffolds. The resulting BG-based scaffolds coated with the MCM-41 particles were heat-treated at 60°C (2°C min^{-1}) for 12 h for drying and at 550°C (2°C min^{-1}) for 6 h in air as reported in **Figure 2**.

Drug-Release Test

To load silica particles with a drug, Ibuprofen (>98%, purchased from Sigma-Aldrich) as model drug was dissolved in hexane (33 mg mL^{-1}) and MCM-41 particles were added to the drug solution (33 mg mL^{-1}) at RT following the procedure presented in literature (Vallet-Regí et al., 2001). The samples with the drug solution were then placed in a vacuum hood at RT at 300 mbar for 10 min in order to enhance the drug infiltration inside the mesoporosity. After 12 h, this procedure was repeated, the drug solution was removed and the particles were dried in a vacuum

TABLE 1 | Composition of four different synthesis solutions used for the preparation of mesoporous silica particles.

Sample	H₂O (mL)	EtOH (mL)	NH₃ (mL)	CTAB (g)	TEOS (mL)
MCM-41_A (Zeleňák et al., 2008)	29	–	18.5	0.2	1
MCM-41_B	11	18	18.5	0.2	1
MCM-41_C	4	25	18.5	0.2	1
MCM-41_D (Grün et al., 1999)	11	19	3.3	0.62	1.25

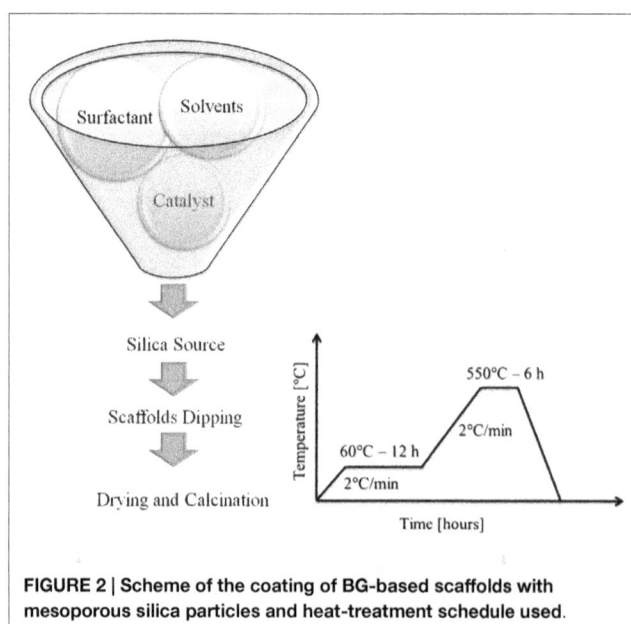

FIGURE 2 | Scheme of the coating of BG-based scaffolds with mesoporous silica particles and heat-treatment schedule used.

hood at RT. All the particle synthesis solutions were tested for their drug-releasing capability.

The scaffolds coated with MCM-41_B were in contact with the drug solution for 3 days (10 mg mL^{-1}) before the starting of the drug-release test, in order to get a better infiltration of the drug. Only the scaffolds coated with MCM-41_B particles were considered for the test, because the resulting particles were still spherical and with ordered mesoporosity and the results were compared with those obtained on scaffolds not coated with MCM-41.

The drug-release kinetics from all samples, particles (10 mg each sample), and scaffolds was assessed by soaking the samples in 4 mL of PBS, kept at 37°C until the complete release of ibuprofen. At every time point, 1 mL of solution was uptake for the drug-release analysis and substituted with 1 mL of fresh PBS. A UV-vis spectrophotometer was used to evaluate the amount of released drug. The calibration curve was calculated using a solution of ibuprofen in PBS with different known concentrations, on the basis of the absorption at 273 nm, typical of this molecule (Vallet-Regí et al., 2001).

Bioactivity and Stability of the Composite System

Simulated body fluid (SBF) was prepared by dissolving reagent-grade 8.035 g L^{-1} NaCl, 0.355 g L^{-1} NaHCO$_3$, 0.225 g L^1 KCl, 0.231 g L^{-1} K$_2$HPO$_4$ (3H$_2$O), 0.311 g L^{-1} MgCl$_2$ (6H$_2$O), 0.292 g L^{-1} CaCl$_2$, and 0.072 g L^{-1} Na$_2$SO$_4$ in deionized water and buffered at pH 7.4 at 36.5°C with 6.118 g L^{-1} tris(hydroxymethyl) aminomethane [(CH$_2$OH)$_3$CNH$_2$] and 1M HCl, as previously reported by Kokubo and Takadama (2007). Cylindrical BG foams coated and not coated with mesoporous silica particles were immersed in SBF at a 1.5 g L^{-1} ratio (Cerruti et al., 2005). The stability of the MCM-41 coating was evaluated in Tris-buffered solution [tris(hydroxymethyl) aminomethane]. Only the scaffolds coated with MCM-41_B were tested, because the silica particles showed suitable features in terms of homogeneous coating, shape, and ordered mesoporosity. In both cases, the solution was kept in a polystyrene container at 37°C in a shaking incubator (90 rpm) up to 1 week. The solution was renewed every 2 days in order to better mimic the *in vivo* behavior, as carried out also in previous studies (Chen et al., 2006). At the end of the incubator period, the foams were washed with deionized water, dried, and stored for further characterizations.

Characterization Techniques

The shape and the surface structure of the resulting MCM-41 particles and BG_MCM-41 were evaluated by means of scanning electron microscope (SEM) (Auriga 0750 from ZEISS). The porous structure of the particles was assessed with high-resolution transmission electron microscopy (HRTEM) (Phillips CM30) operating at an acceleration voltage of 300 kV. For the TEM observation, the samples were dispersed with ethanol on a lacey carbon film. The pore diameter analyses were conducted on HRTEM images with ImageJ analysis software. Small angle X-ray diffraction (SAXRD), carried out using Philips Xpert Diffractometer, was used to analyze the porous structure and the pore diameter of the silica particles. Diffraction data were recorded between 1 and 10° 2θ at an interval of 0.02° 2θ. Nitrogen adsorption desorption analysis was conducted at 77 K in a Quantachrome Autosorb Instrument to assess the specific surface area and the pore size of the particles. Prior to the measurements, the samples were outgassed for 12 h at 300°C under vacuum. The specific surface area and pore size of MCM-41 microspheres were evaluated, respectively, with BET method and BJH method.

RESULTS

MCM-41 Particles

The morphology and the microstructure of the obtained MCM-41 particles were assessed by HRTEM micrographs. HRTEM images of sample MCM-41_A and MCM-41_B showed the existence of highly ordered hexagonal array and streaks structural features (**Figures 3a–d**). The hexagonal array and the streaks are the view of the crystals whose axes are, respectively, parallel and perpendicular to the line of vision. Sample MCM-41_C, which was prepared with a high concentration of ethanol in the synthesis solution, was porous however the porosity was not ordered (**Figures 3e,f**). Moreover MCM-41_D particles were porous but the porosity was not completely ordered, in contrast with the results reported in literature (Grün et al., 1999) (**Figures 3g,h**). From the analysis of the HRTEM images with ImageJ analysis software, the dimension of the pores was evaluated, which was found to be around 3 nm for all samples (**Figure 4**). The analysis has been done applying the Fast Fourier Transform (FFT) and the inverse FFT (**Figure 4A**) to the image, and the plug in plot (**Figure 4B**) has been used to evaluate the distance between the pore channels.

The pore size dimensions were confirmed also by SAXRD analysis. The spectra of sample MCM-41_A exhibited three sharp peaks, called Bragg peaks, indicating the long-range order present in the material, which is typical of MCM-41 materials (Vallet-Regí et al., 2001) (**Figure 5A**) in agreement with literature (Grün et al., 1999). These peaks arise from the quasi-regular arrangement of the mesopores in the bulk material (Grün et al., 1999; Vallet-Regí et al., 2001). The Bragg peaks can be indexed assuming a hexagonal symmetry. *2 theta* values of sample MCM-41_A namely 2.75, 4.65, and 5.10 can be indexed as (100), (110), and (200) reflections, respectively. These values were close to those reported by Grün et al. (1999). The repeating distance, a_0, between two pore centers may be calculated by $a_0 = (2/\sqrt{3})d_{100}$. The pore diameter can be evaluated from a_0 subtracting 1.0 nm, which is approximately the value of the pore wall thickness (Grün et al., 1999). For MCM-41_B particles, it was possible to identify unequivocally only the main peak (100) (**Figure 5B**), meanwhile the 110 and 200 peaks were less pronounced but still visible. The SAXRD results combined with HRTEM results confirm thus the mesoporous ordered structures of MCM-41_A and MCM-41_B particles.

For samples MCM-41_C and MCM-41_D, only the main peak (100) was identified, in agreement with the HRTEM analysis (**Figures 5C,D**). The first peak is in fact an indicator of the presence of mesoporosity in the sample. Also in this case, it was

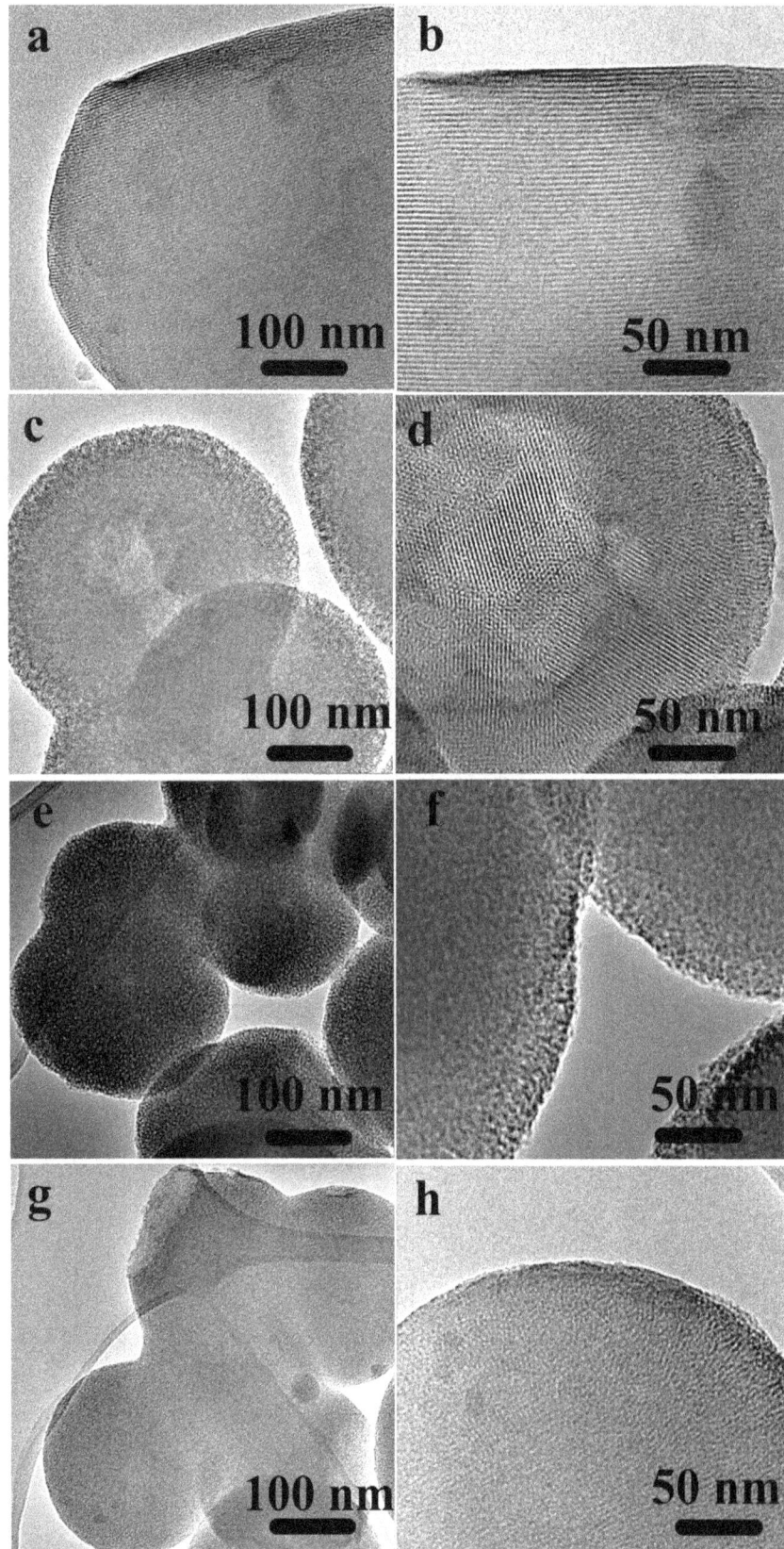

FIGURE 3 | HRTEM images of sample MCM-41_A (a,b) and sample MCM-41_B (c,d), which are characterized by ordered mesoporosity, sample MCM-41_C (e,f) and MCM-41_D (g,h), which are characterized by a disordered porosity.

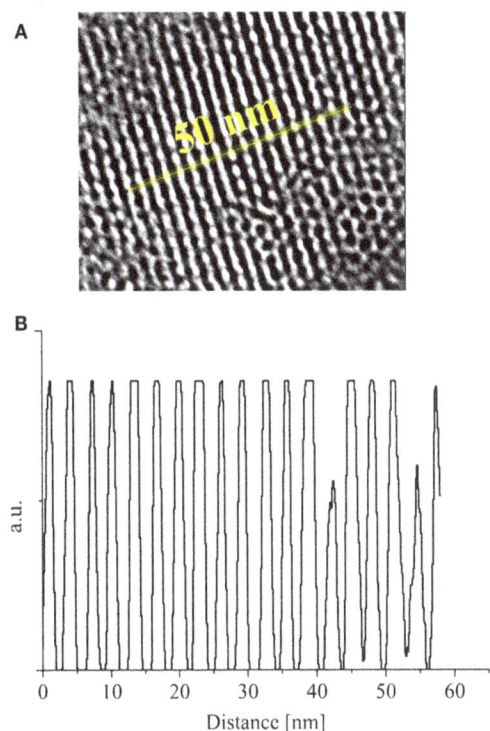

FIGURE 4 | High-resolution image of the ordered mesoporous structure of MCM-41_B after analysis with FFT and inverse FFT (A); plot of the distance between the pore channels obtained with ImageJ plug in plot applied along the yellow line (B).

possible to evaluate the pore diameter with the Bragg's law and the resulting values were in agreement with the ImageJ analysis.

The nitrogen isotherms of sample MCM-41_B are shown in **Figure 6**. The isotherms can be classified as type IV isotherms according to the IUPAC nomenclature for MCM-41 (Vallet-Regí et al., 2012a; Zhao et al., 2013), which is typical of mesoporous material with pore diameter in the range of 2–10 nm. MCM-41_B particles were characterized by a specific surface area of 951 m^2 g^{-1} and a pore volume of 0.24 cm^3 g^{-1}. From **Figure 7**, it was possible to observe how the different amounts of solvent influenced the final shape and mesostructure of the resulting MCM-41 particles. The particles produced with only deionized water (**Figures 7a,b**) as solvent were characterized by hexagonal and not spherical geometry (MCM-41_A). Progressively increasing the amount of ethanol as co-solvent, it was possible to produce spherical particles, which exhibited a fairly homogeneous distribution of particle size but reduced mesoporosity order (**Figures 7e,f**).

Composite Scaffold System

From SEM analysis, it was possible to observe that the surface of scaffolds was completely coated after immersion in the MCM-41 synthesis batch maintaining an open porosity. In the case of the synthesis solution of MCM-41_A (Zeleňák et al., 2008) (**Figures 8a,b**), the one without ethanol as co-solvent, the shape of the resulting MCM-41 particles was seen to be completely changed. The presence of the scaffold affected the formation of the particles, probably due to a reduction in the homogeneity of the solution. Moreover, with this solution,

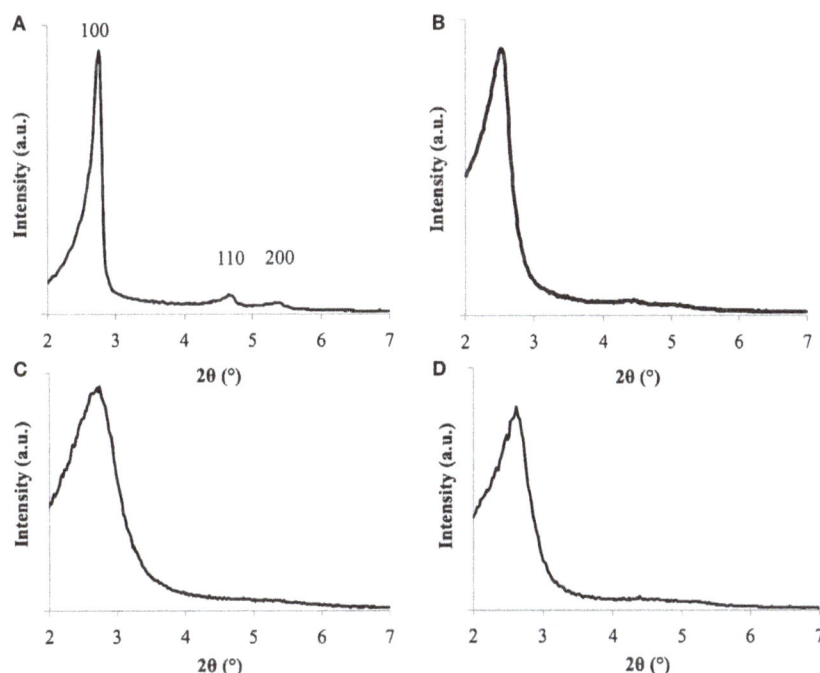

FIGURE 5 | SAXRD of sample MCM-41_A (A), MCM-41_B (B), MCM-41_C (C), and MCM-41_D (D). Sample MCM-41_A is characterized by the three peaks, labeled as 100, 110, and 200.

it was not possible to obtain a homogenous coverage of the BG scaffold surface. With the synthesis solution of samples MCM-41_B (**Figures 8c,d**) and MCM-41_D (Grün et al., 1999) (**Figures 8e,f**), the resulting particles on the surface of the BG scaffolds were still perfectly spherical and they covered completely the surface of the scaffold struts. By means of HRTEM analysis, it was also possible to confirm that the MCM-41_B particles still exhibited ordered mesoporosity, as shown in **Figure 9**.

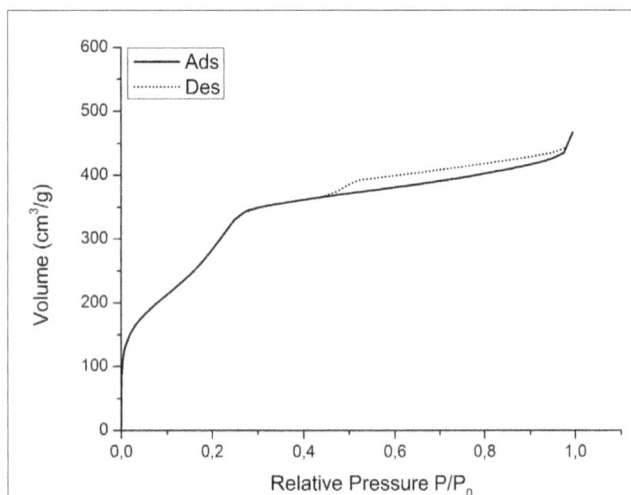

FIGURE 6 | Nitrogen adsorption desorption isotherms on MCM-41_B.

Drug-Release Capability of MCM-41 Particles

The drug-release capability of the different mesoporous silica particles was evaluated and the released profiles are reported in **Figure 10**. Both samples MCM-41_A (**Figure 10A**) and MCM-41_D (**Figure 10D**) were characterized by a burst release and it was confirmed that after 1 h of test, the 80% of the loaded drug was released. The rest 20% of the drug was released within the next 7 days. The particles prepared with solutions MCM-41_B and MCM-41_C showed the best drug-release profile (**Figures 10B,C**), in terms of lack of uncontrolled burst release. Especially MCM-41_B, which was characterized by high-ordered mesoporosity, did not show any burst release during the first hours of the test. Eighty percent of the loaded drug was in fact released only after 30 h and the rest of the ibuprofen was released within the seven following days. It should be pointed out that ibuprofen solubility in water at 25°C is 21 mg L^{-1} (Vallet-Regí et al., 2001). During the present release test, the highest concentrations of ibuprofen were lower than its solubility, also after the first hours of release. At every time point, 1 mL of fresh PBS was added to every sample to keep constant the PBS volume and for this reason the solution was highly diluted.

Drug-Release Capability of Composite Scaffold System

The amounts of released ibuprofen from the BG and BG_MCM-41_B scaffolds are shown in **Figure 11**. The presence of the

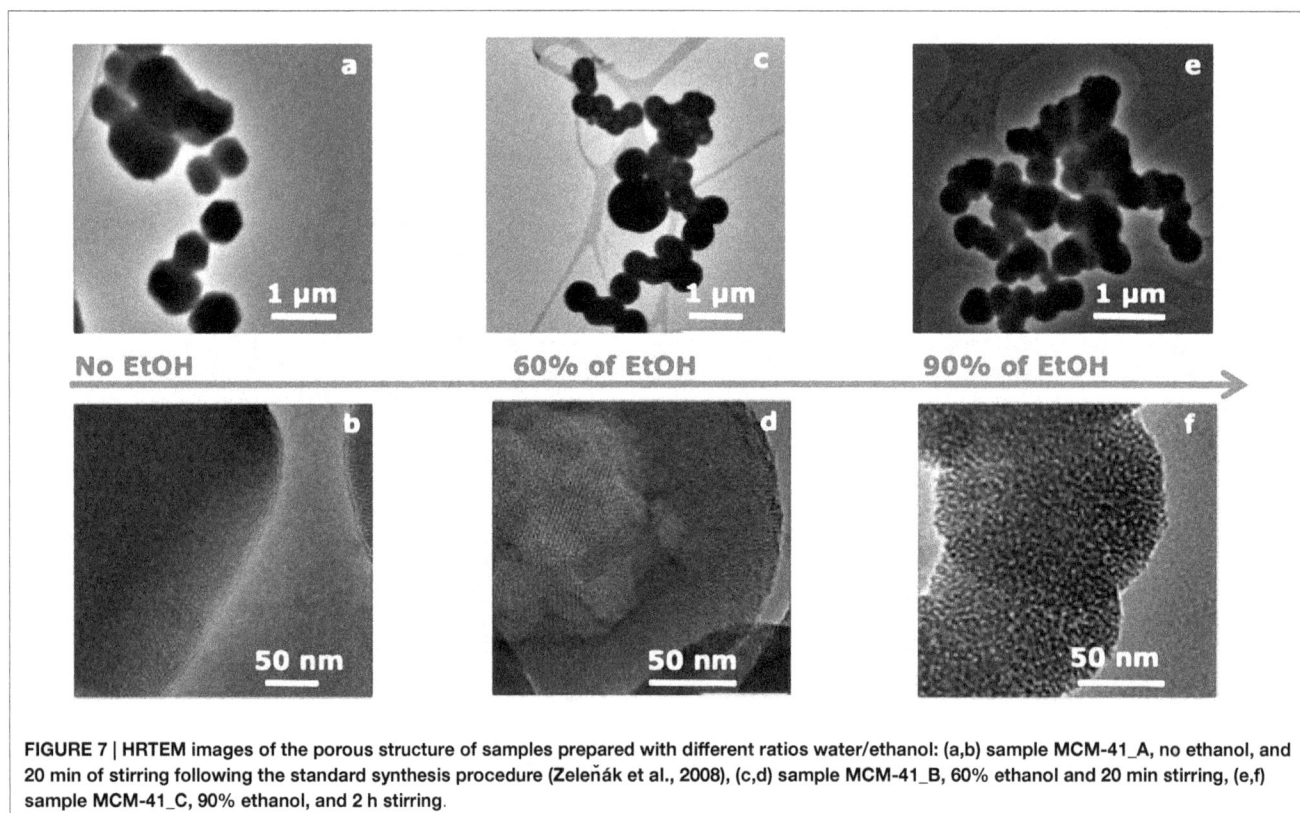

FIGURE 7 | HRTEM images of the porous structure of samples prepared with different ratios water/ethanol: (a,b) sample MCM-41_A, no ethanol, and 20 min of stirring following the standard synthesis procedure (Zeleňák et al., 2008), (c,d) sample MCM-41_B, 60% ethanol and 20 min stirring, (e,f) sample MCM-41_C, 90% ethanol, and 2 h stirring.

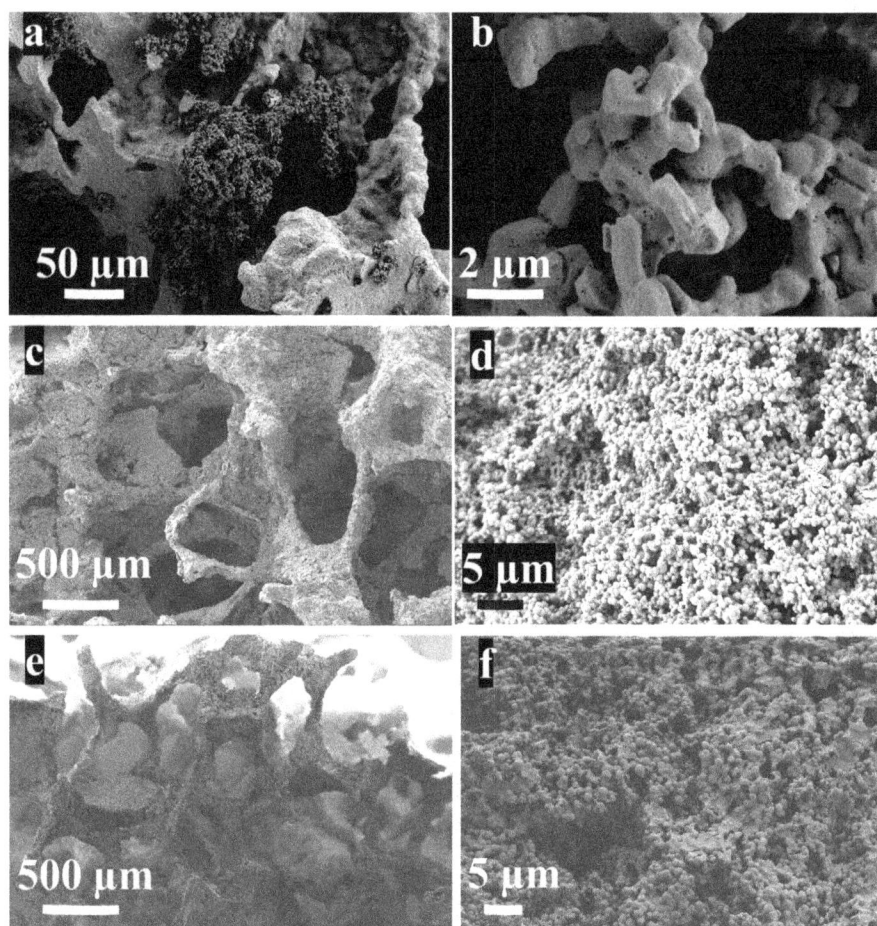

FIGURE 8 | BG-based scaffolds coated with MCM-41_A (Zeleňák et al., 2008) (a,b), MCM-41_B (c,d), and MCM-41_D (Grün et al., 1999) (e,f).

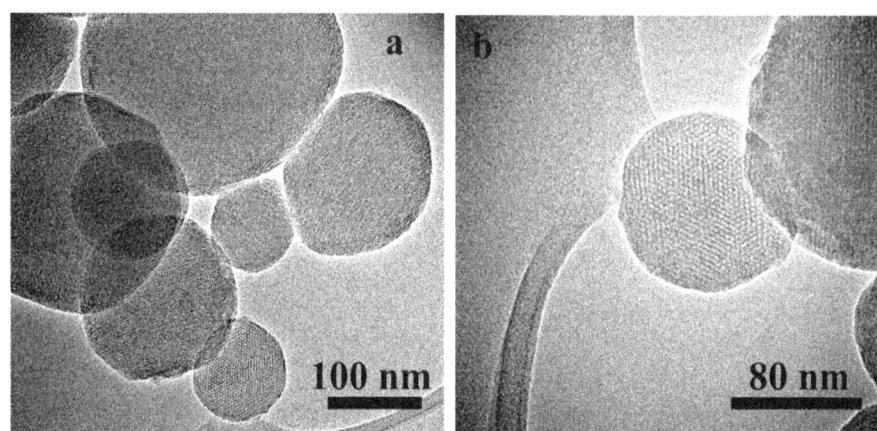

FIGURE 9 | HRTEM images of the MCM-41_B particles coating of BG-based scaffolds at different magnifications. TEM images of few MCM-41_B particles (a) and HRTEM image of a single particle were the ordered mesoporosity was observed (b).

mesoporous silica particles increased the drug incorporation capability, but in both cases most of the drug was released during the first hours of the test. The uncoated BG scaffolds were able to uptake 31 mg$_{IBU}$/g$_{bioglass}$, the scaffolds coated with MCM-41_B could uptake 43 mg$_{IBU}$/g$_{bioglass}$.

Immersion Test

BG-based scaffolds both uncoated and coated with MCM-41_B particles were immersed in SBF at 37°C. After 1 week of immersion, it was possible to observe that the presence of the silica particles did not affect the bioactivity of the (crystallized)

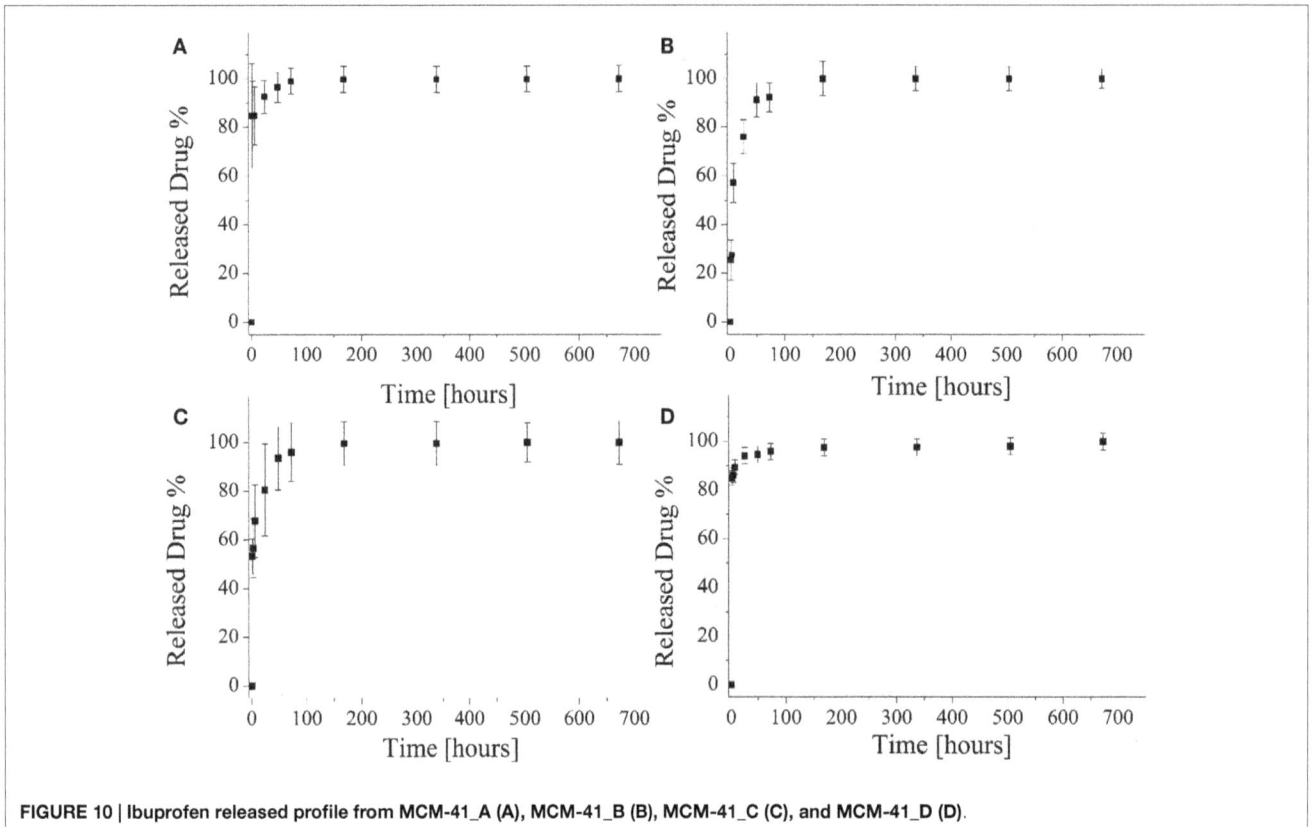

FIGURE 10 | Ibuprofen released profile from MCM-41_A (A), MCM-41_B (B), MCM-41_C (C), and MCM-41_D (D).

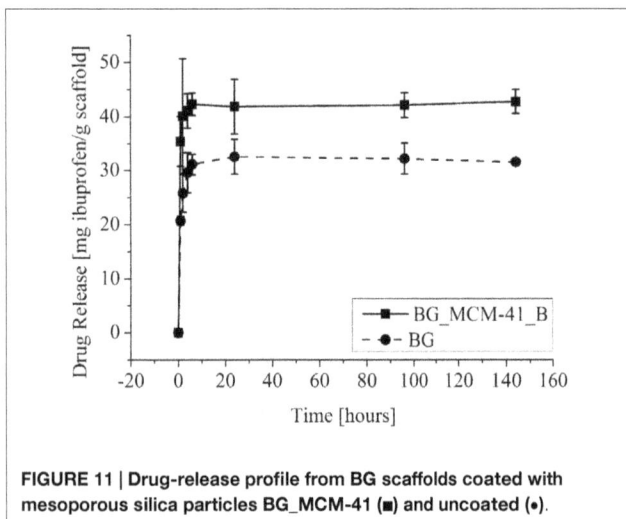

FIGURE 11 | Drug-release profile from BG scaffolds coated with mesoporous silica particles BG_MCM-41 (■) and uncoated (●).

BG struts. In fact on both samples, coated and not coated (**Figure 12a**), a hydroxycarbonate apatite (HCA) layer formation was seen to form (**Figures 12c,d**). Moreover, it was possible to confirm the stability of the MCM-41 coating: after 10 days in Tris buffered solution, it was possible to identify the layer of MCM-41 particles covered with the HCA deposit (**Figure 12e**). The HCA layer was well developed and a deposit was also seen to have formed on the surface of the silica particles (**Figures 12f,g**, black circle).

DISCUSSION

One of the most investigated areas in the bone tissue engineering field is related to the development and characterization of mechanically robust and porous 3D scaffolds. The main challenge is the design of a material able to match at the same time the biological and mechanical properties of the natural bone and also release ions or drugs able to reduce the risk of inflammation and infections after the implantation. In a previous work of Mortera et al. (2008), the possibility to increase the functionality of BG-based porous scaffolds was considered using a coating with MCM-41 particles as drug delivery system. In this way, it was possible to combine in a single system the drug uptake and release capability of mesoporous materials with the bioactivity of BG. In the present work, a further development of this idea was presented, improving the homogeneity of the coating, assessing the bioactivity and stability of the composite system BG_MCM-41. Four different solutions were evaluated for the preparation of mesoporous silica particles, and an optimal synthesis procedure was found (MCM-41_B). In fact, by combining two different synthesis pathways, both well known in literature (Grün et al., 1999; Zeleňák et al., 2008), it was possible to obtain particles characterized by spherical shape and high-ordered mesoporosity as confirmed by HRTEM, SAXRD, and Nitrogen adsorption/desorption analysis (specific surface area 951 m^2 g^{-1}, pore volume 0.24 cm^3 g^{-1}). Moreover, the efficiency of the synthesis was increased and the total amount of produced particles obtained per single batch increased up to 60% compared to the previous

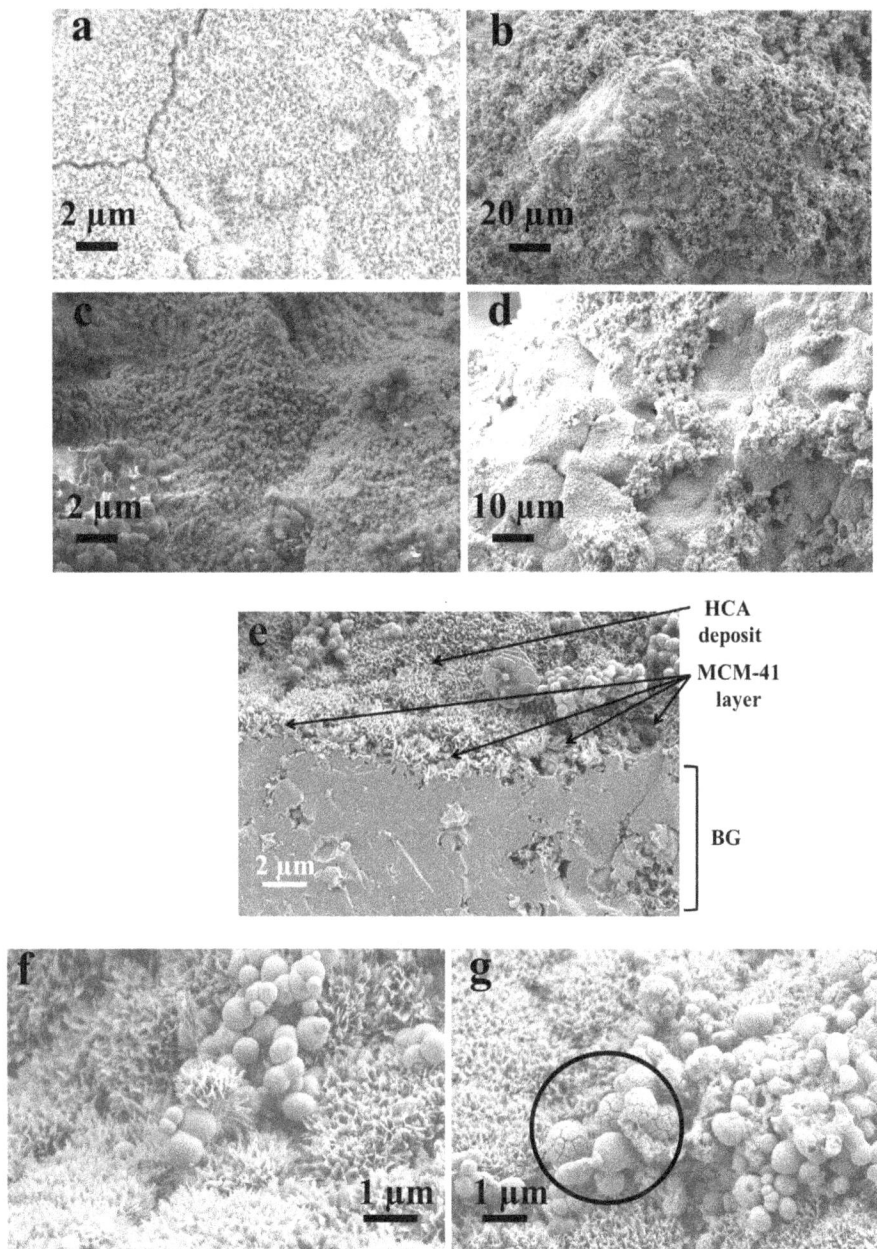

FIGURE 12 | SEM micrographs of BG-based scaffolds uncoated (a) and coated with MCM-41 (b–d) after 1 week in SBF; BG_MCM-41_B scaffolds after immersion in Tris buffered solution for 10 days (e–g).

synthesis procedure: every 500 mL of solution, 4 g of MCM-41_B were produced. MCM-41_B showed the best drug-release profile not exhibiting any burst release during the first hours of the test. The 80% of the loaded drug was in fact released only after 30 h and the rest of the ibuprofen was released within the seven following days. The drug-release times obtained during this work are in agreement with previous studies on drug-release capability of mesoporous silica particles (Vallet-Regí et al., 2001). These novel synthesis solution was used for the coating of 3D BG scaffolds. Due to the high amount of particles produced during

the synthesis, a highly homogeneous coating of the scaffolds was obtained. After the coating procedure, the particles were still spherical in shape and also the ordered mesoporosity was not affected. This was an improvement compared to previous works, in which the coatings were not homogeneously distributed on the surface of the scaffolds and the particles were not characterized by ordered mesoporosity (Mortera et al., 2008). The system BG_MCM-41 was assessed to be bioactive. In fact after 1 week of immersion in SBF on the surface of both coated and not coated scaffolds, a layer of HCA was observed. It has been reported in literature that MCM-41 particles are not bioactive and formation of HCA on their surface was not observed after 2 months of immersion in SBF due to the small pore size and the lower concentration of silanol groups (~2 mmol SiOH m^{-2}) in comparison to other silica particles such as SBA-15 and MCM-48 (Vallet-Regí et al., 2006), which can act as nucleation sites for the apatite layer. This behavior confirms that MCM-41 particles did not have a negative effect on the bioactivity of the BG scaffolds, on the contrary, combined with BG, they seem to enhance the bioactivity. Moreover, most of the MCM-41 particles were still on the surface of the scaffold and some of them are seen to be also coated with HCA in SEM images (**Figures 12f–g**). The MCM-41 particles were in fact adhered to the glass surface due to the thermal treatment: the calcination at 550°C is likely to induce softening of the glass (Lefebvre et al., 2007) which should facilitate adhesion of the MCM-41 spheres. For this reason, the MCM-41 particles coating was stable on the surface of the BG scaffold also after immersion in SBF. Moreover, the presence of the particles on the surface of the BG scaffolds increased the drug uptake capability of the scaffolds compared to the not coated ones. Thanks to the ordered mesoporosity and the pore size in the range of 3 nm, MCM-41 particles were thus confirmed to be an optimal drug delivery carrier.

ACKNOWLEDGMENTS

The authors would like to thank Dipl.-Ing Jürgen Vargas Schmitz (Chair of Separation Science and Technology, University of Erlangen-Nuremberg, Germany) and Dr. Alexandra Inayat (Institute of Chemical Reaction Engineering, University of Erlangen-Nuremberg, Germany) for assistance in N$_2$ physisorption measurements and Lucia Pontiroli (Applied Science and Technology Department, Politecnico di Torino, Italy) for SAXRD analysis.

FUNDING

This research was carried out in the framework of the EU ITN FP-7 project "GlaCERCo." The authors would like to acknowledge its financial support.

REFERENCES

Beck, J. S., Chu, C. T.-W., Johnson, I. D., Kresge, C. T., Leonowicz, M. E., Roth, W. J., (1992). *U.S. Patent* 5 108 725.

Boccardi, E., Philippart, A., Juhasz-Bortuzzo, J. A., Novajra, G., Vitale-Brovarone, C., and Boccaccini, A. R. (2015). Characterisation of Bioglass®-based foams developed via replication of natural marine sponges. *Adv. Appl. Ceram.* doi:10.1179/1743676115Y.0000000036

Cai, Q., Luo, Z., Pang, W., Fan, Y., Chen, X., and Cui, F. (2001). Dilute solution routes to various controllable morphologies of MCM-41 silica with a basic medium. *Chem. Mater.* 10, 258–263. doi:10.1021/cm990661z

Cerruti, M., Greenspan, D., and Powers, K. (2005). Effect of pH and ionic strength on the reactivity of Bioglass® 45S5. *Biomaterials* 26, 1665–1674. doi:10.1016/j.biomaterials.2004.07.009

Chen, Q., Thompson, I., and Boccaccini, A. R. (2006). 45S5 Bioglass-derived glass-ceramic scaffolds for bone tissue engineering. *Biomaterials* 27, 2414–2425. doi:10.1016/j.biomaterials.2005.11.025

Cotí, K. K., Belowich, M. E., Liong, M., Ambrogio, M. W., Lau, Y. A., Khatib, H. A., et al. (2009). Mechanised nanoparticles for drug delivery. *Nanoscale* 1, 16–39. doi:10.1039/b9nr00162j

Grün, M., Lauer, I., and Unger, K. K. (1997). The synthesis of micrometer- and submicrometer-size spheres of ordered mesoporous oxide MCM-41. *Adv. Mater.* 3, 254–257. doi:10.1002/adma.19970090317

Grün, M., Unger, K. K., Matsumoto, A., and Tsutsumi, K. (1999). Novel pathways for the preparation of mesoporous MCM-41 materials: control of porosity and morphology. *Microporous Mesoporous Mater.* 27, 207–216. doi:10.1016/S1387-1811(98)00255-8

Hench, L. L. (2015). Opening paper 2015 – some comments on Bioglass: four eras of discovery and development. *Biomed. Glasses* 1, 1–11. doi:10.1515/bglass-2015-0001

Kokubo, T., and Takadama, H. (2007). How useful is SBF in predicting in vivo bone bioactivity? *Biomaterials* 27, 2907–2915. doi:10.1016/j.biomaterials.2006.01.017

Lefebvre, L., Chevalier, J., Gremillard, L., Zenait, R., Thollet, G., Bernache-Assolant, D., et al. (2007). Structural transformation of bioactive glass 45S5 with thermal treatments. *Acta Biomater.* 55, 3305–3313. doi:10.1016/j.actamat.2007.01.029

Liu, X., Sun, H., Chen, Y., Yang, Y., and Borgna, A. (2009). Preparation of spherical large-particle MCM-41 with a broad particle-size distribution by a modified pseudomorphic transformation. *Microporous Mesoporous Mater.* 121, 73–78. doi:10.1016/j.micromeso.2009.01.018

Mastrogiacomo, M., Scaglione, S., Martinetti, R., Dolcini, L., Beltrame, F., Cancedda, R., et al. (2006). Role of scaffold internal structure on in vivo bone formation in macroporous calcium phosphate bioceramics. *Biomaterials* 27, 3230–3237. doi:10.1016/j.biomaterials.2006.01.031

Misch, K., and Wang, H. L. (2008). Implant surgery complications: etiology and treatment. *Implant Dent.* 17, 159–168. doi:10.1097/ID.0b013e3181752f61

Mortera, R., Onida, B., Fiorilli, S., Cauda, V., Brovarone, C. V., Baino, F., et al. (2008). Synthesis and characterization of MCM-41 spheres inside bioactive glass–ceramic scaffold. *Chem. Eng. J.* 137, 54–61. doi:10.1016/j.cej.2007.07.094

Neut, D., Jim, R., Theo, G., Henny, C., and Henk, J. (2003). Detection of biomaterial-associated infections in orthopaedic joint implants. *Clin. Orthop. Relat. Res.* 413, 261–268. doi:10.1097/01.blo.0000073345.50837.84

Philippart, A., Boccaccini, A. R., Fleck, C., Schubert, D. W., and Roether, J. A. (2015). Toughening and functionalization of bioactive ceramic and glass bone scaffolds by biopolymer coatings and infiltration: a review of the last 5 years. *Expert Rev. Med. Devices* 12, 93–111. doi:10.1586/17434440.2015.958075

Porter, J. R., Ruckh, T. T., and Popat, K. C. (2009). Bone tissue engineering: a review in bone biomimetics and drug delivery strategies. *Biotechnol. Prog.* 25, 1539–1560. doi:10.1002/btpr.246

Slowing, I. I., Trewyn, B. G., Giri, S., and Lin, V. S. Y. (2007). Mesoporous silica nanoparticles for drug delivery and biosensing applications. *Adv. Funct. Mater.* 17, 1225–1236. doi:10.1002/adfm.200601191

Stevens, M. M. (2008). Biomaterials for bone tissue engineering. *Mater. Today* 11, 18–25. doi:10.1016/S1369-7021(08)70086-5

Stober, W., and Fink, A. (1968). Controlled growth of monodisperse silica spheres in the micron size range. *J. Colloid Interface Sci.* 69, 62–69. doi:10.1016/0021-9797(68)90272-5

Vallet-Regí, M. (2006a). Revisiting ceramics for medical applications. *Dalton Trans.* 28, 5211–5220. doi:10.1039/b610219k

Vallet-Regí, M. (2006b). Ordered mesoporous materials in the context of drug delivery systems and bone tissue engineering. *Chemistry* 12, 5934–5943. doi:10.1002/chem.200600226

Vallet-Regí, M., Manzano-García, M., and Colilla, M. (2012a). *Biomedical Applications of Mesoporous Ceramics*. Boca Raton: CRC Press.

Vallet-Regí, M., Izquierdo-Barba, I., and Colilla, M. (2012b). Structure and functionalization of mesoporous bioceramics for bone tissue regeneration and local drug delivery. *Philos. Trans. A Math. Phys. Eng. Sci.* 370, 1400–1421. doi:10.1098/rsta.2011.0258

Vallet-Regí, M., Ramila, A., del Real, R. P., and Perez-Periente, J. (2001). A new property of MCM-41: drug delivery system. *Chem. Mater.* 13, 308–311. doi:10.1021/cm0011559

Vallet-Regí, M., Ruiz-Gonzalez, L., Izquierdo-Barba, I., and Gonzalez-Calbet, J. M. (2006). Revisiting silica based ordered mesoporous materials: medical applications. *J. Mater. Chem.* 16, 26–31. doi:10.1039/B509744D

Vitale-Brovarone, C., Baino, F., Miola, M., Mortera, R., Onida, B., and Verné, E. (2009). Glass-ceramic scaffolds containing silica mesophases for bone grafting and drug delivery. *J. Mater. Sci. Mater. Med.* 20, 809–820. doi:10.1007/s10856-008-3635-7

Wu, C., and Chang, J. (2014). Multifunctional mesoporous bioactive glasses for effective delivery of therapeutic ions and drug/growth factors. *J. Control. Release* 193, 282–295. doi:10.1016/j.jconrel.2014.04.026

Wu, C., Zhou, Y., Chang, J., and Xiao, Y. (2013). Delivery of dimethyloxallyl glycine in mesoporous bioactive glass scaffolds to improve angiogenesis and osteogenesis of human bone marrow stromal cells. *Acta Biomater.* 9, 9159–9168. doi:10.1016/j.actbio.2013.06.026

Zeleňák, V., Badaničová, M., Halamová, D., Čejka, J., Zukal, A., Murafa, N., et al. (2008). Amine-modified ordered mesoporous silica: effect of pore size on carbon dioxide capture. *Chem. Eng. J.* 144, 336–342. doi:10.1016/j.cej.2008.07.025

Zhao, D., Wan, Y., and Zhou, W. (2013). *Ordered Mesoporous Materials*. Wiley-VCH Verlag GmbH & Co. KGaA.

Conflict of Interest Statement: The authors declare that the research was conducted in the absence of any commercial or financial relationships that could be construed as a potential conflict of interest.

6

The long path of human placenta, and its derivatives, in regenerative medicine

Antonietta R. Silini, Anna Cargnoni, Marta Magatti, Stefano Pianta and Ornella Parolini*

Centro di Ricerca "E. Menni", Fondazione Poliambulanza Istituto Ospedaliero, Brescia, Italy

Edited by:
*Martijn Van Griensven,
Technical University Munich,
Germany*

Reviewed by:
*Vasif Nejat Hasirci,
Middle East Technical University,
Turkey
Susanne Wolbank,
Ludwig Boltzmann Institute for
Clinical and Experimental
Traumatology, Austria*

*Correspondence:
*Ornella Parolini
ornella.parolini@poliambulanza.it*

In the 1800s, a baby born with a caul, a remnant of the amniotic sack or fetal membranes, was thought to be lucky, special, or protected. Over time, fetal membranes lost their legendary power and were soon considered nothing more than biological waste after birth. However, placenta tissues have reclaimed their potential and since the early 1900s an increasing body of evidence has shown that these tissues have clinical benefits in a wide range of wound repair and surgical applications. Nowadays, there is a concerted effort to understand the mechanisms underlying the beneficial effects of placental tissues, and, more recently, cells derived thereof. This review will summarize the historical and current clinical applications of human placental tissues, and cells isolated from these tissues, and discuss some mechanisms thought to be responsible for the therapeutic effects observed after tissue and/or cell transplantation.

Keywords: human term placenta, amniotic and chorionic membranes, umbilical cord, stem cells, clinical trials, immunomodulation, paracrine effect, regenerative medicine

A SHORT HISTORY OF THE CLINICAL USES OF HUMAN TERM PLACENTA

Human placenta has been traditionally used in Chinese medicine for centuries. The *Compendium of Materia Medica* was published in *1593* by one of the first and greatest biologists and pharmaceutical experts of China, Li Shi-Zhen (**Figure 1**). This medical text is a Chinese record of substances with medical properties, and it contains a section entirely devoted to the medical uses of human placenta "zi he chi" as a medicine (Young and Benyshek, 2010). At that time, eating the placenta was thought to be beneficial but since then there has been a shift of paradigms in which scientific rationale supports clinical benefit of placental tissues, or derivatives, for treating patients afflicted by a variety of diseases. As discussed below, the earliest reported applications of the placenta (after Li Shi-Zhen's) were focused on fetal membranes. The first reports showing that the placenta also harbors cells, which could have stem/progenitor properties, ultimately giving rise to their potential use in regenerative medicine, were published many years later (**Figure 1**), (Bailo et al., 2004; Fukuchi et al., 2004; Igura et al., 2004; In 't Anker et al., 2004; Soncini et al., 2007; Troyer and Weiss, 2008).

The first documented use of fetal membranes as a surgical material in skin transplantation came more than 3 decades after the placenta was initially reported to possess medicinal properties. In *1910*, Davis (1910) showed that the use of amniotic membrane (AM) in skin grafting gave superior results when compared to xenograft or cadaveric coverings. Shortly afterwards in *1913*, Stern (1913) and Sabella (1913) reported the use of the AM for treating skin wounds. They applied intact amniotic tissues to skin burns and ulcers and then covered them with dressings. Upon removal of the dressings 2 days

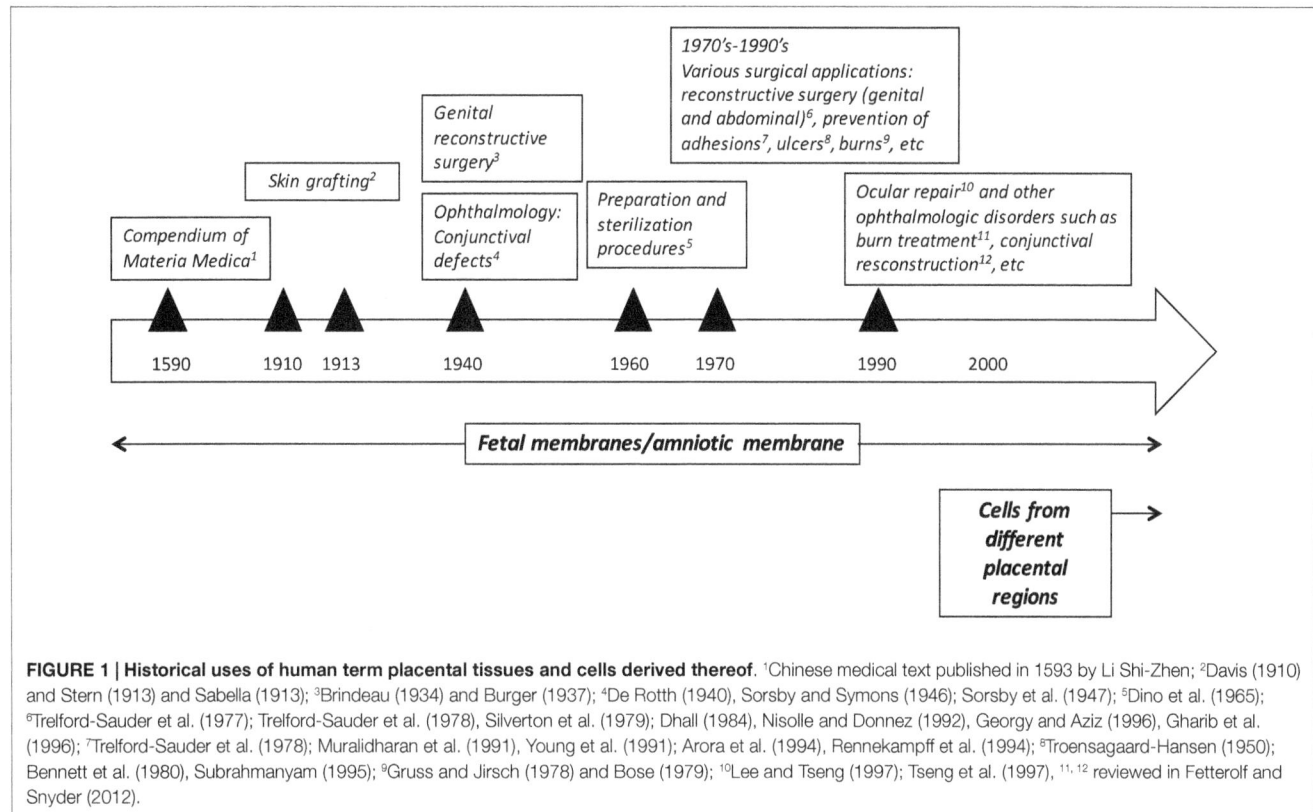

FIGURE 1 | Historical uses of human term placental tissues and cells derived thereof. [1]Chinese medical text published in 1593 by Li Shi-Zhen; [2]Davis (1910) and Stern (1913) and Sabella (1913); [3]Brindeau (1934) and Burger (1937); [4]De Rotth (1940), Sorsby and Symons (1946); Sorsby et al. (1947); [5]Dino et al. (1965); [6]Trelford-Sauder et al. (1977); Trelford-Sauder et al. (1978), Silverton et al. (1979); Dhall (1984), Nisolle and Donnez (1992), Georgy and Aziz (1996), Gharib et al. (1996); [7]Trelford-Sauder et al. (1978); Muralidharan et al. (1991), Young et al. (1991); Arora et al. (1994), Rennekampff et al. (1994); [8]Troensagaard-Hansen (1950); Bennett et al. (1980), Subrahmanyam (1995); [9]Gruss and Jirsch (1978) and Bose (1979); [10]Lee and Tseng (1997); Tseng et al. (1997), [11, 12] reviewed in Fetterolf and Snyder (2012).

later, the authors reported that the amnion had integrated with the patient's tissues. They also reported lack of infection, a significant decrease in pain, and an increased rate of re-epithelialization of the traumatized skin surface in patients treated with amnion.

More than 20 years passed before another study would report the use of amniotic tissues for wound repair or surgery. Around *1940*, the AM was increasingly being used successfully in different applications. In the late 1930s, Brindeau (1934) and Burger (1937) reported the successful use of amnion for vaginal reconstruction surgery in a patient with Mullerian agenesis. Shortly afterwards, the AM was first applied in ophthalmology to repair conjunctival defects (De Rotth, 1940) and burns (Sorsby and Symons, 1946; Sorsby et al., 1947). Ophthalmology would later go on to be one of the most popular applications of the AM to date.

Following these and other studies, between *1940* and *1970,* a number of clinical trials were published reconfirming the successful use of the AM for skin injuries. In *1940*, the first paper was published describing the use of amnion for the prevention of meningocerebral adhesions following head injury. The authors reported lack of adhesions and lack of rejection 60 days after surgery, and "disappearance" of the amnion after 30 days (Chao et al., 1940). Later that decade, and following Burger's work on vaginal reconstruction, Kubanyi (1947) used amnion in patients undergoing abdominal surgery with an enterocutaneus fistula secondary to surgery for lysis of adhesions. After closing the small bowel fistula, the small area of the bowel was wrapped with amnion, and notably, patients were discharged on a regular diet only 12 days after surgery. Importantly, Dino et al. (1965) showed that AM from routine deliveries could be sterilized and kept for

6 weeks at 4°C and safely used on acute second degree burns and on skin donor sites (Dino et al., 1965). This was one of the first reports which suggested handling procedures for the AM, which in turn fueled even more interest among clinicians in using the AM for treating skin lesions.

In *1972*, Trelford et al. (1972) used human amnion in sheep, and confirmed previous findings that as a surface graft, amnion was able to reduce pain, decrease infection, and reduce the loss of fluids. Also in 1972, Robson and his colleagues began to study the use of AM for severe burns and skin injuries. Similar to Trelford, they reported notable pain relief and immediate adherence of the AM dressing to the wound. Interestingly, the membranes were easily peeled off 1 week after application and, according to Robson, spontaneous re-epithelialization had occurred underneath the membranes. Later that decade, in *1977*, Trelford-Sauder et al. (1977) reported the successful use of amnion to replace pelvic peritoneum in patients who had exenterative procedures. Following these and other observations, there was an exponential increase of published clinical studies, which reconfirmed the successful application of fetal membranes in diverse clinical indications, including burns (Gruss and Jirsch, 1978; Bose, 1979), ulcers (Troensagaard-Hansen, 1950; Bennett et al., 1980; Subrahmanyam, 1995), surgical reconstruction of the vagina (Dhall, 1984; Nisolle and Donnez, 1992; Georgy and Aziz, 1996), abdominal surgery (Trelford-Sauder et al., 1978; Silverton et al., 1979; Gharib et al., 1996), and other surgical procedures for the prevention of adhesions (Trelford-Sauder et al., 1978; Muralidharan et al., 1991; Young et al., 1991; Arora et al., 1994; Rennekampff et al., 1994).

The *1990s* can be considered the beginning of modern history on the use of AM in ophthalmology (Dua et al., 2004). In this decade, Dr. Tseng, an ophthalmologist from Miami, applied for Human Cell Tissue Products (HCT/P) regulatory status for the use of amniotic tissues in ocular repair. In 1999, Dr. Tseng's proposal was rejected by the US Food and Drug Administration's (FDA) tissue reference group stating "Amniotic membrane for ocular surface reconstruction is considered a tissue under the current code of federal regulations (CFR) at 21 CFR Part 1270, but the intended use would be non-homologous when 21 CFR Part 1271 becomes effective" (Lee and Tseng, 1997; Tseng et al., 1997). Dr. Tseng appealed the ruling and 1 year later, the FDA reversed the prior ruling stating that "Allogeneic amniotic membrane for ocular repair is considered to be a section 361 HCT/P if the product's advertising is restricted to homologous use for wound covering." The two main points made by the FDA were that it had to be used as a covering and must be acellular, whereas "Amniotic membrane cultured with stem cells for ocular repair is considered to be a biologic product subject to Investigational New Drug and Biologic License Application." From that point on, the use of AM in ophthalmic surgery catapulted. Nowadays, there are over 45,000 applications used by the ophthalmologists, including conjunctival reconstruction, burn treatment, glaucoma surgery, and wound healing (Fetterolf and Snyder, 2012).

CURRENT CLINICAL APPLICATIONS OF PLACENTA

The twenty-first century marks another turning point in which the use of cells isolated from different placental regions are being progressively more investigated and used for their therapeutic potential. These studies have paved the way for what are now considered established clinical uses and investigative clinical trials. Placental tissues, and cells derived thereof, are nowadays interesting therapeutic biomaterials currently used in the clinic. The renewed interest in using the AM in a number of applications has been favored by the development of improved techniques for both membrane cryopreservation (Lee and Tseng, 1997) and advanced isolation and culture procedures for cells derived thereof.

Established Clinical Applications

Recent advances in tissue preservation techniques, accompanied by evidence of therapeutic effects, have resulted in commercially available AM products for use in patients. A repertoire of data shows that these products promote rapid and complete healing of wounds.

Without a doubt, the AM is widely utilized in the field of ophthalmology. The AM is routinely used as a graft, spread onto the ocular surface to treat epithelial defects or ulcers, or as a bandage to cover the ocular surface to promote healing. An infinite number of ocular pathologies are being treated with the AM, such as corneal epithelial defects, corneal ulcers, glaucoma, pterygium, and bullous keratopathy (Dua et al., 2004; Liu et al., 2010; Riau et al., 2010; Kesting et al., 2014). Furthermore, the AM is also making its way in dermatology, where it can be used to cover

burns and to treat chronic ulcers (Lo and Pope, 2009), and in multiple surgical procedures, some of which already mentioned, and others, such as the prevention of post-operative adhesions. The increasing number of case studies will surely support the establishment of a routine use also in the latter two applications.

Clinical Trials

At the time this review was written, 95 clinical trials evaluating placental cells or AM (**Figure 2**; **Tables 1–5**) were registered on the NIH Clinical Trials website (https://clinicaltrials.gov).

Surely, there has been much progress since the first documented use of fetal membranes in the early 1900s, and there have been significant advances in the preparation of amniotic and chorionic membranes for clinical use. In fact, there are many companies which commercialize fetal membranes and/or their derivatives, such as Bio-Tissue®, a subsidiary of TissueTech™ (Prokera®, Amniograft®, Amnioguard®), IOP Ophthalmics (AmbioDisk™, Ambio2™), MiMedx® (Epifix®, Amniofix®), Liventa Bioscience (AmnioClear™), Amniox Medical (NEOX® CORD 1K, Clarix™1K), and NuCel (ReNu™ amniotic allograft), just to name a few.

Recently published reports have provided consistent evidence of the therapeutic benefit of the AM graft. For example, the AM has been successfully used in patients with bullous keratopathy (NCT01926535, completed, **Table 1**), and the results suggested that the technique is safe and represents an efficient alternative to the use of therapeutic contact lenses for the relief of ocular pain in these patients (Venegas et al., 2014). In a different study (NCT00659308, completed, **Table 1**), the AM was shown to be comparable to anterior stromal puncture in the management of pain in patients with bullous keratopathy (Paris Fdos et al., 2013). When tested in patients with scleral thinning, the AM was not as effective as lamellar corneal and scleral transplantation (de Farias et al., 2014), but a phase II/III trial is now enrolling patients for further testing (NCT00801073, **Table 1**).

The use of a dehydrated human amnion/chorion membrane Epifix® (MiMedx®) has been reported to enhance healing and promote complete epithelialization of diabetic foot ulcers (NCT01552499, completed, **Table 2**) (Zelen et al., 2014) and to reduce wound size and improve healing also in patients with venous leg ulcers, both when compared to standard treatment (NCT01552447, completed, **Table 2**) (Serena et al., 2014). This same group also investigated the use of Amniofix® (MiMedx®), a dehydrated human amniotic/chorionic membrane refined by a micronization process, in patients with plantar fasciitis (NCT01659827, completed, **Table 3**) (Zelen et al., 2013). They reported reduced pain and improved physical and mental scores (evaluated by a health survey) versus controls. Interestingly, bovine AM (NCT01895374, completed, **Table 2**) has been tested for the treatment of laser-induced skin wounds, showing once again quicker epithelialization when compared to hydrocolloid-treated wounds (Min et al., 2014), suggesting that xenogenic material can also be used in wound treatment.

As mentioned above, the interest in using cells isolated from different placental regions intensified in the twenty-first century. Different types of placenta-derived cells and factors are being

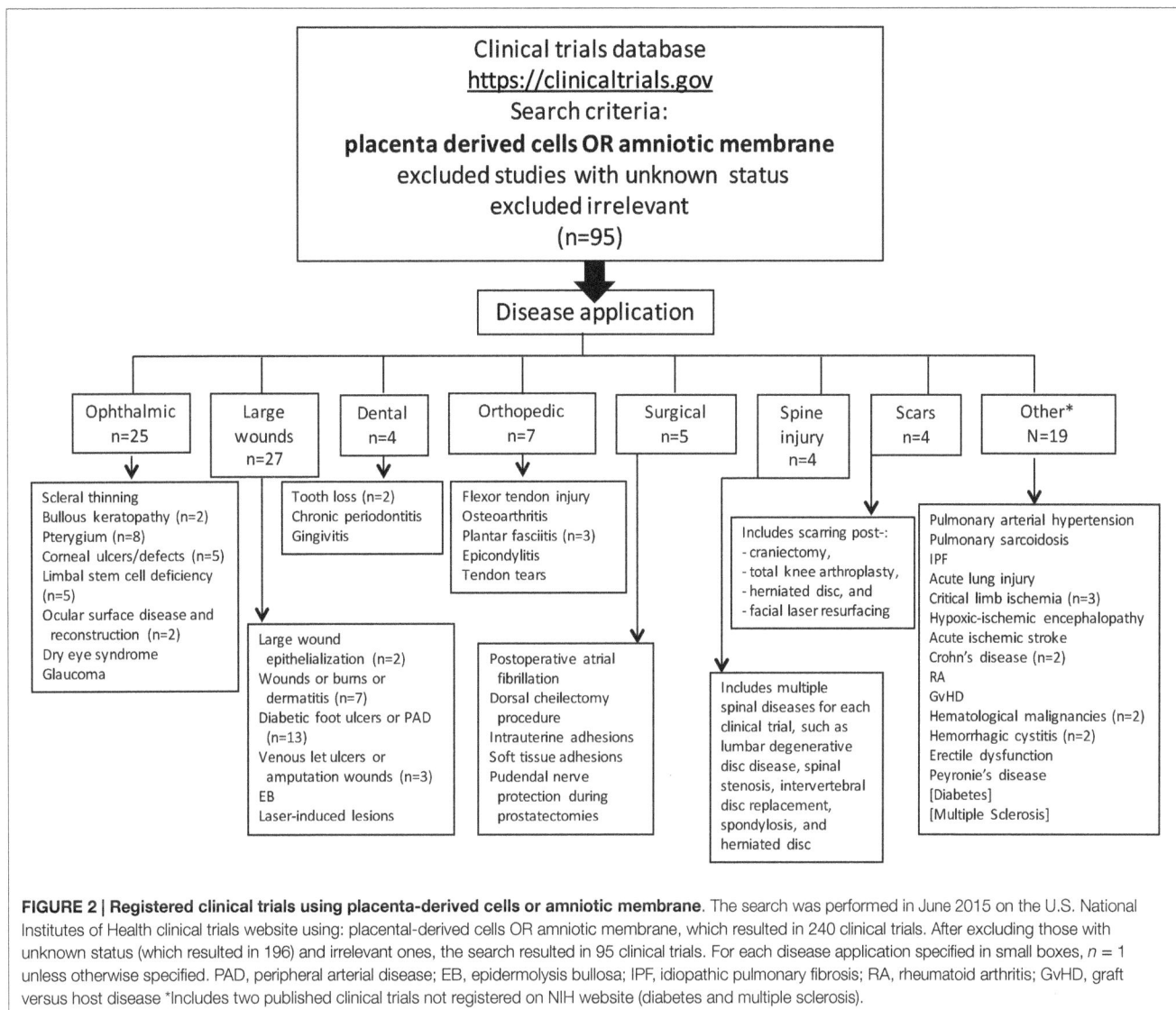

FIGURE 2 | Registered clinical trials using placenta-derived cells or amniotic membrane. The search was performed in June 2015 on the U.S. National Institutes of Health clinical trials website using: placental-derived cells OR amniotic membrane, which resulted in 240 clinical trials. After excluding those with unknown status (which resulted in 196) and irrelevant ones, the search resulted in 95 clinical trials. For each disease application specified in small boxes, *n* = 1 unless otherwise specified. PAD, peripheral arterial disease; EB, epidermolysis bullosa; IPF, idiopathic pulmonary fibrosis; RA, rheumatoid arthritis; GvHD, graft versus host disease *Includes two published clinical trials not registered on NIH website (diabetes and multiple sclerosis).

tested in clinical trials. They come from either fetal placental tissues (such as amnion and chorion) or from maternal tissues (such as decidua). For example, *PLX-PAD* (PLacental eXpanded adherent stromal cells produced by Pluristem Inc.) are isolated from human placenta by enzymatic digestion of both maternal and fetal tissues (Ramot et al., 2009; Kranz et al., 2010). PLX-PAD cells have been used in two clinical trials to treat critical limb ischemia (NCT00919958, completed; NCT00951210, completed), and are now being tested for the treatment of intermittent claudication (NCT01679990, recruiting) and pulmonary arterial hypertension (NCT01795950, active) (**Table 5**). Thus far, no results have been published for the completed trials.

PDA-001/PDA-002 are culture-expanded mesenchymal-like cells produced by Celgene Cellular Therapeutics. The safety and efficacy of PDA001 cells have been studied in patients with Crohn's Disease (Mayer et al., 2013) (NCT01155362, completed; NCT01769755, completed), ischemic stroke (NCT01310114, terminated by sponsor), pulmonary sarcoidosis (NCT01440192,

terminated by sponsor), and active rheumatoid arthritis (NCT01261403, terminated) (**Table 5**). Published results obtained from the Phase I trial (NCT01769755) in patients with Crohn's disease (Mayer et al., 2013) show that out of the six patients treated with low dose and six with high dose, all low dose and two high dose patients responded to the treatment (defined as ≥70 point decrease from baseline in disease activity score). Some minor evidence of infusion-related events, fever, and headache were reported, but no patient withdrew from the study, and PDA001 was well-tolerated (Mayer et al., 2013). A Phase II study (NCT01155362) investigating PDA001 in treatment-resistant Crohn's disease has just been completed, but results are not yet available. PDA001 cells have also been recently tested in patients with multiple sclerosis (Lublin et al., 2014). The published results showed that in all 16 patients, none developed 5 or more new lesions in 2 consecutive monthly MRI scans during a 6-month follow-up. Some infusion-related adverse events, such as hematoma and swelling, occurred and settled without medication. This study is

TABLE 1 | Clinical trials using placenta-derived cells, fetal membranes, or derivatives in ophthalmic disorders.

Condition	Clinical trial ID	Phase	Materials used	Status	Sponsor	Results/status or remarks
Scleral thinning	NCT00801073	II/III	AM graft	Enrolling	Federal University of São Paulo, Brazil	Primary Completion Date: February 2005, last verified December 2008 (de Farias et al., 2014)
Bullous keratopathy	NCT01926535	II	AM graft	Completed	Universidad de Valparaíso, Chile	None available, Study Completion Date: June 2012
	NCT00659308	ns	AM	Completed	Federal University of São Paulo, Brazil	Study Completion Date: June 2007, last verified January 2008 (Paris Fdos et al., 2013)
Pterygium or ocular surface cicatrizing	NCT02102776	ns	AM	Not yet recruiting	Shiyou Zhou, Sun Yat-sen University, China	Estimated Study Completion Date: September 2016
	NCT01319721	ns	AM graft	Completed	Shiyou Zhou, Sun Yat-sen University, China	Results available online (https://clinicaltrials.gov), Study Completion Date: June 2014
diseases or keratitis	NCT00457223	II/III	AM	Completed	Chulalongkorn University, Thailand	None available, study completed in 2007
	NCT00802620	I	AM	Enrolling	Federal University of São Paulo, Brazil	None available, Primary Completion Date: June 2005, last verified December 2008
	NCT02015000	ns	AM	Recruiting	National Taiwan University Hospital, Taiwan	Estimated Study Completion Date: November 2014, last verified December 2013
	NCT00383825	ns	AM	Completed	Baskent University, Ankara, Turkey	None available, Estimated Study Completion Date: December 2004, last verified October 2006
	NCT00344201	I	AM	Completed	Singapore National Eye Centre, Singapore	None available, Study Completion Date: January 2008
	NCT02116062	ns	AM	Recruiting	University Hospital, Strasbourg, France	Estimated Study Completion Date: March 2016
Corneal wounds or ulcers or epithelial defects	NCT00915759	ns	ProKera®	Active	Walter Reed National Military Medical Center, Washington, DC, USA	Estimated Study Completion Date: December 2014, last verified July 2014
	NCT02168790	0	Amnioclip ring system	Completed	Klinikum Chemnitz gGmbH, Germany	None available, Study Completion Date: August 2013
	NCT02388862	ns	AM	Completed	King Khaled Eye Specialist Hospital, Riyadh, Saudi Arabia	None available, study completed in 2007
	NCT02395952	ns	ProKera®, Ambiodisk	Not yet recruiting	Milton S. Hershey Medical Center, PA, USA	Estimated Primary Completion Date: February 2018
	NCT02148016	I/II	AM	Recruiting	Sun Yat-sen University, China	Estimated Study Completion Date: September 2014, last verified May 2014
Limbal stem cell deficiency	NCT01377311	I	AM	Terminated	National Taiwan University Hospital, Taiwan	Study terminated since technique not used in patients, last verified June 2011
	NCT00736307	I/II	AM	Completed	Royan Institute, Tehran, Iran	None available, Study Completion Date: October 2009, last verified April 2010
	NCT01562002	I/II	AM	Completed	Instituto Universitario de Oftalmobiología Aplicada, Spain	None available, Study Completion Date: December 2014, last verified January 2015
	NCT01619189	II	AM	Ongoing	Centre Hospitalier National d'Ophtalmologie des Quinze-Vingts, France	Primary Completion Date: December 2014, last verified February 2015
	NCT00491959	I	AM	Terminated	National Taiwan University Hospital, Taiwan	Study terminated due to unstable cell sheet quality, thus this technique was not used on patients
Ocular surface disease and reconstruction	NCT00348114	II	AM	Completed	Singapore National Eye Centre, Singapore	This study has suspended participant recruitment since 2006
	NCT01341223	ns	AM	Recruiting	National Taiwan University Hospital, Taiwan	Estimated Primary Completion Date: March 2016, last verified March 2012
Dry eye syndrome	NCT02369861	I	ACCS	Recruiting	Stemnion, Inc., Pittsburgh, PA, USA	Estimated Study Completion Date: December 2015
Glaucoma	NCT01551550	II/III	AM graft	Recruiting	Tissue Tech™ Inc., Miami, FL, USA	Estimated Study Completion Date: August 2015

The search status as of June 2015 registered on the ClinicalTrials.gov site of U.S. National Institutes of Health (https://clinicaltrials.gov). ns, not specified; AM, amniotic membrane; ACCS, amnion-derived Cellular Cytokine Solution (Stemnion, Inc.); ProKera® (Tissue Tech™ Inc.) is a device made by a piece of amniotic membrane tissue in between two rings made out of flexible material.

TABLE 2 | Clinical trials using placenta-derived cells, fetal membranes, or derivatives in large wounds.

Condition	Clinical trial ID	Phase	Materials used	Status	Sponsor	Results/status or remarks
Large wound epithelialization	NCT01824381	I	AM	Recruiting	Red de Terapia Cellular, Spain	Estimated Study Completion Date: July 2015, last verified April 2013
	NCT01948934	I	AM	Recruiting	Fundacion para la Formacion e Investigacion Sanitarias de la Region de Murcia, Spain	Estimated Study Completion Date: June 2015, last verified March 2014
Wounds or burns or dermatitis	NCT00674999	II/III	Amnion	Withdrawn	The University of Texas Medical Branch, Galveston, TX, USA	Study was withdrawn prior to enrolling due to skin bank being destroyed by hurricane
	NCT00592189	0	Amnion	Completed	The University of Texas Medical Branch, Galveston, TX, USA	None available, Study Completion Date: June 2014, last verified June 2014
	NCT00886470	I/II	ACCS	Terminated	Stemnion, Inc., Pittsburgh, PA, USA	This study was terminated early due to slow accrual of patients
	NCT01715012	II	ACCS	Terminated	Stemnion, Inc., Pittsburgh, PA, USA	This study was terminated early due to enrollment futility
	NCT02389777	II	ACCS	Not yet recruiting	Stemnion, Inc., Pittsburgh, PA, USA	Estimated Study Completion Date: March 2016
	NCT01714973	I	ACCS	Active	Stemnion, Inc., Pittsburgh, PA, USA	Estimated Study Completion Date: October 2015
	NCT02314416*	IV	Amniotic stem cells	Terminated	Georgia Regents University, Augusta, GA, USA	This study has been withdrawn prior to enrollment
Diabetic foot ulcers or peripheral arterial disease or diabetes	NCT02344329	IV	Amnion	Recruiting	University of North Dakota, USA	Estimated Study Completion Date: August 2016, last verified January 2015
	NCT01859117	I	PDA002	Active	Celgene Corporation, NJ, USA	Ongoing, not recruiting, estimated completion data June 2016
	NCT02460081	II	PDA002	Recruiting	Celgene Corporation, NJ, USA	Estimated Study Completion Date: September 2017
	NCT02264288	II	PDA002	Recruiting	Celgene Corporation, NJ, USA	Estimated Study Completion Date: June 2018
	NCT02399826	ns	AM	Recruiting	Lower Extremity Institute for Research and Therapy, OH, USA	Estimated Study Completion Date: January 2016
	NCT02461641	ns	NuShield, Affinity	Recruiting	NuCel, LLC, Birmingham, AL, USA	Estimated Study Completion Date: September 2016
	NCT02209051	IV	AMNIOEXCEL	Ongoing	Derma Sciences, Inc., NJ, USA	Estimated Study Completion Date: August 2015
	NCT01693133	ns	EpiFix®	Recruiting	MiMedx® Group, Inc., Marietta, GA, USA	Estimated Study Completion Date: July 2015, last verified March 2015
	NCT01552499	ns	EpiFix®	Completed	MiMedx® Group, Inc., Marietta, GA, USA	Study Completion Date: August 2012, last verified September 2012 (Zelen et al., 2014)
	NCT01657474	ns	EpiFix®	Completed	MiMedx® Group, Inc., Marietta, GA, USA	None available, Study Completion Date: November 2013, last verified December 2013
	NCT01921491	ns	EpiFix®	Recruiting	MiMedx® Group, Inc., Marietta, GA, USA	Estimated Primary Completion Date: May 2015
	NCT02120755	IV	AmnioClear™	Not yet recruiting	Liventa Bioscience, Pennsylvania, USA	Estimated Primary Completion Date: January 2015, last verified April 2014
	NCT02166294	ns	NEOX® CORD 1K	Recruiting	Amniox Medical, Inc., Atlanta, GA, USA	Estimated Study Completion Date: June 2015, last verified July 2014
Venous leg ulcers or amputation wounds	NCT01552447	ns	Epifix®	Completed	MiMedx® Group, Inc., Marietta, GA, USA	Study Completion Date: May 2014, last verified November 2013 (Serena et al., 2014)
	NCT02011503	ns	Epifix®	Recruiting	MiMedx® Group, Inc., Marietta, GA, USA	Estimated Study Completion Date: January 2016
	NCT00820274	II	AM	Terminated	University Hospital, Limoges, France	Clinical trial encountered difficulties enrolling a sufficient number of patients
Epidermolysis bullosa	NCT02286427	III	AM	Recruiting	Assistance Publique – Hôpitaux de Paris, France	Estimated Study Completion Date: January 2019
Laser-treatment induced lesions	NCT01895374	ns	Bovine AM	Completed	Seoul National University Hospital, South Korea	Study Completion Date: May 2013, last verified July 2013 (Min et al., 2014)

The search status as of June 2015 registered on the ClinicalTrials.gov site of U.S. National Institutes of Health (https://clinicaltrials.gov).
ns, not specified; AM, amniotic membrane; ACCS, amnion-derived Cellular Cytokine Solution (Stemnion, Inc.); NuShield (NuCel, LLC) is a sterilized dehydrated amnion chorion membrane patch, affinity is an aseptically produced, hypothermically stored amniotic membrane patch. AMNIOEXCEL® (Derma Sciences) is a dehydrated human amnion-derived tissue allograft. EpiFix® (MiMedx®) is a dehydrated Human Amnion/Chorion Membrane. NEOX® CORD (Amniox Medical) is made from cryopreserved human amniotic membrane and umbilical cord. AmnioClear™ (Liventa Bioscience) is an allograft membrane comprising of the amnion and chorion.

TABLE 3 | Clinical trials using placenta-derived cells, fetal membranes, or derivatives in dental and orthopedic defects.

Condition		Clinical trial ID	Phase	Materials used	Status	Sponsor	Results/status or remarks
Dental defects	Tooth loss	NCT01836783	ns	Amnion	Recruiting	University of Alabama at Birmingham, USA	Estimated Study Completion Date: April 2016
		NCT02482987	ns	BioXclude™	Not yet recruiting	Eisenhower Army Medical Center, GA, USA	Estimated Study Completion Date: July 2018
	Chronic periodontitis	NCT02033226	III	AM	Completed	SVS Institute of Dental Sciences, India	None available, Study Completion Date: September 2013; last verified January 2014
	Gingivitis	NCT02071199	I	ACCS	Recruiting	Stemnion, Inc., Pittsburgh, PA, USA	Estimated Study Completion Date: August 2015
Orthopedic defects	Flexor tendon injury	NCT02361814	ns	AM graft	Recruiting	University of Tampere, Finland	Estimated Study Completion Date: December 2016
	Osteoarthritis	NCT02318511	ns	ReNu amniotic allograft	Recruiting	NuCel, LLC, Birmingham, AL, USA	Estimated Study Completion Date: March 2017
	Plantar fasciitis	NCT02427191	II/III	AmnioFix®	Recruiting	MiMedx® Group, Inc., Marietta, GA, USA	Estimated Study Completion Date: December 2017
		NCT01659827	ns	AmnioFix®	Completed	MiMedx® Group, Inc., Marietta, GA, USA	Study Completion Date: March 2013, last verified December 2013 (Zelen et al., 2013)
		NCT01996111	ns	EpiFix®	Terminated	MiMedx® Group, Inc., Marietta, GA, USA	Study terminated due to change in regulatory status
	Epicondylitis	NCT01921569	ns	Micronized dHACM suspension	Terminated	MiMedx® Group, Inc., Marietta, GA, USA	Study terminated by sponsor, used micronized dehydrated human amniotic membrane (dHACM) suspension
	Tendon tears	NCT01708187	ns	Clarix™1k	Terminated	Orthopedic Foot and Ankle Center, OH, USA	Protocol halted due to less than anticipated recruitment

The search status as of June 2015 registered on the ClinicalTrials.gov site of U.S. National Institutes of Health (https://clinicaltrials.gov).
ns, not specified; AM, amniotic membrane; dHACM, dehydrated human amniotic membrane; PAD, peripheral artery disease; ACCS, amnion-derived Cellular Cytokine Solution (Stemnion, Inc.); BioXclude™ (Snoasis Medical, Denver, CO, USA) is a human amnion chorion allograft. ReNu™ (NuTech Medical) is a bioactive suspension derived from human amnion and amniotic fluid. AmnioFix® (MiMedx®) (MiMedx®) is a composite amniotic tissue membrane. PLX-PAD are PLacental eXpanded adherent stromal cells (produced by Pluristem Inc.), Clarix™1k (Amniox Medical), C-HAM is a cryopreserved Human Amniotic Membrane.

TABLE 4 | Clinical trials using placenta-derived cells, fetal membranes, or derivatives in surgery, spinal injuries, and scarring.

Condition		Clinical trial ID	Phase	Materials used	Status	Sponsor	Results/status or remarks
Surgical	Post-operative atrial fibrillation	NCT02193321	I/II	AM patch	Recruiting	University of Arizona, USA	Estimated Study Completion Date: July 2015, last verified July 2014
	Dorsal cheilectomy procedure for Hallux Rigidus	NCT01825356	IV	AM	Recruiting	OrthoCarolina Research Institute, Inc., Charlotte, NC, USA	Estimated Study Completion Date: December 2016, last verified December 2014
	Intrauterine adhesions	NCT02132104	ns	AM graft	Not yet recruiting	Capital Medical University, Beijing, China	Estimated Study Completion Date: November 2016
	Adhesions of soft tissue during the removal of segmental posterior lumbar instrumentation	NCT01357187	ns	AmnioFix®	Completed	MiMedx Group, Inc., Marietta, GA, USA	none available, Study Completion Date: May 2014, last verified June 2014
	Pudendal nerve protection during laparoscopic prostatectomies	NCT01832168	ns	AmnioFix®	Completed	MiMedx Group, Inc., Marietta, GA, USA	None available, Study Completion Date: June 2014, last verified March 2015
Spinal injuries	Various spinal injuries[a]	NCT02070484	ns	NuCel®	Recruiting	OhioHealth, Colombus, OH,USA	Estimated Study Completion Date: February 2016, last verified April 2014
		NCT02381067	ns	NuCel®	Recruiting	NuCel, LLC, Birmingham, AL, USA	Estimated Study Completion Date: September 2016
		NCT02023372	ns	NuCel®	Recruiting	NuCel, LLC, Birmingham, AL, USA	Estimated Study Completion Date: July 2017
	Spinal stenosis and herniated disk	NCT02380456	ns	EpiFix®	Recruiting	Alexander P. Hughes, MD and MiMedx Group, Inc., Marietta, GA, USA	Estimated Study Completion Date: December 2017
Scarring	Scarring post craniectomy	NCT02033824	ns	EpiFix®	Recruiting	MiMedx Group, Inc., Marietta, GA, USA	Estimated Study Completion Date: June 2016
	Scarring post total knee arthroplasty	NCT02088567	ns	EpiFix®	Completed	MiMedx Group, Inc., Marietta, GA, USA	None available, Study Completion Date: October 2014, last verified March 2015
	Scarring/spinal stenosis/herniated disk	NCT02300909	IV	EpiFix®	Recruiting	MiMedx Group, Inc., Marietta, GA, USA	Estimated Study Completion Date: December 2017
	Scarring post laser resurfacing of the face	NCT01995604	ns	EpiFix®	Terminated	MiMedx Group, Inc., Marietta, GA, USA	This study was withdrawn prior to enrollment

The search status as of June 2015 registered on the ClinicalTrials.gov site of U.S. National Institutes of Health (https://clinicaltrials.gov).

ns, not specified; NuCel® (NuCel, LLC) is a bioactive amniotic suspension derived from human amnion and amniotic fluid. EpiFix® (MiMedx®) is a dehydrated Human Amnion/Chorion Membrane (dHACM). AmnioFix® (MiMedx®) is a composite amniotic tissue membrane.

[a]Includes: lumbar degenerative disk disease, spinal stenosis, spondylolisthesis, spondylosis, invertebral disk displacement and degeneration, spinal diseases, bone disease.

TABLE 5 | Clinical trials using placenta-derived cells, fetal membranes, or derivatives in other disorders.

Condition	Clinical trial ID	Phase	Materials used	Status	Sponsor	Results/status or remarks
Lung diseases						
Pulmonary arterial hypertension	NCT01795950	I	PLX-PAD	Recruiting	Pluristem Inc., Haifa, Israel	Estimated Study Completion Date: September 2016
Pulmonary sarcoidosis	NCT01440192	I	PDA001	Terminated	Celgene Corporation, NJ, USA	Study terminated by sponsor
Idiopathic pulmonary fibrosis	NCT01385644	I	Placental MSC	Completed	The Prince Charles Hospital, Brisbane, QLD, Australia	Study Completion Date: May 2013 (Chambers et al., 2014)
Acute lung injury	NCT02175303	I/II	Decidual stromal cells	Recruiting	Karolinska Institutet, Stockholm, Sweden	Estimated Study Completion Date: December 2017
Ischemic diseases						
PAD/peripheral vascular disease/critical limb ischemia	NCT00951210	I	PLX-PAD	Completed	Pluristem Inc., Haifa, Israel	None available, Study Completion Date: October 2011
	NCT01679990	II	PLX-PAD	Recruiting	Pluristem Inc., Haifa, Israel	Estimated Primary Completion Date: December 2015
	NCT00919958	I	PLX-PAD	Completed	Pluristem Inc., Haifa, Israel	None available, Study Completion Date: June 2012
Severe hypoxic–ischemic encephalopathy in neonates	NCT02434965	II	HPDSC	Not yet recruiting	New York Medical College, NY, USA	Estimated Study Completion Date: December 2019
Acute ischemic stroke	NCT01310114	II	PDA001	Terminated	Celgene Corporation, NJ, USA	Study terminated by sponsor
Autoimmune diseases						
Crohn's disease	NCT01155362	II	PDA001	Completed	Celgene Corporation, NJ, USA	None available, Study Completion Date: April 2014, last verified July 2014
	NCT01769755	I	PDA001	Completed	Celgene Corporation, NJ, USA	Study Completion Date: November 2014, last verified April 2015 (Mayer et al., 2013)
Rheumatoid arthritis	NCT01261403	II	PDA001	Terminated	Celgene Corporation, NJ, USA	Enrollment terminated pending additional Phase 1 data
Graft versus host disease	NCT02172924	I/II	Decidual stromal cells	Not yet recruiting	Karolinska Institutet, Stockholm, Sweden	Estimated Study Completion Date: December 2019
Multiple sclerosis	Not applicable	–	PDA001	Published study	–	Lublin et al. (2014)
Diabetes	Not applicable	–	Placenta-derived MSC	Published study	–	Jiang et al. (2011)
Hematological malignancies						
Various[a]	NCT00596999	I	HPDSC	Enrolling	Celgene Corporation, NJ, USA	Estimated Study Completion Date: December 2013, last verified November 2007
Various[b]	NCT01586455	I	HPDSC	Recruiting	New York Medical College, NY, USA	Estimated Study Completion Date: December 2019
Hemorrhagic cystitis						
–	NCT02172963	I/II	Decidual stromal cells	Completed	Karolinska Institutet, Stockholm, Sweden	None available, study completed December 2013
–	NCT02174536	II	Decidual stromal cells	Recruiting	Karolinska Institutet, Stockholm, Sweden	Estimated Study Completion Date: December 2016
Peyronie's disease						
–	NCT02395029	I	PMD-MSC	Completed	Melissa Marchand from Z Urology, Coral Springs, FL, USA	None available, Study completed in March 2015
Erectile dysfunction						
–	NCT02398370	I	PMD-MSC	Completed	Melissa Marchand from Z Urology, Coral Springs, FL, USA	None available, Study completed in March 2015

The search status as of June 2015 registered on the ClinicalTrials.gov site of U.S. National Institutes of Health (https://clinicaltrials.gov).
ns, not specified; AM, amniotic membrane; PMD-MSC, placental matrix-derived mesenchymal stem cells; PLX-PAD are PLacental eXpanded adherent stromal cells (produced by Pluristem Inc.), Clarix™1k (Amniox Medical), HPDSC (human placenta-derived stem cells produced by Celgene Cellular Therapeutics), PDA001 are human placenta-derived adherent cells (Celgene Corporation).
[a]Includes: myelodysplastic syndrome, acute myelogenous/lymphocytic, leukemia, sickle cell disease, beta thalassemia, inborn errors of metabolism, severe combined immunodeficiency disease.
[b]Includes: mucopolysaccharidosis I, mucopolysaccharidosis VI, adrenoleukodystrophy, Niemann–Pick disease, metachromatic leukodystrophy, Wolman disease, Krabbe's disease, Gaucher's disease, fucosidosis, Batten disease, severe aplastic anemia, Diamond–Blackfan anemia, amegakaryocytic thrombocytopenia, myelodysplastic syndrome, acute myelogenous leukemia, acute lymphocytic leukemia.

important in underlining the safety of placental cells in treating patients with multiple sclerosis, and encourages future studies to investigate therapeutic benefit in this physical and mental disabling condition.

PDA002 cells are currently being tested for the treatment of patients with diabetic foot ulcers and peripheral arterial disease (NCT01859117, active; NCT02460081, recruiting; NCT02264288, recruiting) (**Table 2**). Human placenta-derived stem cells (*HPDSC*, also produced by Celgene Cellular Therapeutics) are obtained from placenta perfusion after removal non-viable and red blood cells and tissue debris. These cells are cryopreserved without culture expansion (Kang et al., 2013). HPDSC will soon be investigated for treating neonates with severe hypoxic–ischemic encephalopathy (NCT02434965, not yet recruiting), and patients with hematological malignancies (NCT00596999, enrolling; NCT01586455, recruiting) (**Table 5**).

Placental-derived MSC are isolated from the placental tissues after the removal of umbilical cord and external membranes by enzymatic digestions (Prince Charles Hospital in Brisbane, Australia) (Brooke et al., 2009). The safety of placental-derived MSC has been studied in patients with idiopathic pulmonary fibrosis (IPF, NCT01385644, completed). The results of this study have recently been published and show that intravenous infusion of 2 million cells per kilogram is safe in patients with moderate to severe IPF. Of note, the possibility of embolization of cells in the compromised pulmonary vascular bed, a major concern during this type of treatment, did not lead to major adverse clinical outcomes. Only minor, transient changes in hemodynamics and gas exchange, and only minor adverse events were observed (Chambers et al., 2014).

Placenta-derived decidual stromal cells can be isolated by either trypsin digestion or tissue explants (Karolinska Institutet, Sweden). These cells derive from the decidua parietalis and are of maternal origin (Ringden et al., 2013; Erkers et al., 2015). They have been tested in a pilot study in patients with hemorrhagic cystitis (NCT02172963, completed) and will soon be investigated in a different clinical trial to treat the same disease (NCT02174536, recruiting) (**Table 5**). A clinical trial is also due to begin for the treatment of patients with Graft versus Host Disease (NCT02172924, not yet recruiting). Moreover, a pilot study is currently recruiting patients with acute lung injury to evaluate the safety of placenta DSCs (NCT02175303, recruiting) (**Table 5**).

Remarkably, encouraging results have been published for studies using placenta-derived cells in patients with types II diabetes (**Table 5**) (Jiang et al., 2011). In this Phase I study aimed at evaluating the safety of placenta-derived MSC, 10 patients with type 2 diabetes were given 3 intravenous infusions at the 1-month intervals. The authors reported that the mean insulin requirement was significantly reduced at the 3-month follow-up, and no side effects (fever, chills, liver damage) were documented. This trial could represent a turning point in the use of placental cells, since it is the first to document their use in patients with diabetes. A different study of particular interest was recently published investigating the immunogenicity of placenta decidual stromal cells in combination with AM in an 11-month-old patient with epidermolysis bullosa (Kaipe et al., 2015), showing improved healing of blisters and wounds, but at the same time warranting further investigations on the immunogenicity of these cells.

Notably, other clinical trials have and are currently investigating placental cell derivatives and, in particular *amnion-derived cellular cytokine solution (ACCS)* (Stemnion, Inc., Pittsburgh, PA, USA). ACCS is obtained from amniotic cell culture (Bergmann et al., 2009), and contains factors relevant for wound healing, such as platelet-derived growth factor (PDGF), vascular endothelial growth factor (VEGF), angiogenin, TGF-β2, TIMP-1, and TIMP-2 (Steed et al., 2008). It is currently being tested in patients with radiation-induced dermatitis (NCT01714973, active), and a separate trial is due to begin in patients with UV-induced burns (NCT02389777, not yet recruiting), (**Table 2**). Moreover, other trials are currently recruiting patients to test ACCS in dry eye syndrome (NCT02369861, recruiting, **Table 1**), and gingivitis (NCT02071199, recruiting, **Table 3**). Two trials, the first aimed at investigating ACCS in partial thickness wounds (NCT00886470), and the second in patients with deep burns (NCT01715012), were terminated due to difficulties in enrolling patients (**Table 2**).

Another placenta-derived product, amniotic membrane extract (AMX), which is based on lyophilized human AM for topical application, is under investigation in persistent corneal epithelial defects and has shown promising results for reducing epithelial defects (Kordić et al., 2013).

MECHANISMS OF ACTION: THE QUEST FOR SCIENTIFIC RATIONALE

Evidence of long-term survival with no signs of immune reaction was provided many years ago when the AM was used as an allograft under skin (Douglas et al., 1954) or in the peritoneal cavity (Trelford et al., 1974). Subsequently, a glycoprotein from amnion was reported to be responsible for suppressing "foreign body" reactions by acting on lymphocytes and preventing lymphoblastogenesis (McIntyre and Faulk, 1979).

Since then, numerous mechanisms have been put forth, either to explain the therapeutic effects of the intact or decellularized AM or those of isolated placental cells. Nowadays, the clinical potential of placenta-derived cells essentially relies on their paracrine mechanisms able to induce anti-inflammatory responses and re-epithelialization, and also to possess pro- or anti-angiogenic properties. Below we will briefly discuss these aspects.

Anti-Inflammatory Properties

Among the paracrine actions underlying the anti-inflammatory effect of placenta-derived cells are their interactions with immune cells of innate and adaptive immunity. Indeed, many studies have reported the ability of placenta-derived cells to suppress the proliferation of activated T cells (Bailo et al., 2004; Chang et al., 2006; Wolbank et al., 2007; Prasanna et al., 2010; Kronsteiner et al., 2011a,b), reduce Th1 inflammatory cytokines and induce T regulatory cells (Raicevic et al., 2011; Ohshima et al., 2012; Anam et al., 2013; Parolini et al., 2014; Pianta et al., 2015), and target B lymphocytes (Li et al., 2005; Ma et al., 2012). Furthermore, they can also influence antigen presenting cells by blocking differentiation of monocytes to dendritic cells (Magatti et al., 2009; Tipnis et al., 2010; Kronsteiner et al., 2011a,b; Saeidi et al., 2013; Banas et al., 2014; Abomaray et al., 2015; Donders et al., 2015; Magatti et al., 2015), and induce M2 macrophage differentiation (Manuelpillai et al., 2012; Abumaree et al., 2013; Magatti et al., 2015). Moreover, placenta-derived cells have been shown to inhibit neutrophils (Zhou et al., 2003; Li et al., 2005; Chen et al., 2014), and natural killer cells (Ribeiro et al., 2013; Chatterjee et al., 2014; Li et al., 2015).

Even though the underlying mechanisms are not completely understood, there are numerous studies which have put forth different hypotheses. Herein, we will briefly summarize them, since comprehensive reviews of the interactions between placenta-derived and immune cells have been described elsewhere (Parolini et al., 2009; Parolini et al., 2010; Manuelpillai et al., 2011; Parolini and Caruso, 2011; Prasanna and Jahnavi, 2011; Abumaree et al., 2012; Caruso et al., 2012; La Rocca et al., 2012; Kim et al., 2013; Silini et al., 2013; Insausti et al., 2014). Cells from placental tissues have been shown to produce factors shown to dampen inflammation, such as interleukin (IL)-10 (Kronsteiner et al., 2011a,b; Rossi et al., 2012; Abomaray et al., 2015; Magatti et al., 2015), transforming growth factor (TGF)-β (Liu et al., 2012; Rossi et al., 2012; Pianta et al., 2015), hepatocyte growth factor (HGF) (Najar et al., 2010; Kronsteiner et al., 2011a,b; Raicevic et al., 2011; Yamahara et al., 2014), prostaglandin E2 (PGE2), (Whittle et al., 2000; Chen et al., 2010; Najar et al., 2010; Kronsteiner et al., 2011a,b; Raicevic et al., 2011; Liu et al., 2012; Rossi et al., 2012; Liu et al., 2014; Yamahara et al., 2014; Abomaray et al., 2015), and indoleamine 2,3-dioxygenase (IDO) enzyme (Chang et al., 2006; Rossi et al., 2012; Anam et al., 2013; Donders et al., 2015). Moreover, placenta-derived cells express negative co-signaling proteins B7H3, PD-L1 (CD274), and PD-L2 (CD273), (Petroff and Perchellet, 2010; Tipnis et al., 2010; Kronsteiner et al., 2011a,b; La Rocca et al., 2012; Abumaree et al., 2013; Wu et al., 2014). HLA-G, a molecule known to have immune-regulatory properties through its interactions with immunoglobulin-like transcript (ILT) receptors (ILT-2, ILT-3, ILT-4), (Allan et al., 2000; Hunt et al., 2005), has been reported to be secreted by a variety of placenta-derived cells (Lefebvre et al., 2000; Chang et al., 2006; Banas et al., 2008; Roelen et al., 2009; Kronsteiner et al., 2011a,b; Pratama et al., 2011; Anam et al., 2013; Donders et al., 2015).

On another note, inflammatory cytokines/milieu have been shown to enhance the immunomodulatory properties of placenta-derived cells. For example, interferon (IFN)-γ has been shown to enhance their anti-proliferative properties on PBMC (Chang et al., 2006; Prasanna et al., 2010; Kronsteiner et al., 2011a,b; Donders et al., 2015). IFN-γ has also been shown to increase HLA-G (Lefebvre et al., 2000; Banas et al., 2008; Kronsteiner et al., 2011a,b), PD-L1 and PD-L2 (Banas et al., 2008; Petroff and Perchellet, 2010; Tipnis et al., 2010; Kronsteiner et al., 2011a,b), and PGE2 production by placental cells (Chen et al., 2010). Moreover, IL-1β, a potent inflammatory cytokine, has also been shown to enhance the immune modulatory properties of placental cells, such as through the induction of PGE2 secretion (Mitchell et al., 1993; Fukuda et al.,

1999; Pomini et al., 1999; Chen et al., 2010, Phillips et al., 2011), and by enhancing their suppressive activities toward NK cells (Chatterjee et al., 2014).

Pro- and Anti-Angiogenic Properties

The intact AM has been shown to produce an array of anti-angiogenic factors. This property is epitomized in the use of intact AM for corneal surface reconstruction, where the use of AM decreases vascularization of the ocular surface through the production of anti-angiogenic proteins (Kim and Tseng, 1995; Shao et al., 2004), such as pigment epithelium-derived factor (PEDF), (Kim and Tseng, 1995; Dawson et al., 1999; Shao et al., 2004), tissue inhibitor of metalloproteinase (TIMP)-1 and TIMP-2 (Hao et al., 2000), and thrombospondin-1 (TSP-1), (Zaslavsky et al., 2010). The intact AM has also been reported to have a large amount of ECM proteins (i.e., laminin-1, laminin-5, fibronectin), which are involved in the suppression of neovascularization in the cornea (Fukuda et al., 1999).

Decellularized AM, whereby amniotic epithelial cells are eliminated and the cytokine-rich ECM is retained, has been shown to maintain anti-angiogenic properties (Tseng et al., 2004).

Furthermore, epithelial and mesenchymal cells isolated from the AM have also been shown to produce anti-angiogenic factors, such as TIMP-1, TIMP-2, TSP-1, and endostatin (Rowe et al., 1997; Hao et al., 2000).

On the other hand, pro-angiogenic properties have also been attributed to the AM, which can be considered important contributors to its wound healing and regenerative capabilities. For example, cytokines known to promote angiogenesis have been found in dehydrated human amnion/chorion membrane, such as angiopoietin-2, epidermal growth factor (EGF), basic fibroblast growth factor (bFGF), heparin binding epidermal growth factor (HB-EGF), HGF, platelet-derived growth factor BB (PDGF-BB), placental growth factor (PlGF), and VEGF (Koob et al., 2014b). Recently, pro-angiogenic factors have been found in conditioned medium from MSC isolated from the AM, which was shown to not only limit infarct size but also promote capillary formation at the infarct border zone when injected into infarcted rat hearts (Danieli et al., 2015). These apparently contradictory properties could give rise to the importance of understanding the impact of the microenvironment in determining the pro- or anti-angiogenic abilities of the AM and placental cells.

Promotion of Epithelialization

Another important, and well-documented, property of the intact AM is its ability to promote re-epithelialization. The intact AM has been used as a basement membrane to promote epithelial cell migration, differentiation, and prevent epithelial cell apoptosis (Dua et al., 2004). In addition, it produces factors that can stimulate epithelialization, such as bFGF, HGF, and TGFβ (Dua and Azuara-Blanco, 1999; Koizumi et al., 2000). The intact AM also produces factors that support the growth and differentiation of stem and progenitor cells (Meller et al., 2000; Meller et al., 2002; Insausti et al., 2010), such as keratinocyte growth factor (KGF) (Casey and MacDonald, 1997), supporting its use as a progenitor cell niche (Tseng et al., 2004).

Furthermore, dehydrated human amnion/chorion membrane, which preserves ECM composition and retains an array of cytokines, chemokines, and growth factors naturally present in the native tissue, was found to preserve re-epithelialization properties (Koob et al., 2014a).

Studies performed on the AM denuded of epithelial cells have shown significantly lower levels of bFGF, HGF, EGF, and KGF, when compared to intact AM, suggesting an epithelial origin of these factors (Koizumi et al., 2000). Among other ECM proteins found in AM, fibronectin, laminins, and collagen IV and VII have also been reported, which can in turn promote epithelial adhesion and migration (Fukuda et al., 1999; Lobert et al., 2010).

Cells of the AM have also been suggested to promote epithelialization through secretion/production of factors, which can direct migration, proliferation, and differentiation of keratinocytes. In particular, human amniotic mesenchymal cells (hAMSC) and epithelial cells (hAEC) can secrete factors crucial for wound healing. hAMSC highly express EGF, a factor known for its role in keratinocyte and fibroblast migration, IL-8 that promotes re-epithelialization by increasing keratinocyte proliferation and migration, and IGF-1 that is involved in wound closure by promoting the growth of endothelial cells, dermal fibroblasts, and keratinocytes (Kim et al., 2012).

High expression of EGF and PDGF has also been reported in hAEC, the latter of which stimulates the chemotaxis and proliferation of fibroblasts, and is a critical regulator of ECM deposition in healing wounds (Jin et al., 2015). Both hAMSC and hAEC have been shown to engraft into the wound area thus potentially enhancing their paracrine effects and, furthermore, they could directly participate in re-epithelialization by their trans-differentiation into keratinocytes (Kim et al., 2012; Jin et al., 2015).

CONCLUDING REMARKS

Although there are still many open questions regarding the *sine qua non* conditions for the clinical use of placental cells (Fierabracci et al., 2015), the increasing number of clinical trials underlines the interest in using them. Ongoing and future studies will be crucial in helping define their molecular mechanisms, and establishing the true value of placental derivatives (AM, cells, or molecules they release). These studies will undoubtedly unveil additional applications in the field of regenerative medicine. Studies on placental derivatives available thus far have surely contributed to the vision of regenerative medicine, not only based on cell replacement but also on the importance of their paracrine effects, which could promote endogenous tissue regeneration.

AUTHOR CONTRIBUTIONS

AS, AC, MM, SP, and OP contributed to writing the manuscript, OP gave final approval of the version to be published. All authors read and approved the manuscript.

ACKNOWLEDGMENTS

The authors would like to thank *Fondazione Poliambulanza-Istituto Ospedaliero* of Brescia, and all mothers who donated their baby's placentas for research. This work was supported by Fondazione Poliambulanza-Istituto Ospedaliero, Brescia, Italy, Cariplo Foundation (grant no. 2012-0842), Italian Ministry of Health call "Ricerca Finalizzata" (Project code: RF-2010-2315681), and Competitiveness ROP ERDF 2007-2013 of Lombardy Region (Regional Operational Programme of the European Regional Development Fund – Progetto NUTEC NUove TECnologie ID no. 30263049).

REFERENCES

Abomaray, F. M., Al Jumah, M. A., Kalionis, B., AlAskar, A. S., Al Harthy, S., Jawdat, D., et al. (2015). Human chorionic villous mesenchymal stem cells modify the functions of human dendritic cells, and induce an anti-inflammatory phenotype in CD1+ dendritic cells. Stem Cell. Rev. 11, 423–441. doi:10.1007/s12015-014-9562-8

Abumaree, M., Al Jumah, M., Pace, R. A., and Kalionis, B. (2012). Immunosuppressive properties of mesenchymal stem cells. Stem Cell. Rev. 8, 375–392. doi:10.1007/s12015-011-9312-0

Abumaree, M. H., Al Jumah, M. A., Kalionis, B., Jawdat, D., Al Khaldi, A., Abomaray, F. M., et al. (2013). Human placental mesenchymal stem cells (pMSCs) play a role as immune suppressive cells by shifting macrophage differentiation from inflammatory M1 to anti-inflammatory M2 macrophages. Stem Cell. Rev. 9, 620–641. doi:10.1007/s12015-013-9455-2

Allan, D. S., McMichael, A. J., and Braud, V. M. (2000). The ILT family of leukocyte receptors. Immunobiology 202, 34–41. doi:10.1016/S0171-2985(00)80050-9

Anam, K., Lazdun, Y., Davis, P. M., Banas, R. A., Elster, E. A., and Davis, T. A. (2013). Amnion-derived multipotent progenitor cells support allograft tolerance induction. Am. J. Transplant. 13, 1416–1428. doi:10.1111/ajt.12252

Arora, M., Jaroudi, K. A., Hamilton, C. J., and Dayel, F. (1994). Controlled comparison of interceed and amniotic membrane graft in the prevention of postoperative adhesions in the rabbit uterine horn model. Eur. J. Obstet. Gynecol. Reprod. Biol. 55, 179–182. doi:10.1016/0028-2243(94)90035-3

Bailo, M., Soncini, M., Vertua, E., Signoroni, P. B., Sanzone, S., Lombardi, G., et al. (2004). Engraftment potential of human amnion and chorion cells derived from term placenta. Transplantation 78, 1439–1448. doi:10.1097/01.TP.0000144606.84234.49

Banas, R., Miller, C., Guzik, L., and Zeevi, A. (2014). Amnion-derived multipotent progenitor cells inhibit blood monocyte differentiation into mature dendritic cells. Cell Transplant. 23, 1111–1125. doi:10.3727/096368913X670165

Banas, R. A., Trumpower, C., Bentlejewski, C., Marshall, V., Sing, G., and Zeevi, A. (2008). Immunogenicity and immunomodulatory effects of amnion-derived multipotent progenitor cells. Hum. Immunol. 69, 321–328. doi:10.1016/j.humimm.2008.04.007

Bennett, J. P., Matthews, R., and Faulk, W. P. (1980). Treatment of chronic ulceration of the legs with human amnion. Lancet 1, 1153–1156. doi:10.1016/S0140-6736(80)91616-5

Bergmann, J., Hackl, F., Koyama, T., Aflaki, P., Smith, C. A., Robson, M. C., et al. (2009). The effect of amnion-derived cellular cytokine solution on the epithelialization of partial-thickness donor site wounds in normal and streptozotocin-induced diabetic swine. Eplasty 9, e49.

Bose, B. (1979). Burn wound dressing with human amniotic membrane. Ann. R. Coll. Surg. Engl. 61, 444–447.

Brindeau, A. (1934). Creation d'un vagin artificiel A l'aide des membranes ovulaires d'un oeuf a terme. J. Gynecol. Obstet. Biol. Reprod (Paris) 13, 821–824.

Brooke, G., Rossetti, T., Pelekanos, R., Ilic, N., Murray, P., Hancock, S., et al. (2009). Manufacturing of human placenta-derived mesenchymal stem cells for clinical trials. Br. J. Haematol. 144, 571–579. doi:10.1111/j.1365-2141.2008.07492.x

Burger, K. (1937). Weitere erfahrungen iiber die kunstliche scheidenbildung mit eihauten. Zentralbl. Gynäkol. 69, 1153–1154.

Caruso, M., Evangelista, M., and Parolini, O. (2012). Human term placental cells: phenotype, properties and new avenues in regenerative medicine. *Int. J. Mol. Cell Med.* 1, 64–74.

Casey, M. L., and MacDonald, P. C. (1997). Keratinocyte growth factor expression in the mesenchymal cells of human amnion. *J. Clin. Endocrinol. Metab.* 82, 3319–3323. doi:10.1210/jcem.82.1.3668

Chambers, D. C., Enever, D., Ilic, N., Sparks, L., Whitelaw, K., Ayres, J., et al. (2014). A phase 1b study of placenta-derived mesenchymal stromal cells in patients with idiopathic pulmonary fibrosis. *Respirology* 19, 1013–1018. doi:10.1111/resp.12343

Chang, C. J., Yen, M. L., Chen, Y. C., Chien, C. C., Huang, H. I., Bai, C. H., et al. (2006). Placenta-derived multipotent cells exhibit immunosuppressive properties that are enhanced in the presence of interferon-gamma. *Stem Cells* 24, 2466–2477. doi:10.1634/stemcells.2004-0308

Chao, Y.-C., Humphreys, S., and Penfield, W. (1940). A new method of preventing adhesions. The use of amnioplastin after craniotomy. *Br. Med. J.* 1, 517. doi:10.1136/bmj.1.4134.517

Chatterjee, D., Marquardt, N., Tufa, D. M., Beauclair, G., Low, H. Z., Hatlapatka, T., et al. (2014). Role of gamma-secretase in human umbilical-cord derived mesenchymal stem cell mediated suppression of NK cell cytotoxicity. *Cell Commun. Signal.* 12, 63. doi:10.1186/s12964-014-0063-9

Chen, C. P., Chen, Y. Y., Huang, J. P., and Wu, Y. H. (2014). The effect of conditioned medium derived from human placental multipotent mesenchymal stromal cells on neutrophils: possible implications for placental infection. *Mol. Hum. Reprod.* 20, 1117–1125. doi:10.1093/molehr/gau062

Chen, K., Wang, D., Du, W. T., Han, Z. B., Ren, H., Chi, Y., et al. (2010). Human umbilical cord mesenchymal stem cells hUC-MSCs exert immunosuppressive activities through a PGE2-dependent mechanism. *Clin. Immunol.* 135, 448–458. doi:10.1016/j.clim.2010.01.015

Danieli, P., Malpasso, G., Ciuffreda, M. C., Cervio, E., Calvillo, L., Copes, F., et al. (2015). Conditioned medium from human amniotic mesenchymal stromal cells limits infarct size and enhances angiogenesis. *Stem Cells Transl. Med.* 4, 448–458. doi:10.5966/sctm.2014-0253

Davis, J. (1910). Skin transplantation with a review of 550 cases at the Johns Hopkins hospital. *Johns Hopkins Med. J.* 15, 15.

Dawson, D. W., Volpert, O. V., Gillis, P., Crawford, S. E., Xu, H., Benedict, W., et al. (1999). Pigment epithelium-derived factor: a potent inhibitor of angiogenesis. *Science* 285, 245–248. doi:10.1126/science.285.5425.245

de Farias, C. C., Sterlenich, T., de Sousa, L. B., Vieira, L. A., and Gomes, J. A. (2014). Randomized trial comparing multilayer amniotic membrane transplantation with scleral and corneal grafts for the treatment of scleral thinning after pterygium surgery associated with beta therapy. *Cornea* 33, 1197–1204. doi:10.1097/ICO.0000000000000207

De Rotth, A. (1940). Plastic repair of conjunctival defects with fetal membranes. *Arch. Ophthalmol.* 23, 522. doi:10.1097/ICO.0b013e318156cb08

Dhall, K. (1984). Amnion graft for treatment of congenital absence of the vagina. *Br. J. Obstet. Gynaecol.* 91, 279–282. doi:10.1111/j.1471-0528.1984.tb04768.x

Dino, B., Eufemio, G., De Villa, M., Reysio-Cruz, M., and Jurado, R. (1965). The use of fetal membrane homografts in the local management of burns. *J. Philipp. Med. Assoc.* 41, 890.

Donders, R., Vanheusden, M., Bogie, J. F., Ravanidis, S., Thewissen, K., Stinissen, P., et al. (2015). Human Wharton's jelly-derived stem cells display immunomodulatory properties and transiently improve rat experimental autoimmune encephalomyelitis. *Cell Transplant.* 24, 2077–2098. doi:10.3727/096368914X685104

Douglas, B., Conway, H., Stark, R. B., Joslin, D., and Nieto-Cano, G. (1954). The fate of homologous and heterologous chorionic transplants as observed by the transparent tissue chamber technique in the mouse. *Plast. Reconstr. Surg.* 13, 125–129. doi:10.1097/00006534-195402000-00005

Dua, H. S., and Azuara-Blanco, A. (1999). Amniotic membrane transplantation. *Br. J. Ophthalmol.* 83, 748–752. doi:10.1136/bjo.83.7.885a

Dua, H. S., Gomes, J. A., King, A. J., and Maharajan, V. S. (2004). The amniotic membrane in ophthalmology. *Surv. Ophthalmol.* 49, 51–77. doi:10.1016/j.survophthal.2003.10.004

Erkers, T., Kaipe, H., Nava, S., Mollden, P., Gustafsson, B., Axelsson, R., et al. (2015). Treatment of severe chronic graft-versus-host disease with decidual stromal cells and tracing with (111)indium radiolabeling. *Stem Cells Dev.* 24, 253–263. doi:10.1089/scd.2014.0265

Fetterolf, D. E., and Snyder, R. J. (2012). Scientific and clinical support for the use of dehydrated amniotic membrane in wound management. *Wounds* 24, 299–307.

Fierabracci, A., Lazzari, L., Muraca, M., and Parolini, O. (2015). How far are we from the clinical use of placental-derived mesenchymal stem cells? *Expert Opin. Biol. Ther.* 15, 613–617. doi:10.1517/14712598.2015.1000856

Fukuchi, Y., Nakajima, H., Sugiyama, D., Hirose, I., Kitamura, T., and Tsuji, K. (2004). Human placenta-derived cells have mesenchymal stem/progenitor cell potential. *Stem Cells* 22, 649–658. doi:10.1634/stemcells.22-5-649

Fukuda, K., Chikama, T., Nakamura, M., and Nishida, T. (1999). Differential distribution of subchains of the basement membrane components type IV collagen and laminin among the amniotic membrane, cornea, and conjunctiva. *Cornea* 18, 73–79. doi:10.1097/00003226-199901000-00013

Georgy, M., and Aziz, N. (1996). Vaginoplasty using amnion graft: new surgical technique using the laparoscopic transillumination light. *J. Obstet. Gynaecol.* 16, 262–264. doi:10.3109/01443619609020728

Gharib, M., Ure, B. M., and Klose, M. (1996). Use of amniotic grafts in the repair of gastroschisis. *Pediatr. Surg. Int.* 11, 96–99. doi:10.1007/BF00183734

Gruss, J. S., and Jirsch, D. W. (1978). Human amniotic membrane: a versatile wound dressing. *Can. Med. Assoc. J.* 118, 1237–1246.

Hao, Y., Ma, D. H., Hwang, D. G., Kim, W. S., and Zhang, F. (2000). Identification of antiangiogenic and antiinflammatory proteins in human amniotic membrane. *Cornea* 19, 348–352. doi:10.1097/00003226-200005000-00018

Hunt, J. S., Petroff, M. G., McIntire, R. H., and Ober, C. (2005). HLA-G and immune tolerance in pregnancy. *FASEB J.* 19, 681–693. doi:10.1096/fj.04-2078rev

Igura, K., Zhang, X., Takahashi, K., Mitsuru, A., Yamaguchi, S., and Takashi, T. A. (2004). Isolation and characterization of mesenchymal progenitor cells from chorionic villi of human placenta. *Cytotherapy* 6, 543–553. doi:10.1080/14653240410005366-1

In 't Anker, P. S., Scherjon, S. A., Kleijburg-van der Keur, C., de Groot-Swings, G. M., Claas, F. H., Fibbe, W. E., et al. (2004). Isolation of mesenchymal stem cells of fetal or maternal origin from human placenta. *Stem Cells* 22, 1338–1345. doi:10.1634/stemcells.2004-0058

Insausti, C. L., Alcaraz, A., Garcia-Vizcaino, E. M., Mrowiec, A., Lopez-Martinez, M. C., Blanquer, M., et al. (2010). Amniotic membrane induces epithelialization in massive posttraumatic wounds. *Wound Repair Regen.* 18, 368–377. doi:10.1111/j.1524-475X.2010.00604.x

Insausti, C. L., Blanquer, M., Garcia-Hernandez, A. M., Castellanos, G., and Moraleda, J. M. (2014). Amniotic membrane-derived stem cells: immunomodulatory properties and potential clinical application. *Stem Cells Cloning* 7, 53–63. doi:10.2147/SCCAA.S58696

Jiang, R., Han, Z., Zhuo, G., Qu, X., Li, X., Wang, X., et al. (2011). Transplantation of placenta-derived mesenchymal stem cells in type 2 diabetes: a pilot study. *Front. Med.* 5:94–100. doi:10.1007/s11684-011-0116-z

Jin, E., Kim, T. H., Han, S., and Kim, S. W. (2015). Amniotic epithelial cells promote wound healing in mice through high epithelialization and engraftment. *J. Tissue Eng. Regen. Med.* doi:10.1002/term.2069

Kaipe, H., Carlson, L. M., Erkers, T., Nava, S., Mollden, P., Gustafsson, B., et al. (2015). Immunogenicity of decidual stromal cells in an epidermolysis bullosa patient and in allogeneic hematopoietic stem cell transplantation patients. *Stem Cells Dev.* 24, 1471–1482. doi:10.1089/scd.2014.0568

Kang, L., Voskinarian-Berse, V., Law, E., Reddin, T., Bhatia, M., Hariri, A., et al. (2013). Characterization and ex vivo expansion of human placenta-derived natural killer cells for cancer immunotherapy. *Front. Immunol.* 4:101. doi:10.3389/fimmu.2013.00101

Kesting, M. R., Wolff, K. D., Nobis, C. P., and Rohleder, N. H. (2014). Amniotic membrane in oral and maxillofacial surgery. *Oral Maxillofac. Surg.* 18, 153–164. doi:10.1007/s10006-012-0382-1

Kim, D. W., Staples, M., Shinozuka, K., Pantcheva, P., Kang, S. D., and Borlongan, C. V. (2013). Wharton's jelly-derived mesenchymal stem cells: phenotypic characterization and optimizing their therapeutic potential for clinical applications. *Int. J. Mol. Sci.* 14, 11692–11712. doi:10.3390/ijms140611692

Kim, J. C., and Tseng, S. C. (1995). The effects on inhibition of corneal neovascularization after human amniotic membrane transplantation in severely damaged rabbit corneas. *Korean J. Ophthalmol.* 9, 32–46. doi:10.3341/kjo.1995.9.1.12

Kim, S. W., Zhang, H. Z., Guo, L., Kim, J. M., and Kim, M. H. (2012). Amniotic mesenchymal stem cells enhance wound healing in diabetic NOD/SCID mice through high angiogenic and engraftment capabilities. *PLoS ONE* 7:e41105. doi:10.1371/journal.pone.0041105

Koizumi, N. J., Inatomi, T. J., Sotozono, C. J., Fullwood, N. J., Quantock, A. J., and Kinoshita, S. (2000). Growth factor mRNA and protein in preserved human amniotic membrane. *Curr. Eye Res.* 20, 173–177. doi:10.1076/0271-3683(200003)2031-9FT173

Koob, T. J., Lim, J. J., Massee, M., Zabek, N., and Denoziere, G. (2014a). Properties of dehydrated human amnion/chorion composite grafts: Implications for wound repair and soft tissue regeneration. *J. Biomed. Mater. Res. Part B Appl. Biomater.* 102, 1353–1362. doi:10.1002/jbm.b.33141

Koob, T. J., Lim, J. J., Massee, M., Zabek, N., Rennert, R., Gurtner, G., et al. (2014b). Angiogenic properties of dehydrated human amnion/chorion allografts: therapeutic potential for soft tissue repair and regeneration. *Vasc. Cell* 6, 10. doi:10.1186/2045-824X-6-10

Kordić, R., Suić, S. P., Jandroković, S., Kalauz, M., Kuzman, T., Skegro, I., et al. (2013). Application of the amniotic membrane extract (AMX) for the persistent epithelial defect (PED) of the cornea. *Coll. Antropol.* 37(Suppl. 1), 161–164.

Kranz, A., Wagner, D. C., Kamprad, M., Scholz, M., Schmidt, U. R., Nitzsche, F., et al. (2010). Transplantation of placenta-derived mesenchymal stromal cells upon experimental stroke in rats. *Brain Res.* 1315, 128–136. doi:10.1016/j.brainres.2009.12.001

Kronsteiner, B., Peterbauer-Scherb, A., Grillari-Voglauer, R., Redl, H., Gabriel, C., van Griensven, M., et al. (2011a). Human mesenchymal stem cells and renal tubular epithelial cells differentially influence monocyte-derived dendritic cell differentiation and maturation. *Cell. Immunol.* 267, 30–38. doi:10.1016/j.cellimm.2010.11.001

Kronsteiner, B., Wolbank, S., Peterbauer, A., Hackl, C., Redl, H., Griensven, M. V., et al. (2011b). Human mesenchymal stem cells from adipose tissue and amnion influence T-cells depending on stimulation method and presence of other immune cells. *Stem Cells Dev.* 20, 2115–2126. doi:10.1089/scd.2011.0031

Kubanyi, A. (1947). Prevention of peritoneal adhesions by transplantation of amnion. *Br. Med. J.* 2, 55. doi:10.1136/bmj.2.4514.55-a

La Rocca, G., Corrao, S., Lo Iacono, M., Corsello, T., Farina, F., and Anzalone, R. (2012). Novel immunomodulatory markers expressed by human WJ-MSC: an updated review in regenerative and reparative medicine. *Open Tissue Eng. Regen. Med. J.* 5, 50–58. doi:10.2174/1875043501205010050

Lee, S.-H., and Tseng, S. C. (1997). Amniotic membrane transplantation for persistent epithelial defects with ulceration. *Am. J. Ophthalmol.* 123, 303–312. doi:10.1016/S0002-9394(14)70125-4

Lefebvre, S., Adrian, F., Moreau, P., Gourand, L., Dausset, J., Berrih-Aknin, S., et al. (2000). Modulation of HLA-G expression in human thymic and amniotic epithelial cells. *Hum. Immunol.* 61, 1095–1101. doi:10.1016/S0198-8859(00)00192-0

Li, H., Niederkorn, J. Y., Neelam, S., Mayhew, E., Word, R. A., McCulley, J. P., et al. (2005). Immunosuppressive factors secreted by human amniotic epithelial cells. *Invest. Ophthalmol. Vis. Sci.* 46, 900–907. doi:10.1167/iovs.05-0034

Li, J., Koike-Soko, C., Sugimoto, J., Yoshida, T., Okabe, M., and Nikaido, T. (2015). Human amnion-derived stem cells have immunosuppressive properties on NK cells and monocytes. *Cell Transplant.* 24, 2065–2076. doi:10.3727/09636 8914X685230

Liu, J., Sheha, H., Fu, Y., Liang, L., and Tseng, S. C. (2010). Update on amniotic membrane transplantation. *Expert Rev. Ophthalmol.* 5, 645–661. doi:10.1586/eop.10.63

Liu, W., Morschauser, A., Zhang, X., Lu, X., Gleason, J., He, S., et al. (2014). Human placenta-derived adherent cells induce tolerogenic immune responses. *Clin. Transl. Immunology* 3, e14. doi:10.1038/cti.2014.5

Liu, Y. H., Vaghjiani, V., Tee, J. Y., To, K., Cui, P., Oh, D. Y., et al. (2012). Amniotic epithelial cells from the human placenta potently suppress a mouse model of multiple sclerosis. *PLoS ONE* 7:e35758. doi:10.1371/journal.pone.0035758

Lo, V., and Pope, E. (2009). Amniotic membrane use in dermatology. *Int. J. Dermatol.* 48, 935–940. doi:10.1111/j.1365-4632.2009.04173.x

Lobert, V. H., Brech, A., Pedersen, N. M., Wesche, J., Oppelt, A., Malerod, L., et al. (2010). Ubiquitination of alpha 5 beta 1 integrin controls fibroblast migration through lysosomal degradation of fibronectin-integrin complexes. *Dev. Cell* 19, 148–159. doi:10.1016/j.devcel.2010.06.010

Lublin, F. D., Bowen, J. D., Huddlestone, J., Kremenchutzky, M., Carpenter, A., Corboy, J. R., et al. (2014). Human placenta-derived cells (PDA-001) for the treatment of adults with multiple sclerosis: a randomized, placebo-controlled, multiple-dose study. *Mult. Scler. Relat. Disord.* 3, 696–704. doi:10.1016/j.msard.2014.08.002

Ma, L., Zhou, Z., Zhang, D., Yang, S., Wang, J., Xue, F., et al. (2012). Immunosuppressive function of mesenchymal stem cells from human umbilical cord matrix in immune thrombocytopenia patients. *Thromb. Haemost.* 107, 937–950. doi:10.1160/TH11-08-0596

Magatti, M., Caruso, M., De Munari, S., Vertua, E., De, D., Manuelpillai, U., et al. (2015). Human amniotic membrane-derived mesenchymal and epithelial cells exert different effects on monocyte-derived dendritic cell differentiation and function. *Cell Transplant.* 24, 1733–1752. doi:10.3727/096368914X684033

Magatti, M., De Munari, S., Vertua, E., Nassauto, C., Albertini, A., Wengler, G. S., et al. (2009). Amniotic mesenchymal tissue cells inhibit dendritic cell differentiation of peripheral blood and amnion resident monocytes. *Cell Transplant.* 18, 899–914. doi:10.3727/096368909X471314

Manuelpillai, U., Lourensz, D., Vaghjiani, V., Tchongue, J., Lacey, D., Tee, J. Y., et al. (2012). Human amniotic epithelial cell transplantation induces markers of alternative macrophage activation and reduces established hepatic fibrosis. *PLoS ONE* 7:e38631. doi:10.1371/journal.pone.0038631

Manuelpillai, U., Moodley, Y., Borlongan, C. V., and Parolini, O. (2011). Amniotic membrane and amniotic cells: potential therapeutic tools to combat tissue inflammation and fibrosis? *Placenta* 32(Suppl. 4), S320–S325. doi:10.1016/j.placenta.2011.04.010

Mayer, L., Pandak, W. M., Melmed, G. Y., Hanauer, S. B., Johnson, K., Payne, D., et al. (2013). Safety and tolerability of human placenta-derived cells (PDA001) in treatment-resistant Crohn's disease: a phase I study. *Inflamm. Bowel Dis.* 19, 754–760. doi:10.1097/MIB.0b013e31827f27df

McIntyre, J., and Faulk, W. P. (1979). Antigens of human trophoblast. Effects of heterologous anti-trophoblast sera on lymphocyte responses in vitro. *J. Exp. Med.* 149, 824–836. doi:10.1084/jem.149.4.824

Meller, D., Pires, R. T., Mack, R. J., Figueiredo, F., Heiligenhaus, A., Park, W. C., et al. (2000). Amniotic membrane transplantation for acute chemical or thermal burns. *Ophthalmology* 107, 980–989. doi:10.1016/S0161-6420(00)00024-5

Meller, D., Pires, R. T., and Tseng, S. C. (2002). Ex vivo preservation and expansion of human limbal epithelial stem cells on amniotic membrane cultures. *Br. J. Ophthalmol.* 86, 463–471. doi:10.1136/bjo.86.4.463

Min, S., Yoon, J. Y., Park, S. Y., Kwon, H. H., and Suh, D. H. (2014). Clinical effect of bovine amniotic membrane and hydrocolloid on wound by laser treatment: prospective comparative randomized clinical trial. *Wound Repair Regen.* 22, 212–219. doi:10.1111/wrr.12145

Mitchell, M. D., Edwin, S. S., Lundin-Schiller, S., Silver, R. M., Smotkin, D., and Trautman, M. S. (1993). Mechanism of interleukin-1 beta stimulation of human amnion prostaglandin biosynthesis: mediation via a novel inducible cyclooxygenase. *Placenta* 14, 615–625. doi:10.1016/S0143-4004(05)80426-6

Muralidharan, S., Gu, J., and Laub, G. (1991). A new biological membrane for pericardial closure. *J. Biomed. Mater. Res.* 25, 1201–1209. doi:10.1002/jbm.820251003

Najar, M., Raicevic, G., Boufker, H. I., Fayyad Kazan, H., De Bruyn, C., Meuleman, N., et al. (2010). Mesenchymal stromal cells use PGE2 to modulate activation and proliferation of lymphocyte subsets: combined comparison of adipose tissue, Wharton's jelly and bone marrow sources. *Cell. Immunol.* 264, 171–179. doi:10.1016/j.cellimm.2010.06.006

Nisolle, M., and Donnez, J. (1992). Vaginoplasty using amniotic membranes in cases of vaginal agenesis or after vaginectomy. *J. Gynaecol. Surg.* 8, 25–30. doi:10.1089/gyn.1992.8.25

Ohshima, M., Yamahara, K., Ishikane, S., Harada, K., Tsuda, H., Otani, K., et al. (2012). Systemic transplantation of allogenic fetal membrane-derived mesenchymal stem cells suppresses Th1 and Th17 T cell responses in experimental autoimmune myocarditis. *J. Mol. Cell. Cardiol.* 53, 420–428. doi:10.1016/j.yjmcc.2012.06.020

Paris Fdos, S., Goncalves, E. D., Campos, M. S., Sato, E. H., Dua, H. S., and Gomes, J. A. (2013). Amniotic membrane transplantation versus anterior stromal puncture in bullous keratopathy: a comparative study. *Br. J. Ophthalmol.* 97, 980–984. doi:10.1136/bjophthalmol-2013-303081

Parolini, O., Alviano, F., Bergwerf, I., Boraschi, D., De Bari, C, De Waele, P., et al. (2010). Toward cell therapy using placenta-derived cells: disease mechanisms, cell biology, preclinical studies, and regulatory aspects at the round table. *Stem Cells Dev.* 19, 143–154. doi:10.1089/scd.2009.0404

Parolini, O., and Caruso, M. (2011). Review: preclinical studies on placenta-derived cells and amniotic membrane: an update. *Placenta* 32(Suppl. 2), S186–S195. doi:10.1016/j.placenta.2010.12.016

Parolini, O., Soncini, M., Evangelista, M., and Schmidt, D. (2009). Amniotic membrane and amniotic fluid-derived cells: potential tools for regenerative medicine? *Regen. Med.* 4, 275–291. doi:10.2217/17460751.4.2.275

Parolini, O., Souza-Moreira, L., O'Valle, F., Magatti, M., Hernandez-Cortes, P., Gonzalez-Rey, E., et al. (2014). Therapeutic effect of human amniotic membrane-derived cells on experimental arthritis and other inflammatory disorders. *Arthritis Rheumatol.* 66, 327–339. doi:10.1002/art.38206

Petroff, M. G., and Perchellet, A. (2010). B7 family molecules as regulators of the maternal immune system in pregnancy. *Am. J. Reprod. Immunol.* 63, 506–519. doi:10.1111/j.1600-0897.2010.00841.x

Phillips, R. J., Al-Zamil, H., Hunt, L. P., Fortier, M. A., and ópez Bernal, A. L. (2011). Genes for prostaglandin synthesis, transport and inactivation are differentially expressed in human uterine tissues, and the prostaglandin F synthase AKR1B1 is induced in myometrial cells by inflammatory cytokines. *Mol. Hum. Reprod.* 17, 1–13. doi:10.1093/molehr/gaq057

Pianta, S., Bonassi Signoroni, P., Muradore, I., Rodrigues, M. F., Rossi, D., Silini, A., et al. (2015). Amniotic membrane mesenchymal cells-derived factors skew T cell polarization toward treg and downregulate Th1 and Th17 cells subsets. *Stem Cell. Rev.* 11, 394–407. doi:10.1007/s12015-014-9558-4

Pomini, F., Caruso, A., and Challis, J. R. (1999). Interleukin-10 modifies the effects of interleukin-1beta and tumor necrosis factor-alpha on the activity and expression of prostaglandin H synthase-2 and the NAD+-dependent 15-hydroxyprostaglandin dehydrogenase in cultured term human villous trophoblast and chorion trophoblast cells. *J. Clin. Endocrinol. Metab.* 84, 4645–4651. doi:10.1210/jcem.84.12.6188

Prasanna, S., and Jahnavi, V. (2011). Wharton's jelly mesenchymal stem cells as off-the-shelf cellular therapeutics: a closer look into their regenerative and immunomodulatory properties. *Open Tissue Eng. Regen. Med. J.* 2011, 28–38. doi:10.2174/1875043501104010028

Prasanna, S. J., Gopalakrishnan, D., Shankar, S. R., and Vasandan, A. B. (2010). Pro-inflammatory cytokines, IFNgamma and TNFalpha, influence immune properties of human bone marrow and Wharton jelly mesenchymal stem cells differentially. *PLoS ONE* 5:e9016. doi:10.1371/journal.pone.0009016

Pratama, G., Vaghjiani, V., Tee, J. Y., Liu, Y. H., Chan, J., Tan, C., et al. (2011). Changes in culture expanded human amniotic epithelial cells: implications for potential therapeutic applications. *PLoS ONE* 6:e26136. doi:10.1371/journal.pone.0026136

Raicevic, G., Najar, M., Stamatopoulos, B., De Bruyn, C., Meuleman, N., Bron, D., et al. (2011). The source of human mesenchymal stromal cells influences their TLR profile as well as their functional properties. *Cell. Immunol.* 270, 207–216. doi:10.1016/j.cellimm.2011.05.010

Ramot, Y., Meiron, M., Toren, A., Steiner, M., and Nyska, A. (2009). Safety and biodistribution profile of placental-derived mesenchymal stromal cells (PLX-PAD) following intramuscular delivery. *Toxicol. Pathol.* 37, 606–616. doi:10.1177/0192623309338383

Rennekampff, H. O., Dohrmann, P., Fory, R., and Fandrich, F. (1994). Evaluation of amniotic membrane as adhesion prophylaxis in a novel surgical gastroschisis model. *J. Invest. Surg.* 7, 187–193. doi:10.3109/08941939409018285

Riau, A. K., Beuerman, R. W., Lim, L. S., and Mehta, J. S. (2010). Preservation, sterilization and de-epithelialization of human amniotic membrane for use in ocular surface reconstruction. *Biomaterials* 31, 216–225. doi:10.1016/j.biomaterials.2009.09.034

Ribeiro, A., Laranjeira, P., Mendes, S., Velada, I., Leite, C., Andrade, P., et al. (2013). Mesenchymal stem cells from umbilical cord matrix, adipose tissue and bone marrow exhibit different capability to suppress peripheral blood B, natural killer and T cells. *Stem Cell Res. Ther.* 4, 125. doi:10.1186/scrt336

Ringden, O., Erkers, T., Nava, S., Uzunel, M., Iwarsson, E., Conrad, R., et al. (2013). Fetal membrane cells for treatment of steroid-refractory acute graft-versus-host disease. *Stem Cells* 31, 592–601. doi:10.1002/stem.1314

Roelen, D. L., van der Mast, B. J., in 't Anker, P. S., Kleijburg, C., Eikmans, M., van Beelen, E., et al. (2009). Differential immunomodulatory effects of fetal versus maternal multipotent stromal cells. *Hum. Immunol.* 70, 16–23. doi:10.1016/j.humimm.2008.10.016

Rossi, D., Pianta, S., Magatti, M., Sedlmayr, P., and Parolini, O. (2012). Characterization of the conditioned medium from amniotic membrane cells: prostaglandins as key effectors of its immunomodulatory activity. *PLoS ONE* 7:e46956. doi:10.1371/journal.pone.0046956

Rowe, T. F., King, L. A., MacDonald, P. C., and Casey, M. L. (1997). Tissue inhibitor of metalloproteinase-1 and tissue inhibitor of metalloproteinase-2 expression in

human amnion mesenchymal and epithelial cells. *Am. J. Obstet. Gynecol.* 176, 915–921. doi:10.1016/S0002-9378(97)70621-5

Sabella, N. (1913). Use of fetal membranes in skin grafting. *Med. Rec.* 83, 478–480.

Saeidi, M., Masoud, A., Shakiba, Y., Hadjati, J., Mohyeddin Bonab, M., Nicknam, M. H., et al. (2013). Immunomodulatory effects of human umbilical cord Wharton's jelly-derived mesenchymal stem cells on differentiation, maturation and endocytosis of monocyte-derived dendritic cells. *Iran. J. Allergy Asthma Immunol.* 12, 37–49. doi:012.01/ijaai.3749

Serena, T. E., Carter, M. J., Le, L. T., Sabo, M. J., DiMarco, D. T., and Group, E. V. S. (2014). A multicenter, randomized, controlled clinical trial evaluating the use of dehydrated human amnion/chorion membrane allografts and multilayer compression therapy vs. multilayer compression therapy alone in the treatment of venous leg ulcers. *Wound Repair Regen.* 22, 688–693. doi:10.1111/wrr.12227

Shao, C., Sima, J., Zhang, S. X., Jin, J., Reinach, P., Wang, Z., et al. (2004). Suppression of corneal neovascularization by PEDF release from human amniotic membranes. *Invest. Ophthalmol. Vis. Sci.* 45, 1758–1762. doi:10.1167/iovs.04-0554

Silini, A., Parolini, O., Huppertz, B., and Lang, I. (2013). Soluble factors of amnion-derived cells in treatment of inflammatory and fibrotic pathologies. *Curr. Stem Cell Res. Ther.* 8, 6–14. doi:10.2174/1574888X11308010003

Silverton, J., Trelford, J., and Roussere, J. (1979). The use of amniotic membrane in acute massive full-thickness loss of the abdominal wall from clostridial myonecrosis. *Ann. Plast. Surg.* 3, 558–566. doi:10.1097/00000637-197912000-00012

Soncini, M., Vertua, E., Gibelli, L., Zorzi, F., Denegri, M., Albertini, A., et al. (2007). Isolation and characterization of mesenchymal cells from human fetal membranes. *J. Tissue Eng. Regen. Med.* 1, 296–305. doi:10.1002/term.40

Sorsby, A., Haythorne, J., and Reed, H. (1947). Further experience with amniotic membrane grafts in caustic burns of the eye. *Br. J. Ophthalmol.* 31, 409–418. doi:10.1136/bjo.31.7.409

Sorsby, A., and Symons, H. M. (1946). Amniotic membrane grafts in caustic burns of the eye (burns of the second degree). *Br. J. Ophthalmol.* 30, 337–345. doi:10.1136/bjo.30.1.64

Steed, D. L., Trumpower, C., Duffy, D., Smith, C., Marshall, V., Rupp, R., et al. (2008). Amnion-derived cellular cytokine solution: a physiological combination of cytokines for wound healing. *Eplasty* 8, e18.

Stern, M. (1913). The grafting of preserved amniotic membranes to burned and ulcerated surfaces, substituting skin grafts. *JAMA* 60, 973. doi:10.1001/jama.1913.04340130021008

Subrahmanyam, M. (1995). Amniotic membrane as a cover for microskin grafts. *Br. J. Plast. Surg.* 48, 477–478. doi:10.1016/0007-1226(95)90123-X

Tipnis, S., Viswanathan, C., and Majumdar, A. S. (2010). Immunosuppressive properties of human umbilical cord-derived mesenchymal stem cells: role of B7-H1 and IDO. *Immunol. Cell Biol.* 88, 795–806. doi:10.1038/icb.2010.47

Trelford, J., Anderson, D., Hanson, F., Mendel, V., and Sawyer, R. (1972). Amnion autografts and allografts as a cover for skin defects in sheep. A preliminary report. *J. Med.* 3, 81.

Trelford, J., Hanson, F., Anderson, D., and Mendel, V. (1974). Implanted amniotic membrane as an autograft and as an allograft. *J. Med.* 6, 169–180.

Trelford-Sauder, M., Dawe, E. J., and Trelford, J. D. (1978). Use of allograft amniotic membrane for control of intra-abdominal adhesions. *J. Med.* 9, 273–284.

Trelford-Sauder, M., Trelford, J., and Matolo, N. (1977). Replacement of the peritoneum with amnion following pelvic exenteration. *Surg. Gynecol. Obstet.* 145, 699–701.

Troensagaard-Hansen, E. (1950). Amniotic grafts in chronic skin ulceration. *Lancet* 1, 859–860. doi:10.1016/S0140-6736(50)90693-3

Troyer, D. L., and Weiss, M. L. (2008). Wharton's jelly-derived cells are a primitive stromal cell population. *Stem Cells* 26, 591–599. doi:10.1634/stemcells.2007-0439

Tseng, S. C., Espana, E. M., Kawakita, T., Di Pascuale, M. A., Li, W., He, H., et al. (2004). How does amniotic membrane work? *Ocul. Surf.* 2, 177–187. doi:10.1016/S1542-0124(12)70059-9

Tseng, S. C., Prabhasawat, P., and Lee, S.-H. (1997). Amniotic membrane transplantation for conjunctival surface reconstruction. *Am. J. Ophthalmol.* 124, 765–774. doi:10.1016/S0002-9394(14)71693-9

Venegas, L., Hettich, M., Villena, J., Aris, R., Párraga, M., Parolini, O., et al. (2014). Comparative analysis of human amniotic membrane graft versus contact lenses in symptomatic bullous keratopathy. *J. Stem Cell Res. Ther.* 4, 250. doi:10.4172/2157-7633.1000250

Whittle, W. L., Gibb, W., and Challis, J. R. (2000). The characterization of human amnion epithelial and mesenchymal cells: the cellular expression, activity and glucocorticoid regulation of prostaglandin output. *Placenta* 21, 394–401. doi:10.1053/plac.1999.0482

Wolbank, S., Peterbauer, A., Fahrner, M., Hennerbichler, S., van Griensven, M., Stadler, G., et al. (2007). Dose-dependent immunomodulatory effect of human stem cells from amniotic membrane: a comparison with human mesenchymal stem cells from adipose tissue. *Tissue Eng.* 13, 1173–1183. doi:10.1089/ten.2006.0313

Wu, W., Lan, Q., Lu, H., Xu, J., Zhu, A., Fang, W., et al. (2014). Human amnion mesenchymal cells negative co-stimulatory molecules PD-L1 expression and its capacity of modulating microglial activation of CNS. *Cell Biochem. Biophys.* 69, 35–45. doi:10.1007/s12013-013-9763-9

Yamahara, K., Harada, K., Ohshima, M., Ishikane, S., Ohnishi, S., Tsuda, H., et al. (2014). Comparison of angiogenic, cytoprotective, and immunosuppressive properties of human amnion- and chorion-derived mesenchymal stem cells. *PLoS ONE* 9:e88319. doi:10.1371/journal.pone.0088319

Young, R. L., Cota, J., Zund, G., Mason, B. A., and Wheeler, J. M. (1991). The use of an amniotic membrane graft to prevent postoperative adhesions. *Fertil. Steril.* 55, 624–628.

Young, S. M., and Benyshek, D. C. (2010). In search of human placentophagy: a cross-cultural survey of human placenta consumption, disposal practices, and cultural beliefs. *Ecol. Food Nutr.* 49, 467–484. doi:10.1080/03670244.2010.524106

Zaslavsky, A., Baek, K. H., Lynch, R. C., Short, S., Grillo, J., Folkman, J., et al. (2010). Platelet-derived thrombospondin-1 is a critical negative regulator and potential biomarker of angiogenesis. *Blood* 115, 4605–4613. doi:10.1182/blood-2009-09-242065

Zelen, C. M., Poka, A., and Andrews, J. (2013). Prospective, randomized, blinded, comparative study of injectable micronized dehydrated amniotic/chorionic membrane allograft for plantar fasciitis – a feasibility study. *Foot Ankle Int.* 34, 1332–1339. doi:10.1177/1071100713502179

Zelen, C. M., Serena, T. E., and Snyder, R. J. (2014). A prospective, randomised comparative study of weekly versus biweekly application of dehydrated human amnion/chorion membrane allograft in the management of diabetic foot ulcers. *Int. Wound J.* 11, 122–128. doi:10.1111/iwj.12242

Zhou, S., Chen, J., and Feng, J. (2003). The effects of amniotic membrane on polymorphonuclear cells. *Chin. Med. J. (Engl).* 116, 788–790.

Conflict of Interest Statement: The authors declare that the research was conducted in the absence of any commercial or financial relationships that could be construed as a potential conflict of interest.

7

Use of mesothelial cells and biological matrices for tissue engineering of simple epithelium surrogates

Edited by:
Cornelia Kasper,
University of Natural Resources and
Life Sciences, Austria

Reviewed by:
Darja Marolt Presen,
Ludwig Boltzmann Institute for
Experimental and Clinical
Traumatology, Austria
Enrico Lucarelli,
Istituto Ortopedico Rizzoli, Italy
Wolfgang Holnthoner,
Ludwig Boltzmann Institute for
Experimental and Clinical
Traumatology, Austria

*Correspondence:
Abdelkrim Hmadcha and
Bernat Soria,
Department of Stem Cells,
Andalusian Center for Molecular
Biology and Regenerative Medicine
(CABIMER), Avda. Américo Vespucio
s/n, Parque Científico y Tecnológico
Cartuja, Seville 41092,
Spain
karim.hmadcha@cabimer.es;
bernat.soria@cabimer.es

Christian Claude Lachaud [1,2], Berta Rodriguez-Campins [3,4], Abdelkrim Hmadcha [1,2]* and Bernat Soria [1,2]*

[1] Andalusian Center for Molecular Biology and Regenerative Medicine – Centro Andaluz de Biología Molecular y Medicina Regenerativa (CABIMER), Seville, Spain, [2] Centro de Investigación en Red sobre Diabetes y Enfermedades Metabólicas (CIBERDEM), Madrid, Spain, [3] Departamento de I+D, New Biotechnic S.A., Seville, Spain, [4] Fundación Andaluza de Investigación y Desarrollo (FAID), Seville, Spain

Tissue-engineering technologies have progressed rapidly through last decades resulting in the manufacture of quite complex bioartificial tissues with potential use for human organ and tissue regeneration. The manufacture of avascular monolayered tissues such as simple squamous epithelia was initiated a few decades ago and is attracting increasing interest. Their relative morphostructural simplicity makes of their biomimetization a goal, which is currently accessible. The mesothelium is a simple squamous epithelium in nature and is the monolayered tissue lining the walls of large celomic cavities (peritoneal, pericardial, and pleural) and internal organs housed inside. Interestingly, mesothelial cells can be harvested in clinically relevant numbers from several anatomical sources and not less important, they also display high transdifferentiation capacities and are low immunogenic characteristics, which endow these cells with therapeutic interest. Their combination with a suitable scaffold (biocompatible, degradable, and non-immunogenic) may allow the manufacture of tailored serosal membranes biomimetics with potential spanning a wide range of therapeutic applications, principally for the regeneration of simple squamous-like epithelia such as the visceral and parietal mesothelium vascular endothelium and corneal endothelium among others. Herein, we review recent research progresses in mesothelial cells biology and their clinical sources. We make a particular emphasis on reviewing the different types of biological scaffolds suitable for the manufacture of serosal mesothelial membranes biomimetics. Finally, we also review progresses made in mesothelial cells-based therapeutic applications and propose some possible future directions.

Keywords: tissue engineering, epithelial surrogates, biological matrices, biomaterials, simple epithelia, mesothelial cells, serosal membranes, corneal endothelium

Introduction

Tissue engineering has emerged as a promising alternative to conventional medicine to achieve the healing and regeneration of human damaged tissues and organs. The manufacture of functionally optimal bioartificial tissues is an extremely complex process relying on a comprehensive stepwise combination of cells with scaffolds, extracellular matrices (ECM), and molecular signals. The achievement of such objective usually relies on the combination of advanced knowledge and skills from interdisciplinary specialists, making tissue engineering one of the most challenging fields of biomedical research.

Elaborated bioartificial soft tissues and inclusively some bioartificial organs are under current experimental development and evaluation in laboratories (Mikos et al., 2006; Atala, 2009; Atala et al., 2012). Unfortunately, their clinical application in humans is still far away from being accessible and to date only a limited number of bioartificial tissues including skin substitutes (Debels et al., 2015) or bioprosthetic aortic valves (Brown et al., 2009) have been successfully transferred to clinical practice in humans.

The majority of tissue-engineering applications aiming at regenerating complex human tissues remain still a great challenge, principally because they should be functionally prevascularized to be efficiently integrated into the host (Nomi et al., 2002; Novosel et al., 2011). This has been principally the case for large 3D bioartificial tissues performed so far and that acquired only superficial neovascularization by the surrounding host tissues vasculature during their initial stage of implantation in animal models (Nomi et al., 2002; Park and Gerecht, 2014). To solve this issue, a host of experimental therapeutic angiogenic strategies involving endothelial progenitor cells, proangiogenic growth factors, bioactive microcarriers, or preformed bioartificial vascular networks among others are currently under intense research to achieve the generation of functional prevascularized neotissues [for specific review, see Kaully et al. (2009), Lovett et al. (2009), Roy et al. (2011), and Park and Gerecht (2014)].

In sharp contrast with complex 3D vascularized tissues are avascular monolayered tissues such as simple epithelia, which are made up of a single layer of simple epithelial cells anchored onto a thin basement membrane. Simple epithelia are basically subclassified as columnar, cuboidal, or squamous depending on the size and shape of their cellular component. Simple squamous epithelia are highly distributed within the adult body. Its major form, the mesothelium is the monolayered tissue lining the walls of the largest celomic cavities (pleural, pericardial, and peritoneal) and the surface of celomic visceral organs (Mutsaers, 2002). A layer of mesothelial cells is additionally found lining the side of the Reissner's membrane facing the scala vestibuli within the cochlea. Interestingly, other tissues such as the vascular endothelium, corneal endothelium, and also the synovial membrane lining display in diverse degrees morphological hallmarks as well as structural and biochemical markers consistent with simple epithelial cells (reviewed in **Table 1**).

There has been a growing consensus about the concept that these distinct tissues could somehow be considered other forms of simple squamous epithelia. The synovial membrane lining, mesothelium, vascular endothelium, and corneal endothelium are each of them endowed with specific functions and distinct endogenous regenerative capacities, which is high for the mesothelium (Mutsaers et al., 2007), intermediate for the vascular endothelium (Toya and Malik, 2012) and barely inexistent for the corneal endothelium (Bourne, 2003). Despite such divergences, the inherent regenerative capacity of some forms of simple epithelia is however strongly linked to the extent of their damage. In some instances, accidents, surgical trauma, or diseases can lead to their irreparable damage and ultimately to their loss of function. Their reconstruction or substitution can be eventually achieved through transplantation of autologous or allogeneic native tissues, the accessibility of which is however limited by the important shortage of suitable donor tissues. Tissue engineering of artificial tissues biomimetics has emerged as a promising alternative to the lack of native replacement tissues. The use of mesothelial cells in tissue engineering of simple epithelial-like tissues such as the vascular endothelium or the corneal endothelium has been already initiated and is technically accessible. Sources of mesothelial cells and appropriate biological scaffolds for these applications have been already identified. Additionally, the transdifferentiative capacity of mesothelial cells is also better understood and controlled and should be taken in account in the tissue-engineering procedures of these bioartificial tissues.

Herein, we provide an overview of the main biological and biochemical properties of mesothelial cells and detail their different clinical sources. A particular emphasis is done on reviewing biological scaffolds suitable for tissue engineering of simple epithelial-like tissues. Finally, we review the use of mesothelial cells in different tissue-engineering applications and also suggest some possible future directions.

Mesothelium: Structure and Functions

The single layer of flattened cells covering celomic serous membranes was first described by Bichat in 1827 and later on termed "mesothelium" by Minot in 1880 in reference to its mesodermal origin. Although the mesothelium cells layer appears to be morphostructurally similar between different anatomical locations at a macroscopic level, posterior studies however led to the evidence that parietal mesothelial cells show morphological and biochemical differences with visceral mesothelial cells when examined at an ultrastructural level (Michailova et al., 1999). Parietal mesothelial cells which are the cells lining the walls of celomic cavities are rather large and flattened polygonal cells with low-to-intermediate intracellular organelles, whereas visceral mesothelial cells lining celomic organs are by contrast more tightly compacted and cuboidal and rich in intracellular organelles, principally mitochondria and rough endoplasmic reticulum (RER), indicative of their higher metabolic state (Mutsaers and Wilkosz, 2007).

Biostructurally, the mesothelium represents a semi-permeable laminar interface that separate fluid-filled body cavities from blood vessels and lymphatics running within the underneath submesothelial connective tissue layers. Besides its property of physical barrier, the mesothelium acts also as bioactive interface regulating fluid flows interchanges across its surface to maintain an optimal osmolarity and ionic activity of body cavity fluids; these functions are mainly accomplished by transmembrane ion pumps (Na^+/K^+-ATPase) and water channels (aquaporins) (Witowski et al., 1997; Ji and Nie, 2008). Among other main functions, mesothelial cells also secrete lubricants that stay electrochemically entrapped between their numerous surface microvilli to create a lubricated thin film or glycocalyx allowing

TABLE 1 | Phenotypic marker profiles of different types of simple epithelial-like cells.

Markers	Vascular endothelial cells	Corneal endothelial cells	Fibroblast-like synoviocytes	Mesothelial cells
Vimentin	++ (Chung-Welch et al., 1997b)	++ (Vazquez et al., 2015)	++ (Bartok and Firestein, 2010)	++ (Lachaud et al., 2014a)
N-cadherin	++ (Chung-Welch et al., 1997b)	++ (Zhu et al., 2008b; Lachaud et al., 2014b)	++ (Agarwal et al., 2008)	++ (Lachaud et al., 2014b)
Pan-Cytokeratin	− (Chung-Welch et al., 1997b)	?	?	++ (Yanez-Mo et al., 2003)
Cytokeratin 18	− (Chung-Welch et al., 1997b)	++ (Merjava et al., 2009)	?	++ (Chung-Welch et al., 1997b)
Mesothelin	?	++ (Lachaud et al., 2014b)	?	+ (Lachaud et al., 2014b)
WT1	−/+* (Wagner et al., 2008; Duim et al., 2015)	?	?	++ (Lachaud et al., 2014a)
E-cadherin	−	+ (Zhu et al., 2008b)	− (Agarwal et al., 2008)	−/+* (Lachaud et al., 2014a)
VE-cadherin	++ (Tsai et al., 2007; Chlupac et al., 2014)	+*/+ (Zhu et al., 2008b; Huang et al., 2010b)	?	−
ZO-1	++ (Medina et al., 2010; Shao et al., 2011)	++ (Zhu et al., 2008b; Lachaud et al., 2014b)	++	++ (Lachaud et al., 2013, 2014a)
β-catenin	++ (Medina et al., 2010)	++ (Zhu et al., 2008b; Lachaud et al., 2014b)	++ (Xiao et al., 2011)	++ (Lachaud et al., 2013, 2014a)
Aquaporin 1	++ (Mobasheri and Marples, 2004)	++ (Chng et al., 2013)	+ (Mobasheri and Marples, 2004)	+ (Lai et al., 2001; Ji and Nie, 2008)
COL8A1	+ (Muragaki et al., 1991)	++ (Chng et al., 2013)	?	?
COL8A2	+ (Muragaki et al., 1991)	++ (Chng et al., 2013; Lachaud et al., 2014b)	?	++ (Lachaud et al., 2014b)
SLC4A4	− (Romero et al., 2013)	++ (Chng et al., 2013; Lachaud et al., 2014b)	?	++ (Lachaud et al., 2014b)
SLC4A11	?	++ (Damkier et al., 2007)	?	?
CA-II	++ (Su et al., 2004)	++ (Chng et al., 2013; Lachaud et al., 2014b)	?	++ (Lachaud et al., 2014b)
NA+/K+-ATPase	++ (Trevisi et al., 2006)	++ (Lachaud et al., 2014b; Vazquez et al., 2015)	?	++ (Witowski et al., 1997; Lachaud et al., 2014b)
CD166 (ALCAM)	++ (Swart, 2002)	++ (Okumura et al., 2014)	++ (Joo et al., 2000)	++ (Ross et al., 1998)
vWF (Factor VIII)	++ (Tsai et al., 2007; Chlupac et al., 2014)	−/+ (Shamsuddin et al., 1986)	− (Schwachula et al., 1994)	+* (Chung-Welch et al., 1997b)
CD31 (PECAM-1)	++ (Tsai et al., 2007; Chlupac et al., 2014)	− (Shamsuddin et al., 1986; Huang et al., 2010b)	− (Schwachula et al., 1994)	− (Lachaud et al., 2013, 2014a)
Dil-Ac-LDL	++ (Chung-Welch et al., 1997b; Medina et al., 2010)	− (Huang et al., 2010b)	+ (Schwachula et al., 1994)	+* (Chung-Welch et al., 1997b)
CD45 (LCA)	− (Medina et al., 2010)	− (Huang et al., 2010b)	− (Tran et al., 2008)	− (Lachaud et al., 2013, 2014a)
CD29 (integrin β1)	++ (Chlupac et al., 2014; Kawasaki et al., 2015)	?	?	++ (Lachaud et al., 2013, 2014a)
CD106 (VCAM-1)	++ (Su et al., 2004)	− (Foets et al., 1992)	+*/+ (Bombara et al., 1993; Bartok and Firestein, 2010)	− (Lachaud et al., 2013, 2014a)
CD44 (HCAM)	+ (Su et al., 2004)	− (Foets et al., 1992)	++ (Schwarting et al., 1996)	+ (Lachaud et al., 2013, 2014a)
CD90 (Thy-1)	++ (Su et al., 2004)	?	++ (Bartok and Firestein, 2010)	+/++ (Lachaud et al., 2014a)
CD54 (ICAM-1)	++ (Murohara et al., 1999)	+ (Foets et al., 1992)	++ (Bartok and Firestein, 2010)	++ (Lachaud et al., 2013, 2014a)

Markers expression levels: −, negative; +*, very weak; +, intermediate; ++, strong. /, this symbol is used when expression varies between distinct published works. For example, −/+* indicates a variation in reported expression ranging from negative to weak. ?, this symbol is used for unknown expression levels.

ALCAM, activated leukocyte cell adhesion molecule; CA-II, carbonic anhydrase II; COL8A1, collagen type VIII, alpha 1; COL8A2, collagen type VIII, alpha 2; HCAM, homing cell adhesion molecule; ICAM-1, intercellular cell adhesion molecule 1; NA+/K+-ATPase, sodium-potassium adenosine triphosphatase; PECAM-1, platelet endothelial cell adhesion molecule 1; SLC4A4, electrogenic sodium bicarbonate cotransporter 1; SLC4A11, sodium bicarbonate transporter-like protein 11; VCAM-1, vascular cell adhesion molecule 1; vWF, von Willebrand factor; WT1, Wilms tumor protein; ZO-1, zona occludens 1.

the free sliding of opposite parietal and visceral mesotheliums with minimal abrasion (Mutsaers, 2002). The mesothelial glycocalyx is mainly composed by glycosaminoglycans, especially hyaluronan, a large anionic polymer of disaccharides with high hydrophilicity which forms a highly hydrated gel layer (Yung and Chan, 2007). Mesothelial cells also actively regulate celomic cavities homeostasis and inflammatory status via their secretion of numerous pro- and anti-inflammatory cytokines (Lanfrancone et al., 1992; Mutsaers and Wilkosz, 2007; Ji and Nie, 2008). It has also been evidenced that mesothelial cells are actively recruited during serosal regeneration, through processes of proliferation, migration or delamination, and secretion of a large variety of growth factors or cytokines (Foley-Comer et al., 2002; Mutsaers, 2002; Herrick and Mutsaers, 2004; Mutsaers, 2004; Mutsaers and Wilkosz, 2007; Carmona et al., 2011).

Plasticity of Mesothelial Cells

Mesothelial cells are intriguing cells, because they are mesodermal in origin but however display phenotypic properties rather consistent with simple epithelial cells, an ambiguous phenotype that is reflected by their coexpression of both mesenchymal and epithelial lineage markers (Mutsaers, 2002; Herrick and Mutsaers, 2004; Mutsaers and Wilkosz, 2007).

The concept that the mesothelium may represent a primitive mesoderm was first postulated by Donna and Betta, based on their observation of areas of cartilaginous and osseous differentiation in malignant mesotheliomas (Donna and Betta, 1981; Debels et al., 2015), a tumor arising from mesothelial cells [for review, see Carbone et al. (2012)]. This concept was further reinforced by several lineage tracing studies conducted in the mouse embryo where mesothelial cells were found to originate stromal VSMCs and fibroblasts through a process of epithelial-to-mesenchymal transition in the developing heart, lung, gut, and liver (Dettman et al., 1998; Wilm et al., 2005; Cai et al., 2008; Que et al., 2008; Zhou et al., 2008; Asahina et al., 2011). Furthermore, embryonic mesothelial cells were also shown to generate stellate cells and a subset of cardiomyocytes in the developing liver and heart, respectively (Cai et al., 2008; Zhou et al., 2008; Asahina et al., 2011). Additionally, several in vitro differentiation studies demonstrated that adult mesothelial cells isolated from human and adult rodents could recapitulate an epithelial-to-mesenchymal transition and differentiate along the VSMCs, fibroblasts, chondrocytes, osteocytes, and adipocytes lineages when cultured upon adequate inductive conditions (van Tuyn et al., 2007; Lansley et al., 2011; Lachaud et al., 2013; Lachaud et al., 2014a). Consistent with these in vitro findings, a recent in vivo mesothelial lineage tracing study, conducted in the postnatal mouse, demonstrated that mesothelial cells covering the visceral adipose tissue are the precursor cells giving rise to white adipocytes (Chau et al., 2014). Furthermore, the ability of adult mesothelial cells to adopt myofibroblasts or inclusively macrophage-like features in response to pathological conditions of the peritoneal cavity may represent another evidence of their inherent plasticity and ability to switch their phenotype upon the microenvironment milieu (Yanez-Mo et al., 2003; Katz et al., 2011). Altogether, these studies provide converging evidence supporting the concept that adult mesothelial cells retain embryonic mesodermal multilineage differentiation capacity and could represent a population of primitive mesodermal stem cells. Their inherent plasticity is strongly supporting their use as cellular surrogate for tissue engineering of different types of specialized simple squamous epithelia.

Immunomodulatory and Anti-Inflammatory Properties of Mesothelial Cells

The capacity of a cellular phenotype to reverse or ameliorate the clinical course of inflammatory diseases is of critical therapeutic relevance. Such capacity has been first described in mesenchymal stromal cells (MSCs) used in experimental animal models for human inflammatory diseases. Their protective effects was found to be largely attributed to their hypoimmunogenicity and capacity to regulate innate immune cells functions through secretion of soluble and membrane-bound factors with potent immunosuppressive and/or immunomodulatory activities [for review, see Glenn and Whartenby (2014)].

This major discovery has prompted a general interest in elucidating whether other cell types are endowed with similar properties. The first evidence that cells of the mesothelial lineage could display anti-inflammatory and immunosuppressive properties arose from studies of human malignant mesotheliomas, where it was found that mesothelial tumorigenic cells escape from the control of the immune system through suppression of the proliferation and functions of T lymphocytes and increased recruitment of immunosuppressive regulatory T cells (Hegmans et al., 2006). Later on, normal human omental mesothelial cells were found capable to potently suppress the proliferation of proinflammatory γδ T cells as well as of CD4+ and CD8+ T lymphocytes (T cells), through their secretion of the immunosuppressor TGF-β (Lin et al., 2013). A recent work also indicated that CD90+/CD45- human mesothelial cells belonging to peritoneal fluid could immunosuppress CD4+ T cells in vitro through their potent expression of arginase I and consequent depletion of L-arginine, a major molecule required for T cells activation (Kitayama et al., 2014). Taking in account these in vitro results, it may therefore be expected that bioengineered artificial tissues performed with heterologous mesothelial cells should be globally hypoimmunogenic with a prognostic of good host-tissue integration.

Clinical Sources of Mesothelial Cells

A critical issue in autologous cellular therapies is the identification of accessible anatomical sources from which can be harvested cells in therapeutically relevant numbers and with minimal health impact. In this way, the presence of several celomic cavities in the adult human body offers a large range of approaches (anatomical sources and procedures) to harvest mesothelial cells. Due to its largest size, the abdominal cavity is the predominant anatomical source from where mesothelial cells are harvested. Specific peritoneal sources and isolation procedures are reviewed below.

Greater Omentum
The greater omentum is broadly considered as an optimal and reliable source of mesothelial cells, principally because large pieces of

this tissue can be surgically harvested with minimal health concerns and can provide clinically relevant numbers of mesothelial cells (Riera et al., 2006). In humans, the greater omentum or epiploon is the largest fold of peritoneum filled with abundant visceral adipose tissue with a surface area ranging from 300 to 1500 cm^2. Like other visceral mesotheliums, the omental mesothelium displays a high cellularity and can provide around one million mesothelial cells from each square centimeter of omental tissue (Pronk et al., 1993). Furthermore, laparoscopy represents an effective minimal invasive approach to collect reduced pieces of omental tissue.

Mesenteric Membrane

The peritoneal cavity harbors several portions of serous membranes connecting parietal and visceral components. The mesentery is found to fully meet with such characteristics, and the mesentery is a reticular laminar structure resulting from a fold of the dorsal parietal mesothelium that enwraps in its extremity the overall length of the intestinal tract (Coffey, 2013). The mesenteric membrane acts as a connective supportive structure to hold the reticular network of intestinal vasculature, lymphatics, and nerves. Interestingly, some portions of the mesenteric membrane lack vasculature and associated perivascular adipose tissue, thus appearing as a transparent sheet composed of a double layer of mesothelium enclosing loosely arranged collagenous and elastic fibers (Coffey, 2013). Although previous studies already reported the isolation of rat and human mesenteric mesothelial cells for experimental research procedures (Chailley-Heu et al., 1997; Takazawa et al., 2005), their application in tissue engineering has not been reported. Despite this, it is reasonable to believe that laparoscopic surgery could allow the excision of small areas of avascular mesenteric membrane with minimal clinical impact and from which a relevant number of autologous or heterologous mesothelial cells could be isolated for tissue engineering of serosal membranes biomimetics.

Peritoneal Fluid

The peritoneal serosal fluid harbors a quite relevant population of free-floating cells, which were initially described as corresponding to resident macrophages and in lower extent to polymorphonuclear leukocytes and lymphocytes. Later studies however indicated that a significant subset of free-floating mesothelial cells normally coexists within the peritoneal fluid of healthy humans and rodents (Bercovici and Gallily, 1978; Stauffer et al., 1978). Interestingly, the prevalence of free-floating mesothelial cells strongly increases in the peritoneal fluid of patients undergoing continuous ambulatory peritoneal dialysis (CAPD) (Fok et al., 1989) and during serosal regeneration processes (Foley-Comer et al., 2002; Mutsaers et al., 2007).

Cultures of human peritoneal mesothelial cells could be successfully established from peritoneal lavage cells collected through laparoscopic needle aspiration in healthy humans (Ivarsson et al., 1998). This minimal invasive approach to collect mesothelial cells will however require further improvements to obtain clinically relevant numbers of cells for regenerative medicine applications. Additionally, the effluent peritoneal dialysis fluid from CAPD patients may also be considered as an alternative source of mesothelial cells, principally for heterologous cell therapies

and tissue-engineering applications. However, in some instances these cells may have undergone partial to advanced myofibroblastic transdifferentiation, particularly when they are collected from long-term CAPD patients (Yanez-Mo et al., 2003; Zhang et al., 2013). The ability of mesothelial cells to transit between epithelial and mesenchymal phenotypes under specific in vitro culture conditions indicates that "myofibroblastic mesothelial cells" could be forced back to their original mesothelial phenotype and therefore potentially useful for the manufacture of bioartificial serosal mesothelial membranes.

Parietal Tunica Vaginalis

The parietal tunica vaginalis (lamina parietalis), which is the parietal mesothelium of the testicular cavity, has been identified as another reliable source of mesothelial cells (Asano et al., 2005; Asano et al., 2006; Asano et al., 2007). It originates from an invagination of the peritoneum mesothelium that posteriorly descends into the scrotum. The parietal tunica vaginalis is a quite extensible membrane from which small pieces could be easily excised with minimal health concerns. The authors demonstrated the feasibility to harvest portions of 3.5×4.0 cm^2 of tissue from each testis of beagles. Around 4.0×10^5 mesothelial cells were obtained from each portion by using enzymatic digestion with Dispase I and could be successfully expanded in vitro to generate a confluent cobblestone-type monolayer of cells. Their subculture onto a fibrin gel could allow the generation of autologous mesothelial cells sheets. Interestingly, their apposition onto the surface of injured peritoneum areas (lacking mesothelium) could significantly improve their healing and reduce the score of peritoneal adhesions (Asano et al., 2006). On this basis, the authors suggested that small biopsies of parietal tunica vaginalis offer the advantage of representing an easy accessing and attractive therapeutic source of mesothelial cells, principally for patients with abdominal complications.

Biomaterials Useful for Tissue Engineering of Simple Squamous Epithelia

Animal tissue-derived ECM proteins or purified natural polymeric molecules (proteins or polysaccharides) derived from plants or animals are highly sophisticated molecules that emerged from millions of years of natural evolution. They are usually endowed with desirable properties such as high degradability, excellent biocompatibility, and biomechanical properties such as elasticity, tensile strength, and transparency, which make them excellent candidate materials in biomedical engineering applications (Shin et al., 2003; Badylak, 2007; Ma, 2008).

Of further relevance, biopolymers-based scaffolds or acellular tissues usually provide a highly porous environment for cell invasion and excellent cell adhesion and growth properties (Velema and Kaplan, 2006). In many instances, natural polymers are also easy accessible and cheap to manufacture. Furthermore, and not less important, natural polymeric molecules are also usually rich in chemical side groups to which functionalizing molecules can be bound through chemical post treatments to generate hybrid biological scaffolds with improved cells adhesion, growth, and colonization outcomes.

To date, biological materials have been already used to manufacture biomimetics of the mesothelium, the vascular endothelium, or the corneal endothelium (detailed in further sections). We below review different types of biologic materials that have been previously proposed or used in tissue engineering of diverse types of simple squamous epithelia or related tissues (see also **Table 2**, for summary).

Decellularized Animal Tissues

The manufacture of humanized tissues with biological scaffolds derived from the decellularization of animal tissues has gained increased interest in recent years, principally because they provide many advantages over the use of artificial biomaterial scaffolds (Fu et al., 2014). Indeed, animal tissues of porcine, ovine, or bovine origin are easily available and cheap, and their decellularized forms are low immunogenic, bioactive, and biocompatible, and retain mostly original mechanical properties of native tissues. Not less important, animal tissues and most particularly those of porcine origin usually display similarities in size and histoarchitecture with their human counterparts. In light of this evidence are several studies that reported the usefulness of decellularized porcine tissues such as heart valves, arteries, dermis,

tendons, or cornea in human clinical applications or in animal models research (Hoshiba et al., 2010; Klopsch and Steinhoff, 2012; Yoeruek et al., 2012).

The manufacture of humanized serosal membranes biomimetics is still in its early stages of development and as such only a limited number of works have already reported the use of animal-derived decellularized tissues for their manufacture. It may however be expected that they will be focus of broader interest in next future, particularly regarding to the use of the decellularized porcine epicardium, omental mesothelium, and mesentery. In support of this concept, a previous study indicated that a decellularized porcine mesothelium represents an optimal biological laminar scaffold, which preserves in most extent its original mechanical and biochemical properties (Hoganson et al., 2010). The decellularized porcine pericardium has also been proposed as potential biological scaffold for tissue engineering of heart valves (Dong et al., 2013). Additionally, the use of a decellularized porcine small intestinal submucosa has been focus of intense research for a variety of experimental tissue-engineering applications including skin, esophageal, cardiovascular, gastrointestinal, and musculotendinous regeneration [for review, see Andree et al. (2013)]. Its application in combination with human

TABLE 2 | Biological laminar scaffolds potentially applicable for tissue engineering of human simple epithelia.

Scaffolds	Basic component	Reference	Application
Native tissues [decellularized]			
Animal	Amniotic membrane	Tsai et al. (2007)	VTE
	Omental mesothelium	Hoganson et al. (2010)	RM
	Small intestinal mucosa	Andree et al. (2013)	VTE, SE
	Pericardium	Dong et al. (2013)	VTE
	Cornea	Feng et al. (2014)	Cornea, CE
Human	Amniotic membrane	Wilshaw et al. (2006) and Kuriu et al. (2009)	VTE, PA
	Cornea	Feng et al. (2014)	Cornea, CE
	Lens Capsule	Lachaud et al. (2014b)	CE.
Bioengineered sheets	Chitosan	Grolik et al. (2012)	CE
	Alginate	d'Ayala et al. (2008)	SE
	Silk fibroin+gelatin	Taddei et al. (2013)	SE
Hydrogels [compressed and/or cross-linked]	Gelatin	Lai and Li (2010), Watanabe et al. (2011), and Lai et al. (2013)	CE, Cornea
	Silk Fibroin+Gelatin	Grolik et al. (2012)	C. Epi.
	Chitosan	Rafat et al. (2008) and Lai and Li (2010)	CE, Cornea
	Chitosan+Collagen	Rafat et al. (2008)	CE, Cornea
Fibrous meshes [electrospun fibers]			
Simple	Silk Fibroin	Liu et al. (2011), Madden et al. (2011), and Lv et al. (2014)	VTE, SE, CE
	Collagen	Jiang et al. (2013)	SE
	Laminin I	Neal et al. (2009)	SE
Hybrid biologic	SF+Gelatin	Feng et al. (2014)	CE, Cornea
	SF+Chitosan	Guan et al. (2013a,b)	Cornea
	SF+Collagen IV	Madden et al. (2011)	CE
	SF+Fibronectin	Madden et al. (2011)	CE
	SF+Chondroitin–Laminin	Madden et al. (2011)	CE
	Keratin+Chitosan	Vazquez et al. (2015)	Cornea
	Chitosan+Laminins peptides	Yamada et al. (2011)	SE
	Alginate+Laminins peptides	Yamada et al. (2011)	SE
Hybrid bio-synthetic	SF+poly (ε-caprolactone)	Lv et al. (2014)	SE

CE, corneal endothelium; C.Epi, corneal epithelium; ECM, extracellular matrix; SF, silk fibroin; PA, peritoneal adhesions; RM, regenerative medicine; SE, simple epithelia; VTE, vascular tissue engineering.

mesothelial cells should facilitate the manufacture of biomimetics of the vascular endothelium, the corneal endothelium or inclusively of the synovial intimal lining.

It is therefore reasonable to hypothesize that the use of porcine decellularized tissues such as the mesenteric membrane could be successfully combined with human mesothelial cells and potentially useful for the regeneration of simple squamous epithelia. This consideration will remain to be experimentally addressed.

Decellularized Amniotic Membrane

The human amniotic membrane is a thin avascular membrane composed of a stromal layer and a basement membrane on which is anchored a layer of amniotic cells that are bath in amniotic fluid. The use of the amniotic membrane as potential scaffold in tissue engineering has attracted growing interest since many decades ago, principally because of its wide availability, large surface, and remarkable biological and mechanical properties of its matrix. At term, the human amniotic membrane reaches a total surface area ranging between 1300 and 1500 cm^2 (Niknejad et al., 2008). An adequate decellularization process of the amniotic membrane could strongly minimizes the loss of its original bioactivity (growth factors) and mechanical properties of its stromal matrix and particularly those of its basement membrane, which is critical for an optimal cells adhesion and growth (Hopkinson et al., 2008). However, and soon before parturition, the ECM proteins of amniotic and chorionic membranes are rapidly broken down by matrix metalloproteinases (MMPs) to facilitate their mechanical rupture. The loss of their original mechanical properties may therefore potentially compromise their use for tissue-engineering applications where tensile strength is a critical factor. Amniotic membranes obtained from cesarean will overcome these limitations.

Decellularized amnion has been already used to build grafts that were experimentally applied for wound dressing, skin regeneration (Wilshaw et al., 2006), peritoneal adhesions (Kuriu et al., 2009; Yetkin et al., 2009), peritoneum reconstruction, vascular endothelium replacement (Tsai et al., 2007), or even more for corneal epithelium and endothelium replacement (Xu et al., 2012; Fan et al., 2013; Feng et al., 2014). Technical advances in decellularization processes have permit the generation of a commercially available decellularized and dehydrated human amniotic membrane (DDHAM) allograft which demonstrated positive clinical outcomes for healing of chronic wounds in humans (Smiell et al., 2015) and potential use in ocular surface surgery (Lim et al., 2010).

Natural Polymers and Extracellular Matrix Proteins

Polymeric biomolecules produced either by plants or animals have attracted increasing interest for many tissue-engineering applications. Technological progresses made in the field of biomaterials have permitted that many of these natural polymeric molecules were better isolated, purified, chemically modified, and processed in the form of biological scaffolds (Shin et al., 2003; Ma, 2008). A host of natural biopolymers have been already tested to create thin laminar scaffolds applicable to tissue engineering of serosal membranes biomimetics. Cellulose is the best example of plant biopolymer potentially useful in biomedical research. Alginate, a large polysaccharide principally extracted from brown algae is also another good example of useful plant-derived biopolymer for biomedical applications. Regarding animal-derived biopolymers, the suitability of native polymeric ECM such as collagen, chitosan, or inclusively hyaluronic acid used alone or in combination in order to build biological laminar scaffolds is under intense focus and is detailed below.

Collagen

Collagen proteins are the predominant structural matrix components in connective animal tissues, representing an average of 25–35% of the total body weight. Collagen proteins are very diverse, and each of them endowed with unique properties [for review, see Kadler et al. (2007)]. Their excellent biocompatibility, bioactivity, degradability, and processing capacities into diverse solid formats (sheets, tubes, gels, or porous sponges) make of collagens excellent biomaterials to engineer tailored biological scaffolds and produce them on a large scale. Collagen type I is the predominant type of collagen used in tissue engineering, allowing the formation of rope-like structures that confer strength to bioengineered scaffolds. Collagen-based scaffolds used in tissue engineering of simple squamous epithelium biomimetics should be thin membranes with high collagen density and tensile strength to minimize their contraction by cell shrinkage. Ideally, this limitation can be strongly overcome by reinforcing collagen fibers cohesion by physical or chemical post-crosslinking (Fathima et al., 2010; Jiang et al., 2013) or through combination with other biological materials conferring additional strength such as silk fibroin (SF) (Madden et al., 2011). Collagen-based scaffolds subjected to post-crosslinking have been already used to bioengineer corneal endothelium biomimetics (Mimura et al., 2012).

Fibronectin

Fibronectin is a multifunctional glycoprotein actively involved in a variety of cells–cells and cells–matrix interactions through distinct classes of binding domains specific to integrins, growth factors, fibrin, heparin, collagen, glycosaminoglycans, and proteoglycans (Zhu and Clark, 2014). Fibronectin is a significant ECM component of the basal lamina in native simple epithelial tissues and in the endothelium (Laurie et al., 1982; Yen et al., 1997; Witz et al., 2001). Its role in tissue engineering has gained increasing force as functionalizing molecule increasing the bioactivity of biological scaffolds, principally since the discovery of its RGD binding domain, a tripeptide composed of L-arginine, glycine, and L-aspartic acid, also present in other ECM proteins such as collagen, that could be synthetically used as substitution of fibronectin for coating of material scaffolds and increase their cellular adhesion capacity (Pierschbacher and Ruoslahti, 1984).

Laminins

Laminins are key protein components of the basal lamina layer of basement membranes of distinct types simple epithelia (Laurie et al., 1982). As such, different tissue-engineering applications already integrated a laminin coating treatment of biological scaffolds as a critical step to enhance cells adhesion. Laminin coating of collagen compressed gels was already performed to create a bioartificial cornea (Mi and Connon, 2013). In a similar way, coating of prosthetic vascular small conduit grafts with laminin alone or in combination with collagen, considerably increased endothelial cells adhesion on the luminal graft surface (Chlupac et al., 2014). Of particular interest is the generation of a fibrillar mesh with electrospun laminin that under adequate conditions could generate a thin basement membrane-like carrier for cells adhesion and growth (Neal et al., 2009). The identification of laminin's peptide sequences with cell-binding activities is of particular interest to develop synthetic basement membrane by covalently binding synthetic laminin peptides with polysaccharides such as chitosan or alginate (Yamada et al., 2011).

Gelatin

Gelatin is obtained through partial hydrolysis of collagen, leading to a mixture of peptides and amino acids. As gelatinous substance, gelatin is a highly malleable substance that could be cast in a large variety of 3D scaffold molds. Given to its excellent biocompatibility and malleability, gelatin is also commonly used in combination with solid biomaterials providing strength, while gelatin is used as complement to increase cell adhesion and growth, by providing a soft substrate closer to native ECM (Santoro et al., 2014). Gelatin is particularly useful to generate thin laminar scaffolds somehow mimicking native basement membranes and also to provide a carrier for cells sheet establishment and transplantation. In this way, gelatin hydrogels have been demonstrated useful for tissue engineering of a basement membrane biomimetic for the vascular endothelium (Bruggeman et al., 2012) and also for the corneal endothelium, through establishment of porous gelatin disk generated through cross-linking with carbodiimide (Lai and Li, 2010; Lai et al., 2013).

Alginate

Alginate or alginic acid is an anionic polysaccharide with high hydration capacity and which is widely distributed into brown algae (d'Ayala et al., 2008). Hydrated alginate can form a viscous gel highly compatible for cells and with high biodegradability. By controlling its processing, purified alginate powder can form a solid gel that is mainly useful for cells encapsulation procedures (d'Ayala et al., 2008). Alginate gels have however the downsides of displaying reduced mechanical strength and limited cell adhesion capacities. Like gelatin or inclusively collagens, alginate is generally mixed with other types of biomaterials with higher strength and cell adhesion properties such as chitosan or SF (Lai et al., 2007; Watanabe et al., 2011).

Chitosan

Chitosan is a long-chain polysaccharide derived by deacetylation of chitin, a polymer of N-acetylglucosamine, the structural component of the exoskeleton of arthropods and insects. Commercial chitosan is generally obtained from crustacean shells, mainly from shrimps and crabs. The high-abundance of chitin in nature, makes of its derivative, chitosan a very easy accessible and cheap biomaterial with several desired biological properties for tissue engineering of biological scaffolds, such as a high biocompatibility, easily processable by only pH modification, highly malleable (molding, casting) to generate scaffold with a desired form, porosity, and stiffness. Furthermore, and not less important, the polymer chitosan is particularly rich in chemical side groups, that allow covalent binding with other biomaterials to produce biodegradable biocomposites with increased strength and cell adhesion potential (d'Ayala et al., 2008). Mixtures of chitosan with other biopolymers such as SF or collagen represent useful biocomposites to create laminar biological scaffolds (Grolik et al., 2012; Guan et al., 2013a; Guan et al., 2013b). Additionally, chitosan has also been combined with synthetic polymers such as polyethylene glycol (PEG) for corneal tissue engineering (Rafat et al., 2008).

Silk Fibroin

Silk fibroin obtained from the silkworm (bombyx mori) is considered as a new bioengineering treasure by a majority of the biomedical community. Its outstanding biophysical and biochemical properties such as robustness, flexibility, biocompatibility, biodegradability, and processing properties have prompted a general interest for its use in tissue-engineering applications [for review, see Chen et al. (2011)]. The process of electrospinning allows the production of nano/micro SF fibers and their arrangement in a large varieties of scaffolds including aligned biofunctional nanofibers (Wittmer et al., 2011) and fibrous meshworks mimicking closely native ECM of a given type of tissue [for review, see Zhang et al. (2009)]. Interestingly, electrospun SF nanofibers can provide a high surface area improving cells surface adhesion, while maintaining high porosity for oxygen and molecules permeation, two of the properties provided by the basal lamina in serous membranes. Electrospun SF fibers can be alternatively post-treated with either synthetic or biologic compounds [hyaluronic acid, gelatin, chitosan, polycaprolactone (PC), polypyrrole, etc.] to generate hybrid scaffolds with increased properties or inclusively newly acquired functions (Huang et al., 2013; Yan et al., 2013).

Bioartificial functionalized SF fibrous scaffolds have been yet applied for tissue engineering of vascular endothelium and corneal endothelium biomimetics (Liu et al., 2011; Madden et al., 2011). In these works, the authors described how vascular and corneal endothelial cells (CECs) could readily adhere onto these constructs, proliferate, and form confluent monolayers of cells retaining original phenotypic characteristics. Despite such interesting results, SF-based fibrous meshes have still not been applied to the manufacture a mesothelial tissue biomimetic. Similar positive outcomes with the use of mesothelial cells are likely to be expected, given their close phenotypic similarities with vascular endothelial cells (Chung-Welch et al., 1989, 1997a,b) and CECs (Jirsova et al., 2010; Lachaud et al., 2014b).

Mesothelialization Processes of Biological Scaffolds

The fabrication of a scaffold and its subsequent cellularization are critical steps conditioning the success of the resulting bioengineered tissue. Usually, different type of artificial biological scaffolds may be eventually post-treated with combined proteins generating an artificial basement membrane with are critical for the establishment of artificial simple epithelia. Their subsequent cellularization process is also complex and should basically take into account the phenotypic properties of the cells to be seeded and the cellular architecture of native tissues to be replaced.

The manufacture of simple squamous epithelia biomimetics with the use of mesothelial cells can be roughly achieved by using two distinct cellularization approaches, which can be either through classical static cell-seeding and culture of the scaffold or alternatively through culture of harvestable mesothelial cells sheets that are further layered on top of the scaffold (Asano et al., 2006).

Precoating of Biological Scaffolds with an Artificial Basement Membrane

The basement membrane is a thin multilayered matrix that acts as an anchoring substrate for the epithelium, mesothelium, and endothelium and represents a separating barrier from the underlying connective tissue. In some instances, some hybrid biological scaffolds (i.e., hybrid electrospun SF/polycaprolactone meshes), or scaffolds subjected to posterior treatments (cross-linking) to improve their mechanical properties, can however lose biological properties such as poor cells adhesion index and may require surface treatments with basement membrane proteins. In that sense, different tissue-engineering applications aimed at reproducing and fixing a synthetic basement membrane on top of biologic or synthetic scaffolds to improve adhesive and functional properties of their surface. As example, a study demonstrated that electrospun SF/polycaprolactone meshes posteriorly coated with major basement membrane proteins such as collagen IV, laminins, entactins, and proteoglycans could improve *in vivo* esophageal epithelium regeneration (Lv et al., 2014).

Static Cell-Seeding

The cellular homogeneity and density achieved in a bioengineered mesothelium or in other types of simple squamous epithelial-like tissues are two critical parameters. The static cell-seeding technique, which basically consists in the manual pipetting of a concentrated cells suspension onto the scaffold, has been shown to be a convenient approach for the establishment of mesothelial cells layers (Takazawa et al., 2005; Asano et al., 2006; Kawanishi et al., 2013). Additionally, our laboratory recently reported that a suspension of mesothelial cells adequately dropped on top of human lens capsules, followed by their subsequent culture for a short period in a media enhancing their proliferation and blocking their epithelial-to-mesenchymal transition is reliable procedure to generate an efficient (homogeneous and cellularity) mesothelialization of their surface (Lachaud et al., 2014b).

Cell Sheet-Based Tissue Engineering

The generation of non-invasive methods to detach intact cells monolayer with its deposited ECM has been made possible thanks to the development of thermoresponsive cell culture dishes, which are classical polystyrene Petri culture dishes grafted with the thermoresponsive polymer poly-*N*-isopropylacrylamide (PNIPAAm), this "smart polymer" is capable of hydrophobic to hydrophilic reversible transition in response to temperature changes. By only decreasing the culture temperature below its lower critical solution temperature (LCST) that is around 32°C in pure water, PNIPAAm become hydrophobic, and consequently force the release of cells monolayer from the dishes (Takezawa et al., 1990; Okano et al., 1995). The cell sheet technology (CST)

is particularly useful to obtain intact cells monolayer along with their underlying organized extracellular matrix (ECM) without the need to use a supportive scaffold. Not less important, this technique provides monolayered cells with intact plasma membrane proteins (e.g., cell-surface receptors and ion channels) that otherwise should be severely damaged by the proteolytic activity of trypsin required for classical subculture of adherent cells (Huang et al., 2010a). Of further importance, cells in the detaching monolayer can self-retract, a process which leads to a certain compaction of cells sheets. This issue is particularly important for certain therapeutic applications such as corneal endothelium regeneration where the density of the replacement cells monolayer is a critical factor related to tissue functionality.

The generation of mesothelial cells sheets with thermoresponsive dishes has already been reported (Asano et al., 2006; Kawanishi et al., 2013; Inagaki et al., 2015). Additionally, this technology was also employed to manufacture corneal epithelium and corneal endothelium biomimetics (Hsiue et al., 2006; Lai et al., 2007; Kobayashi et al., 2013). The possibility to manufacture sandwiched layers of cultured cells may inclusively facilitate tissue engineering of complex multilayered artificial tissues such as artificial blood vessels or a bioartificial cornea, through applications of corneal epithelium and endothelium biomimetics on opposite sides of a bioartificial corneal stroma.

Therapeutic Applications of Mesothelial Serosal Membranes Biomimetics

The use of mesothelial cells in regenerative medicine has gained increased interest over the course of the last decades. The clinical accessibility and plasticity of mesothelial cells, among other properties of these cells, have stimulated the interest of a significant number of researchers in evaluating their usefulness for diverse regenerative applications, which are reviewed below.

Prevention of Peritoneal Adhesions

The secretion of lubricants by mesothelial cells provides a slippery, non-adhesive, and protective surface enabling visceral organs to freely move inside celomic cavities (Mutsaers and Wilkosz, 2007). A loss of mesothelium lining provoked either by surgery, ischemia, infection, and foreign bodies or by trauma can lead to adhesions between opposite injured surfaces and the formation of a connective band of fibrous tissue (diZerega and Campeau, 2001).

Post-operative peritoneal adhesions are very frequent in patients undergoing open abdominal surgery and can frequently provoke critical intestinal obstructions. In women, endometriosis is a major cause of pelvic adhesion that could lead to chronic pelvic pain and infertility. Peritoneal adhesions are generally very painful since they strongly limit organs from moving freely. The physical separation of damaged serosal with biodegradable adhesion barriers such as Seprafilm (hyaluronic acid + carboxymethylcellulose) represents the main clinical strategy to prevent or reduce post-operative peritoneal adhesions [for review, see Caglayan et al. (2014)].

The development of new adhesion barriers remains however under current research due to the partial effectiveness of the commercially available adhesion barriers. A host of experimental approaches involving pharmacologic treatments and anti-adhesive polymers or molecules promoting endogenous mesothelialization are also under intense research (Arung et al., 2011; Brochhausen et al., 2012). There is a clear consensus among researchers about the idea that an instantaneous regeneration of the injured mesothelial cells layer represents the ideal anti-adhesive strategy to avoid serosal membranes adhesions. Working in this direction, several studies showed the effectiveness of tissue-engineered mesothelial cells sheets in preventing experimentally induced intraperitoneal adhesions in animals (Takazawa et al., 2005; Asano et al., 2006; Kawanishi et al., 2013; Inagaki et al., 2015).

Vascular Grafts

Coronary and peripheral vascular occlusive diseases are among leading health problems worldwide. They currently require vascular bypass procedures, being autogenous veins the ideal replacement option as they show optimal engraftment and do not require immunosuppressive therapies (Thomas et al., 1988). Unfortunately, patients do not always present suitable healthy vascular tissues and are therefore subjected to an interposition of a prosthetic vascular graft. These artificial conduits are however prone to thrombotic occlusion as the materials [mainly polyethylene terephthalate, or Dacron, and polytetrafluorethylene (PTFE)] by which they are made cannot properly avoid platelet adhesion and they usually develop neointimal hyperplasia. Their poor patency is particularly increased in synthetic conduits with a luminal diameter lower than 8–10 μm [for review, see Kapadia et al. (2008) and Palumbo et al. (2014)]. None of the experimental antithrombogenic strategies tested so far could generate artificial small-diameter vascular grafts displaying successful long-term patency (Seifu et al., 2013). Ideally, prosthetic vascular grafts should be lined with autologous vascular endothelial cells to provide an optimal antithrombogenic luminal surface. However, autologous healthy vascular endothelial cells are not always easily accessible or available. These limitations have prompted a general interest in identifying whether other cellular phenotypes could display similar antithrombogenic activities.

Almost quite similar to the vascular endothelium (Tsuzuki, 2009; Hagensen et al., 2012), the mesothelium is also a specialized simple squamous epithelium that retains intrinsic regenerative capacities (Foley-Comer et al., 2002). The initial misidentification of human omentum-derived mesothelial cells cultures with microvascular endothelial cells (Knedler et al., 1989; Takahashi et al., 1989) led to the evidence that mesothelial and endothelial cells are not only morphologically similar but also display phenotypic similarities as evidenced by their common expression of specific endothelial and simple epithelial cells markers (Chung-Welch et al., 1989; Potzsch et al., 1990; Takahashi et al., 1991; Chung-Welch et al., 1997a,b). It was concluded that only the use of a comprehensive panel of endothelial and mesothelial cells markers could readily allow the distinction of one cell phenotype from another. Not less important, it has also become evident that human mesothelial cells partially display some of the functional features specific to endothelial cells such as the ability to produce the fibrinolytic enzyme tissue-type

plasminogen activator (t-PA), urokinase plasminogen activator (Chlupac et al.), plasminogen activator inhibitor type-1 and type-2 (PAI-1 and PAI-2), and the procoagulant protein tissue factor (TF) (Sitter et al., 1996; Chung-Welch et al., 1997a; Ivarsson et al., 1998). Furthermore, and similar to vascular endothelial cells, mesothelial cells similarly synthesize prostacyclin (prostaglandin I2), a molecule inhibiting platelet activation and acting also as vasodilator (Van de Velde et al., 1986). The close similarities between both cell phenotypes thus led some researchers to test whether the mesothelial cell is a good cellular surrogate for vascular endothelium tissue engineering (Louagie et al., 1986; Bull et al., 1988; Bearn et al., 1992; Theuer et al., 1996; Verhagen et al., 1998; Sparks et al., 2002).

Interestingly, the work of Louagie et al. indicated that patches of mesothelium grafted into the anterior wall of the common iliac vein in dogs did not suffer major damage after several weeks of implantation. Two canine transplantation studies using prosthetic (Dacron) arterial grafts seeded with mesothelial cells however generated markedly divergent outcomes, suggesting that the adhesion capacity of mesothelial cells on this type of synthetic material is reduced and thus strongly influences their long-term patency (Bull et al., 1988; Bearn et al., 1992; Bearn et al., 1993). Other study inclusively indicated the luminal mesothelialization of small-diameter ePTFE vascular prostheses with omental mesothelial cells decreased their patency and increased neointimal formation respective to control unseeded prostheses interposed in the same dogs (Verhagen et al., 1998).

Despite these diverging results regarding the potential of mesothelial cells in vascular tissue engineering, it should be considered that Dacron- or ePTFE-based vascular scaffolds display limited adhesive properties for cells attachment (Sarkar et al., 2007). Therefore, mesothelial cells should be rather preferentially combined with vascular scaffolds of biological origin. Porcine decellularized arteries or veins represent useful candidates as they display morphometric similarity to their human counterparts. Furthermore, efficiently decellularized animal arteries retain almost intact native ECM and basement membrane ensuring optimal adhesion of cells onto their luminal surface, which consequently minimize their delamination in response to the strong shear stress variation proper to the arterial blood flow (Zhu et al., 2008a; Quint et al., 2011).

Corneal Endothelium

The corneal endothelium is the innermost layer of the cornea bathed in the aqueous humor of the eye's anterior chamber. It is made up of a monolayer of CECs anchored on top of a basal membrane, the Descemet membrane. The corneal endothelium layer is critically required for the functionality of the cornea, since CECs are the cells that actively regulate the hydration state of the cornea by pumping out the excess of water in the cornea stroma into the aqueous humor (Bourne, 2003). At the same time, the corneal endothelium is a semi-permeable barrier allowing the transit of solute and nutrients from the aqueous humor toward more superficial layers of the cornea to nourish corneal stromal fibroblasts and corneal epithelial cells. Adult CECs are postmitotic cells that almost lack endogenous regenerative capacities. Diverse studies have shown that the healthy corneal endothelium suffers an inexorable age-related decline in cellularity, which is compensated through hypertrophy of preexisting cells (Senoo and Joyce, 2000; Bourne, 2003). The corneal endothelium could suffer a critical loss of cellularity as a result of either physical or chemical damages or genetic disorders. A loss of corneal endothelium cellularity below a critical threshold leads to an inevitable loss of functionality and a subsequent accumulation of water into the corneal stroma and ultimately to the loss of vision (Bourne, 2003). The only effective clinical treatment available so far is the transplantation of a donor whole cornea or corneal endothelium layer. The important shortage of suitable donor corneas has stimulated the development of host of experimental tissue-engineering strategies to create a bioartificial corneal endothelium or inclusively to achieve the manufacturing of a whole bioartificial cornea [for review, see Mimura et al. (2013)]. Although the majority of these experimental approaches were performed with human CECs, several other studies also reported that CECs-like cells could be obtained through directed differentiation of stem cells populations such as neural crest stem cells, mesenchymal stem cells, and embryonic stem cells [for review, see Yuan and Fan (2015)]. Our laboratory recently reported that mesothelial cells isolated from the mouse visceral adipose tissue sharing many phenotypical similarities with mouse CECs (Lachaud et al., 2014b). Furthermore, we found that mesothelial cells could readily adhere onto decellularized epithelial side surface of human lens capsules. Mesothelial could actively proliferate and generate a compact cell monolayer mimicking some of the main morphological features of the native corneal endothelium (Lachaud et al., 2014b).

Further studies remain to address whether a mesothelial cells monolayer could also be established on other types of biological scaffolds fulfilling the main biophysical characteristics of the Descemet membrane such are transparency, strength, elasticity, and permeability to small molecules (i.e., nutrients). Thin membranes created from electrospun bombyx mori silk fibroin (BMSF) are transparent and were shown to support the growth of human corneal epithelial (HCE) cells (Hogerheyde et al., 2014). Additionally, biological scaffolds that were already tested with human CECs may also be suitable to establish a mesothelial cells monolayer. Among them are found chitosan-based membranes, donor Descemet's membrane, cross-linked collagen matrix, human corneal stromal disks, gelatin hydrogel disks, acellular porcine corneal matrix, plastic compressed collagen, and decellularized human amniotic membrane [for review, see Mimura et al. (2012), Mimura et al. (2013), and Zavala et al. (2013)].

Potential Therapeutic Applications of Mesothelial Serosal Membranes Biomimetics

The evidence that mesothelial cells share structural and biochemical markers with other types of simple epithelial-like cells (see **Table 1**) supports the idea that these cells might be useful for the regeneration of other types of simple epithelial-like tissues. Some possible applications are suggested below.

Synovial Membrane

The synovial membrane is a thin membrane lining the inner surface of the fibrous joint capsule, tendon sheaths, and bursae. The healthy synovium surface layer of cells (intima) is made up of two types of synoviocytes: "phagocytic or absorptive" macrophage-like cells (Type A) and "secretory" fibroblast-like synoviocytes (Type B), these later accounting for around 80% of the total intimal cells (Smith, 2011). Synovial cavities are filled with synovial fluid, a viscous lubricating fluid which forms from an ultrafiltrate of plasma and the secretion of lubricant molecules (mainly proteoglycan-4 and hyaluronan) secreted by fibroblast-like synoviocytes and chondrocytes (Smith, 2011). Distinct to a true epithelium, intimal surface synoviocytes are not tightly adhered to each other by junctional complexes and do not rest on a clearly well developed and continuous basement membrane, even if some basement membrane proteins such as collagen IV and laminin are expressed beneath the basal membrane of fibroblast-like synoviocytes (Pollock et al., 1990; Smith, 2011).

Interestingly, a careful revision of the literature provides evidence of phenotypic similarities between fibroblast-like synoviocytes and mesothelial cells. Hence, both cellular phenotypes are mesodermal epithelial-like cells which display abundant microvilli on their apical membrane, a structural feature that is commonly found in cells secreting fluid (Smith, 2011). In addition, they both abundantly secrete hyaluronan (Hesseldahl and Larsen, 1969; Yung and Chan, 2007; Koyama et al., 2008). Furthermore, both cell phenotypes also express the pan mesenchymal marker vimentin and the intercellular adhesion molecule β-catenin, CD54 (ICAM-1), N-cadherin, and cadherin-11 (Shibata et al., 1996; Agarwal et al., 2008; Kato et al., 2013; Lee et al., 2013; Lachaud et al., 2014a; Lachaud et al., 2014b). Similar to mesothelial cells, fibroblast-like synoviocytes are also antigen-presenting cells and as such they express detectable levels of MHC-II and costimulatory molecule CD40 (Valle et al., 1995; Yang et al., 2004; Kato et al., 2013).

The evidence of phenotypic similarities between fibroblast-like synoviocytes and mesothelial cells stated above could lead to the suggestion that mesothelial cells may represent a putative cellular surrogate of fibroblast-like synoviocytes and suggest thus that mesothelial cells could be potentially useful for the regeneration of the synovial membrane lining.

Mesothelium Lining of the Reissner's Membrane

The vestibular duct (scala vestibuli) is a small cavity filled with perilymph inside the cochlea of the inner ear. The scala vestibuli is separated from the scala media by a very thin membrane termed vestibular membrane or Reissner's membrane. The Reissner's membrane facing the scala vestibuli is covered by a monolayer of mesothelial cells. The opposite side facing the cochlear duct a cavity filled by endolymph is covered by an epithelium. A thin basal lamina separates the mesothelium and epithelium layers (Qvortrup et al., 1994). The Reissner's membrane acts principally as permeable barrier to separate the perilymph from the endolymph. It allows a selective diffusion of solutes and nutrients from the perilymph to the endolymph that tightly controls endolymph/perilymph homeostasis. The rupture of the Reissner's membrane caused either by physical trauma or inclusively due to an increased endolymph pressure (endolymphatic hydrops in Ménières disease) leads to severe hearing loss. To date, no experimental cell-based therapies or tissue-engineering applications have been proposed to reconstruct or substitute the damaged Reissner's membrane. The use of autologous peritoneal mesothelial cells in combination with adequate biological matrices may hypothetically allow the development of tissue-engineered surrogates of the Reissner's membrane.

Acknowledgments

Authors are supported by Fondos FEDER, Fundación Progreso y Salud, Consejería de Salud, Junta de Andalucía (Grants PI-0246-2008 to AH), INNPACTO Program (INP-2011-1615-900000) and SUDOE Program-BIOREG (Intereg SOE3/P1/E750) to BS; Consejería de Innovación Ciencia y Empresa, Junta de Andalucía (Grants CTS-6505 to BS); Ministry of Science and Innovation (Red TerCel-FEDER Grant RD12/0019/0028 to BS; Instituto de Salud Carlos III Grant PI14/01015 to BS) and the Ministry of Health and Consumer Affairs "Advanced Therapies Program Grant TRA-120" to BS. CIBERDEM is an initiative of the Instituto de Salud Carlos III.

Glossary

Allograft: The transplant of an organ or tissue from one individual to another of the same species with a different genotype.

Autologous cells: Cells isolated from and transferred to the same individual's body.

Autologous transplantation: Transplantation of cells or tissues, which are derived, stored, and later given back to the same person.

Bioartificial tissue: Biological tissue manufactured *in vitro* and mimicking the properties and functions of the native tissue to be replaced.

Biocompatible material: A material that is biologically tolerated by the surrounding tissue or organ in which it is transplanted.

Biological scaffold: A structural support of biologic origin that serves for cell attachment and subsequent tissue development.

Biomaterials: Materials used to construct artificial organs, rehabilitation devices, or prostheses and replace natural body tissues.

Bioprosthetic: Referring to prosthesis of biological origin that can be either native tissues or prosthesis manufactured from biological materials.

Coelomic cavities: Fluid-filled body cavities, which are lined by an epithelium derived from the mesoderm.

Peritoneal dialysis: Process by which the peritoneal membrane is used as ultrafiltration interface to eliminate blood waste products through the use of a hypertonic solution flowing into and out of the peritoneal cavity through.

Corneal endothelium: The single layer of simple squamous epithelial-like cells lining the inner surface of the cornea.

Decellularization: The process by which cells are removed from tissues or organs to obtain their extracellular components. It is mainly achieved through perfusion or immersion and the use of enzymes and/or detergents.

Epithelial-to-mesenchymal transition: The process by which epithelial cells undergo a transformation into cells with mesenchymal characteristics.

Extracellular matrix (ECM): Structural molecules produced by cells and excreted to the extracellular space within the tissues and that provide cohesive structure to hold tissues together.

Great omentum: A large fold of the peritoneum hanging down from the stomach and containing abundant vasculature and perivascular adipose tissue.

Heterologous transplant: Cells, grafts, or tissues derived from an individual of a different species in which they are transplanted, being therefore antigenically dissimilar.

Immunomodulation: The adjustment of the immune response to a desired level through immunopotentiation, immunosuppression, or induction of immunologic tolerance.

Immunosuppression: Reduction of the immune response, generally through the use of drugs, active molecules, or cells to prevent grafts rejection or control autoimmune diseases.

Lineage tracing study: Identification and follow-up of all progeny of a single cell using different experimental strategies available for lineage tracing such as live-cell imaging, fluorescent reporter constructs, inducible gene expression, and inducible recombinases.

Matrix: The intercellular substance of a tissue or the tissue from which a structure develops.

Mesoderm: One of the three primary germ layers developing in the early embryo.

Mesothelial cells: A type of simple squamous epithelial cells lining the walls of celomic body cavities and visceral organs located inside.

Mesothelioma: Tumor arising from malignant transformation of mesothelial cells.

Myofibroblast: A fibroblastic cell with some contractile properties and that is usually considered an intermediate cell between fibroblasts and smooth muscle cells.

Parietal mesothelial cells: The mesothelial cells lining the parietal surface of serous body cavities.

Polymeric molecules: Molecules of high molecular weight generated through polymerization of smaller molecules (monomers). They are produced either by living organisms or chemically.

Regulatory T cells: A subtype of T lymphocytes with immunosuppressive properties and capacities to abrogate autoimmune diseases.

Serosal membranes: Membranes lining serous cavities and composed of a single layer of simple squamous epithelial resting on a basement membrane underneath.

Simple squamous epithelium: A simple epithelium composed by a single layer of thin and flat polygonal epithelial cells with secretive properties.

Transdifferentiation: The transformation of a differentiated somatic cell into another type without the need of reverting into an intermediate pluripotent state.

Vascular endothelium: The monolayer of cells lining the lumen of blood vessels.

Visceral mesothelial cells: Mesothelial cells covering visceral organs inside body cavities.

Visceral organs: Organs located within internal body cavities, especially those located within the abdomen.

References

Agarwal, S. K., Lee, D. M., Kiener, H. P., and Brenner, M. B. (2008). Coexpression of two mesenchymal cadherins, cadherin 11 and N-cadherin, on murine fibroblast-like synoviocytes. *Arthritis Rheum.* 58, 1044–1054. doi:10.1002/art.23369

Andree, B., Bar, A., Haverich, A., and Hilfiker, A. (2013). Small intestinal submucosa segments as matrix for tissue engineering: review. *Tissue Eng. Part B Rev.* 19, 279–291. doi:10.1089/ten.TEB.2012.0583

Arung, W., Meurisse, M., and Detry, O. (2011). Pathophysiology and prevention of postoperative peritoneal adhesions. *World J. Gastroenterol.* 17, 4545–4553. doi:10.3748/wjg.v17.i41.4545

Asahina, K., Zhou, B., Pu, W. T., and Tsukamoto, H. (2011). Septum transversum-derived mesothelium gives rise to hepatic stellate cells and perivascular mesenchymal cells in developing mouse liver. *Hepatology* 53, 983–995. doi:10.1002/hep.24119

Asano, T., Takazawa, R., Yamato, M., Kageyama, Y., Kihara, K., and Okano, T. (2005). Novel and simple method for isolating autologous mesothelial cells from the tunica vaginalis. *BJU Int.* 96, 1409–1413. doi:10.1111/j.1464-410X.2005.05816.x

Asano, T., Takazawa, R., Yamato, M., Kihara, K., and Okano, T. (2007). Mesothelial cells from tunica vaginalis, a practical source for mesothelial transplantation. *Int. J. Artif. Organs* 30, 495–500.

Asano, T., Takazawa, R., Yamato, M., Takagi, R., Iimura, Y., Masuda, H., et al. (2006). Transplantation of an autologous mesothelial cell sheet prepared from tunica vaginalis prevents post-operative adhesions in a canine model. *Tissue Eng.* 12, 2629–2637. doi:10.1089/ten.2006.12.2629

Atala, A. (2009). Engineering organs. *Curr. Opin. Biotechnol.* 20, 575–592. doi:10.1016/j.copbio.2009.10.003

Atala, A., Kasper, F. K., and Mikos, A. G. (2012). Engineering complex tissues. *Sci. Transl. Med.* 4, 160rv112. doi:10.1126/scitranslmed.3004890

Badylak, S. F. (2007). The extracellular matrix as a biologic scaffold material. *Biomaterials* 28, 3587–3593. doi:10.1016/j.biomaterials.2007.04.043

Bartok, B., and Firestein, G. S. (2010). Fibroblast-like synoviocytes: key effector cells in rheumatoid arthritis. *Immunol. Rev.* 233, 233–255. doi:10.1111/j.0105-2896.2009.00859.x

Bearn, P. E., Miller, K., Bull, H., Seddon, A. M., Mccollum, C. N., and Marston, A. (1992). An immunohistochemical study of mesothelial cell seeding for knitted Dacron. *Int. J. Exp. Pathol.* 73, 801–808.

Bearn, P. E., Seddon, A. M., Mccollum, C. N., and Marston, A. (1993). Mesothelial seeding of knitted Dacron. *Br. J. Surg.* 80, 587–591. doi:10.1002/bjs.1800800512

Bercovici, B., and Gallily, R. (1978). The cytology of the human peritoneal fluid. *Acta Cytol.* 22, 194–197.

Bombara, M. P., Webb, D. L., Conrad, P., Marlor, C. W., Sarr, T., Ranges, G. E., et al. (1993). Cell contact between T cells and synovial fibroblasts causes induction of adhesion molecules and cytokines. *J. Leukoc. Biol.* 54, 399–406.

Bourne, W. M. (2003). Biology of the corneal endothelium in health and disease. *Eye (Lond.)* 17, 912–918. doi:10.1038/sj.eye.6700559

Brochhausen, C., Schmitt, V. H., Planck, C. N., Rajab, T. K., Hollemann, D., Tapprich, C., et al. (2012). Current strategies and future perspectives for intraperitoneal adhesion prevention. *J. Gastrointest. Surg.* 16, 1256–1274. doi:10.1007/s11605-011-1819-9

Brown, J. M., O'brien, S. M., Wu, C., Sikora, J. A., Griffith, B. P., and Gammie, J. S. (2009). Isolated aortic valve replacement in North America comprising 108,687 patients in 10 years: changes in risks, valve types, and outcomes in the Society of Thoracic Surgeons National Database. *J. Thorac. Cardiovasc. Surg.* 137, 82–90. doi:10.1016/j.jtcvs.2008.08.015

Bruggeman, L. A., Doan, R. P., Loftis, J., Darr, A., and Calabro, A. (2012). A cell culture system for the structure and hydrogel properties of basement membranes; application to capillary walls. *Cell. Mol. Bioeng.* 5, 194–204. doi:10.1007/s12195-012-0221-3

Bull, H. A., Pittilo, R. M., Drury, J., Pollock, J. G., Clarke, J. M., Woolf, N., et al. (1988). Effects of autologous mesothelial cell seeding on prostacyclin production within Dacron arterial prostheses. *Br. J. Surg.* 75, 671–674. doi:10.1002/bjs.1800750716

Caglayan, E. K., Caglayan, K., Erdogan, N., Cinar, H., and Gungor, B. (2014). Preventing intraperitoneal adhesions with ethyl pyruvate and hyaluronic acid/carboxymethylcellulose: a comparative study in an experimental model. *Eur. J. Obstet. Gynecol. Reprod. Biol.* 181, 1–5. doi:10.1016/j.ejogrb.2014.07.004

Cai, C. L., Martin, J. C., Sun, Y., Cui, L., Wang, L., Ouyang, K., et al. (2008). A myocardial lineage derives from Tbx18 epicardial cells. *Nature* 454, 104–108. doi:10.1038/nature06969

Carbone, M., Ly, B. H., Dodson, R. F., Pagano, I., Morris, P. T., Dogan, U. A., et al. (2012). Malignant mesothelioma: facts, myths, and hypotheses. *J. Cell. Physiol.* 227, 44–58. doi:10.1002/jcp.22724

Carmona, R., Cano, E., Grueso, E., Ruiz-Villalba, A., Bera, T. K., Gaztambide, J., et al. (2011). Peritoneal repairing cells: a type of bone marrow derived progenitor cells involved in mesothelial regeneration. *J. Cell. Mol. Med.* 15, 1200–1209. doi:10.1111/j.1582-4934.2010.01087.x

Chailley-Heu, B., Rubio, S., Rougier, J. P., Ducroc, R., Barlier-Mur, A. M., Ronco, P., et al. (1997). Expression of hydrophilic surfactant proteins by mesentery cells in rat and man. *Biochem. J.* 328(Pt 1), 251–256.

Chau, Y. Y., Bandiera, R., Serrels, A., Martinez-Estrada, O. M., Qing, W., Lee, M., et al. (2014). Visceral and subcutaneous fat have different origins and evidence supports a mesothelial source. *Nat. Cell Biol.* 16, 367–375. doi:10.1038/ncb2922

Chen, L., Zhu, Y., Li, Y., Liu, Y., and Yu, J. (2011). [Progress and prospect of electrospun silk fibroin in construction of tissue-engineering scaffold]. *Sheng Wu Gong Cheng Xue Bao* 27, 831–837.

Chlupac, J., Filova, E., Havlikova, J., Matejka, R., Riedel, T., Houska, M., et al. (2014). The gene expression of human endothelial cells is modulated by subendothelial extracellular matrix proteins: short-term response to laminar shear stress. *Tissue Eng. Part A* 20, 2253–2264. doi:10.1089/ten.TEA.2013.0153

Chng, Z., Peh, G. S., Herath, W. B., Cheng, T. Y., Ang, H. P., Toh, K. P., et al. (2013). High throughput gene expression analysis identifies reliable expression markers of human corneal endothelial cells. *PLoS ONE* 8:e67546. doi:10.1371/journal.pone.0067546

Chung-Welch, N., Patton, W. F., Shepro, D., and Cambria, R. P. (1997a). Human omental microvascular endothelial and mesothelial cells: characterization of two distinct mesodermally derived epithelial cells. *Microvasc. Res.* 54, 108–120. doi:10.1006/mvre.1997.2038

Chung-Welch, N., Patton, W. F., Shepro, D., and Cambria, R. P. (1997b). Two-stage isolation procedure for obtaining homogenous populations of microvascular endothelial and mesothelial cells from human omentum. *Microvasc. Res.* 54, 121–134. doi:10.1006/mvre.1997.2039

Chung-Welch, N., Patton, W. F., Yen-Patton, G. P., Hechtman, H. B., and Shepro, D. (1989). Phenotypic comparison between mesothelial and microvascular endothelial cell lineages using conventional endothelial cell markers, cytoskeletal protein markers and in vitro assays of angiogenic potential. *Differentiation* 42, 44–53. doi:10.1111/j.1432-0436.1989.tb00606.x

Coffey, J. C. (2013). Surgical anatomy and anatomic surgery – clinical and scientific mutualism. *Surgeon.* 11, 177–182. doi:10.1016/j.surge.2013.03.002

Damkier, H. H., Nielsen, S., and Praetorius, J. (2007). Molecular expression of SLC4-derived Na+-dependent anion transporters in selected human tissues. *Am. J. Physiol. Regul. Integr. Comp. Physiol.* 293, R2136–R2146. doi:10.1152/ajpregu.00356.2007 d'Ayala, G. G., Malinconico, M., and Laurienzo, P. (2008). Marine derived poly-saccharides for biomedical applications: chemical modification approaches. *Molecules* 13, 2069–2106. doi:10.3390/molecules13092069

Debels, H., Hamdi, M., Abberton, K., and Morrison, W. (2015). Dermal matrices and bioengineered skin substitutes: a critical review of current options. *Plast. Reconstr. Surg. Glob. Open* 3, e284. doi:10.1097/GOX.0000000000000219

Dettman, R. W., Denetclaw, W. Jr., Ordahl, C. P., and Bristow, J. (1998). Common epicardial origin of coronary vascular smooth muscle, perivascular fibroblasts, and intermyocardial fibroblasts in the avian heart. *Dev. Biol.* 193, 169–181. doi:10.1006/dbio.1997.8801

diZerega, G. S., and Campeau, J. D. (2001). Peritoneal repair and post-surgical adhesion formation. *Hum. Reprod. Update* 7, 547–555. doi:10.1093/humupd/7.6.547

Dong, J., Li, Y., and Mo, X. (2013). The study of a new detergent (octyl-glucopyra-noside) for decellularizing porcine pericardium as tissue engineering scaffold. *J. Surg. Res.* 183, 56–67. doi:10.1016/j.jss.2012.11.047

Donna, A., and Betta, P. G. (1981). Mesodermomas: a new embryological approach to primary tumours of coelomic surfaces. *Histopathology* 5, 31–44. doi:10.1111/j.1365-2559.1981.tb01764.x

Duim, S. N., Kurakula, K., Goumans, M. J., and Kruithof, B. P. (2015). Cardiac endothelial cells express Wilms' tumor-1: Wt1 expression in the developing, adult and infarcted heart. *J. Mol. Cell. Cardiol.* 81, 127–135. doi:10.1016/j.yjmcc.2015.02.007

Fan, T., Ma, X., Zhao, J., Wen, Q., Hu, X., Yu, H., et al. (2013). Transplantation of tissue-engineered human corneal endothelium in cat models. *Mol. Vis.* 19, 400–407.

Fathima, N. N., Baias, M., Blumich, B., and Ramasami, T. (2010). Structure and dynamics of water in native and tanned collagen fibers: effect of crosslinking. *Int. J. Biol. Macromol.* 47, 590–596. doi:10.1016/j.ijbiomac.2010.08.003

Feng, Y., Borrelli, M., Reichl, S., Schrader, S., and Geerling, G. (2014). Review of alternative carrier materials for ocular surface reconstruction. *Curr. Eye Res.* 39, 541–552. doi:10.3109/02713683.2013.853803

Foets, B. J., Van Den Oord, J. J., Volpes, R., and Missotten, L. (1992). In situ immunohistochemical analysis of cell adhesion molecules on human corneal endothelial cells. *Br. J. Ophthalmol.* 76, 205–209. doi:10.1136/bjo.76.4.205

Fok, F. K., Bewtra, C., and Hammeke, M. D. (1989). Cytology of peritoneal fluid from patients on continuous ambulatory peritoneal dialysis. *Acta Cytol.* 33, 595–598.

Foley-Comer, A. J., Herrick, S. E., Al-Mishlab, T., Prele, C. M., Laurent, G. J., and Mutsaers, S. E. (2002). Evidence for incorporation of free-floating mesothelial cells as a mechanism of serosal healing. *J. Cell. Sci.* 115, 1383–1389.

Fu, R. H., Wang, Y. C., Liu, S. P., Shih, T. R., Lin, H. L., Chen, Y. M., et al. (2014). Decellularization and recellularization technologies in tissue engineering. *Cell Transplant.* 23, 621–630. doi:10.3727/096368914X678382

Glenn, J. D., and Whartenby, K. A. (2014). Mesenchymal stem cells: emerging mechanisms of immunomodulation and therapy. *World J. Stem Cells* 6, 526–539. doi:10.4252/wjsc.v6.i5.526

Grolik, M., Szczubialka, K., Wowra, B., Dobrowolski, D., Orzechowska-Wylegala, B., Wylegala, E., et al. (2012). Hydrogel membranes based on genipin-cross-linked chitosan blends for corneal epithelium tissue engineering. *J. Mater. Sci. Mater. Med.* 23, 1991–2000. doi:10.1007/s10856-012-4666-7

Guan, L., Ge, H., Tang, X., Su, S., Tian, P., Xiao, N., et al. (2013a). Use of a silk fibroin-chitosan scaffold to construct a tissue-engineered corneal stroma. *Cells Tissues Organs* 198, 190–197. doi:10.1159/000355944

Guan, L., Tian, P., Ge, H., Tang, X., Zhang, H., Du, L., et al. (2013b). Chitosan-functionalized silk fibroin 3D scaffold for keratocyte culture. *J. Mol. Histol.* 44, 609–618. doi:10.1007/s10735-013-9508-5

Hagensen, M. K., Raarup, M. K., Mortensen, M. B., Thim, T., Nyengaard, J. R., Falk, E., et al. (2012). Circulating endothelial progenitor cells do not contribute to regeneration of endothelium after murine arterial injury. *Cardiovasc. Res.* 93, 223–231. doi:10.1093/cvr/cvr278

Hegmans, J. P., Hemmes, A., Hammad, H., Boon, L., Hoogsteden, H. C., and Lambrecht, B. N. (2006). Mesothelioma environment comprises cytokines and T-regulatory cells that suppress immune responses. *Eur. Respir. J.* 27, 1086–1095. doi:10.1183/09031936.06.00135305

Herrick, S. E., and Mutsaers, S. E. (2004). Mesothelial progenitor cells and their potential in tissue engineering. *Int. J. Biochem. Cell Biol.* 36, 621–642. doi:10.1016/j.biocel.2003.11.002

Hesseldahl, H., and Larsen, J. F. (1969). Ultrastructure of human yolk sac: endo-derm, mesenchyme, tubules and mesothelium. *Am. J. Anat.* 126, 315–335. doi:10.1002/aja.1001260306

Hoganson, D. M., Owens, G. E., O'doherty, E. M., Bowley, C. M., Goldman, S. M., Harilal, D. O., et al. (2010). Preserved extracellular matrix components and retained biological activity in decellularized porcine mesothelium. *Biomaterials* 31, 6934–6940. doi:10.1016/j.biomaterials.2010.05.026

Hogerheyde, T. A., Suzuki, S., Stephenson, S. A., Richardson, N. A., Chirila, T. V., Harkin, D. G., et al. (2014). Assessment of freestanding membranes prepared from *Antheraea pernyi* silk fibroin as a potential vehicle for corneal epithelial cell transplantation. *Biomed. Mater.* 9, 025016. doi:10.1088/1748-6041/9/2/025016

Hopkinson, A., Shanmuganathan, V. A., Gray, T., Yeung, A. M., Lowe, J., James, D. K., et al. (2008). Optimization of amniotic membrane (AM) denuding for tissue engineering. *Tissue Eng. Part C Methods* 14, 371–381. doi:10.1089/ten.tec.2008.0315

Hoshiba, T., Lu, H., Kawazoe, N., and Chen, G. (2010). Decellularized matrices for tissue engineering. *Expert Opin. Biol. Ther.* 10, 1717–1728. doi:10.1517/14712598.2010.534079

Hsiue, G. H., Lai, J. Y., Chen, K. H., and Hsu, W. M. (2006). A novel strategy for cor-neal endothelial reconstruction with a bioengineered cell sheet. *Transplantation* 81, 473–476. doi:10.1097/01.tp.0000194864.13539.2c

Huang, H. L., Hsing, H. W., Lai, T. C., Chen, Y. W., Lee, T. R., Chan, H. T., et al. (2010a). Trypsin-induced proteome alteration during cell subculture in mam-malian cells. *J. Biomed. Sci.* 17, 36. doi:10.1186/1423-0127-17-36

Huang, L., Harkenrider, M., Thompson, M., Zeng, P., Tanaka, H., Gilley, D., et al. (2010b). A hierarchy of endothelial colony-forming cell activity displayed by bovine corneal endothelial cells. *Invest. Ophthalmol. Vis. Sci.* 51, 3943–3949. doi:10.1167/iovs.09-4970

Huang, L., Li, C., Yuan, W., and Shi, G. (2013). Strong composite films with layered structures prepared by casting silk fibroin-graphene oxide hydrogels. *Nanoscale* 5, 3780–3786. doi:10.1039/c3nr00196b

Inagaki, N. F., Inagaki, F. F., Kokudo, N., and Miyajima, A. (2015). Use of mouse liver mesothelial cells to prevent postoperative adhesion and promote liver regenera-tion after hepatectomy. *J. Hepatol.* 62, 1141–1147. doi:10.1016/j.jhep.2014.12.010

Ivarsson, M. L., Holmdahl, L., Falk, P., Molne, J., and Risberg, B. (1998). Characterization and fibrinolytic properties of mesothelial cells iso-lated from peritoneal lavage. *Scand. J. Clin. Lab. Invest.* 58, 195–203. doi:10.1080/00365519850186580

Ji, H. L., and Nie, H. G. (2008). Electrolyte and fluid transport in mesothelial cells. *J. Epithel. Biol. Pharmacol.* 1, 1–7. doi:10.2174/1875044300801010001

Jiang, Q., Reddy, N., Zhang, S., Roscioli, N., and Yang, Y. (2013). Water-stable electrospun collagen fibers from a non-toxic solvent and crosslinking system. *J. Biomed. Mater. Res. A.* 101, 1237–1247. doi:10.1002/jbm.a.34422

Jirsova, K., Neuwirth, A., Kalasova, S., Vesela, V., and Merjava, S. (2010). Mesothelial proteins are expressed in the human cornea. *Exp. Eye Res.* 91, 623–629. doi:10.1016/j.exer.2010.08.002

Joo, Y. S., Singer, N. G., Endres, J. L., Sarkar, S., Kinne, R. W., Marks, R. M., et al. (2000). Evidence for the expression of a second CD6 ligand by synovial fibroblasts. *Arthritis Rheum.* 43, 329–335. doi:10.1002/1529-0131(200002)43:2<329::AID-ANR12>3.0.CO;2-Y

Kadler, K. E., Baldock, C., Bella, J., and Boot-Handford, R. P. (2007). Collagens at a glance. *J. Cell. Sci.* 120, 1955–1958. doi:10.1242/jcs.03453

Kapadia, M. R., Popowich, D. A., and Kibbe, M. R. (2008). Modified prosthetic vascular conduits. *Circulation* 117, 1873–1882. doi:10.1161/CIRCULATIONAHA.107.714170

Kato, H., Endres, J., and Fox, D. A. (2013). The roles of IFN-gamma versus IL-17 in pathogenic effects of human Th17 cells on synovial fibroblasts. *Mod. Rheumatol.* 23, 1140–1150. doi:10.1007/s10165-012-0811-x

Katz, S., Balogh, P., and Kiss, A. L. (2011). Mesothelial cells can detach from the mesentery and differentiate into macrophage-like cells. *APMIS* 119, 782–793. doi:10.1111/j.1600-0463.2011.02803.x

Kaully, T., Kaufman-Francis, K., Lesman, A., and Levenberg, S. (2009). Vascularization – the conduit to viable engineered tissues. *Tissue Eng. Part B Rev.* 15, 159–169. doi:10.1089/ten.teb.2008.0193

Kawanishi, K., Yamato, M., Sakiyama, R., Okano, T., and Nitta, K. (2013). Peritoneal cell sheets composed of mesothelial cells and fibroblasts prevent intra-abdominal adhesion formation in a rat model. *J Tissue Eng. Regen. Med.* doi:10.1002/term.1860

Kawasaki, H., Kosugi, I., Sakao-Suzuki, M., Meguro, S., Arai, Y., Tsutsui, Y., et al. (2015). Cytomegalovirus initiates infection selectively from high-level beta1 integrin-expressing cells in the brain. *Am. J. Pathol.* 185, 1304–1323. doi:10.1016/j.ajpath.2015.01.032

Kitayama, J., Emoto, S., Yamaguchi, H., Ishigami, H., Yamashita, H., Seto, Y., et al. (2014). CD90(+)CD45(-) intraperitoneal mesothelial-like cells inhibit T cell activation by production of arginase I. *Cell. Immunol.* 288, 8–14. doi:10.1016/j.cellimm.2014.01.008

Klopsch, C., and Steinhoff, G. (2012). Tissue-engineered devices in cardiovascular surgery. *Eur. Surg. Res.* 49, 44–52. doi:10.1159/000339606

Knedler, A., Eckel, R. H., Kern, P. A., and Ham, R. G. (1989). Microvascular endothelial cell cultures from human omental adipose tissue. *In vitro Cell. Dev. Biol.* 25, 863–864. doi:10.1007/BF02623995

Kobayashi, T., Kan, K., Nishida, K., Yamato, M., and Okano, T. (2013). Corneal regeneration by transplantation of corneal epithelial cell sheets fabricated with automated cell culture system in rabbit model. *Biomaterials* 34, 9010–9017. doi:10.1016/j.biomaterials.2013.07.065

Koyama, E., Shibukawa, Y., Nagayama, M., Sugito, H., Young, B., Yuasa, T., et al. (2008). A distinct cohort of progenitor cells participates in synovial joint and articular cartilage formation during mouse limb skeletogenesis. *Dev. Biol.* 316, 62–73. doi:10.1016/j.ydbio.2008.01.012

Kuriu, Y., Yamagishi, H., Otsuji, E., Nakashima, S., Miyagawa, K., Yoshikawa, T., et al. (2009). Regeneration of peritoneum using amniotic membrane to prevent postoperative adhesions. *Hepatogastroenterology* 56, 1064–1068.

Lachaud, C. C., Lopez-Beas, J., Soria, B., and Hmadcha, A. (2014a). EGF-induced adipose tissue mesothelial cells undergo functional vascular smooth muscle differentiation. *Cell Death Dis.* 5, e1304. doi:10.1038/cddis.2014.271

Lachaud, C. C., Soria, F., Escacena, N., Quesada-Hernandez, E., Hmadcha, A., Alio, J., et al. (2014b). Mesothelial cells: a cellular surrogate for tissue engineering of corneal endothelium. *Invest. Ophthalmol. Vis. Sci.* 55, 5967–5978. doi:10.1167/iovs.14-14706

Lachaud, C. C., Pezzolla, D., Dominguez-Rodriguez, A., Smani, T., Soria, B., and Hmadcha, A. (2013). Functional vascular smooth muscle-like cells derived from adult human uterine mesothelial cells. *PLoS ONE* 8:e55181. doi:10.1371/journal.pone.0055181

Lai, J. Y., Chen, K. H., and Hsiue, G. H. (2007). Tissue-engineered human corneal endothelial cell sheet transplantation in a rabbit model using functional biomaterials. *Transplantation* 84, 1222–1232. doi:10.1097/01.tp.0000287336.09848.39

Lai, J. Y., and Li, Y. T. (2010). Functional assessment of cross-linked porous gelatin hydrogels for bioengineered cell sheet carriers. *Biomacromolecules* 11, 1387–1397. doi:10.1021/bm100213f

Lai, J. Y., Ma, D. H., Lai, M. H., Li, Y. T., Chang, R. J., and Chen, L. M. (2013). Characterization of cross-linked porous gelatin carriers and their interaction with corneal endothelium: biopolymer concentration effect. *PLoS ONE* 8:e54058. doi:10.1371/journal.pone.0054058

Lai, K. N., Li, F. K., Lan, H. Y., Tang, S., Tsang, A. W., Chan, D. T., et al. (2001). Expression of aquaporin-1 in human peritoneal mesothelial cells and its upregulation by glucose in vitro. *J. Am. Soc. Nephrol.* 12, 1036–1045.

Lanfrancone, L., Boraschi, D., Ghiara, P., Falini, B., Grignani, F., Peri, G., et al. (1992). Human peritoneal mesothelial cells produce many cytokines (granulocyte colony-stimulating factor [CSF], granulocyte-monocyte-CSF, macrophage-CSF, interleukin-1 [IL-1], and IL-6) and are activated and stimulated to grow by IL-1. *Blood* 80, 2835–2842.

Lansley, S. M., Searles, R. G., Hoi, A., Thomas, C., Moneta, H., Herrick, S. E., et al. (2011). Mesothelial cell differentiation into osteoblast- and adipocyte-like cells. *J. Cell. Mol. Med.* 15, 2095–2105. doi:10.1111/j.1582-4934.2010.01212.x

Laurie, G. W., Leblond, C. P., and Martin, G. R. (1982). Localization of type IV collagen, laminin, heparan sulfate proteoglycan, and fibronectin to the basal lamina of basement membranes. *J. Cell Biol.* 95, 340–344. doi:10.1083/jcb.95.1.340

Lee, B. L., Tang, Z., Wang, A., Huang, F., Yan, Z., Wang, D., et al. (2013). Synovial stem cells and their responses to the porosity of microfibrous scaffold. *Acta Biomater.* 9, 7264–7275. doi:10.1016/j.actbio.2013.03.009

Lim, L. S., Poh, R. W., Riau, A. K., Beuerman, R. W., Tan, D., and Mehta, J. S. (2010). Biological and ultrastructural properties of acelagraft, a freeze-dried gamma-irradiated human amniotic membrane. *Arch. Ophthalmol.* 128, 1303–1310. doi:10.1001/archophthalmol.2010.222

Lin, C. Y., Kift-Morgan, A., Moser, B., Topley, N., and Eberl, M. (2013). Suppression of pro-inflammatory T-cell responses by human mesothelial cells. *Nephrol. Dial. Transplant.* 28, 1743–1750. doi:10.1093/ndt/gfs612

Liu, H., Li, X., Zhou, G., Fan, H., and Fan, Y. (2011). Electrospun sulfated silk fibroin nanofibrous scaffolds for vascular tissue engineering. *Biomaterials* 32, 3784–3793. doi:10.1016/j.biomaterials.2011.02.002

Louagie, Y., Legrand-Monsieur, A., Remacle, C., Maldague, P., Lambotte, L., and Ponlot, R. (1986). Morphology and fibrinolytic activity of canine autogenous mesothelium used as venous substitute. *Res. Exp. Med. (Berl.)* 186, 239–247. doi:10.1007/BF01852301

Lovett, M., Lee, K., Edwards, A., and Kaplan, D. L. (2009). Vascularization strategies for tissue engineering. *Tissue Eng. Part B Rev.* 15, 353–370. doi:10.1089/ten.TEB.2009.0085

Lv, J., Chen, L., Zhu, Y., Hou, L., and Liu, Y. (2014). Promoting epithelium regeneration for esophageal tissue engineering through basement membrane reconstitution. *ACS Appl. Mater. Interfaces* 6, 4954–4964. doi:10.1021/am4059809

Ma, P. X. (2008). Biomimetic materials for tissue engineering. *Adv. Drug Deliv. Rev.* 60, 184–198. doi:10.1016/j.addr.2007.08.041

Madden, P. W., Lai, J. N., George, K. A., Giovenco, T., Harkin, D. G., and Chirila, T. V. (2011). Human corneal endothelial cell growth on a silk fibroin membrane. *Biomaterials* 32, 4076–4084. doi:10.1016/j.biomaterials.2010.12.034

Medina, R. J., O'neill, C. L., Humphreys, M. W., Gardiner, T. A., and Stitt, A. W. (2010). Outgrowth endothelial cells: characterization and their potential for reversing ischemic retinopathy. *Invest. Ophthalmol. Vis. Sci.* 51, 5906–5913. doi:10.1167/iovs.09-4951

Merjava, S., Neuwirth, A., Mandys, V., and Jirsova, K. (2009). Cytokeratins 8 and 18 in adult human corneal endothelium. *Exp. Eye Res.* 89, 426–431. doi:10.1016/j.exer.2009.04.009

Mi, S., and Connon, C. J. (2013). The formation of a tissue-engineered cornea using plastically compressed collagen scaffolds and limbal stem cells. *Methods Mol. Biol.* 1014, 143–155. doi:10.1007/978-1-62703-432-6_9

Michailova, K., Wassilev, W., and Wedel, T. (1999). Scanning and transmission electron microscopic study of visceral and parietal peritoneal regions in the rat. *Ann. Anat.* 181, 253–260. doi:10.1016/S0940-9602(99)80040-5

Mikos, A. G., Herring, S. W., Ochareon, P., Elisseeff, J., Lu, H. H., Kandel, R., et al. (2006). Engineering complex tissues. *Tissue Eng.* 12, 3307–3339. doi:10.1089/ten.2006.12.3307

Mimura, T., Yamagami, S., and Amano, S. (2013). Corneal endothelial regeneration and tissue engineering. *Prog. Retin. Eye Res.* 35, 1–17. doi:10.1016/j.preteyeres.2013.01.003

Mimura, T., Yokoo, S., and Yamagami, S. (2012). Tissue engineering of corneal endothelium. *J. Funct. Biomater.* 3, 726–744. doi:10.3390/jfb3040726

Mobasheri, A., and Marples, D. (2004). Expression of the AQP-1 water channel in normal human tissues: a semiquantitative study using tissue microarray technology. *Am. J. Physiol. Cell Physiol.* 286, C529–C537. doi:10.1152/ajpcell.00408.2003

Muragaki, Y., Mattei, M. G., Yamaguchi, N., Olsen, B. R., and Ninomiya, Y. (1991). The complete primary structure of the human alpha 1 (VIII) chain and assignment of its gene (COL8A1) to chromosome 3. *Eur. J. Biochem.* 197, 615–622. doi:10.1111/j.1432-1033.1991.tb15951.x

Murohara, T., Witzenbichler, B., Spyridopoulos, I., Asahara, T., Ding, B., Sullivan, A., et al. (1999). Role of endothelial nitric oxide synthase in endothelial cell migration. *Arterioscler. Thromb. Vasc. Biol.* 19, 1156–1161. doi:10.1161/01.ATV.19.5.1156

Mutsaers, S. E. (2002). Mesothelial cells: their structure, function and role in serosal repair. *Respirology* 7, 171–191. doi:10.1046/j.1440-1843.2002.00404.x

Mutsaers, S. E. (2004). The mesothelial cell. *Int. J. Biochem. Cell Biol.* 36, 9–16. doi:10.1016/S1357-2725(03)00242-5

Mutsaers, S. E., Prele, C. M., Lansley, S. M., and Herrick, S. E. (2007). The origin of regenerating mesothelium: a historical perspective. *Int. J. Artif. Organs* 30, 484–494.

Mutsaers, S. E., and Wilkosz, S. (2007). Structure and function of mesothelial cells. *Cancer Treat. Res.* 134, 1–19.

Neal, R. A., Mcclugage, S. G., Link, M. C., Sefcik, L. S., Ogle, R. C., and Botchwey, E. A. (2009). Laminin nanofiber meshes that mimic morphological properties and bioactivity of basement membranes. *Tissue Eng. Part C Methods* 15, 11–21. doi:10.1089/ten.tec.2007.0366

Niknejad, H., Peirovi, H., Jorjani, M., Ahmadiani, A., Ghanavi, J., and Seifalian, A. M. (2008). Properties of the amniotic membrane for potential use in tissue engineering. *Eur. Cell. Mater.* 15, 88–99.

Nomi, M., Atala, A., Coppi, P. D., and Soker, S. (2002). Principals of neovascularization for tissue engineering. *Mol. Aspects Med.* 23, 463–483. doi:10.1016/S0098-2997(02)00008-0

Novosel, E. C., Kleinhans, C., and Kluger, P. J. (2011). Vascularization is the key challenge in tissue engineering. *Adv. Drug Deliv. Rev.* 63, 300–311. doi:10.1016/j.addr.2011.03.004

Okano, T., Yamada, N., Okuhara, M., Sakai, H., and Sakurai, Y. (1995). Mechanism of cell detachment from temperature-modulated, hydrophilic-hydrophobic polymer surfaces. *Biomaterials* 16, 297–303. doi:10.1016/0142-9612(95)93257-E

Okumura, N., Hirano, H., Numata, R., Nakahara, M., Ueno, M., Hamuro, J., et al. (2014). Cell surface markers of functional phenotypic corneal endothelial cells. *Invest. Ophthalmol. Vis. Sci.* 55, 7610–7618. doi:10.1167/iovs.14-14980

Palumbo, V. D., Bruno, A., Tomasello, G., Damiano, G., and Lo Monte, A. I. (2014). Bioengineered vascular scaffolds: the state of the art. *Int. J. Artif. Organs* 37, 503–512. doi:10.5301/ijao.5000343

Park, K. M., and Gerecht, S. (2014). Harnessing developmental processes for vascular engineering and regeneration. *Development* 141, 2760–2769. doi:10.1242/dev.102194

Pierschbacher, M. D., and Ruoslahti, E. (1984). Cell attachment activity of fibronectin can be duplicated by small synthetic fragments of the molecule. *Nature* 309, 30–33. doi:10.1038/309030a0

Pollock, L. E., Lalor, P., and Revell, P. A. (1990). Type IV collagen and laminin in the synovial intimal layer: an immunohistochemical study. *Rheumatol. Int.* 9, 277–280. doi:10.1007/BF00541324

Potzsch, B., Grulich-Henn, J., Rossing, R., Wille, D., and Muller-Berghaus, G. (1990). Identification of endothelial and mesothelial cells in human omental tissue and in omentum-derived cultured cells by specific cell markers. *Lab. Invest.* 63, 841–852.

Pronk, A., Leguit, P., Hoynck Van Papendrecht, A. A., Hagelen, E., Van Vroonhoven, T. J., and Verbrugh, H. A. (1993). A cobblestone cell isolated from the human omentum: the mesothelial cell; isolation, identification, and growth characteristics. *In vitro Cell. Dev. Biol.* 29A, 127–134. doi:10.1007/BF02630943

Que, J., Wilm, B., Hasegawa, H., Wang, F., Bader, D., and Hogan, B. L. (2008). Mesothelium contributes to vascular smooth muscle and mesenchyme during lung development. *Proc. Natl. Acad. Sci. U.S.A.* 105, 16626–16630. doi:10.1073/pnas.0808649105

Quint, C., Kondo, Y., Manson, R. J., Lawson, J. H., Dardik, A., and Niklason, L. E. (2011). Decellularized tissue-engineered blood vessel as an arterial conduit. *Proc. Natl. Acad. Sci. U.S.A.* 108, 9214–9219. doi:10.1073/pnas.1019506108

Qvortrup, K., Rostgaard, J., and Bretlau, P. (1994). Ultrastructure of Reissner's membrane in the rabbit. *Eur. Arch. Otorhinolaryngol.* 251, 249–256. doi:10.1007/BF00181879

Rafat, M., Li, F., Fagerholm, P., Lagali, N. S., Watsky, M. A., Munger, R., et al. (2008). PEG-stabilized carbodiimide crosslinked collagen-chitosan hydrogels for corneal tissue engineering. *Biomaterials* 29, 3960–3972. doi:10.1016/j.biomaterials.2008.06.017

Riera, M., Mcculloch, P., Pazmany, L., and Jagoe, T. (2006). Optimal method for isolation of human peritoneal mesothelial cells from clinical samples of omentum. *J. Tissue Viability* 16, 22–24. doi:10.1016/S0965-206X(06)64005-9

Romero, M. F., Chen, A. P., Parker, M. D., and Boron, W. F. (2013). The SLC4 family of bicarbonate (HCO(3)(-)) transporters. *Mol. Aspects Med.* 34, 159–182. doi:10.1016/j.mam.2012.10.008

Ross, J. A., Ansell, I., Hjelle, J. T., Anderson, J. D., Miller-Hjelle, M. A., and Dobbie, J. W. (1998). Phenotypic mapping of human mesothelial cells. *Adv. Perit. Dial.* 14, 25–30.

Roy, R. S., Roy, B., and Sengupta, S. (2011). Emerging technologies for enabling proangiogenic therapy. *Nanotechnology* 22, 494004. doi:10.1088/0957-4484/22/49/494004

Santoro, M., Tatara, A. M., and Mikos, A. G. (2014). Gelatin carriers for drug and cell delivery in tissue engineering. *J. Control Release* 190, 210–218. doi:10.1016/j.jconrel.2014.04.014

Sarkar, S., Sales, K. M., Hamilton, G., and Seifalian, A. M. (2007). Addressing thrombogenicity in vascular graft construction. *J. Biomed. Mater. Res. Part B Appl. Biomater.* 82, 100–108. doi:10.1002/jbm.b.30710

Schwachula, A., Riemann, D., Kehlen, A., and Langner, J. (1994). Characterization of the immunophenotype and functional properties of fibroblast-like synoviocytes in comparison to skin fibroblasts and umbilical vein endothelial cells. *Immunobiology* 190, 67–92. doi:10.1016/S0171-2985(11)80284-6

Schwarting, A., Schlaak, J., Lotz, J., Pfers, I., Meyer Zum Buschenfelde, K. H., and Mayet, W. J. (1996). Endothelin-1 modulates the expression of adhesion molecules on fibroblast-like synovial cells (FLS). *Scand. J. Rheumatol.* 25, 246–256. doi:10.3109/03009749609069994

Seifu, D. G., Purnama, A., Mequanint, K., and Mantovani, D. (2013). Small-diameter vascular tissue engineering. *Nat. Rev. Cardiol.* 10, 410–421. doi:10.1038/nrcardio.2013.77

Senoo, T., and Joyce, N. C. (2000). Cell cycle kinetics in corneal endothelium from old and young donors. *Invest. Ophthalmol. Vis. Sci.* 41, 660–667.

Shamsuddin, A. K., Nirankari, V. S., Purnell, D. M., and Chang, S. H. (1986). Is the corneal posterior cell layer truly endothelial? *Ophthalmology* 93, 1298–1303. doi:10.1016/S0161-6420(86)33573-5

Shao, C., Fu, Y., Lu, W., and Fan, X. (2011). Bone marrow-derived endothelial progenitor cells: a promising therapeutic alternative for corneal endothelial dysfunction. *Cells Tissues Organs* 193, 253–263. doi:10.1159/000319797

Shibata, T., Ochiai, A., Gotoh, M., Machinami, R., and Hirohashi, S. (1996). Simultaneous expression of cadherin-11 in signet-ring cell carcinoma and stromal cells of diffuse-type gastric cancer. *Cancer Lett.* 99, 147–153. doi:10.1016/0304-3835(95)04047-1

Shin, H., Jo, S., and Mikos, A. G. (2003). Biomimetic materials for tissue engineering. *Biomaterials* 24, 4353–4364. doi:10.1016/S0142-9612(03)00339-9

Sitter, T., Toet, K., Fricke, H., Schiffl, H., Held, E., and Kooistra, T. (1996). Modulation of procoagulant and fibrinolytic system components of mesothelial cells by inflammatory mediators. *Am. J. Physiol.* 271, R1256–R1263.

Smiell, J. M., Treadwell, T., Hahn, H. D., and Hermans, M. H. (2015). Real-world experience with a decellularized dehydrated human amniotic membrane allograft. *Wounds* 27, 158–169.

Smith, M. D. (2011). The normal synovium. *Open Rheumatol. J.* 5, 100–106. doi:10.2174/1874312901105010100

Sparks, S. R., Tripathy, U., Broudy, A., Bergan, J. J., Kumins, N. H., and Owens, E. L. (2002). Small-caliber mesothelial cell-layered polytetraflouroethylene vascular grafts in New Zealand white rabbits. *Ann. Vasc. Surg.* 16, 73–76. doi:10.1007/s10016-001-0133-5

Stauffer, J. L., Potts, D. E., and Sahn, S. A. (1978). Cellular content of the normal rabbit pleural space. *Acta Cytol.* 22, 570–574.

Su, A. I., Wiltshire, T., Batalov, S., Lapp, H., Ching, K. A., Block, D., et al. (2004). A gene atlas of the mouse and human protein-encoding transcriptomes. *Proc. Natl. Acad. Sci. U.S.A.* 101, 6062–6067. doi:10.1073/pnas.0400782101

Swart, G. W. (2002). Activated leukocyte cell adhesion molecule (CD166/ALCAM): developmental and mechanistic aspects of cell clustering and cell migration. *Eur. J. Cell Biol.* 81, 313–321. doi:10.1078/0171-9335-00256

Taddei, P., Chiono, V., Anghileri, A., Vozzi, G., Freddi, G., and Ciardelli, G. (2013). Silk fibroin/gelatin blend films crosslinked with enzymes for biomedical applications. *Macromol. Biosci.* 13, 1492–1510. doi:10.1002/mabi.201300156

Takahashi, K., Goto, T., Mukai, K., Sawasaki, Y., and Hata, J. (1989). Cobblestone monolayer cells from human omental adipose tissue are possibly mesothelial, not endothelial. *In Vitro Cell. Dev. Biol.* 25, 109–111. doi:10.1007/BF02626165

Takahashi, K., Hata, J., Mukai, K., and Sawasaki, Y. (1991). Close similarity between cultured human omental mesothelial cells and endothelial cells in cytochemical markers and plasminogen activator production. *In Vitro Cell. Dev. Biol.* 27A, 542–548. doi:10.1007/BF02631284

Takazawa, R., Yamato, M., Kageyama, Y., Okano, T., and Kihara, K. (2005). Mesothelial cell sheets cultured on fibrin gel prevent adhesion formation in an intestinal hernia model. *Tissue Eng.* 11, 618–625. doi:10.1089/ten.2005.11.618

Takezawa, T., Mori, Y., and Yoshizato, K. (1990). Cell culture on a thermo-responsive polymer surface. *Biotechnology (N. Y.)* 8, 854–856. doi:10.1038/nbt0990-854

Theuer, C. J., Bergamini, T. M., Theuer, H. H., Burns, C. D., Proctor, M. L., and Garrison, R. N. (1996). Vena cava replacement with a peritoneum-lined vascular graft. *ASAIO J.* 42, 266–270. doi:10.1097/00002480-199642040-00007

Thomas, J. H., Pierce, G. E., Iliopoulos, J. I., and Hermreck, A. S. (1988). Vascular graft selection. *Surg. Clin. North Am.* 68, 865–874.

Toya, S. P., and Malik, A. B. (2012). Role of endothelial injury in disease mechanisms and contribution of progenitor cells in mediating endothelial repair. *Immunobiology* 217, 569–580. doi:10.1016/j.imbio.2011.03.006

Tran, C. N., Thacker, S. G., Louie, D. M., Oliver, J., White, P. T., Endres, J. L., et al. (2008). Interactions of T cells with fibroblast-like synoviocytes: role of the B7 family costimulatory ligand B7-H3. *J. Immunol.* 180, 2989–2998. doi:10.4049/jimmunol.180.5.2989

Trevisi, L., Pighin, I., and Luciani, S. (2006). Vascular endothelium as a target for endogenous ouabain: studies on the effect of ouabain on human endothelial cells. *Cell. Mol. Biol. (Noisy-le-grand)* 52, 64–70.

Tsai, S. H., Liu, Y. W., Tang, W. C., Zhou, Z. W., Hwang, C. Y., Hwang, G. Y., et al. (2007). Characterization of porcine arterial endothelial cells cultured on amniotic membrane, a potential matrix for vascular tissue engineering. *Biochem. Biophys. Res. Commun.* 357, 984–990. doi:10.1016/j.bbrc.2007.04.047

Tsuzuki, M. (2009). Bone marrow-derived cells are not involved in reendothelialized endothelium as endothelial cells after simple endothelial denudation in mice. *Basic Res. Cardiol.* 104, 601–611. doi:10.1007/s00395-009-0021-7

Valle, M. T., Degl'innocenti, M. L., Bertelli, R., Facchetti, P., Perfumo, F., Fenoglio, D., et al. (1995). Antigen-presenting function of human peritoneum mesothelial cells. *Clin. Exp. Immunol.* 101, 172–176. doi:10.1111/j.1365-2249.1995.tb02294.x

Van de Velde, V. J., Herman, A. G., and Bult, H. (1986). Effects of dexamethasone on prostacyclin biosynthesis in rabbit mesothelial cells. *Prostaglandins* 32, 169–178. doi:10.1016/0090-6980(86)90122-X

van Tuyn, J., Atsma, D. E., Winter, E. M., Van Der Velde-Van Dijke, I., Pijnappels, D. A., Bax, N. A., et al. (2007). Epicardial cells of human adults can undergo an epithelial-to-mesenchymal transition and obtain characteristics of smooth muscle cells in vitro. *Stem Cells* 25, 271–278. doi:10.1634/stemcells.2006-0366

Vazquez, N., Chacon, M., Meana, A., Menendez-Menendez, Y., Ferrero-Gutierrez, A., Cereijo-Martin, D., et al. (2015). Keratin-chitosan membranes as scaffold for tissue engineering of human cornea. *Histol. Histopathol.* 30, 813–821. doi:10.14670HH-11-585

Velema, J., and Kaplan, D. (2006). Biopolymer-based biomaterials as scaffolds for tissue engineering. *Adv. Biochem. Eng. Biotechnol.* 102, 187–238.

Verhagen, H. J., Blankensteijn, J. D., De Groot, P. G., Heijnen-Snyder, G. J., Pronk, A., Vroom, T. M., et al. (1998). In vivo experiments with mesothelial cell seeded ePTFE vascular grafts. *Eur. J. Vasc. Endovasc. Surg.* 15, 489–496. doi:10.1016/S1078-5884(98)80108-1

Wagner, N., Michiels, J. F., Schedl, A., and Wagner, K. D. (2008). The Wilms' tumour suppressor WT1 is involved in endothelial cell proliferation and migration: expression in tumour vessels in vivo. *Oncogene* 27, 3662–3672. doi:10.1038/sj.onc.1211044

Watanabe, R., Hayashi, R., Kimura, Y., Tanaka, Y., Kageyama, T., Hara, S., et al. (2011). A novel gelatin hydrogel carrier sheet for corneal endothelial transplantation. *Tissue Eng. Part A* 17, 2213–2219. doi:10.1089/ten.TEA.2010.0568

Wilm, B., Ipenberg, A., Hastie, N. D., Burch, J. B., and Bader, D. M. (2005). The serosal mesothelium is a major source of smooth muscle cells of the gut vasculature. *Development* 132, 5317–5328. doi:10.1242/dev.02141

Wilshaw, S. P., Kearney, J. N., Fisher, J., and Ingham, E. (2006). Production of an acellular amniotic membrane matrix for use in tissue engineering. *Tissue Eng.* 12, 2117–2129. doi:10.1089/ten.2006.12.2117

Witowski, J., Breborowicz, A., Topley, N., Martis, L., Knapowski, J., and Oreopoulos, D. G. (1997). Insulin stimulates the activity of Na+/K(+)-ATPase in human peritoneal mesothelial cells. *Perit. Dial. Int.* 17, 186–193.

Wittmer, C. R., Claudepierre, T., Reber, M., Wiedemann, P., Garlick, J. A., Kaplan, D., et al. (2011). Multifunctionalized electrospun silk fibers promote axon regeneration in central nervous system. *Adv. Funct. Mater.* 21, 4202. doi:10.1002/adfm.201190103

Witz, C. A., Montoya-Rodriguez, I. A., Cho, S., Centonze, V. E., Bonewald, L. F., and Schenken, R. S. (2001). Composition of the extracellular matrix of the peritoneum. *J. Soc. Gynecol. Investig.* 8, 299–304. doi:10.1016/S1071-5576(01)00122-8

Xiao, C. Y., Pan, Y. F., Guo, X. H., Wu, Y. Q., Gu, J. R., and Cai, D. Z. (2011). Expression of beta-catenin in rheumatoid arthritis fibroblast-like synoviocytes. *Scand. J. Rheumatol.* 40, 26–33. doi:10.3109/03009742.2010.486767

Xu, B., Fan, T. J., Zhao, J., Sun, A., Wang, R. X., Hu, X. Z., et al. (2012). Transplantation of tissue-engineered human corneal epithelium in limbal stem cell deficiency rabbit models. *Int. J. Ophthalmol.* 5, 424–429. doi:10.3980/j.issn.2222-3959.2012.04.04

Yamada, Y., Hozumi, K., and Nomizu, M. (2011). Construction and activity of a synthetic basement membrane with active laminin peptides and polysaccharides. *Chemistry* 17, 10500–10508. doi:10.1002/chem.201101064

Yan, S., Zhang, Q., Wang, J., Liu, Y., Lu, S., Li, M., et al. (2013). Silk fibroin/chondroitin sulfate/hyaluronic acid ternary scaffolds for dermal tissue reconstruction. *Acta Biomater.* 9, 6771–6782. doi:10.1016/j.actbio.2013.02.016

Yanez-Mo, M., Lara-Pezzi, E., Selgas, R., Ramirez-Huesca, M., Dominguez-Jimenez, C., Jimenez-Heffernan, J. A., et al. (2003). Peritoneal dialysis and epithelial-to-mesenchymal transition of mesothelial cells. *N. Engl. J. Med.* 348, 403–413. doi:10.1056/NEJMoa020809

Yang, X., Ye, R., Kong, Q., Yang, Q., Dong, X., and Yu, X. (2004). CD40 is expressed on rat peritoneal mesothelial cells and upregulates ICAM-1 production. *Nephrol. Dial. Transplant.* 19, 1378–1384. doi:10.1093/ndt/gfh144

Yen, C. J., Fang, C. C., Chen, Y. M., Lin, R. H., Wu, K. D., Lee, P. H., et al. (1997). Extracellular matrix proteins modulate human peritoneal mesothelial cell behavior. *Nephron* 75, 188–195. doi:10.1159/000189530

Yetkin, G., Uludag, M., Citgez, B., Karakoc, S., Polat, N., and Kabukcuoglu, F. (2009). Prevention of peritoneal adhesions by intraperitoneal administration of vitamin E and human amniotic membrane. *Int. J. Surg.* 7, 561–565. doi:10.1016/j.ijsu.2009.09.007

Yoeruek, E., Bayyoud, T., Maurus, C., Hofmann, J., Spitzer, M. S., Bartz-Schmidt, K. U., et al. (2012). Reconstruction of corneal stroma with decellularized porcine xenografts in a rabbit model. *Acta Ophthalmol.* 90, e206–e210. doi:10.1111/j.1755-3768.2011.02300.x

Yuan, S., and Fan, G. (2015). Stem cell-based therapy of corneal epithelial and endothelial diseases. *Regen. Med.* 10, 495–504. doi:10.2217/rme.15.3

Yung, S., and Chan, T. M. (2007). Hyaluronan – regulator and initiator of peritoneal inflammation and remodeling. *Int. J. Artif. Organs* 30, 477–483.

Zavala, J., Lopez Jaime, G. R., Rodriguez Barrientos, C. A., and Valdez-Garcia, J. (2013). Corneal endothelium: developmental strategies for regeneration. *Eye (Lond.)* 27, 579–588. doi:10.1038/eye.2013.15

Zhang, L., Liu, F., Peng, Y., Sun, L., and Chen, G. (2013). Changes in expression of four molecular marker proteins and one microRNA in mesothelial cells of the peritoneal dialysate effluent fluid of peritoneal dialysis patients. *Exp. Ther. Med.* 6, 1189–1193. doi:10.3892/etm_2013.1281

Zhang, X., Reagan, M. R., and Kaplan, D. L. (2009). Electrospun silk biomaterial scaffolds for regenerative medicine. *Adv. Drug Deliv. Rev.* 61, 988–1006. doi:10.1016/j.addr.2009.07.005

Zhou, B., Ma, Q., Rajagopal, S., Wu, S. M., Domian, I., Rivera-Feliciano, J., et al. (2008). Epicardial progenitors contribute to the cardiomyocyte lineage in the developing heart. *Nature* 454, 109–113. doi:10.1038/nature07060

Zhu, C., Ying, D., Mi, J., Li, L., Zeng, W., Hou, C., et al. (2008a). Development of anti-atherosclerotic tissue-engineered blood vessel by A20-regulated endothelial progenitor cells seeding decellularized vascular matrix. *Biomaterials* 29, 2628–2636. doi:10.1016/j.biomaterials.2008.03.005

Zhu, Y. T., Hayashida, Y., Kheirkhah, A., He, H., Chen, S. Y., and Tseng, S. C. (2008b). Characterization and comparison of intercellular adherent junctions expressed by human corneal endothelial cells in vivo and in vitro. *Invest. Ophthalmol. Vis. Sci.* 49, 3879–3886. doi:10.1167/iovs.08-1693

Zhu, J., and Clark, R. A. (2014). Fibronectin at select sites binds multiple growth factors and enhances their activity: expansion of the collaborative ECM-GF paradigm. *J. Invest. Dermatol.* 134, 895–901. doi:10.1038/jid.2013.484

Conflict of Interest Statement: Christian Claude Lachaud, Abdelkrim Hmadcha, and Bernat Soria are inventors of the Patent (use of mesothelial cells in tissue engineering and artificial tissues, PCT/EP2014/061746) filed by the Fundación Progreso y Salud, Vissum Corporation and NewBiotechnic SA. Berta Rodriguez-Campins is an employee of NBT SA.

8

Projection stereolithographic fabrication of human adipose stem cell-incorporated biodegradable scaffolds for cartilage tissue engineering

Edited by:
Cornelia Kasper,
University of Natural Resources and
Life Sciences Vienna, Austria

Reviewed by:
Sourabh Ghosh,
Indian Institute of Technology Delhi,
India
Enrico Lucarelli,
Istituto Ortopedico Rizzoli, Italy
Brian O'Callaghan Diekman,
University of North Carolina at Chapel
Hill, USA

*Correspondence:
Rocky S. Tuan,
Department of Orthopaedic Surgery,
Center for Cellular and
Molecular Engineering, University of
Pittsburgh School of Medicine,
450 Technology Drive,
Pittsburgh, PA 15219, USA
rst13@pitt.edu

† Aaron X. Sun and Hang Lin have
contributed equally to this work.

Aaron X. Sun[1,2†], Hang Lin[1†], Angela M. Beck[1,3], Evan J. Kilroy[1,3] and Rocky S. Tuan[1,3]*

[1] Center for Cellular and Molecular Engineering, Department of Orthopaedic Surgery, University of Pittsburgh School of Medicine, Pittsburgh, PA, USA, [2] Medical Scientist Training Program, University of Pittsburgh School of Medicine, Pittsburgh, PA, USA, [3] Department of Bioengineering, University of Pittsburgh Swanson School of Engineering, Pittsburgh, PA, USA

The poor self-healing ability of cartilage necessitates the development of methods for cartilage regeneration. Scaffold construction with live stem cell incorporation and subsequent differentiation presents a promising route. Projection stereolithography (PSL) offers high resolution and processing speed as well as the ability to fabricate scaffolds that precisely fit the anatomy of cartilage defects using medical imaging as the design template. We report here the use of a visible-light-based PSL (VL-PSL) system to encapsulate human adipose-derived stem cells (hASCs) into a biodegradable polymer [poly-D,L-lactic acid/polyethylene glycol/poly-D,L-lactic acid (PDLLA-PEG)]/hyaluronic acid (HA) matrix to produce live cell constructs with customized architectures. After fabrication, hASCs showed high viability (84%) and were uniformly distributed throughout the constructs, which possessed high mechanical properties with a compressive modulus of 780 kPa. The hASC-seeded constructs were then cultured in control or TGF-β3-containing chondrogenic medium for up to 28 days. In chondrogenic medium-treated group (TGF-β3 group), hASCs maintained 77% viability and expressed chondrogenic genes Sox9, collagen type II, and aggrecan at 11, 232, and 2.29×10^5 fold increases, respectively compared to levels at day 0 in non-chondrogenic medium. The TGF-β3 group also produced a collagen type II and glycosaminoglycan-rich extracellular matrix, detected by immunohistochemistry, Alcian blue staining, and Safranin O staining suggesting robust chondrogenesis within the scaffold. Without chondroinductive addition (Control group), cell viability decreased with time (65% at 28 days) and showed poor cartilage matrix deposition. After 28 days, mechanical strength of the TGF-β3 group remained high at 240 kPa. Thus, the PSL and PDLLA-PEG/HA-based fabrication method using adult stem cells is a promising approach in producing mechanically competent engineered cartilage for joint cartilage resurfacing.

Keywords: adipose stem cells, cartilage tissue engineering, PDLLA-PEG, projection stereolithography, live cell-scaffold fabrication

Introduction

Cartilage damaged by trauma, disease, or aging demonstrates very limited capabilities for self-regeneration and ultimately results in osteoarthritis (OA) (Tuan et al., 2013). Given the high prevalence of OA in the United States (27 million affected) (Zhang and Jordan, 2010), which is projected to increase due to population aging as well as the obesity epidemic, methods toward managing and treating these cartilage defects are critical. While there exist procedures to treat these defects, such as microfracture and osteochondral grafting, they either finally lead to the formation of fibrocartilage or are limited by tissue availability (Moriya et al., 2007; Gigante et al., 2011; Ye et al., 2013). In addition, allografting bone and cartilage have the potential risk of infection and disease transmission. Severe cartilage defects ultimately require total joint arthroplasty to reduce pain and improve mobility, but this involves a major surgery and ends the biological life of cartilage (Moran and Horton, 2000; Nashi et al., 2014). As such, a regenerative approach that can restore the native properties of cartilage represents an attractive alternative.

Recently, regenerative medicine has garnered high interest, which involves the development of cartilage-like constructs through the use of cells, growth factors, scaffolds, and combinations (Tuan et al., 2013; Demoor et al., 2014). For example, autologous chondrocyte implantation (ACI) and matrix-induced ACI (MACI) are popular procedures that harvest and expand chondrocytes *in vitro* from the patient's own tissue, which are then grafted into the cartilage defect site with or without accompanying extracellular matrix (ECM). However, this source of healthy chondrocytes is limited and requires several weeks of cell culturing to obtain adequate cell numbers for transplantation, which results in chondrocyte dedifferentiation (Kuo et al., 2006). Thus, adult tissue-derived stem/progenitor cells, such as mesenchymal stem cells (MSCs), that have been shown to have the ability to differentiate into a variety of cell lines including chondrocytes (Pittenger et al., 1999) offer a promising substitute for the primary chondrocytes. In particular, adipose tissue-derived MSCs (ASCs) have attracted recent attention because they are isolated in higher quantities than stem cells found from other sources, such as bone marrow, and are obtainable through minimally invasive procedures, thus offering the advantage of reducing or even eliminating *in vitro* expansion to allow point-of-care application (Roux et al., 2013). In addition, ASCs have been shown to be beneficial in cartilage healing, including reducing pain and improving function for aging patients with knee OA after intra-articular injection (Koh et al., 2013).

A key component in cartilage tissue engineering is a biomaterial scaffold to deliver the candidate cells, such as MSCs, to the defect site and to also temporarily fill the defect to facilitate cell growth. In addition to biocompatibility, the ideal scaffold for cartilage tissue engineering should possess viscoelastic hydrogel-like characteristics that mimic the mechanical properties and functions of native cartilage. Optimally, the biomaterial will also be biodegradable such that as the stem cells differentiate into chondrocytes and produce a cartilaginous ECM, the scaffold degrades and the newly secreted ECM remodels the construct into a cartilage-like tissue. In addition, precise fitting of the scaffold into the local

structural geometry of the defect and the host tissue anatomy is critical for enhancing the repair process such that the absence of gaps will optimize integration between implants and native tissue and allow continuous load distribution (Da Silva et al., 2012). To date, many technologies have been developed in the fabrication of scaffolds with different geometry and internal architecture. Traditional technologies, such as solvent casting, particulate leaching, and electrospinning, do allow for limited control of structure, but they are not able to perform the fabrication of highly detailed structures on a patient by patient basis (Yang et al., 2001). In addition, these methods require the use of either organic solvents or conditions unfavorable for cell survival, thereby limiting their ability to seed cells directly within scaffolds (Yang et al., 2002; Derby, 2012).

Solid free-form fabrication (SFF) methods have been shown to offer the ability to control both the macrostructure as well as the microstructure of scaffolds. With the utilization of medical imaging and computer-aided design (CAD) model guided scaffold fabrication, SFF methods can create scaffolds with precise architectures (Bajaj et al., 2012). Different SFF methods have been applied in the fabrication of a variety of biomaterials, including laser sintering, stereolithography, fused deposition modeling, and 3D printing. Of these techniques, stereolithography is the most accurate and is based on light-induced photopolymerization of derivatized monomers (Melchels et al., 2010). Projection stereolithography (PSL) in particular is a method that has been attracting increased interest due to its high fabrication rate and resolution. By utilizing a layer-by-layer-based image projection of defined thickness, fabrication times are drastically reduced from conventional stereolithography. Recently, in our laboratory, PSL using visible-light illumination (VL-PSL) has been applied in a one-step live cell-scaffold fabrication in which highly viable human adipose-derived stem cells (hASCs) were uniformly incorporated within polyethylene glycol diacrylate (PEGDA) scaffolds (Lin et al., 2013). While this procedure for the first time allows live cell-scaffold fabrication using VL-PSL, it is currently limited by the monomer that is used because PEG is not biodegradable and does not provide cell-binding ligands. In addition, Percoll was used to suspend the cells during the fabrication, which introduces additional non-native molecules into the final construct. The extent to which chondrogenesis of hASCs is supported in the PEG scaffold was also not investigated.

A number of properties are desirable for a biomaterial suitable for implantation for cartilage repair, including biodegradability, biocompatibility, strong compressive modulus, and presence of cell-binding ligands. Most importantly, the material must also be water-soluble in order to not interfere with cell survival during the photo-crosslinking scaffold fabrication process. We report here the identification of a novel hybrid matrix in which the synthetic polymer, poly-D,L-lactic acid/polyethylene glycol/poly-D,L-lactic acid (PDLLA-PEG), served as the structural component (Seck et al., 2010), and hyaluronic acid (HA) as the co-polymer to supply cell-binding ligands and to inhibit cell settlement during PSL fabrication owing to its viscous property. HA is a glycosaminoglycan (GAG) present in abundance in the cartilage ECM and synovial fluid and has been shown to promote hASC chondrogenesis through interaction with its surface receptor, CD44 (Wu et al., 2013; Chopra et al., 2014).

In this study, hASCs were suspended in a methacrylated PDLLA-PEG and HA (mPDLLA-PEG) solution and subjected to VL-PSL with different CAD architectures. The cell-seeded fabricated scaffolds were cultured in control medium or TGF-β3-containing chondrogenic medium for up to 4 weeks. Cell viability was examined at different time points and the progression of chondrogenesis of hASCs within the scaffolds was assessed by mechanical testing, real time reverse transcription polymerase chain reaction (RT-PCR) analysis of gene expression, and histological staining. Our results showed that the VL-PSL produced hybrid scaffolds precisely mimicked the CAD structure and maintained high cell viability during the fabrication process. In addition, mPDLLA-PEG/HA scaffolds supported efficient hASC chondrogenesis upon induction. Thus, the method described in this report represents a promising method for the development of personalized stem cell-based repair of articular cartilage defect.

Materials and Methods

All chemicals were purchased from Sigma-Aldrich (St. Louis, MO, USA) unless otherwise stated.

Human Adipose Stem Cell Isolation

Human adipose-derived stem cells were isolated from lipoaspirate with Institutional Review Board approval (University of Pittsburgh and University of Washington) using an automated cell isolation system from Tissue Genesis, Inc. (Honolulu, HI, USA). The isolated cell pellets were re-suspended in expansion medium (EM: DMEM-high glucose, 10% MSC-certified fetal bovine serum (FBS), 100 U/ml penicillin, 100 µg/ml streptomycin; Invitrogen, Carlsbad, CA, USA) and plated on tissue culture flask. After 3 days, the non-attached cells were washed out with Hank's Balanced Salt Solution (HBSS). The medium was changed every 3 days. At 80% confluence, cells were detached with 0.25% trypsin in 1 mM EDTA (Invitrogen) and passaged. All experiments were performed with hASCs obtained at passage 3 (P3). hASCs used in this study were pooled from two patients (36- and 28-year females).

Synthesis of Methacrylated PDLLA-PEG and HA

Preparation of the mPDLLA-PEG was performed as described by Seck et al. (2010). Briefly, 50 g of PEG (4 kDa molecular weight) was placed into a 250 ml Erlenmeyer flask and subjected to 600 W microwave irradiation for 3 min. Subsequently, 3.5 g (2.80 ml) of stannous octoate [Sn(Oct)$_2$] was added to the molten PEG followed by addition of 7.2 g poly-D,L-lactide. The mixture was subjected to 600 W microwave irradiation for 1 min. The initial PDLLA-PEG polymer was precipitated in 500 ml cold isopropanol, and was dried under vacuum for 2 days. Dry polymer was dissolved in 100 ml dichloromethane (DCM), followed by addition of three equivalents of triethylamine (TEA, ~5.25 ml) and three equivalents of methacrylic anhydride (MA, ~5.60 ml). The reaction mixture was covered with punctured Parafilm and allowed to stir at room temperature for 7 days. After completion of the reaction, the mixture was precipitated into diethyl ether. For

further purification, the macromer was redissolved in minimal amounts of chloroform and reprecipitated in diethyl ether.

Methacrylated hyaluronic acid was prepared by reacting MA with sodium hyaluronate (research grade, MW ~700 kDa, Lifecore, Chaska, MN) (Chung et al., 2009).

Synthesis of Photoinitiator LAP

The visible-light sensitive initiator lithium phenyl-2,4,6-trimethylbenzoylphosphinate (LAP) was synthesized as described by Fairbanks et al. (2009).

PSL Fabrication of Live Cell Constructs

The PSL apparatus was purchased from EnvisionTec (Perfactory Standard, Gladbeck, Germany) equipped with digital light processing (DLP) technology. Visible-light mode (Hg illumination utilizing a UV barrier filter) was used, with the curing depth of each layer set at 50 µm.

Solutions of polymer, LAP, and phenol red dye were prepared in 50 ml tubes. Thirty percent PDLLA-PEG was chosen because it not only maintained the fabrication fidelity of VL-PSL but also formed a scaffold with mechanical properties more similar to that of cartilage. HA was used at 0.5% concentration because it yielded sufficient specific gravity to suspend cells but did not compromise routine cell mixing by trituration, for example, by repeated pipetting. For instance, the preparation of mPDLLA-PEG (30% w/v), mHA (0.5% w/v), LAP (0.6% w/v), and phenol red (0.025% w/v) was carried out as follows: polymer (12 g mPDLLA-PEG and 0.2 g mHA) was placed in the 50 ml tube followed by slow addition of HBSS close to the 40 ml mark and subsequent addition of LAP (240 mg) and phenol red (10 mg). The solution was titrated to pH 7.4 with 10 N NaOH and adjusted to 40 ml using HBSS.

P3 hASCs were pelleted by centrifugation, and the supernatant was completely removed. The polymer solution prepared above was added on top of the pellets and mixed with cells thoroughly by gently pipetting up and down 20 times. The final hASC density was 4×10^6 cells/ml. After the bubbles were removed by aspiration, the cell-polymer solution was immediately poured into the basement plate of the PSL device for printing with different 3D models as the template, using our recently described procedure (Lin et al., 2013).

The fabricated constructs were detached from the platform and washed three times to remove uncured polymer solution. The constructs were cultured in control medium [CM, DMEM with 1% L-alanyl-L-glutamine (GlutaMAX), 55 µM sodium pyruvate, 1× antibiotic-antimycotic, and 1% insulin–transferrin–selenium (ITS) (Invitrogen, Carlsbad, CA, USA)] or chondrogenic medium [CGM, CM supplemented with 10 ng/ml transforming growth factor-β3 (TGF-β3; PeproTech, Rocky Hill, NJ, USA], 100 nM dexamethasone, 50 µM L-ascorbic acid 2-phosphate, and 23 µM L-proline) up to 28 days, which were designated as control or TGF-β3 group, respectively.

Degradation Test

Fabricated scaffolds (5 mm diameter and 2 mm height) produced as described above but without cells were immersed in 5 ml HBSS and maintained in cell culture incubator at 37°C. HBSS was changed every 3 days. Since our ultimate goal was to apply the engineered tissue constructs for articular cartilage repair *in vivo*, their functional characteristics, particularly in terms of mechanical property, were of critical importance. Therefore, the degradation of polymer was estimated by measuring the mechanical property of scaffolds at different times.

Mechanical testing of scaffolds was conducted with a mechanical tester (Bose Electroforce model 3230 Series II). Briefly, the cylindrical scaffolds were placed between the compressive motor and load cell and subjected to 10% compression (0.2 mm) at 0.01 mm/s. The stress–strain curve was then plotted, and the linear area was used to calculate the compressive modulus of scaffolds.

Live/Dead Staining

At various time points post-fabrication, cell viability was assessed with the live/dead viability/cytotoxicity kit (Invitrogen) as examined by epifluorescence microscopy following the product manual. The percentage of live cells was calculated as the number of green-staining cells divided by the total number of cells (green and red staining cells).

MTS Assay

On days 0 and 28, cell metabolic activity was assessed with CellTiter 96® AQueous One Solution Cell Proliferation Assay [3-(4,5-dimethylthiazol-2-yl)-5-(3-carboxymethoxyphenyl)-2-(4-sulfophenyl)-2H-tetrazolium, inner salt; MTS, Promega, Madison, WI, USA]. The constructs with cells were cultured with MTS solution for 4 h, and absorbance at 492 nm was measured using a microplate reader (BioTek, Winooski, VT, USA).

Analysis of Gene Expression by Real-Time RT-PCR

Total RNA of the cells within the constructs was isolated using TRIZOL reagent (Invitrogen) and purified using RNeasy Plus Mini Kit (Qiagen, Germantown, MD, USA). Reverse transcription reactions were performed using SuperScript® VILO™ cDNA Synthesis Kit (Invitrogen) according to manufacturer's manual. Real-time PCR was performed using the SYBR Green Reaction Mix (Applied Biosystems, Foster City, CA, USA) with a StepOnePlus thermocycler (Applied Biosystems). All sample values were normalized to 18S rRNA using the $2^{-\Delta\Delta Ct}$ method.

Hydroxyproline Quantitation

Total collagen content deposited within the constructs was determined by measuring hydroxyproline levels. The constructs (5 mm diameter and 2 mm thickness) were homogenized in water by grinding and hydrolyzed using the same volume of 12 N HCl (Fisher, Pittsburgh, PA, USA) at 120°C for 3 h. Hydroxyproline content in constructs was quantitated using a Hydroxyproline Colorimetric Assay Kit (BioVision, San Francisco, CA, USA).

Histology

After 28 days culture, constructs were removed from the incubator, washed twice, and fixed in buffered paraformaldehyde (4%, Fisher) for 1 day at room temperature. After washing with PBS three times, they were then cryosectioned using a cryostat

(CM1520, Leica) at 8 μm thickness. For assessment of GAG deposition, the slides were stained with either Alcian Blue or Safranin O/Fast Green following standard protocols. Images were captured with a CKX41 microscope (Olympus, Japan) equipped with a Leica DFC 3200 camera.

Immunohistochemistry

Enzymatic antigen retrieval was performed using chondroitinase/hyaluronidase (1 and 5 mg/ml) at 37°C for 30 min, and was suppressed with 1% horse serum (Vector Labs, Burlingame, CA, USA) in PBS for 45 min. After blocking endogenous peroxidase (3% H_2O_2 in methanol for 10 min) and non-specific binding [1% horse serum (Vector Labs)], slices were incubated with primary antibodies against collagen type II (Abcam, Cambridge, MA, USA) overnight at 4°C. After washing, biotinylated secondary antibodies (Vector Labs) were applied for 30 min. Staining was developed by treating samples with horseradish peroxidase (HRP)-conjugated streptavidin/NovaRED™ peroxidase substrate (Vector Labs).

Mechanical Property Assessment

The mechanical property of constructs at days 0 and 28 were measured using the procedure described before.

Statistical Analysis

All studies were performed with three experimental replicates. Results were expressed as the mean ± SD. Significant differences between control and chondrogenic groups were determined by one-tailed Student's *t*-test. Significance was considered at $p < 0.05^*$ and $p < 0.01^{**}$.

Results

Constructs generated using VL-PSL were first assessed for their ability to faithfully replicate designed architectures. **Figure 1** illustrates the construction of various 3D shapes, including conical, cubic, and cylindrical (**Figures 1A,B**), and more complicated alpha numeric structures (**Figures 1C,D**). In all cases, the structures produced using VL-PSL mimicked the designs with high fidelity upon visual inspection.

Degradation Analysis

Due to the presence of ester bonds in the mPDLLA-PEG/HA co-polymers, the scaffolds are expected to be degraded through hydrolytic cleavage (Seck et al., 2010). To test the degradation behavior, PSL-fabricated mPDLLA-PEG/HA scaffolds were incubated in PBS at 37°C and their mechanical properties tested at different time points up to 4 weeks. As shown in **Figure 2**, the compressive modulus of scaffolds significantly decreased with time, demonstrating structural degradation in aqueous solution. After 4 weeks, scaffolds retained only ~25% of their original mechanical strength but still maintained the original cylindrical structure.

Cell Viability Assessment

Cell viability was determined immediately after fabrication and also at 28 days after culturing in control and chondrogenic

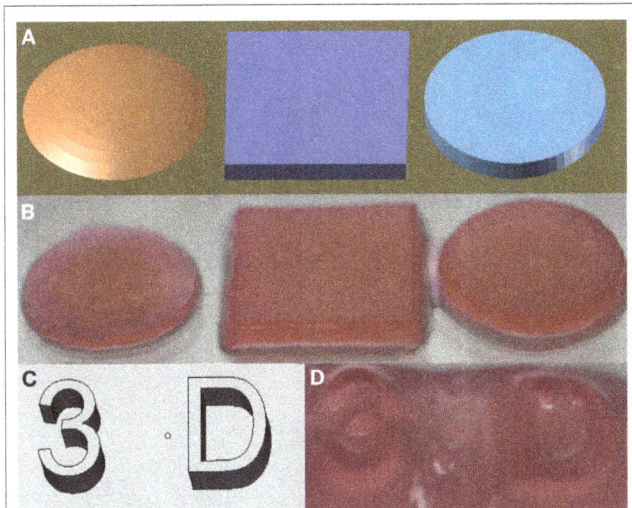

FIGURE 1 | mPDLLA-PEG constructs generated using VL-PSL.
(A,B) PDLLA-PEG hydrogels with spherical, cuboidal, and cylindrical
architecture (B) based on CAD models (A). (C,D) Alphanumeric
mPDLLA-PEG hydrogels (D) based on CAD models (C). Formulation used
includes mPDLLA-PEG (30% w/v), mHA (0.5% w/v), LAP (0.6% w/v), and
phenol red (0.025% w/v).

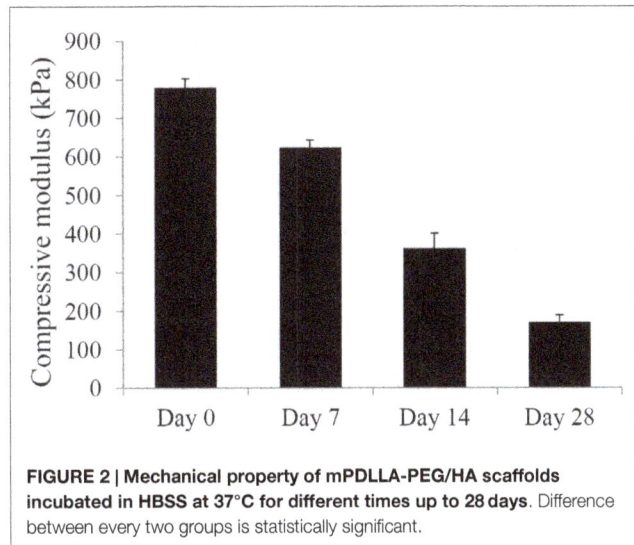

FIGURE 2 | Mechanical property of mPDLLA-PEG/HA scaffolds
incubated in HBSS at 37°C for different times up to 28 days. Difference
between every two groups is statistically significant.

medium. **Figure 3A** shows a surface view of a Calcein-AM stained construct, and **Figure 3B** shows a cross-sectional view of the construct at day 0. Uniform distribution of single cells throughout the construct was clearly seen, suggesting that cells remained suspended and separated from each other in the fabrication solution for at least 30 min. Cell viability was determined to be high at 81% after fabrication (**Figures 3C,D,I**). After 28 days of culture in control medium, cell viability decreased to 65% (**Figures 3E,F,I,J**). In contrast, chondrogenic medium supplemented with TGF-β3 not only maintained higher cell viability (77%, **Figures 3G–I**) but also promoted higher overall cell metabolic activity as indicated by MTS assay (**Figure 3J**). There is a statistically significant difference between the control and the TGF-β3 group in cell number.

Chondrogenesis Analysis

Chondrogenic differentiation of the hASCs seeded within the dense mPDLLA-PEG/HA scaffolds and exposed to TGF-β3-containing chondrogenic medium was analyzed by real time RT-PCR for the expression of genes associated with chondrogenesis. **Figures 4A–D** show the relative levels of gene expression for Sox 9, aggrecan, collagen type II, and Runx2. All three chondrogenic genes, Sox 9, aggrecan, and collagen II, were also considerably higher in the TGF-β3 group. In contrast, Runx2, an osteogenesis marker, expression was found to be higher in the control group. Thus, TGF-β3 chondrogenic medium effectively induced chondrogenesis and concurrently inhibited osteogenesis in hASCs encapsulated within the PSL-fabricated scaffolds.

The chondrogenic activity of the cells within the constructs cultured in the chondrogenic medium was next assessed based on hydroxyproline assay to estimate the content of newly synthesized collagen. The TGF-β3 group showed a hydroxyproline level of 21.16 ± 7.15 μg/construct versus an undetectable level in the control group (**Figure 5**). Since this assay did not differentiate between the different collagen types, we further performed immunohistochemistry (IHC) to examine the presence of collage type II. IHC revealed positive staining for collagen type II, a major ECM component in cartilage, only in the TGF-β3 group (**Figure 6**). GAG and proteoglycan content were also estimated by histological staining with Alcian Blue and Safranin O, respectively. Weak staining was seen in the control group after 28 days culture (**Figures 7A,C**), while dense, strong staining was seen in the TGF-β3 group (**Figures 7B,D**). Taken together, these results clearly demonstrate that with TGF-β3 induction, robust chondrogenic differentiation of the hASCs took place within the PSL-fabricated constructs.

Lastly, the compressive moduli for the constructs containing the mPDLLA-PEG polymer were measured. At day 0, the compressive modulus was 780 ± 23 kPa, which fell to 240 ± 20 kPa in the control group and 238 ± 25 kPa in the TGF-β3 group by day 28 (**Figure 8**), principally due to the degradation of the scaffold material.

Discussion

This study reported the application of a VL-PSL protocol to fabricate live hASC-laden, biodegradable polymeric mPDLLA-PEG/HA constructs with cartilage-like mechanical properties. Within the photocrosslinked constructs, cells were uniformly distributed and underwent robust chondrogenesis upon TGF-β3 stimulation, suggesting the potential application of this technology for cartilage tissue repair.

Tissue engineering has been considered a promising approach to repair degenerated articular cartilage in degenerative joint diseases, such as OA. The goal has been to construct or regenerate tissues that possess the properties of native cartilage, but currently there are many technical challenges. First, articular cartilage is an avascular tissue, which limits the ability of cells of

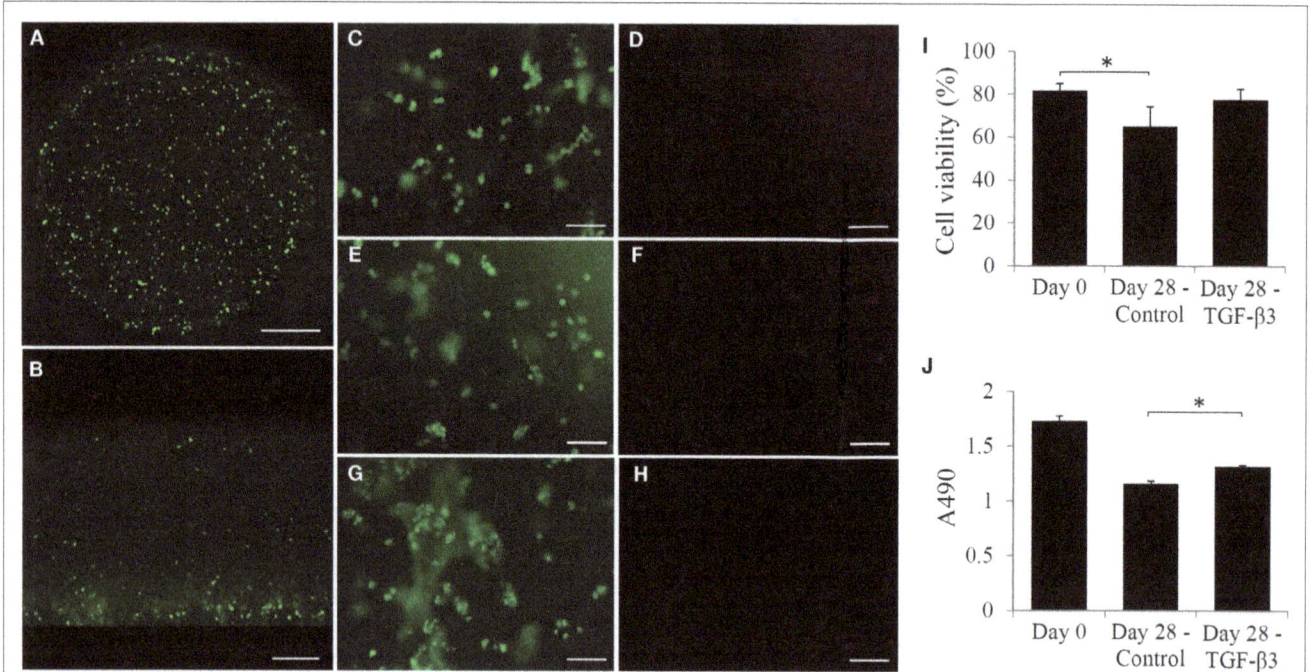

FIGURE 3 | Cell viability in VL-PSL generated mPDLLA-PEG scaffolds at 0 and 28 days after fabrication. **(A–C,E,G)** Calcein-AM staining (green, live cells) and **(D,F,H)** EthD-1 staining (red, dead cells) in scaffold demonstrate the cell viability following fabrication throughout VL-PSL method. Cells were seen to be uniformly distributed at different layers. **(I)** Based on live/dead staining results, cell viability at days 0 and 28 in control as well as TGF-β3 group was calculated. **(J)** MTS assay of constructs at days 0 and 28 in control as well as TGF-β3 group. Scale bars: **(A)** 1 mm; **(B)** 500 μm; and **(C–H)** 100 μm. *$p < 0.05$.

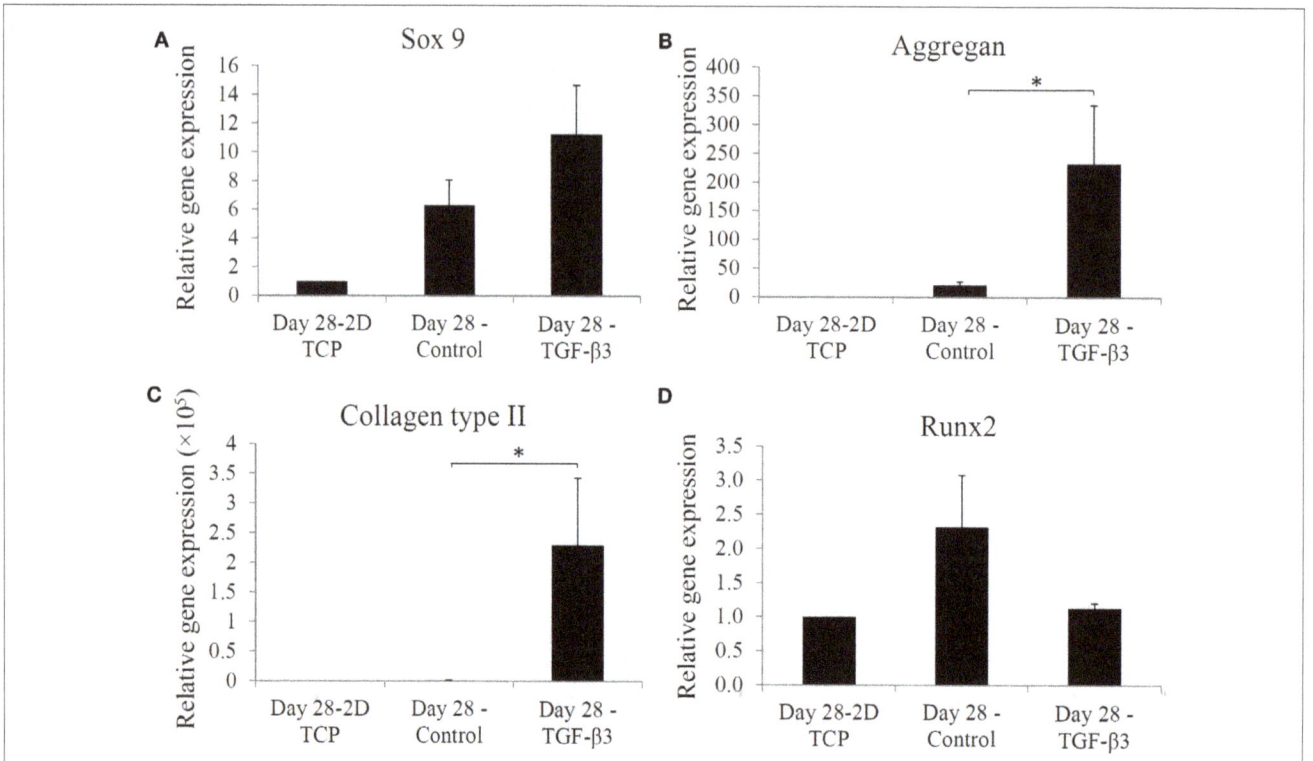

FIGURE 4 | Real time-PCR analysis of gene expression in hASCs at day 28 in 2D tissue culture plate, control group, and TGF-β3 group. Relative gene expression levels of **(A)** Sox 9, **(B)** aggregan, **(C)** collagen type II, and **(D)** Runx2 at day 28, are normalized to gene expression in 2D culture without chondrogenic induction. *$p < 0.05$.

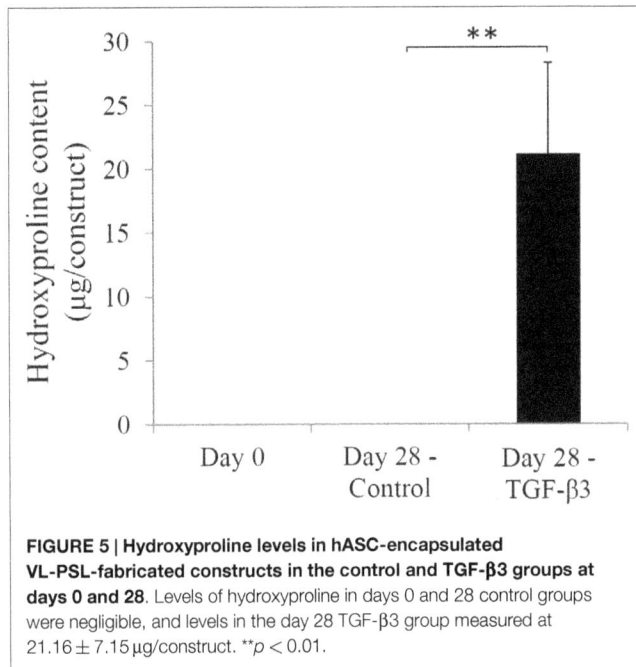

FIGURE 5 | Hydroxyproline levels in hASC-encapsulated VL-PSL-fabricated constructs in the control and TGF-β3 groups at days 0 and 28. Levels of hydroxyproline in days 0 and 28 control groups were negligible, and levels in the day 28 TGF-β3 group measured at $21.16 \pm 7.15 \mu g$/construct. $^{**}p < 0.01$.

surrounding tissues to infiltrate the defect site following implantation of the engineered tissue implant. Thus, a uniform cell distribution throughout the scaffold that makes up the construct is required so that tissue repair can occur within the entire scaffold and not be confined to the superficial zones. A second challenge is the mechanical environment within the articular joint environment, namely the natural high loads that any scaffold or neo-tissue must withstand. The scaffold thus needs to be inherently mechanically stiff immediately following grafting. A third challenge is that articular cartilage defects, by trauma-induced loss or chronic osteoarthritic lesions, are irregular in shape, which makes moldable cell-seeded materials desirable. No currently available hydrogel materials have completely met these requirements.

Recently, our group introduced a visible-light-based PSL method for live cell-scaffold fabrication. Utilizing this technology, live cells were uniformly distributed within scaffolds with designed architectures. While this presented progress toward the first and third challenges, the chondrogenic potential of constructs was not tested. In addition, the PEG material used is non-biodegradable and does not allow for conversion to native cartilage tissue. Given the limitations of the PEG methacrylate hydrogel, we seek to develop a biomaterial that possesses the ability to be applied in VL-PSL (biocompatibility and water-solubility) as well as exhibits both higher mechanical strength and biodegradability. We have identified PDLLA-PEG as a material that possesses these properties. We then further use high MW HA (>700 kDa) to replace Percoll to maintain hASCs in suspension during fabrication, which not only eliminates the presence of Percoll but also provides native cell-binding ligands. The results in **Figure 3B** clearly demonstrate that cells remain sufficiently suspended uniformly throughout the scaffold during the 30-min fabrication time.

Even without TGF-β3 stimulation, hASCs cultured in PDLLA-PEG/HA scaffolds showed increased chondrogenic gene expression (**Figure 4**). Since PDLLA-PEG is an inert material like agarose and alginate, it is reasonable to speculate that this effect resulted from the inclusion of HA and a 3D culture environment (Wu et al., 2010; Schagemann et al., 2013). With TGF-β3 supplementation, hASCs showed robust chondrogenesis indicated by enhanced chondrogenic gene expression and cartilage ECM deposition. Because of the different types of supplemented TGF-β, and variable cell density, culture duration, nature of scaffold, and size of constructs used, no previous data are available for direct comparison to our results. In one study using TGF-β3 treatment for 21 days, collagen type II and aggrecan expression in hASCs encapsulated within fibrin increased 50- and 5-fold, respectively (Park et al., 2011), compared to the 220- and 12-fold increased observed here in PDLLA-PEG/HA, strongly suggesting the chondroinductive property of PDLLA-PEG/HA.

The scaffolds constructed using mPDLLA-PEG/HA are found to rapidly degrade in aqueous solution (**Figure 2**), which agree with previous report (Seck et al., 2010). Currently, there are relatively limited studies investigating the degradation behavior of this material. Yang et al. reported that half of a PDLLA-PEG (4:1, w/w) scaffold was degraded in 5 days (Yang and Kao, 2006). The relative slow degradation rate of scaffold used in our study might be due to lower PDLLA:PEG ratio and inclusion of photocrosslinkable HA. After 12 weeks of culture in HBSS, the scaffolds still maintain the original architecture (data not shown).

Even with slower degradation rates, the scaffolds lose 75% of their strength in 4 weeks (**Figure 2**). However, they are still stronger (160 kPa compressive modulus) than commonly used hydrogels, such as agarose, alginate, and gelatin, which have compressive moduli lower than 30 kPa (Byers et al., 2008; Stojkovska et al., 2010; Lin et al., 2014). While this result indicates good mechanical properties of mPDLLA-PEG/HA, it also suggests relatively limited matrix deposition by the encapsulated hASCs (240 kPa compressive modulus at 28 days). Several reasons could account for this limited matrix deposition: (1) cell death during culture, (2) insufficient cell number, and (3) inadequate ECM synthesis. As shown in **Figure 3J**, cell metabolic activity did decrease after 28 days of culture. In the control group, the cell viability is low (65%), which might be due to limited nutrient exchange through the dense scaffolds, a generic deficiency of hydrogel scaffolds with high mechanical properties. However, the addition of TGF-β3 maintains cell survival (77%). In addition, together with the enhanced levels of gene expression of Sox 9, aggrecan, and collagen type II as well as the presence of collage type II protein, GAGs, and proteoglycan, we conclude that TGF-β3 is able to diffuse into the scaffolds and act to stimulate the encapsulated cells. The observation of metabolic activity reduction in the TGF-β3 group might be due to the relatively low metabolic activity of chondrogenically differentiated hASCs in serum-free environments compared to the naïve hASCs grown in serum-rich conditions without differentiation stimulation (Xu et al., 2008). Therefore, we conclude that the insufficient ECM production in constructs is due to low cell density used during the fabrication process. To optimize deposition of ECM, in future studies, we will use higher initial cell loading density and further optimized

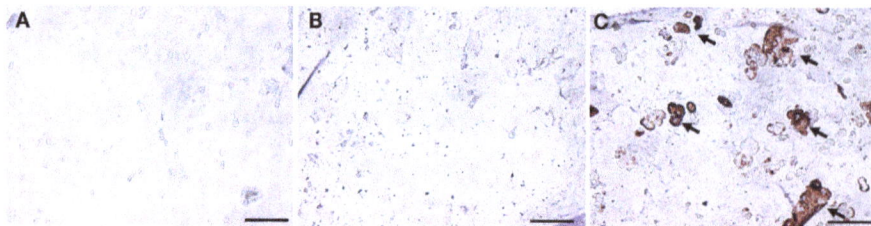

FIGURE 6 | Immunohistochemical staining for collagen type II in hASC-encapsulated VL-PSL-fabricated constructs. (A) Day 0 immediately after fabrication; **(B)** day 28 control group; and **(C)** day 28 TGF-β3 group. Positive collage type II staining (brown) was only seen in the day 28 TGF-β3 treated group as indicated by arrows. Scale bar: 50 μm.

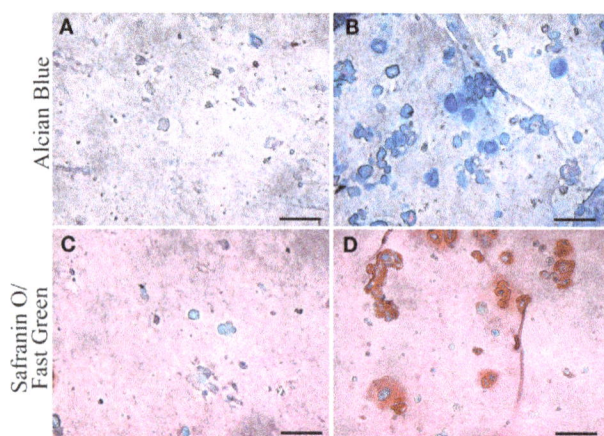

FIGURE 7 | Glycosaminoglycan (GAG) and proteoglycan content in hASC-encapsulated VL-PSL-fabricated constructs visualized by Alcian blue and safranin O/fast green staining at day 28. (A,C) Alcian blue and safranin O staining, respectively, of control group. Negligible amounts of GAG and proteoglycan are detected. **(B,D)** Alcian blue and safranin O staining, respectively, of TGF-β3 group at day 28, showing strong staining. Scale bar: 50 μm.

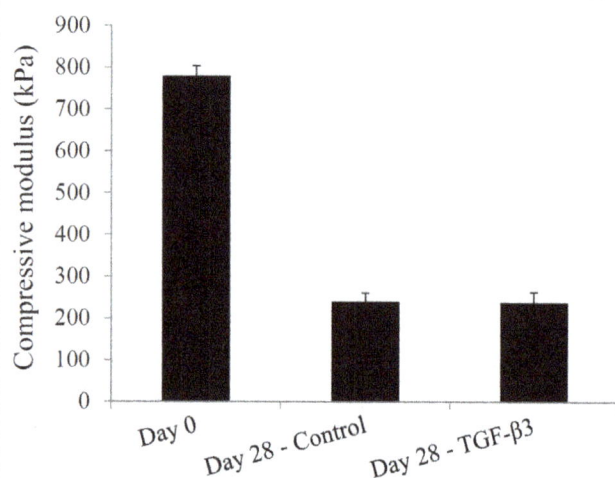

FIGURE 8 | Compressive moduli of hASC-encapsulated VL-PSL-fabricated constructs measured at culture days 0 and 28 in the control and TGF-β3 groups.

chondroinductive conditions. Mauck et al. showed that higher cell density, such as 60×10^6 cells/ml, resulted in considerably higher ECM content than lower cell density culture and contributed to the mechanical property of whole construct (Mauck et al., 2002). Also, it has been reported that the addition of BMP-6 dramatically enhanced the matrix production by hASCs (Puetzer et al., 2010).

In summary, we report here a new combination of biodegradable water-soluble polymers compatible with the VL-PSL fabrication process that has the ability to accommodate seeding as well as chondrogenic differentiation of hASCs and possesses high compressive modulus. Future studies will attempt to: (1) optimize cell density and differentiation conditions to accelerate ECM deposition and (2) address the effect of adding various substituent groups onto the polymer to control its degradation profile, as well as increase and fine-tune the mechanical properties of the scaffold.

Conclusion

Using the degradable mPDLLA-PEG/HA matrix, we have successfully applied VL-PSL to fabricate scaffolds based on CAD models as the template with high fidelity. hASCs were introduced into the scaffolds during the fabrication process and maintained high viability. TGF-β3-containing chondrogenic medium not only enhanced hASC survival but also effectively induced hASC chondrogenesis, as indicated by increased chondrogenic gene expression and cartilage ECM deposition. Live cell-based PSL-fabricated scaffolds developed in this study thus show great potential in the development of customized repair of cartilage in degenerative joint diseases, such as OA.

Acknowledgments

The authors gratefully thank Drs. Joon Paek (Tissue Genesis Institute, LLC) and Paul Manner (University of Washington) for providing adipose tissue, Dr. Jian Tan (University of Pittsburgh) for isolating hASCs, and Dr. Thomas Lozito (University of Pittsburgh) for IHC support. This work supported in part by the National Institutes of Health grant (U18TR000532, T32GM008208), the Commonwealth of Pennsylvania Department of Health (SAP4100050913), and the U.S. Department of Defense (W81XWH-10-1-0850, W81XWH-14-2-0003).

References

Bajaj, P., Chan, V., Jeong, J. H., Zorlutuna, P., Kong, H., and Bashir, R. (2012). 3-D biofabrication using stereolithography for biology and medicine. *Conf. Proc. IEEE Eng. Med. Biol. Soc.* 2012, 6805–6808. doi:10.1109/EMBC.2012. 6347557

Byers, B. A., Mauck, R. L., Chiang, I. E., and Tuan, R. S. (2008). Transient exposure to transforming growth factor beta 3 under serum-free conditions enhances the biomechanical and biochemical maturation of tissue-engineered cartilage. *Tissue Eng. Part A* 14, 1821–1834. doi:10.1089/ten.tea.2007.0222

Chopra, A., Murray, M. E., Byfield, F. J., Mendez, M. G., Halleluyan, R., Restle, D. J., et al. (2014). Augmentation of integrin-mediated mechanotransduction by hyaluronic acid. *Biomaterials* 35, 71–82. doi:10.1016/j.biomaterials.2013.09.066

Chung, C., Beecham, M., Mauck, R. L., and Burdick, J. A. (2009). The influence of degradation characteristics of hyaluronic acid hydrogels on in vitro neocartilage formation by mesenchymal stem cells. *Biomaterials* 30, 4287–4296. doi:10.1016/j.biomaterials.2009.04.040

Da Silva, J. V., Martins, T. A., and Noritomi, P. Y. (2012). Scaffold informatics and biomimetic design: three-dimensional medical reconstruction. *Methods Mol. Biol.* 868, 91–109. doi:10.1007/978-1-61779-764-4_6

Demoor, M., Ollitrault, D., Gomez-Leduc, T., Bouyoucef, M., Hervieu, M., Fabre, H., et al. (2014). Cartilage tissue engineering: molecular control of chondrocyte differentiation for proper cartilage matrix reconstruction. *Biochim. Biophys. Acta* 1840, 2414–2440. doi:10.1016/j.bbagen.2014.02.030

Derby, B. (2012). Printing and prototyping of tissues and scaffolds. *Science* 338, 921–926. doi:10.1126/science.1226340

Fairbanks, B. D., Schwartz, M. P., Bowman, C. N., and Anseth, K. S. (2009). Photoinitiated polymerization of PEG-diacrylate with lithium phenyl-2,4,6-trimethylbenzoylphosphinate: polymerization rate and cytocompatibility. *Biomaterials* 30, 6702–6707. doi:10.1016/j.biomaterials.2009.08.055

Gigante, A., Calcagno, S., Cecconi, S., Ramazzotti, D., Manzotti, S., and Enea, D. (2011). Use of collagen scaffold and autologous bone marrow concentrate as a one-step cartilage repair in the knee: histological results of second-look biopsies at 1 year follow-up. *Int. J. Immunopathol. Pharmacol.* 24, 69–72.

Koh, Y. G., Choi, Y. J., Kwon, S. K., Kim, Y. S., and Yeo, J. E. (2013). Clinical results and second-look arthroscopic findings after treatment with adipose-derived stem cells for knee osteoarthritis. *Knee Surg. Sports Traumatol. Arthrosc.* 23, 1308–1316. doi:10.1007/s00167-013-2807-2

Kuo, C. K., Li, W. J., Mauck, R. L., and Tuan, R. S. (2006). Cartilage tissue engineering: its potential and uses. *Curr. Opin. Rheumatol.* 18, 64–73. doi:10.1097/01.bor.0000198005.88568.df

Lin, H., Chen, A. W., Alexander, P. G., Beck, A. M., and Tuan, R. (2014). Cartilage tissue engineering application of injectable gelatin hydrogel with in situ visible light-activated gelation capability in both air and aqueous solution. *Tissue Eng. Part A* 20, 2402–2411. doi:10.1089/ten.TEA.2013.0642

Lin, H., Zhang, D., Alexander, P. G., Yang, G., Tan, J., Cheng, A. W., et al. (2013). Application of visible light-based projection stereolithography for live cell-scaffold fabrication with designed architecture. *Biomaterials* 34, 331–339. doi:10.1016/j.biomaterials.2012.09.048

Mauck, R. L., Seyhan, S. L., Ateshian, G. A., and Hung, C. T. (2002). Influence of seeding density and dynamic deformational loading on the developing structure/function relationships of chondrocyte-seeded agarose hydrogels. *Ann. Biomed. Eng.* 30, 1046–1056. doi:10.1114/1.1512676

Melchels, F. P., Feijen, J., and Grijpma, D. W. (2010). A review on stereolithography and its applications in biomedical engineering. *Biomaterials* 31, 6121–6130. doi:10.1016/j.biomaterials.2010.04.050

Moran, C. G., and Horton, T. C. (2000). Total knee replacement: the joint of the decade. A successful operation, for which there's a large unmet need. *BMJ* 320, 820. doi:10.1136/bmj.320.7238.820

Moriya, T., Wada, Y., Watanabe, A., Sasho, T., Nakagawa, K., Mainil-Varlet, P., et al. (2007). Evaluation of reparative cartilage after autologous chondrocyte implantation for osteochondritis dissecans: histology, biochemistry, and MR imaging. *J. Orthop. Sci.* 12, 265–273. doi:10.1007/s00776-007-1111-8

Nashi, N., Hong, C. C., and Krishna, L. (2014). Residual knee pain and functional outcome following total knee arthroplasty in osteoarthritic patients. *Knee Surg. Sports Traumatol. Arthrosc.* 23, 1841–1847. doi:10.1007/s00167-014-2910-z

Park, J. S., Shim, M. S., Shim, S. H., Yang, H. N., Jeon, S. Y., Woo, D. G., et al. (2011). Chondrogenic potential of stem cells derived from amniotic fluid, adipose tissue, or bone marrow encapsulated in fibrin gels containing TGF-beta3. *Biomaterials* 32, 8139–8149. doi:10.1016/j.biomaterials.2011.07.043

Pittenger, M. F., Mackay, A. M., Beck, S. C., Jaiswal, R. K., Douglas, R., Mosca, J. D., et al. (1999). Multilineage potential of adult human mesenchymal stem cells. *Science* 284, 143–147. doi:10.1126/science.284.5411.143

Puetzer, J. L., Petitte, J. N., and Loboa, E. G. (2010). Comparative review of growth factors for induction of three-dimensional in vitro chondrogenesis in human mesenchymal stem cells isolated from bone marrow and adipose tissue. *Tissue Eng. Part B Rev.* 16, 435–444. doi:10.1089/ten.teb.2009.0705

Roux, C., Pisani, D. F., Yahia, H. B., Djedaini, M., Beranger, G. E., Chambard, J. C., et al. (2013). Chondrogenic potential of stem cells derived from adipose tissue: a powerful pharmacological tool. *Biochem. Biophys. Res. Commun.* 440, 786–791. doi:10.1016/j.bbrc.2013.10.012

Schagemann, J. C., Paul, S., Casper, M. E., Rohwedel, J., Kramer, J., Kaps, C., et al. (2013). Chondrogenic differentiation of bone marrow-derived mesenchymal stromal cells via biomimetic and bioactive poly-epsilon-caprolactone scaffolds. *J. Biomed. Mater. Res. A.* 101, 1620–1628. doi:10.1002/jbm.a.34457

Seck, T. M., Melchels, F. P., Feijen, J., and Grijpma, D. W. (2010). Designed biodegradable hydrogel structures prepared by stereolithography using poly(ethylene glycol)/poly(D,L-lactide)-based resins. *J. Control Release* 148, 34–41. doi:10.1016/j.jconrel.2010.07.111

Stojkovska, J., Bugarski, B., and Obradovic, B. (2010). Evaluation of alginate hydrogels under in vivo-like bioreactor conditions for cartilage tissue engineering. *J. Mater. Sci. Mater. Med.* 21, 2869–2879. doi:10.1007/s10856-010-4135-0

Tuan, R. S., Chen, A. F., and Klatt, B. A. (2013). Cartilage regeneration. *J. Am. Acad. Orthop. Surg.* 21, 303–311. doi:10.5435/JAAOS-21-05-303

Wu, S. C., Chang, J. K., Wang, C. K., Wang, G. J., and Ho, M. L. (2010). Enhancement of chondrogenesis of human adipose derived stem cells in a hyaluronan-enriched microenvironment. *Biomaterials* 31, 631–640. doi:10.1016/j.biomaterials.2009.09.089

Wu, S. C., Chen, C. H., Chang, J. K., Fu, Y. C., Wang, C. K., Eswaramoorthy, R., et al. (2013). Hyaluronan initiates chondrogenesis mainly via CD44 in human adipose-derived stem cells. *J. Appl. Physiol.* 114, 1610–1618. doi:10.1152/japplphysiol.01132.2012

Xu, J. P., Wang, W., Ludeman, M., Cheng, K. V., Hayami, T., Lotz, J. C., et al. (2008). Chondrogenic differentiation of human mesenchymal stem cells in three-dimensional alginate gels. *Tissue Eng. Part A* 14, 667–680. doi:10.1089/tea.2007.0272

Yang, H., and Kao, W. Y. J. (2006). Thermoresponsive gelatin/monomethoxy poly(ethylene glycol)-poly(D,L-lactide) hydrogels: formulation, characterization, and antibacterial drug delivery. *Pharm. Res.* 23, 205–214. doi:10.1007/s11095-005-8417-z

Yang, S., Leong, K. F., Du, Z., and Chua, C. K. (2001). The design of scaffolds for use in tissue engineering. Part I. Traditional factors. *Tissue Eng.* 7, 679–689. doi:10.1089/107632701753337645

Yang, S., Leong, K. F., Du, Z., and Chua, C. K. (2002). The design of scaffolds for use in tissue engineering. Part II. Rapid prototyping techniques. *Tissue Eng.* 8, 1–11. doi:10.1089/107632702753503009

Ye, K., Di Bella, C., Myers, D. E., and Choong, P. F. (2013). The osteochondral dilemma: review of current management and future trends. *ANZ J. Surg.* 84, 211–217. doi:10.1111/ans.12108

Zhang, Y., and Jordan, J. M. (2010). Epidemiology of osteoarthritis. *Clin. Geriatr. Med.* 26, 355–369. doi:10.1016/j.cger.2010.03.001

Conflict of Interest Statement: The authors declare that the research was conducted in the absence of any commercial or financial relationships that could be construed as a potential conflict of interest.

9

Adenosine Signaling Mediates Osteogenic Differentiation of Human Embryonic Stem Cells on Mineralized Matrices

Vikram Rao[1†], Yu-Ru V. Shih[1†], Heemin Kang[2], Harsha Kabra[1] and Shyni Varghese[1]*

[1] Department of Bioengineering, University of California San Diego, La Jolla, CA, USA, [2] Materials Science and Engineering Program, University of California San Diego, La Jolla, CA, USA

Edited by:
Eric Farrell,
Erasmus University Medical Center,
Netherlands

Reviewed by:
Marie-Noelle Giraud,
University of Fribourg, Switzerland
Cathal O. Flatharta,
NUI Galway, Ireland

*Correspondence:
Shyni Varghese
svarghese@eng.ucsd.edu

†Vikram Rao and Yu-Ru V. Shih have
contributed equally to this work.

Human embryonic stem cells (hESCs) are attractive cell sources for tissue engineering and regenerative medicine due to their self-renewal and differentiation ability. Design of biomaterials with an intrinsic ability that promotes hESC differentiation to the targeted cell type boasts significant advantages for tissue regeneration. We have previously developed biomineralized calcium phosphate (CaP) matrices that inherently direct osteogenic differentiation of hESCs without the need of osteogenic-inducing chemicals or growth factors. Here, we show that CaP matrix-driven osteogenic differentiation of hESCs occurs through A2b adenosine receptor (A2bR). The inhibition of the receptor with an A2bR-specific antagonist attenuated mineralized matrix-mediated osteogenic differentiation of hESCs. In addition, when cultured on matrices in an environment deficient of CaP minerals, exogenous adenosine promoted osteogenic differentiation of hESCs, but was attenuated by the inhibition of A2bR. Such synthetic matrices that intrinsically support osteogenic commitment of hESCs are not only beneficial for bone tissue engineering but can also be used as a platform to study the effect of the physical and chemical cues to the extracellular milieu on stem cell commitment. Insights into the cell signaling during matrix-induced differentiation of stem cells will also help define the key processes and enable discovery of new targets that promote differentiation of pluripotent stem cells for bone tissue engineering.

Keywords: human embryonic stem cells, osteogenic differentiation, mineralized matrix, calcium phosphate, A2b adenosine receptor

INTRODUCTION

Human embryonic stem cells (hESCs) have tremendous potential as a cell source for regenerative medicine due to their self-renewal and differentiation ability (Wobus and Boheler, 2005). One of the major areas of regenerative medicine includes the application of stem cells in tissue engineering and reconstruction (Heng et al., 2004; Marolt et al., 2012). However, a main challenge in using pluripotent stem cells (PSCs) lies in consistently directing them toward a targeted phenotype (Murry and Keller, 2008; De Peppo et al., 2013). This often requires complex stepwise *in vitro* strategies to direct differentiation of PSCs (Levi et al., 2012; Li and Niyibizi, 2012; De Peppo et al., 2013; Hynes et al., 2014; Phillips et al., 2014).

Biomaterials containing calcium phosphate (CaP) moieties have been recognized for their osteoinductive and osteoconductive functions and hence been widely used as a scaffold for bone tissue engineering both *in vitro* and *in vivo* (Yuan et al., 2007; Levi et al., 2012; Eyckmans et al., 2013; Inzana et al., 2014; Kobayashi et al., 2014). Recently, we have engineered biomineralized CaP matrices that intrinsically induce osteogenic differentiation of human mesenchymal stem cells (hMSCs), hESCs, and human-induced pluripotent stem cells (hiPSCs), without the use of osteoinductive soluble factors, such as BMPs or dexamethasone (Phadke et al., 2012; Kang et al., 2014a,b). These biomineralized matrices also support *in vivo* bone tissue formation, even in the absence of any exogenous biologics (Phadke et al., 2013; Kang et al., 2014b; Shih et al., 2015; Wen et al., 2015).

Calcium phosphate-based biomaterials promote osteogenic differentiation of progenitor or stem cells through multiple mechanisms. This involves the ability of CaP minerals to sequester osteoinductive growth factors, such as bone morphogenetic proteins, and/or regulate extracellular Ca^{2+} and PO_4^{3-} concentrations (Autefage et al., 2009; Lee et al., 2011). This is further supported by the findings of significantly increased osteogenic differentiation of stem cells when cultured in medium containing high levels of Ca^{2+} and PO_4^{3-} (Chai et al., 2011; Phadke et al., 2012). Moreover, it has been shown that biomaterials of CaP that can easily dissociate into Ca^{2+} and PO_4^{3-} can contribute to better bone healing (Yuan et al., 2001; Barradas et al., 2013). In addition, a study by Wen et al. (2012) has demonstrated the involvement of L-type Ca^{2+} channels on Ca^{2+}-mediated osteogenic differentiation. Recently, we have shown that the PO_4^{3-} of the CaP minerals can promote osteogenic differentiation through A2b adenosine receptor (A2bR) signaling (Shih et al., 2014). This finding is consistent with other studies that demonstrated the role of adenosine signaling on bone tissue formation and osteogenesis of progenitor cells (Costa et al., 2011; Takedachi et al., 2012). For instance, studies by Evans et al. (2006) have shown the involvement of P1 purinergic adenosine receptor signaling in bone function. Specifically, it has been demonstrated that A2bR is functionally present in osteoprogenitor cells and plays a role in osteoblastic differentiation (Gharibi et al., 2011). Similarly, studies by Carroll et al. (2012) have shown that A2bR knockout mice had MSCs with decreased osteogenic potential, lower bone density, and delayed fracture repair (Carroll et al., 2012). Although it has been shown that osteogenesis of hMSCs is mediated by the activation of A2bR, its role in promoting osteogenic differentiation of PSCs, such as hESCs, remains unclear.

In this study, we determine whether the mineralized matrix-induced osteogenic differentiation of hESCs involves adenosine signaling similar to hMSCs. HESCs exhibit a developmentally naive phenotype as well as possess a vastly different cell machinery compared to hMSCs (Ulloa-Montoya et al., 2007; Aranda et al., 2009; Barbet et al., 2011). Despite the intrinsic differences between both cell types, we find that A2bR is involved in upregulation of genes associated with osteogenesis and increased protein expression of osteocalcin (OCN). This underscores the importance of A2bR signaling during osteogenic differentiation of stem cells with different maturation states.

MATERIALS AND METHODS

PEGDA-*co*-A6ACA Hydrogel Synthesis

Poly(ethylene glycol)-diacrylate (PEGDA; M_n = 6 kDa), N-acryloyl 6-aminocaproic acid (A6ACA), and PEGDA-*co*-A6ACA hydrogels were synthesized, as described previously (Kang et al., 2014b). To summarize, 555 mg of A6ACA was dissolved in 3 mL of 1M NaOH. Upon neutralization, 60 mg of PEGDA was added to yield a precursor solution composed of 1M A6ACA and 2% (wt/vol) PEGDA. Using 0.15% N,N,N′,N′-tetramethylethylenediamine (TEMED) and 0.5% ammonium persulfate (APS) as the initiator and accelerator, respectively, the resulting solution was polymerized within 1-mm glass spacer plates (Bio-Rad, catalog number: 165-3311) for 1 h at room temperature (RT) to yield PEDGA-*co*-A6ACA hydrogels. The 1-mm hydrogel sheets were immersed and equilibrated in phosphate buffered saline (PBS; pH = 7.4) for 30 min, after which circular disks measuring 1 cm^2 in area were punched out and incubated overnight in PBS.

Hydrogel Mineralization and Sterilization

Mineralization of PEGDA-*co*-A6ACA hydrogels was carried out as described elsewhere (Phadke et al., 2012). Briefly, hydrogels were equilibrated in deionized (DI) water for 6 h and subsequently immersed in modified simulated body fluid (m-SBF; pH = 7.4) for 6 h. The ionic concentrations of m-SBF include 142.0 mM Na$^+$, 5.0 mM K$^+$, 2.5 mM Ca^{2+}, 1.5 mM Mg^{2+}, 103.0 mM Cl$^-$, 10.0 mM HCO$_3^-$, 1.0 mM HPO$_4^{2-}$, and 0.5 mM SO$_4^{2-}$ (Oyane et al., 2003). After briefly rinsing in DI water, the hydrogels were immersed in a solution (pH = 5.2) containing 40 mM Ca^{2+} and 24 mM HPO$_4^{2-}$ while rotating on a VWR Mini-shaker at a speed of 200 rpm for 45 min at 25°C. Afterwards, the hydrogels were briefly rinsed in DI water and reimmersed in m-SBF for 48 h at 37°C, during which the solution was changed daily. The hydrogels were then immersed and equilibrated in PBS for 6 h prior to sterilization. Sterilization for both mineralized and non-mineralized PEGDA-*co*-A6ACA hydrogels was carried out by immersion in 70% ethanol for 3 h, followed by five daily washes in sterile PBS for 3 days prior to cell culture.

Scanning Electron Microscopy and Energy Dispersive Spectra

Scanning electron microscopy (SEM) was performed on flat strips of mineralized and non-mineralized matrices. The samples were flash-frozen in liquid nitrogen, lyophilized overnight, and coated with Iridium for 7 s within a sputter (Emitech, K575X). The samples were imaged using scanning electron microscope (Philips XL30 ESEM), and also analyzed for elemental spectra using its integrated energy dispersive spectra (EDS) system. The Ca/P atomic ratio was computed using Oxford Energy Dispersive Spectra with INCA software.

Cell Culture

Human embryonic stem cells (HUES9) were maintained on mitotically inactivated mouse embryonic fibroblast (MEF) feeder cells with culture medium containing Knockout DMEM

(Life Technologies, catalog number: 10829-018) supplemented with 10% (vol/vol) Knockout Serum Replacement (KSR; Life Technologies, catalog number: 10828-028), 10% (vol/vol) human plasmanate (Talecris Biotherapeutics), 1% (vol/vol) non-essential amino acids (NEAA), 1% (vol/vol) Gluta-MAX, 1% (vol/vol) penicillin streptomycin, and 55 μM 2-mercaptoethanol (Chang et al., 2013). The medium was supplemented with basic fibroblast growth factor (bFGF; 30 ng/mL) and exchanged with fresh medium daily. Cells were enzymatically detached using Accutase (Millipore) and regularly passaged upon reaching approximately 80% confluence.

Prior to cell seeding, both mineralized and non-mineralized matrices were coated with Matrigel (Corning, catalog number: 354277) diluted with DMEM (Invitrogen) at a ratio of 1:82 (298 μL Matrigel diluted with 24.5 mL DMEM) and incubated overnight at 4°C. The following day, matrices were incubated in medium containing high glucose DMEM, 20% (vol/vol) fetal bovine serum [Premium (FBS); Atlanta Biologicals, catalog number: S11150], and 1% (vol/vol) penicillin streptomycin for 24 h at 37°C. Cells were seeded at an initial density of 10,000 cells/cm² and cultured in hESC-maintenance medium containing bFGF (30 ng/mL) for 1 day. The hESCs were cultured for an additional 2 days in hESC-maintenance medium without bFGF. The hESCs were subsequently cultured in growth medium (GM) containing high glucose DMEM, 4 mM L-glutamine, 10% (vol/vol) FBS (Gibco), and 1% (vol/vol) penicillin streptomycin. Adenosine and PSB 603 were supplemented into growth media for cell treatment. Adenosine (Sigma Aldrich) was first dissolved in DMEM as 11.2 mM stock solution and filter sterilized by using 0.22-μm syringe filters. The stock solution was further diluted 1,000× in growth media to 11.2 μM as the final concentration for experiments. 8-[4-[4-(4-chlorophenzyl)piperazide-1-sulfonyl) phenyl]]-1-propylxanthine (PSB 603) (Tocris Biosciences, catalog number: 3198) was dissolved in dimethyl sulfoxide (DMSO) as 1 mM stock solution and filter sterilized. The stock solution was further diluted 10,000× in growth media to 100 nM as the final concentration for experiments. All cell cultures were maintained at 37°C and 5% CO_2.

Cell Tracker Staining

To visualize cell attachment in 2-D culture, cells were stained with CellTracker (Life Technologies, catalog number: C34552) at 3, 5, and 8 days postseeding. Cells attached to the matrix were stained in 20 μM CellTracker reagent in DMEM at 37°C for 30 min. The stained cells were imaged using a fluorescence microscope (Carl Zeiss, Axio Observer.A1).

Quantitative Real-Time Polymerase Chain Reaction

Samples from two biological experiments were collected and pooled together using TRIzol Reagent (Life Technologies, catalog number: 15596-018), and RNA extraction was performed using phenol–chloroform extraction method. For each sample, 1 μg of RNA was reverse transcribed to complementary DNA (cDNA) using iScript cDNA Synthesis Kit (Bio-Rad, catalog number: 17-8891) according to the manufacturer's instructions. The synthesized cDNA was analyzed via quantitative

real-time polymerase chain reaction (qRT-PCR) for osteogenic markers, such as OCN, runt-related transcription factor 2 (RUNX2), and secreted phosphoprotein 1 (SPP1) as well as additional genes, including solute carrier family 20 (phosphate transporter), member 1 (SLC20a1), and Nanog homeobox (NANOG). Primer sequences for each analyzed gene are provided in Table S1 in Supplementary Material. Reactions were performed using SYBR Select Master Mix (Life Technologies, catalog number: 4472908) and ABI Prism 7700 Sequence Detection (Applied Biosystems). Fold expression values were determined by $2^{-\Delta\Delta C_t}$ after normalizing each target gene with respect to the housekeeping gene (GAPDH) within the sample, and compared to undifferentiated hESCs as the control that was expressed as 1.

Immunofluorescent Staining

Osteogenic differentiation of hESCs was evaluated by immunofluorescent staining for OCN. Cells were fixed in 4% paraformaldehyde for 10 min at RT, and incubated in blocking buffer composed of 3% (wt/vol) bovine serum albumin (BSA) and 0.1% (vol/vol) Triton™ X-100 in PBS for 45 min. The fixed cells were incubated overnight with primary antibodies (1:50; mouse monoclonal, Santa Cruz Biotechnology, catalog number: sc-74495) in blocking buffer at 4°C. They were then incubated with blocking buffer containing secondary antibody (1:100; goat anti-mouse Alexa Fluor® 568, Life Technologies, catalog number: A-11004) and phalloidin (1:100; Alexa Fluor® 488, Life Technologies, catalog number: A12379). Nuclei were counter-stained using Hoechst 33342 (2 μg/mL; Life Technologies, catalog number: H1399) at RT for 10 min and washed with PBS. The samples were mounted onto glass slides and imaged using a fluorescence microscope. Images were acquired using an A1 Zeiss Inverted microscope and analyzed using ImageJ. Immunofluorescent images of all samples were acquired under the linear mode and at an exposure time of 1 s. The background was uniformly subtracted from all images using a rolling ball radius method and value of 750.0 pixels.

Statistical Analysis

Statistical analyses were carried out using GraphPad Prism® (v. 5.00). One-way analysis of variance (ANOVA) along with Tukey–Kramer *post hoc* test was used to compare multiple groups at the same time point. Two-tailed Student's *t*-test was utilized to compare two groups at the same time point. Two-way ANOVA with Bonferroni *post hoc* test was used to compare multiple groups at different time points. From these tests, the *p*-values were determined and asterisks were assigned to denote statistical significances for *p*-values <0.05.

RESULTS

Synthesis and Characterization of Non-Mineralized and Mineralized PEGDA-co-A6ACA Matrices

Hydrogel matrices were synthesized by cross-linking poly(ethylene glycol)-diacrylate (PEGDA) with *N*-acryloyl

6-aminocaproic acid (A6ACA). Mineralization of matrices occurred with the binding of Ca^{2+} to terminal carboxyl groups along the pendant side chain of A6ACA, leading to the subsequent nucleation and growth of CaP minerals (Phadke et al., 2010). In order to characterize the morphology and elemental composition mineralized matrices, SEM and energy dispersive spectra (EDS) analyses were performed as shown in **Figure 1**. The SEM images showed the mineralized matrices displaying a continuous layer of bound CaP minerals exhibiting a plate-like morphology. The elemental spectra analysis confirmed the presence of calcium and phosphorous elements in the mineralized matrices with a quantified Ca/P ratio of approximately 1:31. As expected, no such moieties or peaks distinguishing such elements were observed for non-mineralized matrices.

Mineralized Matrix-Driven Osteogenic Differentiation of hESCs

The hESCs cultured on non-mineralized and mineralized matrices in GM were able to adhere and grow on the matrices as a function of time (**Figure 2**). Analysis of the gene expression demonstrated a significant upregulation of various osteogenic markers, OCN, RUNX2, and SPP1 for hESCs cultured on mineralized matrices compared to non-mineralized matrices over 21 days (**Figure 3A**). This is consistent with our previous study, which showed significant upregulation of osteogenic markers in hESCs cultured on mineralized matrices (Kang et al., 2014b). Immunofluorescent staining for OCN further

corroborated these findings, where OCN was stained positive in hESCs cultured on mineralized matrices in contrast to those cultured on non-mineralized matrices (**Figure 3B**). OCN staining intensity markedly increased between 14 and 21 days. In addition to osteogenic expression, hESCs exhibited a higher upregulation of the sodium–phosphate symporter, SLC20a1, when cultured on mineralized matrices compared to non-mineralized matrices (Figure S1A in Supplementary Material). Consistent with the differentiation of hESCs, the pluripotency marker, NANOG, was found to be downregulated as a function of time for both non-mineralized and mineralized matrix groups (Figure S1B in Supplementary Material). The hESCs cultured on mineralized matrices showed higher upregulation of A2bR compared to non-mineralized matrices (Figure S2 in Supplementary Material).

Mineralized Matrix-Assisted Osteogenic Differentiation Through A2bR Signaling

To explore whether adenosine signaling through A2bR is involved during osteogenic differentiation of hESCs on mineralized matrices, we used a selective antagonist, 8-[4-[4-(4-chlorophenzyl)piperazide-1-sulfonyl)phenyl]]-1-propylxanthine (PSB 603), to block A2bR. As shown in **Figure 4A**, the presence of PSB 603 in the culture medium abrogated the mineralized matrix-induced upregulation of osteogenic genes (**Figure 4A**). These observations were further supported by analysis of immunofluorescent staining intensity for OCN. The intensity

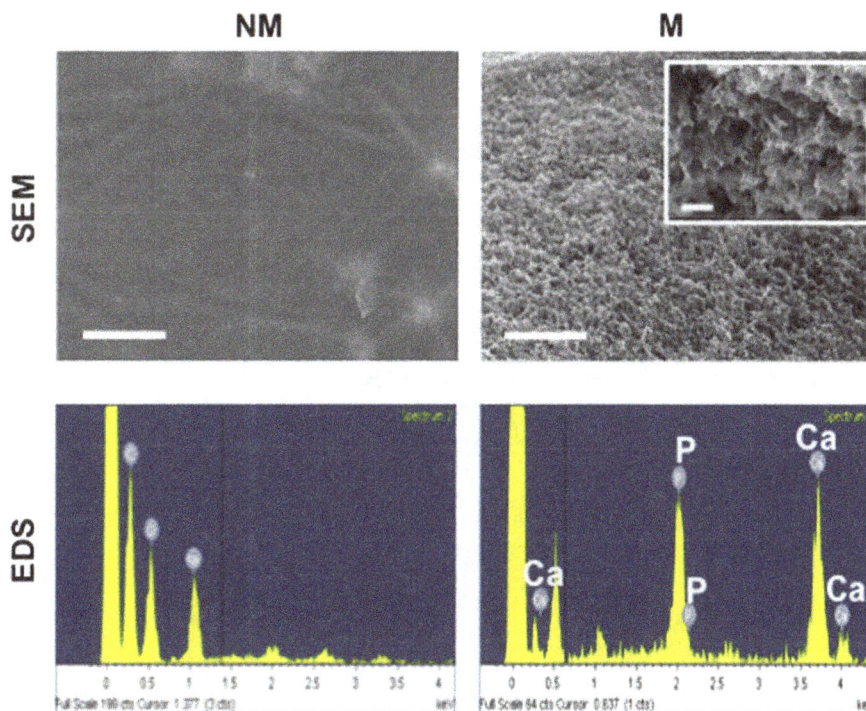

FIGURE 1 | Characterization of non-mineralized and mineralized matrices. Scanning electron microscopy (SEM) images and corresponding energy dispersive spectroscopy (EDS) of non-mineralized (NM) and mineralized (M) matrices. Scale bars represent 5 μm. Inset shows high magnification SEM image. Scale bar represents 500 nm.

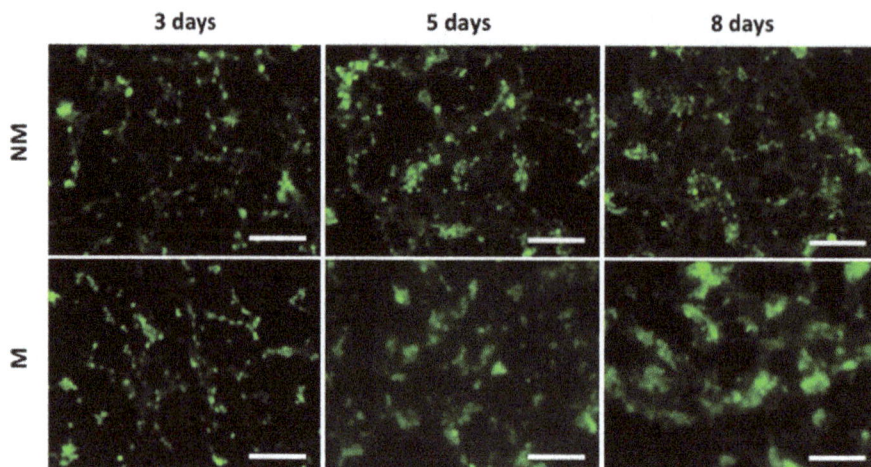

FIGURE 2 | Morphology of hESCs on non-mineralized and mineralized matrices. Fluorescent images of hESCs stained by CellTracker cultured on non-mineralized (NM) and mineralized (M) matrices after 3, 5, and 8 days of culture. Scale bars represent 200 μm.

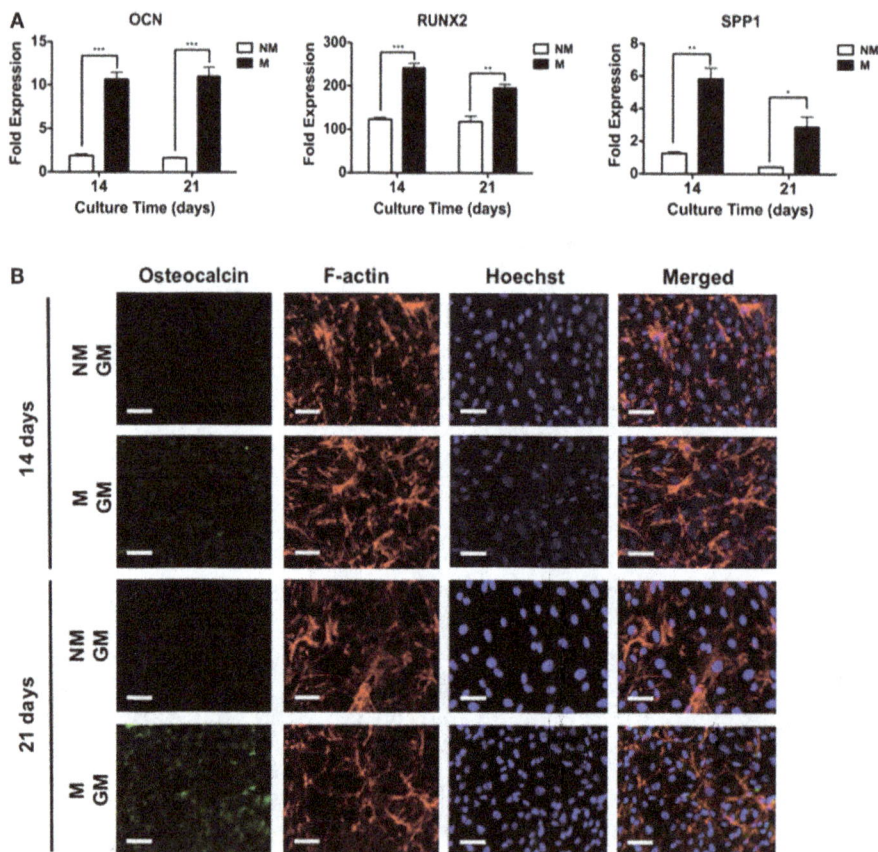

FIGURE 3 | Mineralized matrix-mediated osteogenic differentiation of hESCs. **(A)** Gene expression profiles for OCN, RUNX2, and SPP1 of hESCs on non-mineralized (NM) and mineralized (M) matrices after 14 and 21 days of culture. **(B)** Immunofluorescent staining of osteocalcin, F-actin, and Hoechst for hESCs cultured on NM and M matrices in growth medium (GM) after 14 and 21 days. Data are presented as mean ± SEs ($n = 3$). Two-tailed Student's t-test was used to compare two groups at the same time point. Asterisks denote statistical significances according to p-values (*$p < 0.05$, **$p < 0.01$, ***$p < 0.001$). Scale bars represent 100 μm.

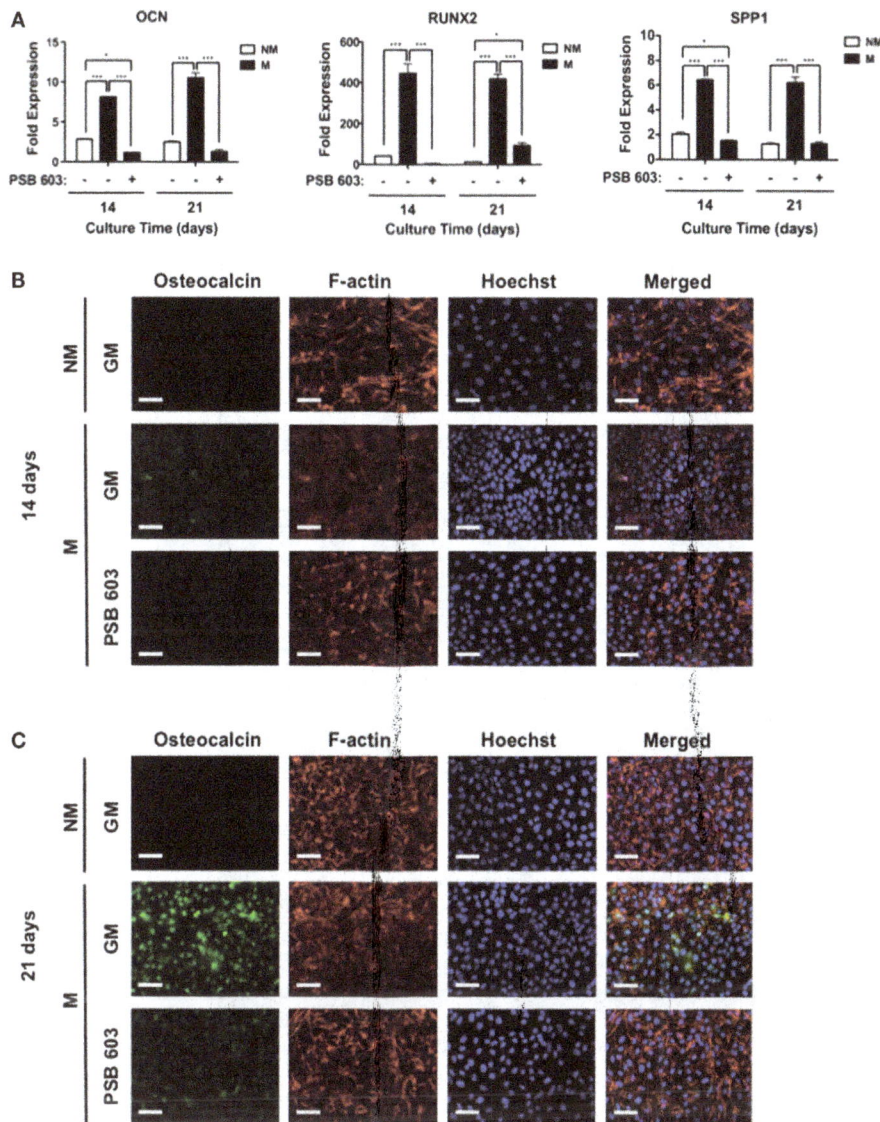

FIGURE 4 | Mineralized matrix-assisted osteogenic differentiation of hESCs involves A2bR. (A) OCN, RUNX2, and SPP1 gene expressions of hESCs on non-mineralized (NM) in growth medium (GM) as well as on mineralized matrices in growth medium (GM) with and without A2bR antagonist, PSB 603. Corresponding immunofluorescent staining of osteocalcin, F-actin, and Hoechst for hESCs cultured on NM and M matrices as well on M matrices in presence of PSB 603 for (B) 14 and (C) 21 days of culture. Data are presented as mean ± SEs (n = 3). Multiple groups at the same time point were compared by one-way ANOVA with Tukey–Kramer post hoc test. Asterisks denote statistical significances according to p-values (*p < 0.05, ***p < 0.001). Scale bars represent 100 μm.

of OCN was increased for hESCs cultured on mineralized matrices after 14 days, but diminished in the presence of PSB 603 (Figure 4B). A similar finding was observed at 21 days post-culture (Figure 4C).

Exogenous Adenosine Promotes Osteogenic Differentiation Through A2bR

To further substantiate the role of adenosine signaling on osteogenic differentiation of hESCs, cells were cultured on non-mineralized matrices, devoid of CaP, and exposed to culture medium containing adenosine. Results showed supplementation of exogenous adenosine-promoted osteogenic differentiation of hESCs on non-mineralized matrices, while inhibition of A2bR with PSB 603 led to a downregulation of the osteogenic genes, OCN, RUNX2, and SPP1 (Figure 5A). In addition, immunofluorescent staining for OCN was highly positive for cells cultured on non-mineralized matrices in the presence of adenosine, whereas a reduction in the staining intensity was observed in other medium conditions after 14 and 21 days (Figures 5B,C).

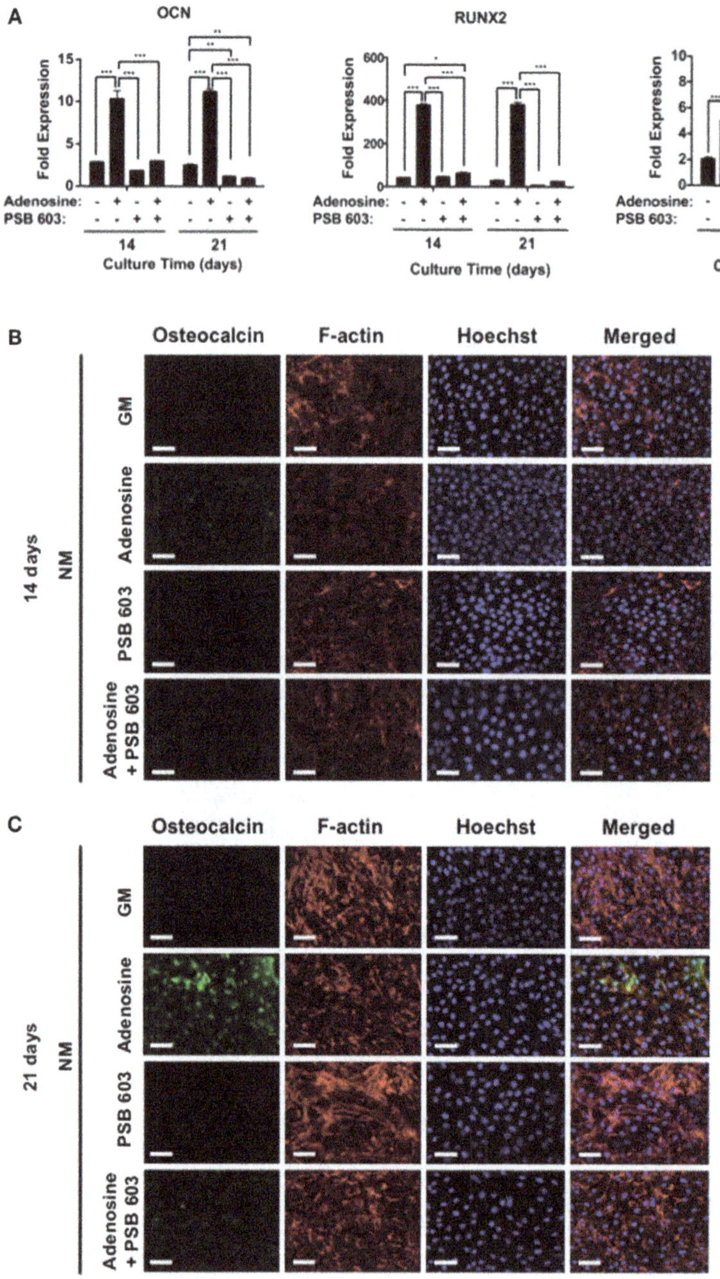

FIGURE 5 | Exogenous adenosine-mediated osteogenic differentiation of hESCs through A2bR signaling. (A) OCN, RUNX2, and SPP1 gene expressions for hESCs on non-mineralized (NM) matrices in growth medium (GM) supplemented with or without adenosine and PSB 603. Corresponding immunofluorescent staining of osteocalcin, F-actin, and Hoechst for hESCs on NM matrices after **(B)** 14 and **(C)** 21 days of culture. Data are presented as mean $\pm$ SEs ($n = 3$). Multiple groups at the same time point were compared by one-way ANOVA with Tukey–Kramer *post hoc* test. Asterisks denote statistical significances according to *p*-values (*$p < 0.05$, **$p < 0.01$, ***$p < 0.001$). Scale bars represent 100 µm.

DISCUSSION

Previously, we have shown that human PSCs, including hESCs, can be differentiated into osteoblasts by using matrix-based cues from the mineralized biomaterials (Kang et al., 2014a,b). Consistent with these findings, the hESCs on mineralized matrices exhibited an upregulation of osteogenic markers in GM even in the absence of any osteogenic-inducing soluble factors. As evident from the NANOG expression, the cells on both mineralized and non-mineralized matrices lost their pluripotency, while only these on mineralized matrices underwent significant osteogenic differentiation. The observed loss of pluripotency on all matrices is due to the culture conditions, which lack components that are known to assist maintenance of pluripotency of hESCs (Chang et al., 2013). Since increased surface roughness at the cell–material interface may increase osteogenic differentiation (Faia-Torres et al., 2014), a limitation to this study is the extent of how the topology of mineralized matrices contributes to osteogenic commitment.

The hESCs on mineralized matrices not only showed an upregulation of gene markers that are relevant to osteogenic differentiation but also exhibited high levels of OCN, a bone-specific protein. The cells on non-mineralized matrices, which lack any intrinsic ability to induce osteogenesis, underwent osteogenic differentiation when cultured in medium supplemented with adenosine. Both mineralized matrix- and exogenous adenosine-assisted osteogenic differentiations of hESCs were annulled in the presence in PSB 603, which is a known pharmacological inhibitor of A2bR. Taken together, these results underscore the influence of adenosine signaling through A2b receptor on osteogenic differentiation of hESCs. These findings are also consistent with our previous reports that showed the role of adenosine signaling on mineralized matrix-induced osteogenic differentiation of hMSCs (Shih et al., 2014). The adenosine signaling mediated by the mineralized matrices not only promotes osteogenic differentiation of hMSCs but also inhibits their adipogenic differentiation (Kang et al., 2015).

The observation that hESCs on the mineralized matrix exhibited upregulation of SLC20a1 implies the potential contribution of PO_4^{3-} ions from the CaP minerals toward this process. SLC20a1, also known as PiT-1, is a sodium–phosphate symporter that transports PO_4^{3-} ions from the extracellular milieu into the cytoplasm. We have previously shown that the extracellular PO_4^{3-} of the CaP minerals play an important role in promoting osteogenic differentiation of hMSCs through adenosine signaling, where the cellular intake of PO_4^{3-} is regulated by SLC20a1 (Shih et al., 2014). Previous studies have also shown the importance of SLC20a1 in mineralization (Yoshiko et al., 2007; Cowan et al., 2012) as well as A2bR in osteogenic differentiation (Gharibi et al., 2011; He et al., 2013). Despite the differences in cell machinery, we find hESCs consistently differentiate into osteoblasts and upregulate the phosphate transporter, SLC20a1, on CaP matrices in a similar manner to hMSCs. Such an upregulation may facilitate PO_4^{3-} to serve as a substrate for the production of adenosine triphosphate (ATP), which has been shown to be essential for osteogenic differentiation (Chen et al., 2008). This production of ATP results in a subsequent increase in extracellular adenosine that requires A2bR signaling during CaP-directed osteogenic differentiation (Shih et al., 2014). Although we did not investigate its role, calcium is required during PO_4^{3-}-induced osteogenic differentiation since this process is blunted in the absence of CaP crystal formation (Khoshniat et al., 2011).

We detected A2bR gene expression in pluripotent hESCs that increased as a function of culture time, possibly demonstrating the increased role of the receptor during the maturation process. Despite the finding that mineralized matrices promote osteogenic differentiation of hESCs through A2bR expression, the downstream signaling following A2bR expression remains unclear. For instance, whether A2bR signaling crosstalks with calcium-responsive ion channels in ESCs remains to be determined. Studies have shown A2bR expression resulted in significant potentiation of P-type Ca^{2+} current (Vacas et al., 2003). A2bR signaling is coupled to the activation of cyclic AMP (cAMP) through G_s proteins, leading to stimulation of downstream signaling molecules (Ham and Evans, 2012). Furthermore, Hsiao et al. (2008) have demonstrated the engineering of a G-protein coupled receptor (GPCR) with constitutive G_s signaling in murine osteoblasts dramatically enhanced bone mass. A study by Siddappa et al. (2008) reported the involvement of protein kinase A (PKA), where cAMP/PKA signaling induced *in vitro* osteogenesis of hMSCs and promoted *in vivo* bone formation with cAMP either stimulating or inhibiting osteogenesis in hMSCs, depending on the duration rather than the strength of the signal (Siddappa et al., 2010). However, cAMP may exert contrasting effects during early versus late stages of osteogenic differentiation of murine ESCs by inhibiting differentiation at early stages, but is required at later stages (Zhang et al., 2012).

To summarize, the results in this study demonstrate that CaP-bearing biomineralized PEGDA-*co*-A6ACA matrices direct osteogenic commitment of hESCs via adenosine signaling. Although this study describes the importance of adenosine signaling through A2bR in directing ESC osteogenic fate, there is warrant for future studies to further elucidate the role of calcium and the signaling network that are involved in mediating osteogenic differentiation of PSCs on CaP matrices. Further efforts to investigate the cellular signaling pathways can shed light on our biological understanding of how cells behave in biomaterials to expose new targets of regulation and aid in the development of novel biomaterials for cell transplantation and bone tissue engineering.

AUTHOR CONTRIBUTIONS

VR, YS, HKang, HKabra, and SV designed the experiments. VR, YS, HKang, and HKabra, performed the experiments. VR, YS, HKang, HKabra, and SV analyzed and interpreted the data. VR, YS, and SV wrote the paper.

ACKNOWLEDGMENTS

The authors gratefully acknowledge the financial support from National Institutes of Health (NIH, Grant 5R01 AR063184-02).

REFERENCES

Aranda, P., Agirre, X., Ballestar, E., Andreu, E. J., Roman-Gomez, J., Prieto, I., et al. (2009). Epigenetic signatures associated with different levels of differentiation potential in human stem cells. *PLoS ONE* 4:e7809. doi:10.1371/journal.pone.0007809

Autefage, H., Briand-Mesange, F., Cazalbou, S., Drouet, C., Fourmy, D., Goncalves, S., et al. (2009). Adsorption and release of BMP-2 on nanocrystalline apatite-coated and uncoated hydroxyapatite/beta-tricalcium phosphate porous ceramics. *J. Biomed. Mater Res. B Appl. Biomater.* 91, 706–715. doi:10.1002/jbm.b.31447

Barbet, R., Peiffer, I., Hatzfeld, A., Charbord, P., and Hatzfeld, J. A. (2011). Comparison of gene expression in human embryonic stem cells, hESC-derived mesenchymal stem cells and human mesenchymal stem cells. *Stem. Cells Int.* 2011, 368192. doi:10.4061/2011/368192

Barradas, A. M., Monticone, V., Hulsman, M., Danoux, C., Fernandes, H., Tahmasebi Birgani, Z., et al. (2013). Molecular mechanisms of biomaterial-driven osteogenic differentiation in human mesenchymal stromal cells. *Integr. Biol.* 5, 920–931. doi:10.1039/c3ib40027a

Carroll, S. H., Wigner, N. A., Kulkarni, N., Johnston-Cox, H., Gerstenfeld, L. C., and Ravid, K. (2012). A2B adenosine receptor promotes mesenchymal stem cell differentiation to osteoblasts and bone formation in vivo. *J. Biol. Chem.* 287, 15718–15727. doi:10.1074/jbc.M112.344994

Chai, Y. C., Roberts, S. J., Schrooten, J., and Luyten, F. P. (2011). Probing the osteoinductive effect of calcium phosphate by using an in vitro biomimetic model. *Tissue Eng. Part A* 17, 1083–1097. doi:10.1089/ten.TEA.2010.0160

Chang, C. W., Hwang, Y., Brafman, D., Hagan, T., Phung, C., and Varghese, S. (2013). Engineering cell-material interfaces for long-term expansion of human pluripotent stem cells. *Biomaterials* 34, 912–921. doi:10.1016/j.biomaterials.2012.10.020

Chen, C. T., Shih, Y. R., Kuo, T. K., Lee, O. K., and Wei, Y. H. (2008). Coordinated changes of mitochondrial biogenesis and antioxidant enzymes during osteogenic differentiation of human mesenchymal stem cells. *Stem Cells* 26, 960–968. doi:10.1634/stemcells.2007-0509

Costa, M. A., Barbosa, A., Neto, E., Sa-E-Sousa, A., Freitas, R., Neves, J. M., et al. (2011). On the role of subtype selective adenosine receptor agonists during proliferation and osteogenic differentiation of human primary bone marrow stromal cells. *J. Cell. Physiol.* 226, 1353–1366. doi:10.1002/jcp.22458

Cowan, C. M., Zhang, X., James, A. W., Kim, T. M., Sun, N., Wu, B., et al. (2012). NELL-1 increases pre-osteoblast mineralization using both phosphate transporter Pit1 and Pit2. *Biochem. Biophys. Res. Commun.* 422, 351–357. doi:10.1016/j.bbrc.2012.04.077

De Peppo, G. M., Marcos-Campos, I., Kahler, D. J., Alsalman, D., Shang, L., Vunjak-Novakovic, G., et al. (2013). Engineering bone tissue substitutes from human induced pluripotent stem cells. *Proc. Natl. Acad. Sci. U.S.A.* 110, 8680–8685. doi:10.1073/pnas.1301190110

Evans, B. A., Elford, C., Pexa, A., Francis, K., Hughes, A. C., Deussen, A., et al. (2006). Human osteoblast precursors produce extracellular adenosine, which modulates their secretion of IL-6 and osteoprotegerin. *J. Bone Miner. Res.* 21, 228–236. doi:10.1359/JBMR.051021

Eyckmans, J., Roberts, S. J., Bolander, J., Schrooten, J., Chen, C. S., and Luyten, F. P. (2013). Mapping calcium phosphate activated gene networks as a strategy for targeted osteoinduction of human progenitors. *Biomaterials* 34, 4612–4621. doi:10.1016/j.biomaterials.2013.03.011

Faia-Torres, A. B., Guimond-Lischer, S., Rottmar, M., Charnley, M., Goren, T., Maniura-Weber, K., et al. (2014). Differential regulation of osteogenic differentiation of stem cells on surface roughness gradients. *Biomaterials* 35, 9023–9032. doi:10.1016/j.biomaterials.2014.07.015

Gharibi, B., Abraham, A. A., Ham, J., and Evans, B. A. (2011). Adenosine receptor subtype expression and activation influence the differentiation of mesenchymal stem cells to osteoblasts and adipocytes. *J. Bone Miner. Res.* 26, 2112–2124. doi:10.1002/jbmr.424

Ham, J., and Evans, B. A. (2012). An emerging role for adenosine and its receptors in bone homeostasis. *Front. Endocrinol.* 3:113. doi:10.3389/fendo.2012.00113

He, W., Mazumder, A., Wilder, T., and Cronstein, B. N. (2013). Adenosine regulates bone metabolism via A1, A2A, and A2B receptors in bone marrow cells from normal humans and patients with multiple myeloma. *FASEB J.* 27, 3446–3454. doi:10.1096/fj.13-231233

Heng, B. C., Cao, T., Stanton, L. W., Robson, P., and Olsen, B. (2004). Strategies for directing the differentiation of stem cells into the osteogenic lineage in vitro. *J. Bone Miner. Res.* 19, 1379–1394. doi:10.1359/JBMR.040714

Hsiao, E. C., Boudignon, B. M., Chang, W. C., Bencsik, M., Peng, J., Nguyen, T. D., et al. (2008). Osteoblast expression of an engineered Gs-coupled receptor dramatically increases bone mass. *Proc. Natl. Acad. Sci. U.S.A.* 105, 1209–1214. doi:10.1073/pnas.0707457105

Hynes, K., Menicanin, D., Mrozik, K., Gronthos, S., and Bartold, P. M. (2014). Generation of functional mesenchymal stem cells from different induced pluripotent stem cell lines. *Stem Cells Dev.* 23, 1084–1096. doi:10.1089/scd.2013.0111

Inzana, J. A., Olvera, D., Fuller, S. M., Kelly, J. P., Graeve, O. A., Schwarz, E. M., et al. (2014). 3D printing of composite calcium phosphate and collagen scaffolds for bone regeneration. *Biomaterials* 35, 4026–4034. doi:10.1016/j.biomaterials.2014.01.064

Kang, H., Shih, Y. R., Hwang, Y., Wen, C., Rao, V., Seo, T., et al. (2014a). Mineralized gelatin methacrylate-based matrices induce osteogenic differentiation of human induced pluripotent stem cells. *Acta Biomater.* 10, 4961–4970. doi:10.1016/j.actbio.2014.08.010

Kang, H., Wen, C., Hwang, Y., Shih, Y. R., Kar, M., Seo, S. W., et al. (2014b). Biomineralized matrix-assisted osteogenic differentiation of human embryonic stem cells. *J. Mater. Chem.* 2, 5676–5688. doi:10.1039/C4TB00714J

Kang, H., Shih, Y. R., and Varghese, S. (2015). Biomineralized matrices dominate soluble cues to direct osteogenic differentiation of human mesenchymal stem cells through adenosine signaling. *Biomacromolecules* 16, 1050–1061. doi:10.1021/acs.biomac.5b00099

Khoshniat, S., Bourgine, A., Julien, M., Petit, M., Pilet, P., Rouillon, T., et al. (2011). Phosphate-dependent stimulation of MGP and OPN expression in osteoblasts via the ERK1/2 pathway is modulated by calcium. *Bone* 48, 894–902. doi:10.1016/j.bone.2010.12.002

Kobayashi, K., Anada, T., Handa, T., Kanda, N., Yoshinari, M., Takahashi, T., et al. (2014). Osteoconductive property of a mechanical mixture of octacalcium phosphate and amorphous calcium phosphate. *ACS Appl. Mater Interfaces* 6, 22602–22611. doi:10.1021/am5067139

Lee, J. S., Suarez-Gonzalez, D., and Murphy, W. L. (2011). Mineral coatings for temporally controlled delivery of multiple proteins. *Adv. Mater.* 23, 4279–4284. doi:10.1002/adma.201100060

Levi, B., Hyun, J. S., Montoro, D. T., Lo, D. D., Chan, C. K., Hu, S., et al. (2012). In vivo directed differentiation of pluripotent stem cells for skeletal regeneration. *Proc. Natl. Acad. Sci. U.S.A.* 109, 20379–20384. doi:10.1073/pnas.1218052109

Li, F., and Niyibizi, C. (2012). Cells derived from murine induced pluripotent stem cells (iPSC) by treatment with members of TGF-beta family give rise to osteoblasts differentiation and form bone in vivo. *BMC Cell Biol.* 13:35. doi:10.1186/1471-2121-1113-1135

Marolt, D., Campos, I. M., Bhumiratana, S., Koren, A., Petridis, P., Zhang, G., et al. (2012). Engineering bone tissue from human embryonic stem cells. *Proc. Natl. Acad. Sci. U.S.A.* 109, 8705–8709. doi:10.1073/pnas.1201830109

Murry, C. E., and Keller, G. (2008). Differentiation of embryonic stem cells to clinically relevant populations: lessons from embryonic development. *Cell* 132, 661–680. doi:10.1016/j.cell.2008.02.008

Oyane, A., Kim, H. M., Furuya, T., Kokubo, T., Miyazaki, T., and Nakamura, T. (2003). Preparation and assessment of revised simulated body fluids. *J. Biomed. Mater Res.* 65, 188–195. doi:10.1002/jbm.a.10482

Phadke, A., Hwang, Y., Kim, S. H., Kim, S. H., Yamaguchi, T., Masuda, K., et al. (2013). Effect of scaffold microarchitecture on osteogenic differentiation of human mesenchymal stem cells. *Eur. Cell Mater.* 25, 114–129. doi:10.1002/jbm.a.10482

Phadke, A., Shih, Y. R., and Varghese, S. (2012). Mineralized synthetic matrices as an instructive microenvironment for osteogenic differentiation of human mesenchymal stem cells. *Macromol. Biosci.* 12, 1022–1032. doi:10.1002/mabi.201100289

Phadke, A., Zhang, C., Hwang, Y., Vecchio, K., and Varghese, S. (2010). Templated mineralization of synthetic hydrogels for bone-like composite materials: role of matrix hydrophobicity. *Biomacromolecules* 11, 2060–2068. doi:10.1021/bm100425p

Phillips, M. D., Kuznetsov, S. A., Cherman, N., Park, K., Chen, K. G., Mcclendon, B. N., et al. (2014). Directed differentiation of human induced pluripotent stem cells toward bone and cartilage: in vitro versus in vivo assays. *Stem Cells Transl. Med.* 3, 867–878. doi:10.5966/sctm.2013-0154

Shih, Y. R., Hwang, Y., Phadke, A., Kang, H., Hwang, N. S., Caro, E. J., et al. (2014). Calcium phosphate-bearing matrices induce osteogenic differentiation of stem cells through adenosine signaling. *Proc. Natl. Acad. Sci. U.S.A.* 111, 990–995. doi:10.1073/pnas.1321717111

Shih, Y. R., Phadke, A., Yamaguchi, T., Kang, H., Inoue, N., Masuda, K., et al. (2015). Synthetic bone mimetic matrix-mediated in situ bone tissue formation through host cell recruitment. *Acta Biomater.* 19, 1–9. doi:10.1016/j.actbio.2015.1003.1017

Siddappa, R., Doorn, J., Liu, J., Langerwerf, E., Arends, R., Van Blitterswijk, C., et al. (2010). Timing, rather than the concentration of cyclic AMP, correlates to osteogenic differentiation of human mesenchymal stem cells. *J. Tissue Eng. Regen. Med.* 4, 356–365. doi:10.1002/term.246

Siddappa, R., Martens, A., Doorn, J., Leusink, A., Olivo, C., Licht, R., et al. (2008). cAMP/PKA pathway activation in human mesenchymal stem cells in vitro results in robust bone formation in vivo. *Proc. Natl. Acad. Sci. U.S.A.* 105, 7281–7286. doi:10.1073/pnas.0711190105

Takedachi, M., Oohara, H., Smith, B. J., Iyama, M., Kobashi, M., Maeda, K., et al. (2012). CD73-generated adenosine promotes osteoblast differentiation. *J. Cell Physiol.* 227, 2622–2631. doi:10.1002/jcp.23001

Ulloa-Montoya, F., Kidder, B. L., Pauwelyn, K. A., Chase, L. G., Luttun, A., Crabbe, A., et al. (2007). Comparative transcriptome analysis of embryonic and adult stem cells with extended and limited differentiation capacity. *Genome Biol.* 8, R163. doi:10.1186/gb-2007-1188-1188-r1163

Vacas, J., Fernandez, M., Ros, M., and Blanco, P. (2003). Adenosine modulation of [Ca2+]i in cerebellar granular cells: multiple adenosine receptors involved. *Brain Res.* 992, 272–280. doi:10.1016/j.brainres.2003.08.055

Wen, C., Kang, H., Shih, Y. V., Hwang, Y., and Varghese, S. (2015). In vivo comparison of biomineralized scaffold-directed osteogenic differentiation of human embryonic and mesenchymal stem cells. *Drug Deliv. Transl. Res.* 1–11. doi:10.1007/s13346-13015-10242-13342

Wen, L., Wang, Y., Wang, H., Kong, L., Zhang, L., Chen, X., et al. (2012). L-type calcium channels play a crucial role in the proliferation and osteogenic differentiation of bone marrow mesenchymal stem cells. *Biochem. Biophys. Res. Commun.* 424, 439–445. doi:10.1016/j.bbrc.2012.06.128

Wobus, A. M., and Boheler, K. R. (2005). Embryonic stem cells: prospects for developmental biology and cell therapy. *Physiol. Rev.* 85, 635–678. doi:10.1152/physrev.00054.2003

Yoshiko, Y., Candeliere, G. A., Maeda, N., and Aubin, J. E. (2007). Osteoblast autonomous Pi regulation via Pit1 plays a role in bone mineralization. *Mol. Cell Biol.* 27, 4465–4474. doi:10.1128/MCB.00104-07

Yuan, H., De Bruijn, J. D., Li, Y., Feng, J., Yang, Z., De Groot, K., et al. (2001). Bone formation induced by calcium phosphate ceramics in soft tissue of dogs: a comparative study between porous alpha-TCP and beta-TCP. *J. Mater. Sci. Mater. Med.* 12, 7–13. doi:10.1023/A:1026792615665

Yuan, J., Cui, L., Zhang, W. J., Liu, W., and Cao, Y. (2007). Repair of canine mandibular bone defects with bone marrow stromal cells and porous beta-tricalcium phosphate. *Biomaterials* 28, 1005–1013. doi:10.1016/j.biomaterials.2006.10.015

Zhang, S., Kaplan, F. S., and Shore, E. M. (2012). Different roles of GNAS and cAMP signaling during early and late stages of osteogenic differentiation. *Horm. Metab. Res.* 44, 724–731. doi:10.1055/s-0032-1321845

Conflict of Interest Statement: The authors declare that the research was conducted in the absence of any commercial or financial relationships that could be construed as a potential conflict of interest.

10

Distribution and viability of fetal and adult human bone marrow stromal cells in a biaxial rotating vessel bioreactor after seeding on polymeric 3D additive manufactured scaffolds

Anne M. Leferink[1,2], Yhee-Cheng Chng[3], Clemens A. van Blitterswijk[1,2] and Lorenzo Moroni[1,2]*

[1] Department of Tissue Regeneration, MIRA Institute, University of Twente, Enschede, Netherlands, [2] Department of Complex Tissue Regeneration, Faculty of Health, Medicine and Life Sciences, Maastricht University, Maastricht, Netherlands, [3] Quintech Life Sciences Pte Ltd., Singapore, Singapore

Edited by:
Alessandro Polini,
Radboud University Medical Centre,
Netherlands

Reviewed by:
Y. Shrike Zhang,
Harvard Medical School, USA
Ljupcho Prodanov,
Nottingham University, UK

*Correspondence:
Lorenzo Moroni
l.moroni@maastrichtuniversity.nl

One of the conventional approaches in tissue engineering is the use of scaffolds in combination with cells to obtain mechanically stable tissue constructs in vitro prior to implantation. Additive manufacturing by fused deposition modeling is a widely used technique to produce porous scaffolds with defined pore network, geometry, and therewith defined mechanical properties. Bone marrow-derived mesenchymal stromal cells (MSCs) are promising candidates for tissue engineering-based cell therapies due to their multipotent character. One of the hurdles to overcome when combining additive manufactured scaffolds with MSCs is the resulting heterogeneous cell distribution and limited cell proliferation capacity. In this study, we show that the use of a biaxial rotating bioreactor, after static culture of human fetal MSCs (hfMSCs) seeded on synthetic polymeric scaffolds, improved the homogeneity of cell and extracellular matrix distribution and increased the total cell number. Furthermore, we show that the relative mRNA expression levels of indicators for stemness and differentiation are not significantly changed upon this bioreactor culture, whereas static culture shows variations of several indicators for stemness and differentiation. The biaxial rotating bioreactor presented here offers a homogeneous distribution of hfMSCs, enabling studies on MSCs fate in additive manufactured scaffolds without inducing undesired differentiation.

Keywords: bone marrow stromal cells, scaffolds, biaxial rotating bioreactor, perfusion-flow bioreactor, cellular distribution

INTRODUCTION

The field of tissue engineering aims at applying the fundamentals of cell biology and materials engineering to construct replacements for damaged, diseased, or lost tissue (Langer and Vacanti, 1993). One of the conventional approaches is based on three-dimensional (3D) mechanically stable scaffolds in combination with multipotent cell types. Scaffolds with a highly defined geometry, porosity, and tailored mechanical properties can be obtained by additive manufacturing (Moroni et al., 2005). These scaffolds provide the necessary support for cells to attach, proliferate, and differentiate, and define the overall shape of the tissue engineered transplant. Several researchers already showed successful application of such scaffolds in, for example, bone and cartilage tissue engineering *in vivo* (Woodfield et al., 2004; Kim et al., 2012; Reichert et al., 2012). Woodfield et al. found a rapid attachment and a homogenous distribution of both bovine and human chondrocytes on poly (ethylene oxide terephthalate)-co-poly (butylene terephthalate) (PEOT/PBT) based scaffolds after spinner flask culture *in vitro*. Subsequently, scaffolds seeded with bovine chondrocytes were implanted subcutaneously in mice for 21 days and formed cartilaginous tissue *in vivo* as demonstrated by the presence of articular extracellular matrix (ECM) components (Woodfield et al., 2004). Despite successes in regenerating tissues with additive manufactured scaffolds optionally combined with different bioreactors, the highly organized open structure of such scaffolds poses still challenges in homogenously distributing cells and controlling their proliferation and differentiation capacities. This is even more important when mesenchymal stromal cell (MSCs) are used, as their capacity to adhere and be homogeneously distributed in 3D scaffolds has shown to be more demanding (Griffon et al., 2011).

To gain control over cell seeding efficiency, distribution and fate on additive manufactured 3D scaffolds *in vitro* prior to implantation or as a study model, several hurdles have to be overcome. First, the cell seeding process has to be optimized per scaffold geometry, scaffold material, and cell type to achieve proper cell attachment and distribution throughout the construct (Sobral et al., 2011). Several studies showed the influence of scaffold geometry or culture conditions in cell and tissue distribution after *in vitro* culture (Wang et al., 2005; Leferink et al., 2013). Papadimitropoulos et al. (2013) introduced a collagen-network in porous PCL–TCP scaffolds, which resulted in a 2.5-fold increase in MSCs seeding efficiency under perfusion flow compared to the bare PCL–TCP scaffolds. Despite an increased cell seeding efficiency in the presence of a collagen-network, no obvious qualitative differences were found after 19 days of culture among the experimental groups with respect to cell viability and distribution, and ECM formation. Although the incorporation of a collagenous matrix in additive manufactured scaffolds seemed to have a beneficial effect on cell seeding efficiency, control over cell fate remains to be further elucidated.

A second hurdle to overcome is the supply of oxygen and nutrients as well as the clearance of metabolic products which showed to become critically limiting for cells cultured under static conditions (Schantz et al., 2012). Bioreactor systems, based on convection, such as rotating vessels and stirrer flasks, or based on perfusion, such as a directional flow-through bioreactor, are used to overcome these mass transfer limitations (Grayson et al., 2011). These systems do not only enhance nutrient and waste product exchange but can also exert mechanical stimuli on the cells to proliferate,

migrate, or differentiate (Martin et al., 2004; Grayson et al., 2011). Although most of these commercially available rotating vessel bioreactors are uniaxial in design, Singh et al. (2005) have shown with *in silico* simulations that a biaxial design, which rotates simultaneously in two independent orthogonal axes, resulted in improved fluidics over an uniaxial design. Therefore, we investigated the use of a biaxial bioreactor system for the *in vitro* culture of highly porous PEOT/PBT scaffolds seeded with human fetal MSCs (hfMSCs) or human adult MSCs (haMSCs).

Previous work showed the differentiation potential of hfMSCs into the adipogenic (Jo et al., 2008), osteogenic (Guillot et al., 2008; Abarrategi et al., 2012; Brady et al., 2014), and chondrogenic (Abarrategi et al., 2012; van Gool et al., 2012) lineages and maintenance of telomerase activity during *in vitro* monolayer culture (Jo et al., 2008). Also for haMSCs, multipotency is traditionally shown by studying the differentiation capacity into the adipogenic (Pittenger et al., 1999), chondrogenic (Mackay et al., 1998; Pittenger et al., 1999), and osteogenic (Pittenger et al., 1999) lineages in the presence of soluble factors in monolayer or pellet culture *in vitro*. Yet, the differentiation of haMSCs into multiple other lineages, such as the neurogenic (Zaim et al., 2012), endothelial (Janeczek Portalska et al., 2012), and myogenic lineages (Muguruma et al., 2003; Bossolasco et al., 2004), has been reported as well. The multipotent differentiation capacity of haMSCs is donor and age dependent and decreases upon increasing population doublings *in vitro* (Zaim et al., 2012). Zhang et al. (2009a) reported a superior proliferative and osteogenic differentiation capacity of hfMSCs over haMSCs after comparative studies *in vitro* in static monolayer culture. In addition, both hfMSCs and haMSCs showed osteogenic differentiation on a composite bioactive PCL–TCP scaffold in static culture *in vitro* and ectopic bone formation in the scaffold after implantation *in vivo*. Yet, osteogenic differentiation of hfMSCs was found superior to haMSCs.

We hypothesize that by the introduction of a biaxial rotating bioreactor, higher cell numbers and a more homogeneous distribution of cells throughout 3D scaffolds could be achieved compared to static culture in a well plate. It is well-known that shear forces due to medium flow can affect cell fate. Therefore, in this study, the effect of bioreactor culture on cell and ECM distribution as well as on cellular phenotype was assessed for both hfMSCs and haMSCs cultured on scaffolds in two different bioreactor systems and compared to the results from static culture on scaffolds in a well plate. In our study, we chose PEOT/PBT as a biomaterial to fabricate 3D additive manufactured scaffolds. This family of copolymers has shown successful applications in tissue regeneration applications (Beumer et al., 1994; Claase et al., 2007; Moroni et al., 2008), due to the flexibility to change their physico-chemical and mechanical properties (Deschamps et al., 2002). These results in the possibility to control cell adhesion, morphology, and ultimately phenotype at the interface with 3D scaffolds made of these biomaterials, which is of particular interest for stem cell-driven tissue regeneration strategies.

MATERIALS AND METHODS

Isolation and Culture of hfMSCs and haMSCs

Bone marrow-derived hfMSCs were isolated as described before, from 17 weeks and 1-day-old fetuses after clinically indicated termination of pregnancy (Chan et al., 2007; Zhang et al., 2009b). Pregnant women gave separate written consent for the clinical procedure and for the use of fetal tissue for research purposes. Briefly, fetal bone marrow cells were retrieved by flushing the bone marrow cells out of the humeri and femurs into Dulbecco's modified eagle's medium (DMEM, Sigma, USA) with Glutamax (GIBCO, USA) supplemented with 10% heat-inactivated fetal bovine serum (FBS, Hyclone, USA), 50 U/mL penicillin, and 50 µg/mL streptomycin (GIBCO, USA), which will be referred to as fMSC medium. Medium was refreshed twice per week and cells were used for further subculturing or cryopreservation on reaching near confluence.

Bone marrow-derived haMSCs (donor 1 female, 77 years old; donor 2 female, 55 years old) were isolated and proliferated, as described previously (de Bruijn et al., 1999). Bone marrow aspirates were obtained from patients who had given written informed consent. Briefly, aspirates were cultured in minimal essential medium (alpha-MEM; Life Technologies, USA) supplemented with 10% heat-inactivated fetal bovine serum (FBS; Lonza, USA), 0.2 mM L-Ascorbic acid 2-phosphate magnesium salt (ASAP, Sigma-Aldrich, the Netherlands), 2 mM L-glutamine (L-glut, Invitrogen, the Netherlands), 100 U/mL penicillin (Life Technologies, USA), 100 µg/mL streptomycin (Life Technologies, USA), and 1 ng/mL basic fibroblast growth factor (bFGF; Instruchemie, The Netherlands), which will be referred to as proliferation medium. Cells were cultured at 37°C in a humidified atmosphere with 5% CO_2. Medium was refreshed twice per week and cells were used for further subculturing or cryopreservation on reaching near confluence.

Fabrication of PEOT/PBT Scaffolds

Scaffold were fabricated of PolyActive™ 300/55/45 (PolyVation, the Netherlands), a block copolymer is composed of poly(ethylene oxide terephthalate) (PEOT) and poly(butylene terephthalate) (PBT) with a weight ratio of 55:45 for the two components, respectively, and a molecular weight of the starting poly(ethylene glycol) (PEG) segments of 300 Da used in the co-polymerization process (Deschamps et al., 2002). Fused deposition modeling was used with a bioscaffolder (SysENG, Germany) to fabricate 3D cylindrical scaffolds as described before (Moroni et al., 2005), with a diameter of 8 mm and a height of 3 mm. For the additive manufacturing process, the fiber spacing was set to 1000 µm, the layer thickness to 150 µm, and a needle with an internal diameter of approximately 250 µm was used, which resulted in fiber diameters of approximately 200 µm. Scaffolds were treated in Argon plasma for 30 min with a pressure of 0.1–0.2 mBar and a power of 30 W. Sterilization of all scaffolds was performed in 70% ethanol twice for 30 min, subsequently washed in PBS first for 5 min and additionally twice for another 30 min each time, and finally incubated in culture medium overnight prior to cell culture.

Cell Seeding on PEOT/PBT Scaffolds

For studies with hfMSCs, scaffolds were transferred from a tube with culture medium to a non-treated 24-well plate (Greiner bio-one, Germany). Passage 3 hfMSCs were harvested from monolayer expansion, and seeded on the scaffolds with a density of 750,000 cells in 30 µL of fMSC medium. After 15 min of incubation, the scaffolds were flipped and allowed to incubate for another 45 min before 10 µL of fMSC medium was added. Subsequently, for the next 5 h, 10 µL of proliferation medium was added for each seeded scaffolds at an interval of 75 min for each addition. Scaffolds were then transferred to a non-treated 24-well plate (Greiner bio-one, Germany) with 750 µL of proliferation medium and cultured for 3 days either in static culture conditions or in a biaxial rotating vessel bioreactor for which the culture parameters are specified in the next section.

For studies with haMSCs, scaffolds were transferred from a tube with culture medium to a non-treated 24-well plate (NUNC, Fisher Scientific, the Netherlands). Passage 3 haMSCs were harvested from monolayer expansion, and seeded on the scaffolds with a density of 750,000 cells in 100 µL of proliferation medium. After 1.5 h incubation, the medium was filled up to 1 mL and cell culture was continued for 3 days in static culture condition before transferring the samples to a new culture well, to the biaxial bioreactor system, or to a bioreactor perfusion culture. The culture parameters in the bioreactors are specified in the next section.

In the results section, the legends of the figures refer to the total culture time, including the static incubation period on the scaffolds placed in a well plate (in most figures this period was 3 days, unless specified differently).

Bioreactor Culture

After static culture, some of the scaffolds were transferred to the biaxial bioreactor system or the chamber of the perfusion bioreactor, whereas a control group was maintained under static culture conditions (**Figure 1**). The perfusion bioreactor consisted of a small chamber in which the scaffold was press-fitted to ensure the medium to be flown through the longitudinal pores of the scaffold. The set-up of the perfusion bioreactor was constructed, as described before (Janssen et al., 2006). Medium was ran with a flow speed of 0.1 mL/min in a home-made incubator at 37°C with a controlled flow of mixed gas containing 5% CO_2 and 21% O_2.

The biaxial bioreactor system consisted of a cylindrical vessel for culture (volume 40 mL), in which the cellular-scaffold constructs are mounted to the lid of the bioreactor by pins, and a medium reservoir to ensure continuous replacement of the medium in the culture vessel. Gaseous exchange was enabled through a special membrane incorporated into the medium reservoir. The bioreactor was ran with a medium flow speed of 1 rpm (corresponding to 1.5 mL/min), a biaxial rotation with an arm rotational speed of 2 rpm, and a chamber rotation speed of 3 rpm at 37°C in a humidified atmosphere with 5% CO_2.

Proliferation medium was used to fill the 40 mL medium reservoir of the perfusion bioreactor containing 1 scaffold seeded with haMSCs per circuitry. Proliferation medium was used to fill the 40 mL bioreactor chamber and the 300 mL reservoir of the

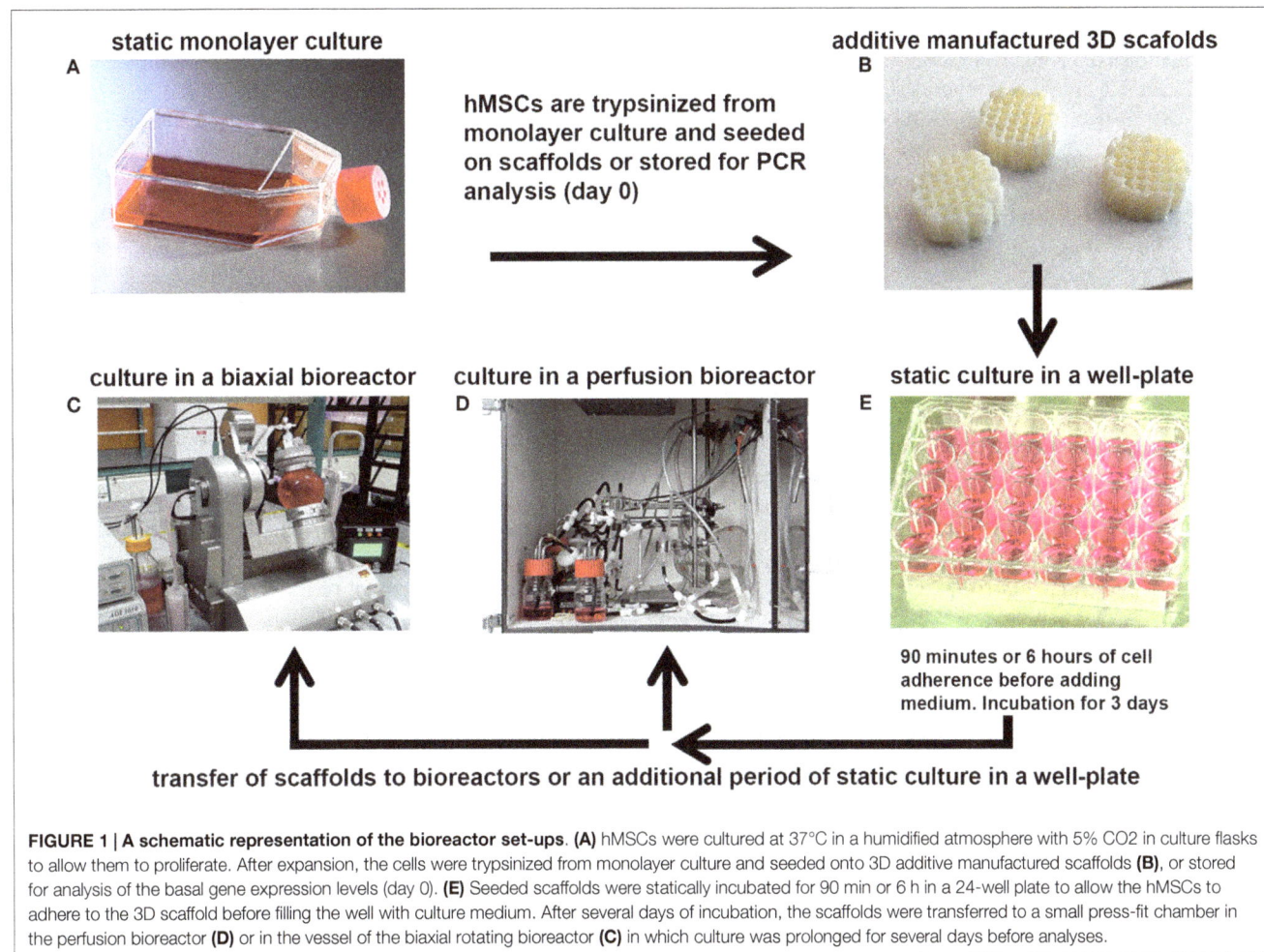

FIGURE 1 | A schematic representation of the bioreactor set-ups. (A) hMSCs were cultured at 37°C in a humidified atmosphere with 5% CO2 in culture flasks to allow them to proliferate. After expansion, the cells were trypsinized from monolayer culture and seeded onto 3D additive manufactured scaffolds **(B)**, or stored for analysis of the basal gene expression levels (day 0). **(E)** Seeded scaffolds were statically incubated for 90 min or 6 h in a 24-well plate to allow the hMSCs to adhere to the 3D scaffold before filling the well with culture medium. After several days of incubation, the scaffolds were transferred to a small press-fit chamber in the perfusion bioreactor **(D)** or in the vessel of the biaxial rotating bioreactor **(C)** in which culture was prolonged for several days before analyses.

biaxial bioreactor containing 4 scaffolds seeded with haMSCs. fMSC medium was used to fill the 500 mL bioreactor chamber and the 300 mL reservoir of the biaxial bioreactor containing 12 scaffolds seeded with hfMSCs. As a control, static culture was continued on the scaffolds that were transferred to a new well in a non-treated 24-well plate.

Viability Staining

Cell viability was assessed by 4 μg/mL fluorescein diacetate (FDA, Sigma-Aldrich, the Netherlands) and 40 μg/mL propidium iodide (PI, Sigma-Aldrich, the Netherlands) staining, where FDA stains viable cells green, and PI stains necrotic and apoptotic cell nuclei red. Scaffolds were cut in half, stained with FDA and PI, as previously described (Zhang et al., 2009a), and viewed under a confocal laser microscope (Olympus, FV1000Fluoview, Japan). Cellular scaffolds were examined in both planar view and cross-sectional view after 3 and 9 days of culture.

DNA Assay

The total DNA from scaffolds cultured with hfMSCs was extracted from each scaffold by incubating the constructs in 0.4 mL of enzymatic cocktail [consisting of 0.1% collagenase A

(Roche, Switzerland) with 0.1% Trypsin mixed in PBS] at 37°C for 2 h, with vortex every 30 min followed by three cycles of freeze and thaw. For haMSCs, after culture all scaffolds were washed gently in PBS, dried by aspirating the PBS, cut in pieces and stored at −80°C for at least 24 h. After thawing, the constructs were digested for 16 h at 56°C with 1 mg/mL proteinase K (Sigma-Aldrich, the Netherlands) in Tris/EDTA buffer (pH 7.6). This solution contained 18.5 μg/mL iodoacetamine (Sigma-Aldrich, the Netherlands) and 1 μg/mL Pepstatin A (Sigma-Aldrich, the Netherlands). Quantification of total DNA was done using the CyQuant® DNA assay (Molecular Probes, Fisher Scientific, the Netherlands) and a spectrophotometer (excitation 480 nm, emission 520 nm) (Victor 3, Perkin Elmer, the Netherlands).

Hydroxyproline Assay

Hydroxyproline colorimetric assay kit (Biovision, USA) was performed according to the manufacturer's protocol to determine the total collagen amount on the same samples as used for DNA quantification. In brief, from the digested sample, 30 μL was transferred to a Teflon® capped glass bottle. Another 30 μL of concentrated hydrochloric acid (HCl, 12M, Sigma-Aldrich, the Netherlands) was added and samples were hydrolyzed at 120°C for 3 h. The complete supernatant was transferred to a 96-well plate and left to evaporate at 60°C. Subsequently, 100 µL of chloramine T/Oxidation buffer mix (Biovision, USA) was added to each well and incubated at room temperature for 5 min. Finally, 100 µL of DMAB Reagent (Biovision, USA) was added to each well including the hydroxyproline standard and incubated for 90 min at 60°C. A micro plate reader (Multiskan GO, Thermo Fisher, the Netherlands) was used to determine the absorbance at 560 nm.

Gene Expression Analysis of hfMSCs and haMSCs

For gene expression analysis of hfMSCs, samples were seeded ($n = 4$ for static cultures; $n = 5$ for the biaxial bioreactor system) at different time points. After culture, medium was aspirated from the scaffolds, the samples were transferred to 2 mL Eppendorf tubes and stored at −80°C. Prior to RNA isolation from the samples by using a Bioke RNA II nucleospin RNA isolation kit (Macherey-Nagel, Germany), first 500 µL of TRIzol® (Invitrogen, the Netherlands) was added. The scaffolds were disrupted by crushing with RNA isolation pestles (Kimble Kontes, Fisher Scientific, the Netherlands). Samples for basal gene expression analysis, referred to as T25 day 0, were retrieved from two-dimensional (2D) culture in T25 tissue culture flasks (NUNC, Fisher Scientific, the Netherlands) by adding 500 µL of TRIzol® (Invitrogen, the Netherlands) upon reaching 70% confluence. Subsequently, the cell/TRIzol® suspension was transferred to an Eppendorf tube and 200 µL of CHCl₃ was added to each sample and mixed by vigorously shaking the tubes. The TRIzol®/CHCl₃ mixture was centrifuged at 12,000 × g for 15 min at 4°C. The aqueous phase was transferred to a new Eppendorf tube and mixed 1:1 with 70% ethanol. The mixture was transferred to filter columns from the kit and the RNA isolation was continued following the manufacturer's protocol. RNA concentrations and purity were determined by using an ND1000 spectrophotometer (Nanodrop Technologies, USA). The cDNA was synthesized from 630 ng of RNA, using iScript™ (BIO-RAD, Bio-rad Laboratories, the Netherlands) according to the manufacturer's protocol. Quantitative polymerase chain reaction (qPCR) was performed on cDNA samples by using the iQ SYBR® Green Supermix (Bio-Rad, the Netherlands) on the primers as listed in **Table 1**. PCR reactions were carried out on the MyiQ2 Two-Color Real-Time PCR Detection System (Bio-Rad, the Netherlands) under the following conditions: cDNA was denatured for 10 min at 95°C, followed by 40 cycles, consisting of 15 s at 95°C, 30 s at 60°C, and 30 s at 72°C. For each reaction, a melting curve was generated to test primer dimer formation and non-specific priming. The cycle threshold (Ct) values were determined with the Bio-RadiQ5 optical system software, in which a threshold value was set for the fluorescent signal at the lower log-linear part above the baseline. Ct values were normalized to the B2M housekeeping gene and ΔCt ((average of $Ct_{control}$) − Ct_{value}). Results are expressed as relative mRNA expression normalized to the gene expression levels of hfMSCs from T25 day 0 and calculated as $2^{-\Delta Ct}$.

For gene expression analysis of haMSCs, samples were seeded statically for 3 days followed by another 6 days of static culture or 6 days of dynamic culture in the biaxial bioreactor system or in the perfusion-flow bioreactor. After culture, medium was aspirated from the scaffolds, the samples were transferred to 2 mL Eppendorf tubes and stored at −80°C. Samples for basal gene expression analysis (referred to as day 0 static culture) were retrieved from 2D culture in T25 tissue culture asks (NUNC, Fisher Scientific, the Netherlands) by adding 500 µL of TRIzol® (Invitrogen, the Netherlands) upon reaching 70% confluence. RNA isolation, cDNA synthesis, and RT-PCR were carried out as described for hfMSCs. Results are expressed as relative mRNA expression normalized to the gene expression levels of haMSCs from T25 day 0 and calculated as $2^{-\Delta Ct}$.

Scanning Electron Microscopy Analysis

Cell morphology, attachment, and distribution were characterized by scanning electron microscopy (SEM) analysis with a Philips XL 30 ESEM-FEG (FEI, the Netherlands). Samples were fixed for 30 min in 10% formalin. Subsequently, the samples were dehydrated in sequential ethanol series and critical point dried from liquid carbon dioxide using a Balzers CPD 030 Critical Point Dryer (Leica, Germany). The constructs were gold sputter coated (Cressington, UK) prior to SEM analysis. SEM images were obtained under high vacuum with an acceleration voltage of 30 kV and a working distance of 10 mm.

Methylene Blue Staining

Cell morphology, attachment, and distribution of haMSCs were qualitatively assessed by methylene blue staining. Samples were fixed for 30 min in 10% formalin, washed with PBS twice, and stained with methylene blue (Sigma, the Netherlands) for 30 s immediately followed by extensive washing with DI-water until the water remained colorless. The samples were imaged using a stereomicroscope (Nikon SMZ800 with Q-imaging Retiga 1300 camera, Nikon Instruments Europe, the Netherlands).

Histological Analysis

Samples were fixed after live/dead imaging or directly after culture for 30 min in 10% formalin and stored in PBS at 5°C until further processing. Samples were dehydrated using a sequential ethanol series (60, 70, 80, 90, 96, and 100% ethanol, 30 min for each step), and subsequently embedded in glycol methacrylate (GMA). The obtained blocks were sectioned at 5 µm intervals, and stained with hematoxylin and eosin (H&E, Sigma, the Netherlands) for visualization of the nuclei and cytoplasm, and Masson Trichrome (Merck, Germany) to stain for collagen-like ECM formation.

Statistical Analyses

Results are presented as mean ± SD, and compared using either one-way ANOVA (multiple conditions) with a Bonferroni post-test or Student's t-test (two conditions). Statistical significance was set to p-value <0.05 (*).

TABLE 1 | Primer sequences.

Gene	Forward primer	Reverse primer
B2M	GACTTGTCTTTCAGCAAGGA	ACAAAGTCACATGGTTCACA
ALCAM	ACGATGAGGCAGACGAGATAAGT	CAGCAAGGAGGAGACCAACAA
CD-63	GCCCTTGGAATTGCTTTTGTCG	CATCACCTCGTAGCCACTTCT
f-Actin	GGCATCCTCACCCTGAAGTA	GGTGTGGTGCCAGATTTTC
Runx2	GGAGTGGACGAGGCAAGAGTTT	AGCTTCTGTCTGTGCCTTCTGG
ALP	ACAAGCACTCCCACTTCATC	TTCAGCTCGTACTGCATGTC
ACAN	AGGCAGCGTGATCCTTACC	GGCCTCTCCAGTCTCATTCTC
Sox9	TGGGCAAGCTCTGGAGACTTC	ATCCGGGTGGTCCTTCTTGTG
Col-1	GTCACCCACCGACCAAGAAACC	AAGTCCAGGCTGTCCAGGGATG
Col-2	CGTCCAGATGACCTTCCTACG	TGAGCAGGGCCTTCTTGAG

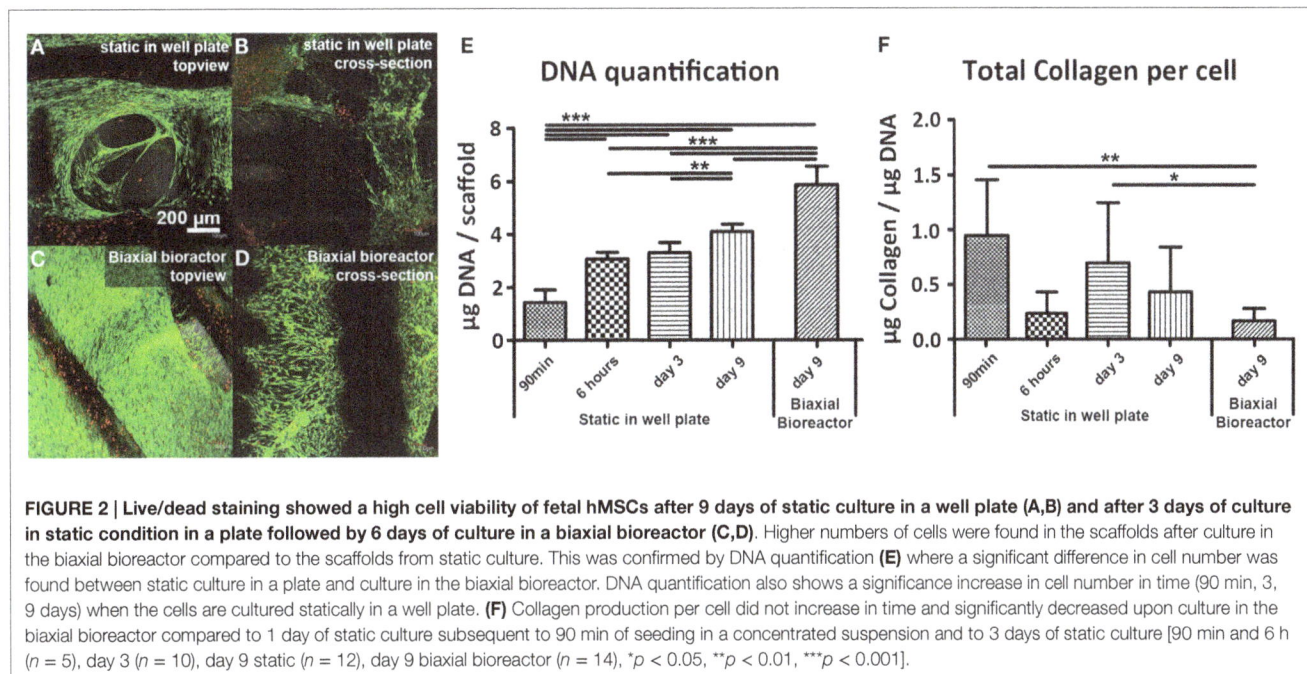

FIGURE 2 | Live/dead staining showed a high cell viability of fetal hMSCs after 9 days of static culture in a well plate (A,B) and after 3 days of culture in static condition in a plate followed by 6 days of culture in a biaxial bioreactor (C,D). Higher numbers of cells were found in the scaffolds after culture in the biaxial bioreactor compared to the scaffolds from static culture. This was confirmed by DNA quantification **(E)** where a significant difference in cell number was found between static culture in a plate and culture in the biaxial bioreactor. DNA quantification also shows a significance increase in cell number in time (90 min, 3, 9 days) when the cells are cultured statically in a well plate. **(F)** Collagen production per cell did not increase in time and significantly decreased upon culture in the biaxial bioreactor compared to 1 day of static culture subsequent to 90 min of seeding in a concentrated suspension and to 3 days of static culture [90 min and 6 h ($n = 5$), day 3 ($n = 10$), day 9 static ($n = 12$), day 9 biaxial bioreactor ($n = 14$), $*p < 0.05$, $**p < 0.01$, $***p < 0.001$].

RESULTS

Viability, Distribution, and Gene Expression Profile of hfMSCs

Scaffolds seeded with hfMSCs showed comparable viability after 9 days of culture in both well plate (static) and in the biaxial bioreactor (**Figures 2A,C**, respectively). A high viability was also found 6 h after seeding (Figures S1A,B in Supplementary Material) and after 3 days of static culture (Figures S1C,D in Supplementary Material). In the cross-sectional view of the scaffolds, it could be observed that the number of hfMSCs and their distribution seemed to be enhanced when the constructs were cultured in the biaxial bioreactor (**Figure 2D**) compared to the scaffolds with hfMSCs cultured statically in a well plate (**Figure 2B**). Also, the morphology of the cells in the pores of the scaffolds appeared more spread after culture in the biaxial bioreactor (Figures S1E–H in Supplementary Material). The difference in cell number was confirmed by DNA quantification (**Figure 2E**). Both the scaffolds in static culture and in the biaxial bioreactor showed an increase in cell number over time; yet, the increase in the biaxial bioreactor was significantly higher than in static culture.

Furthermore, allowing the cells to adhere to the scaffold initially for 6 h before adding medium resulted in a significant higher cell seeding efficiency than when the medium was added already after 1.5 h of incubation. A hydroxyproline assay was performed to determine the total amount of intra and extracellular collagen, which is a measure for cells activity and ECM formation (**Figure 2F**). A small increase in total collagen production per cell was observed between 6 h and 3 days of static culture, whereas the DNA content remained similar. At later timepoints, the DNA content increased, whereas the total collagen content per scaffold remained constant for these conditions, resulting in a decrease of collagen production per cell. This suggests that hfMSCs were mainly proliferating.

Gene expression levels of ALCAM (CD166, activated leukocyte cell adhesion molecule) and CD63, both indicators for stemness (Jeannet et al., 2013) (**Figures 3A,B** respectively), fluctuated over time in static culture. ALCAM and CD63 were

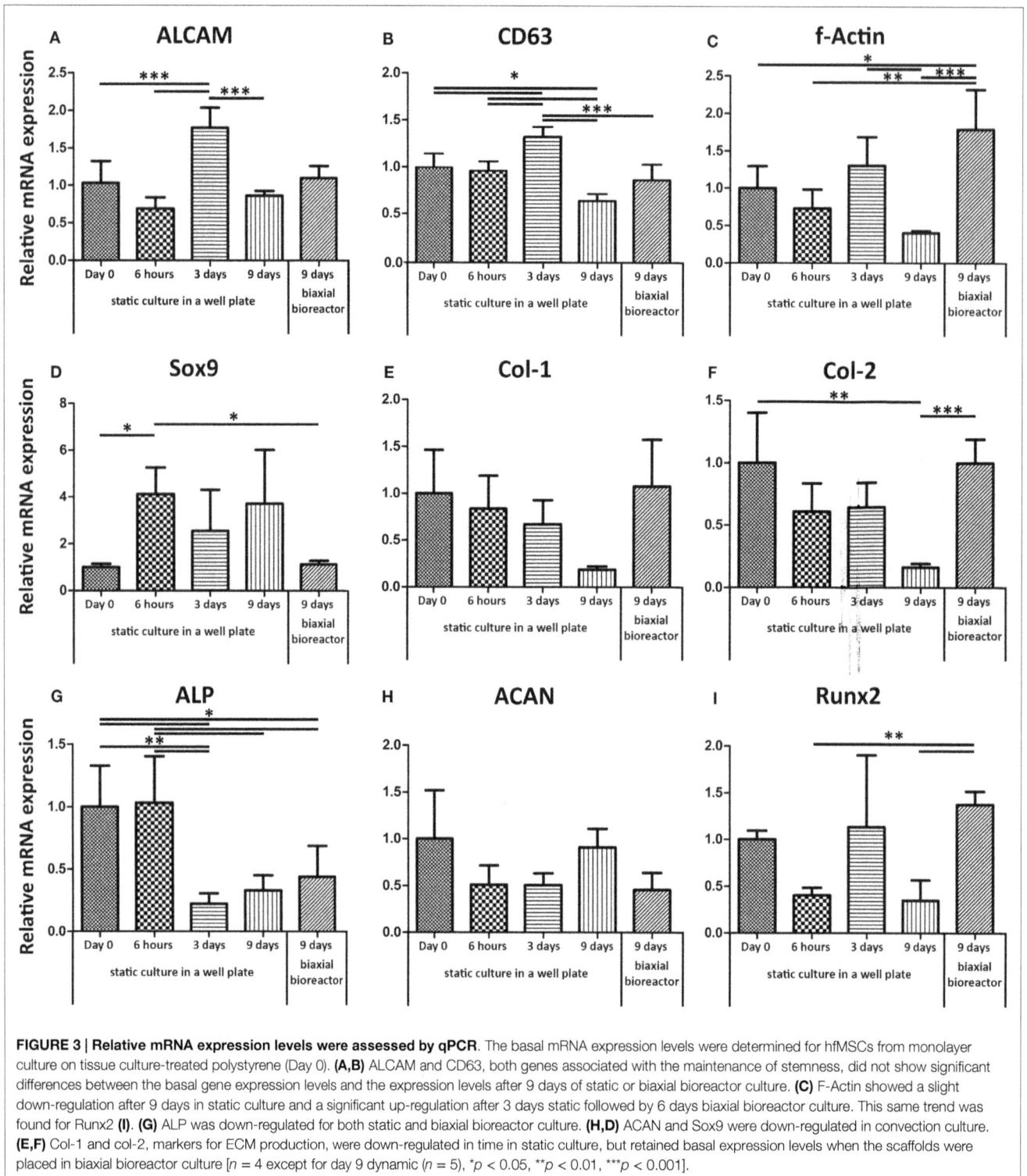

FIGURE 3 | Relative mRNA expression levels were assessed by qPCR. The basal mRNA expression levels were determined for hfMSCs from monolayer culture on tissue culture-treated polystyrene (Day 0). (A,B) ALCAM and CD63, both genes associated with the maintenance of stemness, did not show significant differences between the basal gene expression levels and the expression levels after 9 days of static or biaxial bioreactor culture. (C) F-Actin showed a slight down-regulation after 9 days in static culture and a significant up-regulation after 3 days static followed by 6 days biaxial bioreactor culture. This same trend was found for Runx2 (I). (G) ALP was down-regulated for both static and biaxial bioreactor culture. (H,D) ACAN and Sox9 were down-regulated in convection culture. (E,F) Col-1 and col-2, markers for ECM production, were down-regulated in time in static culture, but retained basal expression levels when the scaffolds were placed in biaxial bioreactor culture [$n = 4$ except for day 9 dynamic ($n = 5$), $^*p < 0.05$, $^{**}p < 0.01$, $^{***}p < 0.001$].

similarly expressed after 9 days in both static cultures in a well plate and after 9 days of culture in the biaxial bioreactor compared to their basal level measured in cells trypsinized from monolayer culture at a confluence of approximately 70% (day 0 static). F-actin mRNA expression showed a significant twofold up-regulation in dynamic culture and a twofold

down-regulation in static culture after 9 days. A similar but less robust trend was found for Runt-related transcription factor 2 (Runx2), associated with early osteogenic differentiation. Alkaline phosphatase (ALP) expression, involved in osteogenesis, was down-regulated over time both for static and bioreactor culture.

Aggrecan (ACAN), a marker for chondrogenesis, did not show any significant differences between any of the conditions. Yet, Sox9, an early marker for chondrogenesis, was up-regulated in static culture in a well plate, whereas the biaxial bioreactor system restored the mRNA expression levels similar to the basal levels (day 0 static culture). Collagen type-1 (col-1) and collagen type-2 (col-2) markers for ECM proteins, abundantly present in bone and cartilage, respectively, were both down-regulated over time in static culture, whereas their expression levels were restored upon culture in the biaxial bioreactor system.

Scanning electron microscopy analysis was performed on cross-sections of the scaffolds after 9 days of culture to assess cell distribution, morphology, and tissue formation (**Figure 4**). Statically cultured scaffolds (**Figures 4A,C,E**) showed lower cell numbers compared to scaffolds cultured in the biaxial bioreactor (**Figures 4B,D,F**). The cellular distribution appeared more homogeneous and the cells invaded the longitudinal pores of the scaffold more profoundly after culture in the biaxial bioreactor system compared to culture in static conditions. There were no large differences observed in ECM formation and cell morphology between static culture and culture in the biaxial bioreactor system. In both conditions, the cells were spread while partly attached to the scaffold material or the secreted ECM. The formed tissue appeared relatively open inside the pores of the scaffolds, whereas the outer layer of tissue found at the bottom or top of the scaffold appeared as a more dense and closed layer.

From the SEM analysis after 6 h (Figures S2A–C in Supplementary Material) and 3 days of static culture (Figures S2D–F in Supplementary Material), it could be seen that the cell morphology changed over time from a rounded shape to a more spread morphology. Similar cell-shape changes were observed in 2D culture where hfMSCs showed a more spread morphology upon attachment to the substrate material. This change in cellular morphology could also be observed in histological analysis by H&E staining (Figure S3 in Supplementary Material). Further analysis with Masson Trichrome staining showed collagen-like materials stained green, which did not show any differences between 9 days of static culture in a well plate and 9 days of culture in the biaxial bioreactor (Figure S4 in Supplementary Material).

The Cell Adherence, Distribution, and Gene Expression Profile of haMSCs

Comparing the methylene blue staining of haMSCs after 3 days of static culture followed by 6 days of culture in a biaxial bioreactor (Figure S5B in Supplementary Material) to the staining after 9 days of static culture in a well plate (Figure S5A in Supplementary Material), no improvement on cell number and cellular distribution was found upon bioreactor culture. In static culture, haMSCs adhered to the fibers and partly filled the pores of the scaffold probably upon proliferation and ECM production (Figure S5A in Supplementary Material). In the biaxial bioreactor culture, the cells did not fill the pores of the scaffold to the same extend as the cells in static culture. From the cross-sectional view,

it could be observed that the distribution of the cells throughout the scaffold was still limited in both conditions. Donor 2 showed limited cell adherence after 3 days of static culture in a well plate followed by 6 days of culture in the perfusion bioreactor (Figure S5C in Supplementary Material).

The DNA content was quantified for two donors in triplicate (Figure S6 in Supplementary Material). The results showed on average a relatively low DNA content (about a threefold less compared to hfMSCs) in both bioreactors. For donor 1, a slight increase in DNA content was found upon bioreactor culture compared to static culture. Donor 2, however, showed a significant difference between static and perfusion culture, and between the biaxial bioreactor and the perfusion bioreactor culture. For this same donor, higher cell numbers were also observed in static culture compared to culture in the biaxial bioreactor or in the perfusion bioreactor when the constructs were cultured statically in a well plate for 31 days prior to a 14 days culture in the two bioreactor systems (Figure S7 in Supplementary Material). These findings were confirmed by DNA assay in which a significant drop in DNA content was observed after the scaffolds were cultured in the biaxial bioreactor or perfusion bioreactor culture compared to the DNA content after 31 and 45 days of static culture (Figure S8 in Supplementary Material).

The gene expression profile of haMSCs was assessed for the same genes as hfMSCs (**Figure 5**). The gene expression levels were determined after 9 days of static culture and compared to gene expression levels of haMSCs after 3 days of static culture followed by 6 days of dynamic culture in the biaxial bioreactor or in the perfusion bioreactor. A significant twofold down-regulation of ALCAM was found for haMSCs cultured in a perfusion bioreactor compared to static culture and culture in the biaxial bioreactor. F-Actin, col-1, and col-2 showed a significant down-regulation in both dynamic culture systems compared to static culture. Sox-9 was significantly down-regulated in the biaxial bioreactor and ACAN was up-regulated a 10-fold in perfusion culture compared to static culture. However, this change was not statistically significant.

DISCUSSION

Mesenchymal stromal cells derived from bone marrow have been used as a cellular source in several tissue engineering applications due to their availability, ease of isolation from autologous source and therewith reduced immunological-related risks upon re-implantation. Moreover, MSCs have shown a certain degree of plasticity by the ability to differentiate and transdifferentiate after differentiation into several well-defined cell lineages both *in vitro* and *in vivo* (Phinney et al., 1999; Grove et al., 2004; Song and Tuan, 2004; Phinney, 2007; Russell et al., 2010; Ullah et al., 2013).

The multipotency of MSCs is often assessed by soluble factor-induced differentiation in which the results of histological or biochemical assays are used to characterize cell fate. However, instead of focusing on changes in MSCs phenotype by quantifying the expression of differentiation-related genes, it could be also of interest to assess to what extent the cellular phenotype of MSCs can be maintained by investigating genes related to multipotency.

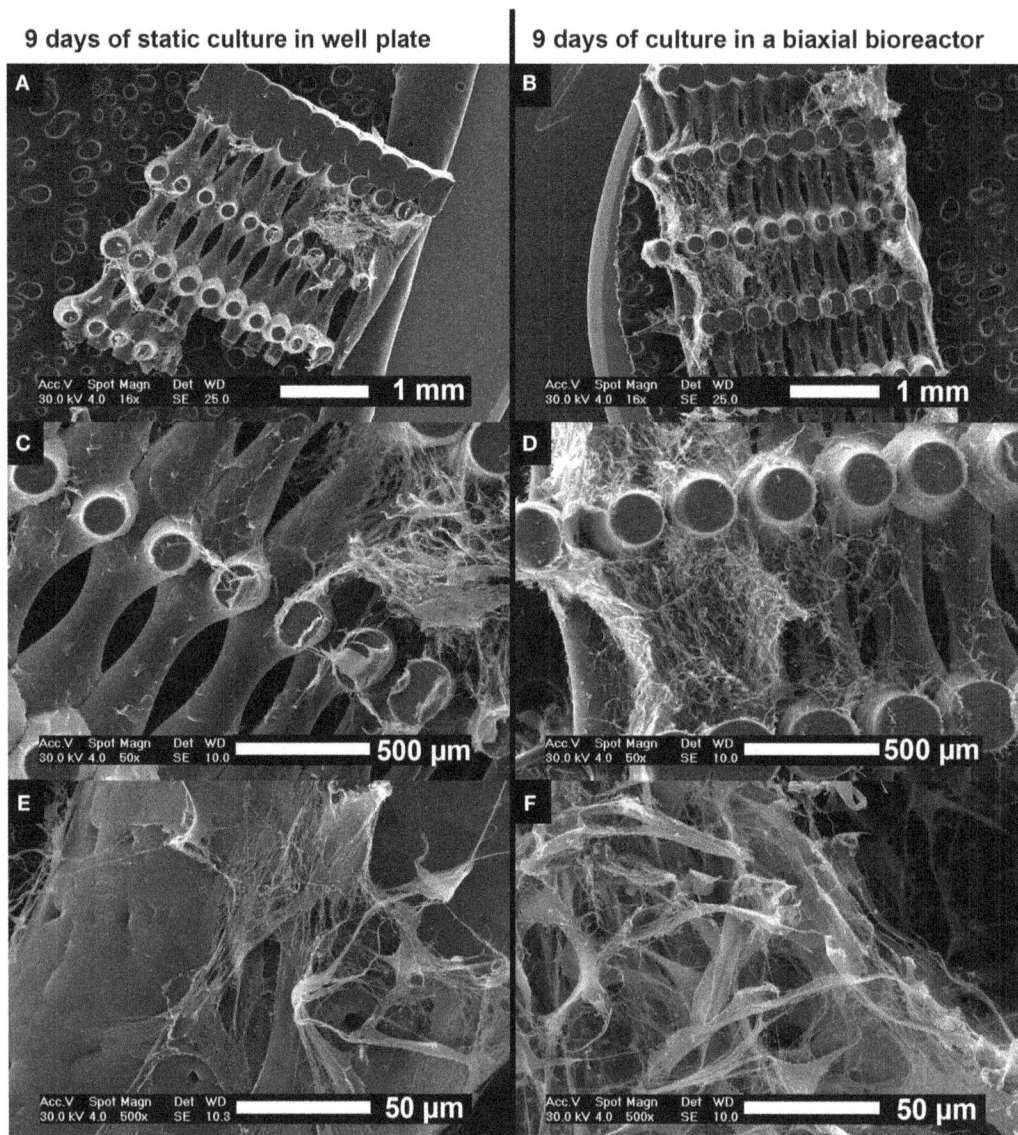

FIGURE 4 | Scanning electron microscopy images of the distribution of hfMSCs throughout the scaffolds after 9 days of static culture in a well plate (A,C,E) and after 3 days of static followed by 6 days of dynamic culture in a biaxial rotating bioreactor (B,D,F). A slightly more homogeneous distribution of cells and ECM was found after culture in the biaxial bioreactor compared to static culture in a well plate. Scale bars represent **(A,B)** 1 mm, **(C,D)** 500 μm, and **(E,F)** 50 μm.

In the past decades, researchers focused on defining stemness and identifying stemness markers to be able to more directly assess the potency of patient-derived MSC populations (Menicanin et al., 2009).

A known drawback in the use of haMSC is their slow proliferation time and generally limited proliferation capacity. More recently, hfMSCs have been characterized showing a higher proliferation and osteogenic differentiation capacity and reduced immunogenicity when compared to mesenchymal stem cell populations derived from the umbilical cord, adult adipose tissue, or adult bone marrow in 3D culture systems both *in vitro* and

in vivo (Zhang et al., 2009a). Here, we have assessed hfMSCs and haMSCs behavior in 3D scaffolds with respect to cell attachment, proliferation, and genetic profile.

Static and bioreactor culture conditions both resulted in similar cell viability on the PEOT/PBT scaffolds (**Figures 2A–D**). However, the number of hfMSCs in the biaxial bioreactor culture was higher (**Figure 2E**) and the distribution of the cells throughout the scaffolds seemed to be improved with respect to the scaffolds in static culture in a well plate (**Figures 2A–D** and **Figure 4**). With respect to the gene expression levels, it could be concluded that 6 days of biaxial bioreactor culture subsequent to 3 days of static

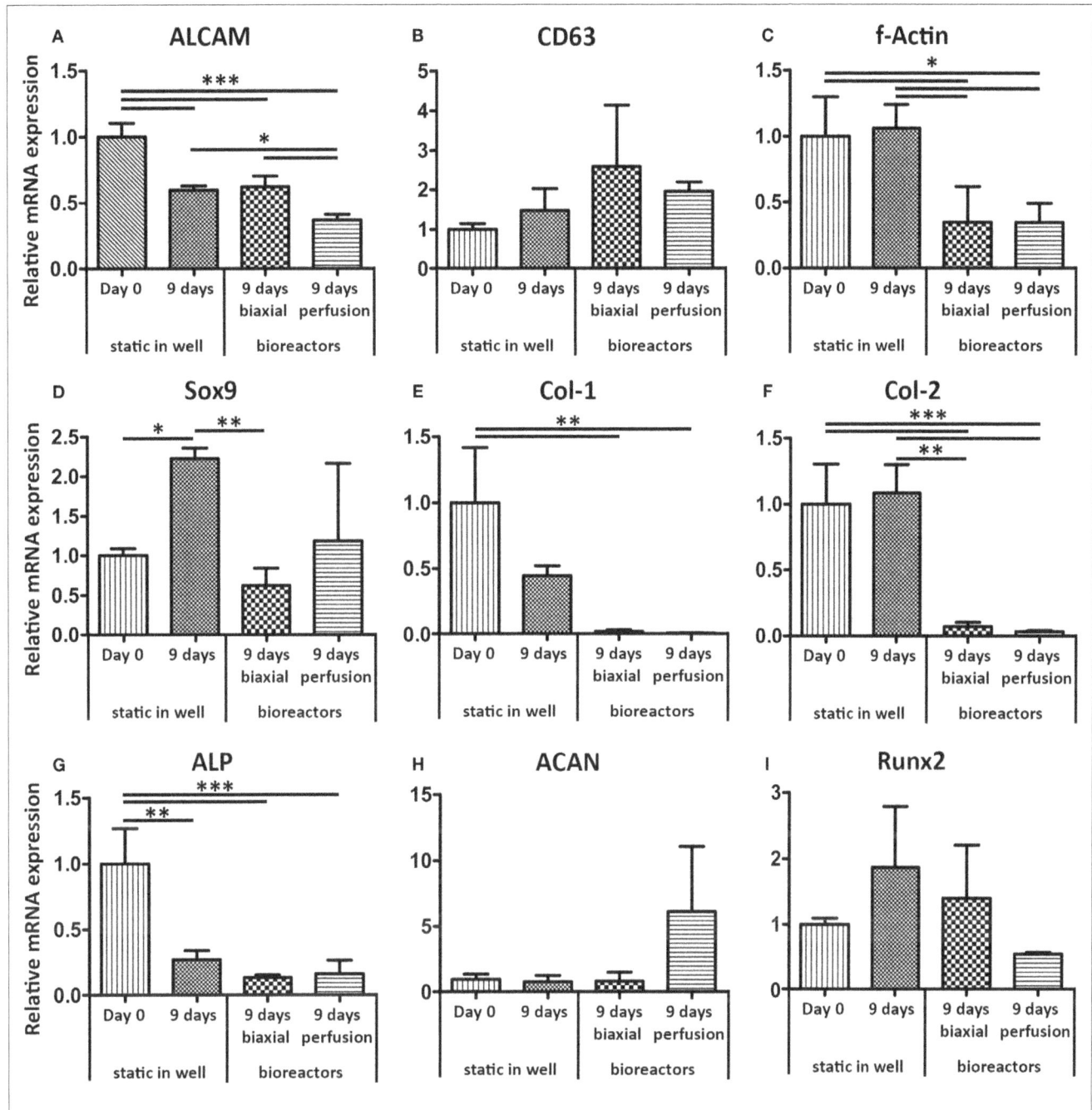

FIGURE 5 | Relative mRNA expression levels of haMSCs in static, biaxial bioreactor, and perfusion bioreactor culture were assessed by qPCR.
(A) ALCAM showed a twofold significant down-regulation after 9 days of perfusion culture compared to static and biaxial bioreactor cultures. **(B)** CD63 showed no significant differences between the different culture systems. **(C)** F-Actin showed a down-regulation after 9 days in both dynamic culture systems compared to static culture. **(D)** Sox9 was significantly up-regulated in static culture in a well plate, whereas the bioreactor systems restored the mRNA expression levels similar to the basal levels (day 0 static culture). **(E,F)** Col-1 and Col-2, markers for extra-cellular matrix production, were down-regulated in both dynamic culture systems. **(G)** ALP showed a significant down-regulation in all conditions after 9 days of culture compared to day 0 in static culture. **(H)** ACAN showed a 10-fold up-regulation after perfusion culture compared to static and biaxial bioreactor culture; however, this change was not statistically significant. **(I)** For Runx2, no significant differences between the different culture conditions were found ($n = 3$, $*p < 0.05$, $**p < 0.01$, $***p < 0.001$).

culture restored the basal gene expression levels, found at day 0 in static monolayer culture, for all genes except ALP and f-actin. Similar results were found by a study of Katayama et al. (2013), in which no change in gene expression levels of stem cell markers, such as ALCAM, was found in adult hMSCs cultured on collagen sheets under perfusion flow.

Considering the genes involved in ECM production, such as f-actin, col-1, and col-2, static culture seemed to provide insufficient cues to the cells to activate ECM formation-related pathways. Col-1 and col-2 expressions were maintained in the biaxial bioreactor culture and down-regulated in static culture. This indicated that the hfMSCs in the biaxial bioreactor probably experienced shear forces, due to a sort of convection flow, resulting in activation of the f-actin pathway among others, which could subsequently lead to an increase in tissue formation (Sansores-Garcia et al., 2011). Furthermore, shear forces have been known to induce osteogenic differentiation, which could explain the initial significant decrease of ALP expression in static culture and the subsequent small increase in ALP in the biaxial bioreactor (**Figure 3**) (Yeatts et al., 2012). On the other hand, a recent study of Kock et al. (2014) has shown a negative influence of perfusion flow on cartilage-like ECM production of chondrogenic pre-differentiated hMSCs, although these changes were not evident from gene expression analysis (Kock et al., 2014).

Scanning electron microscopy analysis (**Figures 4E,F**) showed an increase in tissue formation and tissue density was observed for dynamically cultured samples compared to statically cultured scaffolds. Although 6 days of culture in the biaxial bioreactor may have altered the gene expression levels compared to static culture, no difference was found on total collagen production by biochemical and histological analysis (**Figure 2F** and Figures S4E–H in Supplementary Material, respectively). However, the number of cells in the interior of the scaffold in the biaxial bioreactor was higher than in static culture conditions, indicating that bioreactor culture did improve cellular distribution.

Although hfMSCs have shown some beneficial properties over haMSCs in previous studies, the application of haMSCs remained of interest due to their more immediate clinical relevance. Fetal MSCs cannot be used from autologous source and their use involves more ethical issues. Therefore, the use of haMSCs on these scaffolds in the biaxial bioreactor was evaluated as well. A perfusion-flow bioreactor was introduced in parallel to be able to compare the results obtained in the biaxial bioreactor culture to both static and perfusion culture conditions. The cell number of haMSCs per scaffold assessed by DNA assay after 9 days of static culture was found to be significantly lower for both haMSC donors (Figure S6 in Supplementary Material) compared to hfMSCs (**Figure 2E**). Cell seeding efficiency of haMSCs has already shown to be limited and donor dependent in one of our previous studies, in which several seeding parameters were optimized to decrease cell loss after seeding (Leferink et al., 2013).

For the two haMSCs donors, no difference in the number of cells was found upon culture in the biaxial bioreactor compared to static culture conditions. Similar results were found in a study of Stiehler et al. (2009), in which hMSCs seeded on PLGA-based scaffolds did not show any difference in cell number after 7 days of convection culture compared to static culture. In other studies, perfusion culture was applied on porous 3D scaffolds and showed to improve cell proliferation and scaffold colonization (Alvarez-Barreto et al., 2007; Bjerre et al., 2008; Grayson et al., 2008, 2011; Schumacher et al., 2010). In our study, however, perfusion culture showed to significantly decrease the number of haMSCs from donor 2 compared to static culture or culture in the biaxial bioreactor. This could be due to the highly interconnected and organized pore network of additive manufactured scaffolds compared to more conventional sponges and non-woven scaffolds with random fiber organization used in previous studies. A similar negative effect was reported in a study by Bjerre et al.

(2011) in which perfusion culture unfavorably changed the morphology and vitality of haMSCs (Bjerre et al., 2011).

Differences in initial cell attachment between the two donors could be an effect of differences in heterogeneity of cell populations due to donor variation (DiGirolamo et al., 1999; Phinney et al., 1999; Siddappa et al., 2007; Leferink et al., 2013; Siegel et al., 2013). Changes in cell response to the introduction of perfusion flow could also be related to several other factors such as the amount of ECM produced at the moment of transfer from static culture to the perfusion-flow system and the distribution of the cells and ECM throughout the scaffold. Upon closure of the longitudinal pores of the scaffold due to the presence of the formed ECM in static culture, the pressure, or the perfusion flow is expected to be increased, which could have led to tissue detachment. We hypothesized that prolonging the static culture period prior to applying bioreactor culture could result in more ECM with stronger binding and entanglement to the scaffold material (Griffon et al., 2011). Therefore, the scaffolds were cultured statically for 31 days followed by 14 days of culture in the biaxial bioreactor or in the perfusion bioreactor. From cross-sectional views on methylene blue stained scaffolds (Figure S7 in Supplementary Material), it could be observed that the cells and tissues indeed seemed to be detached from the scaffold upon dynamic culture, whereas in static conditions, a homogeneous distribution of cells and tissue throughout the scaffold was found. These results were confirmed by DNA quantification, which showed a significant loss of cells upon transferring the constructs from static to bioreactor culture (Figure S8 in Supplementary Material). In both the biaxial bioreactor and the perfusion bioreactor, loosened cell sheets were found in the longitudinal pores of the scaffolds. A difference between the two bioreactor systems was found with respect to the adherence sites of the cells. In perfusion culture conditions, cells were found on the outer layer of scaffold material, whereas in the biaxial bioreactor, lesser cells were found to reside on the outer layer of the scaffold.

The gene expression levels of f-actin, col-1, and col-2 previously showed to be significantly up-regulated in hfMSCs, whereas a significant down-regulation was found in haMSCs when comparing the basal gene expression levels and the levels after 9 days of static culture to the levels after 3 days of static culture followed by 6 days of culture in the biaxial bioreactor. For Sox-9, a similar response was found for hfMSCs compared to haMSCs. ALCAM, CD63, and ACAN did not show any significant differences in hfMSCs and haMSCs cultured statically or dynamically in the biaxial bioreactor. Larger differences in gene expression levels were found between perfusion culture and static culture than between culture in the biaxial bioreactor and static culture. ALCAM, f-Actin, col-1, and col-2 were significantly down-regulated in perfusion culture compared to static culture after 9 days. This could have been related to the lower cell number as a consequence of relatively high shear forces involved in a perfusion culture system.

Overall, the results presented in this study suggested that a more homogeneous cell distribution could be obtained for fetal MSCs compared to adult ones in all conditions, and that the benefit of applying bioreactor culture over static culture was not obvious for adult MSCs. Although the experiments with haMSCs were not as successful as with hfMSCs with respect to cell number and distribution, we believe that there is still the potential for a bioreactor system in a later stage of tissue culture with haMSCs. When static cultures lead to complete filling of the scaffold with closure of the pores, cells in the scaffold interior might undergo necrosis by mass transfer limitations. At that stage, a dynamic system, such as the biaxial rotating vessel presented in this study, might become favorable over static culture. Furthermore, in our study, the complex influence of rotational speed and medium perfusion speed on the fluid dynamics was not modeled. Screening the influence of these parameters on MSC fate in additive manufactured scaffolds might result in optimal culture conditions in which a homogeneous distribution throughout the scaffold can be achieved without compromising cells viability or altering MSCs phenotype.

CONCLUSION

The biaxial rotating vessel bioreactor used in this study has shown to improve hfMSCs distribution and proliferation in 3D additive manufactured PEOT/PBT scaffolds. The hfMSCs in the biaxial bioreactor produced ECM while retaining a comparable gene expression profile as the basal levels of hfMSCs seeded statically in 2D. Static culture on 3D scaffolds with hfMSCs showed downregulation of f-actin, col-1, col-2, ALP, and runx2 gene expression levels and also resulted in less ECM production and lower cell numbers than in the biaxial bioreactor, thus suggesting a more quiescent state of hfMSCs. As a third well-known dynamic culture system, a perfusion bioreactor was introduced for the experiments

with a more clinically relevant haMSCs population. No increase in cell number and cellular distribution upon culture in the biaxial or the perfusion bioreactor was observed for haMSCs, even after an extended period of static culture prior to culture in the biaxial bioreactors. In addition, the gene expression profile of haMSCs showed a different response to the culture in the biaxial bioreactor than the profile of hfMSCs. There were no consistent significant differences in cell number between 9 days of static culture and 3 days of static culture followed by 6 days of bioreactor culture in both the biaxial bioreactor and the perfusion-flow bioreactor. Overall, the biaxial rotating vessel bioreactor introduced in this study has shown to maintain hfMSCs viability and distribution throughout the scaffold, without inducing differentiation. Therefore, this system could serve as a tool to study cell activity in distinct 3D scaffolds.

ACKNOWLEDGMENTS

The authors gratefully acknowledge the funding from the Netherlands Institute for Regenerative Medicine (NIRM) through the grant number FES0908. This project/research has been made possible also with the support of the Dutch Province of Limburg. The authors would like to acknowledge Hui-Lun Soh from Quintech Life Sciences Pte Ltd. Singapore for her help in the experiments regarding hfMSCs.

REFERENCES

Abarrategi, A., Fernandez-Valle, M. E., Desmet, T., Castejon, D., Civantos, A., Moreno-Vicente, C., et al. (2012). Label-free magnetic resonance imaging to locate live cells in three-dimensional porous scaffolds. *J. R. Soc. Interface* 9, 2321–2331. doi:10.1098/rsif.2012.0068

Alvarez-Barreto, J. F., Linehan, S. M., Shambaugh, R. L., and Sikavitsas, V. I. (2007). Flow perfusion improves seeding of tissue engineering scaffolds with different architectures. *Ann. Biomed. Eng.* 35, 429–442. doi:10.1007/s10439-006-9244-z

Beumer, G. J., van Blitterswijk, C. A., and Ponec, M. (1994). Biocompatibility of a biodegradable matrix used as a skin substitute: an in vivo evaluation. *J. Biomed. Mater. Res.* 28, 545–552. doi:10.1002/jbm.820280504

Bjerre, L., Bunger, C., Baatrup, A., Kassem, M., and Mygind, T. (2011). Flow perfusion culture of human mesenchymal stem cells on coralline hydroxyapatite scaffolds with various pore sizes. *J. Biomed. Mater. Res.* 97, 251–263. doi:10.1002/jbm.a.33051

Bjerre, L., Bunger, C. E., Kassem, M., and Mygind, T. (2008). Flow perfusion culture of human mesenchymal stem cells on silicate-substituted tricalcium phosphate scaffolds. *Biomaterials* 29, 2616–2627. doi:10.1016/j.biomaterials.2008.03.003

Bossolasco, P., Corti, S., Strazzer, S., Borsotti, C., Del Bo, R., and Fortunato, F. (2004). Skeletal muscle differentiation potential of human adult bone marrow cells. *Exp. Cell Res.* 295, 66–78. doi:10.1016/j.yexcr.2003.12.015

Brady, K., Dickinson, S. C., Guillot, P. V., Polak, J., Blom, A. W., Kafienah, W., et al. (2014). Human fetal and adult bone marrow-derived mesenchymal stem cells use different signaling pathways for the initiation of chondrogenesis. *Stem Cells Dev.* 23, 541–554. doi:10.1089/scd.2013.0301

Chan, J., Waddington, S. N., O'Donoghue, K., Kurata, H., Guillot, P. V., Gotherstrom, C., et al. (2007). Widespread distribution and muscle differentiation of human

fetal mesenchymal stem cells after intrauterine transplantation in dystrophic MDX mouse. *Stem Cells* 25, 875–884. doi:10.1634/stemcells.2006-0694

Claase, M. B., de Bruijn, J. D., Grijpma, D. W., and Feijen, J. (2007). Ectopic bone formation in cell-seeded poly(ethylene oxide)/poly(butylene terephthalate) copolymer scaffolds of varying porosity. *J. Mater. Sci. Mater. Med.* 18, 1299–1307. doi:10.1007/s10856-006-0077-y

de Bruijn, J. D., van den Brink, I., Mendes, S., Dekker, R., Bovell, Y. P., and van Blitterswijk, C. A. (1999). Bone induction by implants coated with cultured osteogenic bone marrow cells. *Adv. Dent. Res.* 13, 74–81. doi:10.1177/08959374990130011801

Deschamps, A. A., Claase, M. B., Sleijster, W. J., de Bruijn, J. D., Grijpma, D. W., and Feijen, J. (2002). Design of segmented poly(ether ester) materials and structures for the tissue engineering of bone. *J. Control. Release* 78, 175–186. doi:10.1016/S0168-3659(01)00497-7

DiGirolamo, C. M., Stokes, D., Colter, D., Phinney, D. G., Class, R., and Prockop, D. J. (1999). Propagation and senescence of human marrow stromal cells in culture: a simple colony-forming assay identifies samples with the greatest potential to propagate and differentiate. *Br. J. Haematol.* 107, 275–281. doi:10.1046/j.1365-2141.1999.01715.x

Grayson, W. L., Bhumiratana, S., Cannizzaro, C., Chao, P. H., Lennon, D. P., Caplan, A. I., et al. (2008). Effects of initial seeding density and fluid perfusion rate on formation of tissue-engineered bone. *Tissue Eng.* 14, 1809–1820. doi:10.1089/ten.tea.2007.0255

Grayson, W. L., Marolt, D., Bhumiratana, S., Frohlich, M., Guo, X. E., and Vunjak-Novakovic, G. (2011). Optimizing the medium perfusion rate in bone tissue engineering bioreactors. *Biotechnol. Bioeng.* 108, 1159–1170. doi:10.1002/bit.23024

Griffon, D. J., Abulencia, J. P., Ragetly, G. R., Fredericks, L. P., and Chaieb, S. (2011). A comparative study of seeding techniques and three-dimensional matrices for mesenchymal cell attachment. *J. Tissue Eng. Regen. Med.* 5, 169–179. doi:10.1002/term.302

Grove, J. E., Bruscia, E., and Krause, D. S. (2004). Plasticity of bone marrow-derived stem cells. *Stem Cells* 22, 487–500. doi:10.1634/stemcells.22-4-487

Guillot, P. V., De Bari, C., Dell'Accio, F., Kurata, H., Polak, J., and Fisk, N. M. (2008). Comparative osteogenic transcription profiling of various fetal and adult mesenchymal stem cell sources. *Differentiation* 76, 946–957. doi:10.1111/j.1432-0436.2008.00279.x

Janeczek Portalska, K., Leferink, A., Groen, N., Fernandes, H., Moroni, L., van Blitterswijk, C., et al. (2012). Endothelial differentiation of mesenchymal stromal cells. *PLoS ONE* 7:e46842. doi:10.1371/journal.pone.0046842

Janssen, F. W., Oostra, J., Oorschot, A., and van Blitterswijk, C. A. (2006). A perfusion bioreactor system capable of producing clinically relevant volumes of tissue-engineered bone: in vivo bone formation showing proof of concept. *Biomaterials* 27, 315–323. doi:10.1016/j.biomaterials.2005.07.044

Jeannet, R., Cai, Q., Liu, H., Vu, H., and Kuo, Y. H. (2013). Alcam regulates long-term hematopoietic stem cell engraftment and self-renewal. *Stem Cells* 31, 560–571. doi:10.1002/stem.1309

Jo, C. H., Kim, O. S., Park, E. Y., Kim, B. J., Lee, J. H., Kang, S. B., et al. (2008). Fetal mesenchymal stem cells derived from human umbilical cord sustain primitive characteristics during extensive expansion. *Cell Tissue Res.* 334, 423–433. doi:10.1007/s00441-008-0696-3

Katayama, A., Arano, T., Sato, T., Ikada, Y., and Yoshinari, M. (2013). Radial-flow bioreactor enables uniform proliferation of human mesenchymal stem cells throughout a three-dimensional scaffold. *Tissue Eng. Part C Methods* 19, 109–116. doi:10.1089/ten.TEC.2011.0722

Kim, J., McBride, S., Tellis, B., Alvarez-Urena, P., Song, Y. H., Dean, D. D., et al. (2012). Rapid-prototyped PLGA/beta-TCP/hydroxyapatite nanocomposite scaffolds in a rabbit femoral defect model. *Biofabrication* 4, 025003. doi:10.1088/1758-5082/4/2/025003

Kock, L. M., Malda, J., Dhert, W. J., Ito, K., and Gawlitta, D. (2014). Flow-perfusion interferes with chondrogenic and hypertrophic matrix production by mesenchymal stem cells. *J. Biomech.* 47, 2122–2129. doi:10.1016/j.jbiomech.2013.11.006

Langer, R., and Vacanti, J. P. (1993). Tissue engineering. *Science* 260, 920–926. doi:10.1126/science.8493529

Leferink, A. M., Hendrikson, W. J., Rouwkema, J., Karperien, M., van Blitterswijk, C. A., and Moroni, L. (2013). Increased cell seeding efficiency in bioplotted three-dimensional PEOT/PBT scaffolds. *J. Tissue Eng. Regen. Med.* doi:10.1002/term.1842

Mackay, A. M., Beck, S. C., Murphy, J. M., Barry, F. P., Chichester, C. O., and Pittenger, M. F. (1998). Chondrogenic differentiation of cultured human mesenchymal stem cells from marrow. *Tissue Eng.* 4, 415–428. doi:10.1089/ten.1998.4.415

Martin, I., Wendt, D., and Heberer, M. (2004). The role of bioreactors in tissue engineering. *Trends Biotechnol.* 22, 80–86. doi:10.1016/j.tibtech.2003.12.001

Menicanin, D., Bartold, P. M., Zannettino, A. C., and Gronthos, S. (2009). Genomic profiling of mesenchymal stem cells. *Stem Cell. Rev.* 5, 36–50. doi:10.1007/s12015-009-9056-2

Moroni, L., de Wijn, J. R., and van Blitterswijk, C. A. (2005). Three-dimensional fiber-deposited PEOT/PBT copolymer scaffolds for tissue engineering: influence of porosity, molecular network mesh size, and swelling in aqueous media on dynamic mechanical properties. *J. Biomed. Mater. Res.* 75, 957–965. doi:10.1002/jbm.a.30499

Moroni, L., Schotel, R., Hamann, D., de Wijn, J. R., and van Blitterswijk, C. A. (2008). 3D fiber-deposited electrospun integrated scaffolds enhance cartilage tissue formation. *Adv. Funct. Mater.* 18, 53–60. doi:10.1002/adfm.200601158

Muguruma, Y., Reyes, M., Nakamura, Y., Sato, T., Matsuzawa, H., Miyatake, H., et al. (2003). In vivo and in vitro differentiation of myocytes from human bone marrow-derived multipotent progenitor cell. *Exp. Hematol.* 31, 1323–1330. doi:10.1016/j.exphem.2003.09.003

Papadimitropoulos, A., Riboldi, S. A., Tonnarelli, B., Piccinini, E., Woodruff, M. A., Hutmacher, D. W., et al. (2013). A collagen network phase improves cell seeding of open-pore structure scaffolds under perfusion. *J. Tissue Eng. Regen. Med.* 7, 183–190. doi:10.1002/term.506

Phinney, D. G. (2007). Biochemical heterogeneity of mesenchymal stem cell populations: clues to their therapeutic efficacy. *Cell Cycle* 6, 2884–2889. doi:10.4161/cc.6.23.5095

Phinney, D. G., Kopen, G., Righter, W., Webster, S., Tremain, N., and Prockop, D. J. (1999). Donor variation in the growth properties and osteogenic potential of human marrow stromal cells. *J. Cell. Biochem.* 75, 424–436. doi:10.1002/(SICI)1097-4644(19991201)75:3<424::AID-JCB8>3.3.CO;2-#

Pittenger, M. F., Mackay, A. M., Beck, S. C., Jaiswal, R. K., Douglas, R., Mosca, J. D., et al. (1999). Multilineage potential of adult human mesenchymal stem cells. *Science* 284, 143–147. doi:10.1126/science.284.5411.143

Reichert, J. C., Cipitria, A., Epari, D. R., Saifzadeh, S., Krishnakanth, P., Berner, A., et al. (2012). A tissue engineering solution for segmental defect regeneration in load-bearing long bones. *Sci. Transl. Med.* 4, 141ra93. doi:10.1126/scitranslmed.3003720

Russell, K. C., Phinney, D. G., Lacey, M. R., Barrilleaux, B. L., Meyertholen, K. E., and O'Connor, K. C. (2010). In vitro high-capacity assay to quantify the clonal heterogeneity in trilineage potential of mesenchymal stem cells reveals a complex hierarchy of lineage commitment. *Stem Cells* 28, 788–798. doi:10.1002/stem.312

Sansores-Garcia, L., Bossuyt, W., Wada, K., Yonemura, S., Tao, C., Sasaki, H., et al. (2011). Modulating F-actin organization induces organ growth by affecting the Hippo pathway. *EMBO J.* 30, 2325–2335. doi:10.1038/emboj.2011.157

Schantz, J. T., Machens, H. G., Schilling, A. F., and Teoh, S. H. (2012). Regenerative medicine: implications for craniofacial surgery. *J. Craniofac. Surg.* 23, 530–536. doi:10.1097/SCS.0b013e318241dc3a

Schumacher, M., Uhl, F., Detsch, R., Deisinger, U., and Ziegler, G. (2010). Static and dynamic cultivation of bone marrow stromal cells on biphasic calcium phosphate scaffolds derived from an indirect rapid prototyping technique. *J. Mater. Sci. Mater. Med.* 21, 3039–3048. doi:10.1007/s10856-010-4153-y

Siddappa, R., Licht, R., van Blitterswijk, C., and de Boer, J. (2007). Donor variation and loss of multipotency during in vitro expansion of human mesenchymal stem cells for bone tissue engineering. *J. Orthop. Res.* 25, 1029–1041. doi:10.1002/jor.20402

Siegel, G., Kluba, T., Hermanutz-Klein, U., Bieback, K., Northoff, H., and Schafer, R. (2013). Phenotype, donor age and gender affect function of human bone marrow-derived mesenchymal stromal cells. *BMC Med.* 11:146. doi:10.1186/1741-7015-11-146

Singh, H., Teoh, S. H., Low, H. T., and Hutmacher, D. W. (2005). Flow modelling within a scaffold under the influence of uni-axial and bi-axial bioreactor rotation. *J. Biotechnol.* 119, 181–196. doi:10.1016/j.jbiotec.2005.03.021

Sobral, J. M., Caridade, S. G., Sousa, R. A., Mano, J. F., and Reis, R. L. (2011). Three-dimensional plotted scaffolds with controlled pore size gradients: effect of scaffold geometry on mechanical performance and cell seeding efficiency. *Acta Biomater.* 7, 1009–1018. doi:10.1016/j.actbio.2010.11.003

Song, L., and Tuan, R. S. (2004). Transdifferentiation potential of human mesenchymal stem cells derived from bone marrow. *FASEB J.* 18, 980–982.

Stiehler, M., Bunger, C., Baatrup, A., Lind, M., Kassem, M., and Mygind, T. (2009). Effect of dynamic 3-D culture on proliferation, distribution, and osteogenic differentiation of human mesenchymal stem cells. *J. Biomed. Mater. Res.* 89, 96–107. doi:10.1002/jbm.a.31967

Ullah, M., Stich, S., Notter, M., Eucker, J., Sittinger, M., and Ringe, J. (2013). Transdifferentiation of mesenchymal stem cells-derived adipogenic-differentiated cells into osteogenic- or chondrogenic-differentiated cells proceeds via dedifferentiation and have a correlation with cell cycle arresting and driving genes. *Differentiation* 85, 78–90. doi:10.1016/j.diff.2013.02.001

van Gool, S. A., Emons, J. A. M., Leijten, J. C. H., Decker, E., Sticht, C., van Houwelingen, J. C., et al. (2012). Fetal mesenchymal stromal cells differentiating towards chondrocytes acquire a gene expression profile resembling human growth plate cartilage. *PLoS ONE* 7:e44561. doi:10.1371/journal.pone.0044561

Wang, H., Pieper, J., Peters, F., van Blitterswijk, C. A., and Lamme, E. N. (2005). Synthetic scaffold morphology controls human dermal connective tissue formation. *J. Biomed. Mater. Res.* 74, 523–532. doi:10.1002/jbm.a.30232

Woodfield, T. B. F., Malda, J., de Wijn, J., Peters, F., Riesle, J., and van Blitterswijk, C. A. (2004). Design of porous scaffolds for cartilage tissue engineering using a three-dimensional fiber-deposition technique. *Biomaterials* 25, 4149–4161. doi:10.1016/j.biomaterials.2003.10.056

Yeatts, A. B., Geibel, E. M., Fears, F. F., and Fisher, J. P. (2012). Human mesenchymal stem cell position within scaffolds influences cell fate during dynamic culture. *Biotechnol. Bioeng.* 109, 2381–2391. doi:10.1002/bit.24497

Zaim, M., Karaman, S., Cetin, G., and Isik, S. (2012). Donor age and long-term culture affect differentiation and proliferation of human bone marrow mesenchymal stem cells. *Ann. Hematol.* 91, 1175–1186. doi:10.1007/s00277-012-1438-x

Zhang, Z. Y., Teoh, S. H., Chong, M. S., Schantz, J. T., Fisk, N. M., Choolani, M. A., et al. (2009a). Superior osteogenic capacity for bone tissue engineering of fetal compared with perinatal and adult mesenchymal stem cells. *Stem Cells* 27, 126–137. doi:10.1634/stemcells.2008-0456

Zhang, Z. Y., Teoh, S. H., Chong, W. S., Foo, T. T., Chng, Y. C., Choolani, M., et al. (2009b). A biaxial rotating bioreactor for the culture of fetal mesenchymal stem cells for bone tissue engineering. *Biomaterials* 30, 2694–2704. doi:10.1016/j.biomaterials.2009.01.028

Conflict of Interest Statement: The authors declare that the research was conducted in the absence of any commercial or financial relationships that could be construed as a potential conflict of interest.

11

Microsphere-based scaffolds carrying opposing gradients of chondroitin sulfate and tricalcium phosphate

Vineet Gupta[1], Neethu Mohan[2], Cory J. Berkland[1,3] and Michael S. Detamore[1,4]*

[1] Bioengineering Graduate Program, University of Kansas, Lawrence, KS, USA, [2] Division of Tissue Engineering and Regeneration Technologies, Biomedical Technology Wing, Sree Chitra Tirunal Institute for Medical Sciences and Technology, Trivandrum, India, [3] Department of Pharmaceutical Chemistry, University of Kansas, Lawrence, KS, USA, [4] Department of Chemical and Petroleum Engineering, University of Kansas, Lawrence, KS, USA

Edited by:
Anna Lagunas,
Instituto de Salud Carlos III, Spain

Reviewed by:
Kyle Douglas Allen,
University of Florida, USA
Jennifer Patterson,
KU Leuven, Belgium
Yi Hong,
University of Texas at Arlington, USA

*Correspondence:
Michael S. Detamore,
Department of Chemical and
Petroleum Engineering, The
University of Kansas, 4149 Learned
Hall, 1530 West 15th Street,
Lawrence, KS 66045-7618, USA
detamore@ku.edu

Extracellular matrix (ECM) components, such as chondroitin sulfate (CS) and tricalcium phosphate, serve as raw materials, and thus spatial patterning of these raw materials may be leveraged to mimic the smooth transition of physical, chemical, and mechanical properties at the bone-cartilage interface. We hypothesized that encapsulation of opposing gradients of these raw materials in high molecular weight poly(D,L-lactic-co-glycolic acid) (PLGA) microsphere-based scaffolds would enhance differentiation of rat bone marrow–derived stromal cells. The raw material encapsulation altered the microstructure of the microspheres and also influenced the cellular morphology that depended on the type of material encapsulated. Moreover, the mechanical properties of the raw material encapsulating microsphere-based scaffolds initially relied on the composition of the scaffolds and later on were primarily governed by the degradation of the polymer phase and newly synthesized ECM by the seeded cells. Furthermore, raw materials had a mitogenic effect on the seeded cells and led to increased glycosaminoglycan (GAG), collagen, and calcium content. Interestingly, the initial effects of raw material encapsulation on a per-cell basis might have been overshadowed by medium-regulated environment that appeared to favor osteogenesis. However, it is to be noted that *in vivo*, differentiation of the cells would be governed by the surrounding native environment. Thus, the results of this study demonstrated the potential of the raw materials in facilitating neo-tissue synthesis in microsphere-based scaffolds and perhaps in combination with bioactive signals, these raw materials may be able to achieve intricate cell differentiation profiles required for regenerating the osteochondral interface.

Keywords: raw materials, chondroitin sulfate, tricalcium phosphate, gradient, microsphere-based scaffolds

Introduction

A scaffold with opposing gradients of physical and chemical signals at the osteochondral interface may trigger simultaneous bone and cartilage regeneration by having a cooperative effect on tissue regeneration. Our previous studies have shown that 3D microsphere-based gradient scaffolds have the potential to guide the chondro- and osteogenic differentiation of cells in different regions of the scaffolds. Moreover, the gradients in signals have the ability to control patterning of cell phenotype and to secrete tissue-specific extracellular matrix (ECM) components to promote osteochondral interface regeneration (Dormer et al., 2010, 2011, 2012b; Mohan et al., 2011).

Chondroitin sulfate (CS), a glycosaminoglycan (GAG) and a key ECM component of cartilage, when incorporated into 3D scaffolds resulted in increased DNA, GAG, and collagen accumulation by the cultured cells (Uygun et al., 2009; Kim et al., 2014). Moreover, CS also enhanced their chondrogenic gene expression (Chen et al., 2013). Likewise, bioactive ceramic beta-tricalcium phosphate (β-TCP) is widely used in bone tissue engineering because of its excellent oseteoconductivity, cellular adhesion, mechanical properties, and faster degradation rate than other crystalline calcium phosphates. Scaffolds incorporating β-TCP have shown better potential for osteogenic differentiation than the scaffolds without it (Takahashi et al., 2005; Liao et al., 2013; Todo and Arahira, 2013). We have previously demonstrated that encapsulation of raw materials, such as CS and bioactive glass (BG possesses the capability to directly bind to bone), in low molecular weight (around 40–45 kDa) poly(D,L-lactic-co-glycolic acid) (PLGA) microsphere-based scaffolds created a favorable environment for cells to create a tissue-specific ECM. Additionally, evident regional variation in newly synthesized ECM indicated that the raw materials could potentially be used to replace growth factors, thus holding tremendous clinical significance by providing a more streamlined path for regulatory approval and greater financial incentive for translation to the clinic (Mohan et al., 2013).

The low molecular weight PLGA microsphere-based scaffolds are well suited for *in vitro* studies as signal release and cellular response to the encapsulated signals can be conveniently studied in these scaffolds because of rapid degradation of microspheres (Tracy, 1999; Alexis, 2004; Singh et al., 2008; Dormer et al., 2010, 2012a; Mohan et al., 2013). Moreover, these low molecular weight scaffolds can also be used to study tissue regeneration in small animal model *in vivo* studies where skeletal changes occur at a faster rate compared to humans (Pearce et al., 2007; Mohan et al., 2011; Dormer et al., 2012b). In order for a scaffold to be clinically effective and commercially successful, it is imperative that its biodegradation rate matches with the tissue regeneration rate in animal models that closely approximate the human regeneration rate. To begin exploring the clinical implications of our raw material microsphere gradient scaffolds, we need to translate our successes with scaffolds *in vitro* and *in vivo* with small animal models to scaffolds that can be employed in preclinical animal models. The foremost step in that direction will be to study cellular response toward encapsulated factors released from a scaffold system that can be employed in translational animal models (such as sheep, dogs, etc.). Therefore, the objective of this study was to investigate the *in vitro* response of raw material encapsulating microsphere-based scaffolds fabricated with high molecular weight PLGA as a first step to establish the clinical efficacy of these scaffolds. PLGA with an intrinsic viscosity (i.v.) of ~0.7 (M_W: 106–112 kDa) was chosen for this study due to its relevance in large animal studies (Fonseca et al., 2014), and to correspond to an ongoing sheep study from our group. The polymer formulation used in the study represents a more translational product, inspired by a Coulter Foundation-funded project and input from Food and Drug Administration (FDA) regulatory consultant and

business advisors. From this study, we hope to gain an insight into parameters that can have profound implications during *in vivo* experiments.

In this study, we investigated whether the encapsulated raw materials (CS and TCP) in high molecular weight PLGA scaffolds can provide building blocks and facilitate differentiation of the seeded cells simultaneously in the direction of bone- and cartilage-like cells. 3D microsphere-based scaffolds were fabricated using high molecular weight PLGA microspheres encapsulating CS (for cartilage regeneration) and TCP (for bone regeneration) as raw materials. Additionally, scaffolds containing gradient of the raw materials were also fabricated via a gradient technology as previously reported (Singh et al., 2008). The response of rat bone marrow-derived stromal cells (rBMSCs) to the raw materials was evaluated when cultured in a medium consisting of exogenous factors. We hypothesized that encapsulation of raw materials, CS and TCP, in high molecular weight PLGA microsphere-based scaffolds would enhance the differentiation of rBMSCs toward chondrogenic and osteogenic lineages, respectively. Moreover, we anticipate rBMSCs in gradient scaffolds to differentiate simultaneously along an osteochondral route as previously seen in low molecular weight scaffolds encapsulating CS and BG (Mohan et al., 2013).

Materials and Methods

Materials

Poly(D,L-lactic-co-glycolic acid) (50:50, lauryl ester end group, $M_W = 106$ kDa) with an i.v. of 0.65 dL/g ("PLGA50:50"), and PLGA (75:25, lauryl ester end group, $M_W = 112$ kDa) with an i.v. of 0.69 dL/g ("PLGA75:25") were obtained from Lakeshore Biomaterials (Birmingham, AL, USA). Murine IGF-I was obtained from Peprotech, Inc. (Rocky Hill, NJ, USA). Chondroitin-4-sulfate (lyophilized powder of CS, a sodium salt from bovine trachea) and TCP powder (<200 nm particle) were obtained from Sigma (St. Louis, MO, USA). All other reagents and organic solvents utilized were of cell culture or ACS grade.

Fabrication of Microspheres

Three different types of microspheres were fabricated for the study: (i) PLGA75:25 microspheres (PLGA), (ii) CS–NaHCO$_3$ encapsulated PLGA50:50 microspheres (CS), and (iii) TCP-encapsulated PLGA75:25 microspheres (TCP). The rationale for choosing PLGA with two different compositions was to correspond to an on going *in vivo* sheep study from our group. The relatively faster degrading polymer (PLGA50:50) was selected for its ability to release the raw materials quickly in the cartilage region to facilitate chondrogenesis, whereas the slower degrading polymer (PLGA75:25) in the bone region was selected to lend more structural stability to the regenerating tissue. The CS–NaHCO$_3$ encapsulated microspheres were fabricated by adding 2% w/v CS and 2% w/v NaHCO$_3$ to 16% w/v PLGA50:50 dissolved in dichloromethane (DCM), and the TCP encapsulated microspheres were fabricated by adding 4% w/v TCP to 16% w/v PLGA75:25 dissolved in DCM. Using the PLGA-CS/TCP emulsions, microspheres were fabricated via our previously reported technology (Berkland et al., 2001; Singh et al., 2008; Dormer et al., 2010, 2011, 2012a,b; Mohan et al., 2011,

2013). Briefly, using acoustic excitation produced by an ultrasonic transducer (Branson Ultrasonics, Danbury, CT, USA), regular jet instabilities were created in the polymer stream, thereby creating uniform polymer droplets. An annular carrier non-solvent stream of 0.5% w/v poly (vinyl alcohol) (PVA, 88% hydrolyzed, 25 kDa, Polysciences, Inc., Warrington, PA, USA) in deionized water (DI H$_2$O) surrounding the polymer droplets was flowed using a coaxial nozzle that carried the emanated polymer droplets into a beaker containing the non-solvent solution at 0.5% w/v in DI H$_2$O, to prevent aggregation of the droplets. The polymer droplets were stirred for 3–4 h to allow for solvent to evaporate, and then filtered and rinsed with DI H$_2$O to remove residual PVA, and stored at -20°C. The particles were lyophilized for 48 h before further use.

Scaffold Fabrication

Gradient scaffolds ("GRADIENT" group) were prepared using our previously established technology (Singh et al., 2008; Dormer et al., 2010; Mohan et al., 2011, 2013). In brief, lyophilized microspheres (50–100 mg) of two different types, CS and TCP, were dispersed in DI H$_2$O and loaded into two separate syringes. The suspensions were then pumped at opposing flow rates using programmable syringe pumps (PHD 22/2000; Harvard Apparatus, Inc., Holliston, MA, USA) into a cylindrical plastic mold (diameter ~ 4 mm) having a filter at the bottom until a height of about 6 mm was reached. The scaffolds were 3.8–4.0 mm in diameter and around 6 mm in height. The profile for these gradient constructs was linear, where the top one-fourth of the total height comprised of CS microspheres (1.5 mm), then the next one-fourth (1.5 mm) was a linear transition from CS to TCP microspheres, and the remaining half (3 mm) contained only TCP microspheres. The stacked microspheres were then sintered with ethanol-acetone (95:5 v/v) for 55 min. The scaffolds were further lyophilized for 48 h and sterilized with ethylene oxide for 12 h prior to cell seeding experiments. The control PLGA and other homogenous scaffolds, abbreviated as CS and TCP, were fabricated by packing the corresponding microspheres into the same molds, followed by sintering for 55 min, except for PLGA scaffolds (sintered for 45 min). The homogeneous scaffolds had dimensions similar to GRADIENT scaffolds (diameter 3.8–4.0 mm and height 6 mm). A total of four different groups were tested in the study and were named according to the composition of microspheres as: PLGA, CS, TCP, and GRADIENT.

Cell Seeding of Scaffolds

Rat bone marrow-derived stromal cells were obtained from the femurs of 10 young male Sprague–Dawley rats (176–200 g, SASCO), following a University of Kansas approved IACUC protocol (175–08) and cultured in medium consisting of α-MEM supplemented with 10% FBS (MSC-Qualified, cat #10437-028) and 1% penicillin–streptomycin (P/S) (all from Invitrogen Life Technologies, Carlsbad, CA, USA). When the cells were 80–90% confluent, they were trypsinized and re-plated at 7,000 cells/cm^2. Seeding was performed when cells reached P4. Scaffolds were sterilized using ethylene oxide for 12 h, allowed to ventilate overnight after sterilization, and placed in a 24-well plate. Cells (P4) were resuspended in culture medium at a concentration of ~10 million/mL. Eighty microliters of this cell suspension (~750 K cells) were

placed directly onto the top of the scaffold, which infiltrated the scaffold via capillary action (Dormer et al., 2012a). Cells were allowed to attach for 1 h after which 2 mL of culture medium was added. After 24 h, the culture medium was replaced by 2 mL of differentiation medium consisting of α-MEM, 1% P/S, 10% FBS, 4 mM β-glycerophosphate (β-GP), 100 nM dexamethasone (DEX) (MP Biomedicals, Santa Ana, CA, USA), 25 mM HEPES buffer (Fisher Scientific, Fairlawn, NJ, USA), and 100 ng/mL murine IGF-I (Peprotech Inc., Rocky Hill, NJ, USA). Every 48 h for 6 weeks, two-thirds of the differentiation medium were replaced with fresh medium.

Scanning Electron Microscopy

Scaffolds in culture were fixed in glutaraldehyde followed by dehydration in ethanol. Afterwards, the scaffolds were lyophilized for 48 h prior to imaging. The PLGA, CS, TCP, and GRADIENT acellular (week 0) and cellular (week 1.5) microsphere-based scaffolds were imaged using a LEO 1550 field emission scanning electron microscope at an accelerating voltage of 10 kV.

Mechanical Testing

Unconfined compression tests of the acellular (week 0) and cellular (week 6) microsphere-based scaffolds ($n = 4$–5) were conducted using a uniaxial testing apparatus (Instron Model 5848, Canton, MA, USA) with a 50 N load cell. A custom-made stainless steel bath and compression-plate assembly were mounted in the apparatus (Singh, 2008). Cylindrical scaffold samples were compressed to 80% strain at a strain rate of 1%/s under phosphate-buffered saline [PBS: 0.138M sodium chloride, 0.0027M potassium chloride] at 37°C. Among all possible testing modalities, compression at a 1%/s strain rate provides the most valuable information in terms of achieving high strain levels to view the entire stress-strain profile, which cyclic testing and stress relaxation/creep testing do not provide, and moreover a reproducible elastic modulus can be obtained without preconditioning as we have done in the past (Detamore and Athanasiou, 2003). Compressive moduli of elasticity were calculated from the initial linear regions, ~5% strain, of the stress–strain curves as described previously (Singh et al., 2008; Dormer et al., 2010, 2012a; Mohan et al., 2013).

Porosity Measurement

We have previously demonstrated a close match between theoretical porosities and porosities measured by porosimetry and microCT (Singh et al., 2008; Jeon et al., 2013). Therefore, a fluid saturation method was used in this study to calculate the porosities of the scaffolds:

$$V_B = 4m \div \pi d^2 h,$$
$$W_{\text{Water}} = W_{\text{W}} - W_{\text{D}},$$
$$V_P = W_{\text{Water}} \div \rho_{\text{Water}},$$
$$\text{Porosity}(\varphi)(\%) = (V_P \div V_B) \times 100$$

where V_B, m, d, h, W_W, W_D, and V_P are the bulk volume, mass, diameter, height, wet weight, dry weight, and pore volume of the scaffolds, respectively. W_{Water} and ρ_{Water} are the weight and density of water. Briefly, wet and dry weights of scaffolds were recorded after fabrication and porosities were determined by the above-described method.

Biochemical Analyses

Engineered constructs ($n = 5$) were analyzed for matrix production at 0, 3, and 6 weeks. The samples were digested in two different types of digestion solution: (i) Papain solution for DNA, GAG, and hydroxyproline (HYP) content analyses, and (ii) Triton-X solution for calcium content and alkaline phosphatase (ALP) activity analyses. The papain digestion solution consisted of 125 mg/mL papain (from papaya latex), 5 mM N-acetyl cysteine, 5 mM ethylenediaminetetraacetic acid, and 100 mM potassium phosphate buffer (20 mM monobasic potassium phosphate, 79 mM dibasic potassium phosphate) (all reagents from Sigma Aldrich) in DI H_2O. Engineered constructs were removed from culture in a sterile manner, placed in microcentrifuge tubes, homogenized with the papain solution (1 mL), and allowed to digest overnight in a 60°C water bath. The digested scaffolds were then centrifuged at 10,000 rpm for 5 min to pellet fragments of polymer and other impurities and stored at -20°C. Later, the supernatant was used to determine DNA, GAG, and HYP contents using the Picogreen (Molecular Probes, Eugene, OR, USA), dimethylmethylene blue (DMMB) (Biocolor, Newtownabbey, Northern Ireland), and HYP (cat #MAK008, Sigma Aldrich, St. Louis, MO, USA) assays, respectively. For calcium and ALP analyses, constructs were digested in 0.05% Triton X-100 and the supernatants were placed in the -20°C before the analyses. Calcium content was assessed using a QuantiChromTM Calcium Assay Kit (DICA-500; QuantiChrom, Hayward, CA, USA). ALP activity was estimated by determining liberated p-nitrophenol (p-NITRO) rate (concentration/µg DNA per minute) as described elsewhere (Boyan et al., 1989). In the cases of GAG and calcium content, the values of acellular controls for CS and TCP groups (listed in Tables S1 and S2 in Supplementary Material), respectively, were subtracted from the corresponding values of the cellular scaffolds at each time point in an effort to distinguish the bioactivity provided by the CS and TCP from the amounts retained in the scaffolds.

Gene Expression Analyses

Reverse transcriptase quantitative polymerase chain reaction (RT-qPCR) was performed for gene expression analyses in microsphere-based constructs ($n = 3$–5) at weeks 0, 1.5, 3, and 6. Certain groups at certain time points (indicated in Section "Results") had insufficient sample size ($n < 3$) because some of the samples were lost during processing. In preparation for RT-qPCR, samples were first homogenized in 1 mL of Trizol reagent (Invitrogen), and the RNA was isolated according to the manufacturer's guidelines. Isolated RNA was cleaned using an RNeasy spin column method (Qiagen, Valencia, CA, USA) and converted to complementary DNA using a TaqMan High Capacity kit (Applied Biosystems, Foster City, CA, USA) in an Eppendorf Realplex Mastercycler. TaqMan Gene expression assays from Applied Biosystems for appropriate genes (**Table 1**) were run in the Eppendorf system. A $2^{-\Delta\Delta Ct}$ method was used to evaluate the relative level of expression for each target gene. For quantification, the PLGA constructs at week 0 were designated as the calibrator group and GAPDH expression as the endogenous control.

TABLE 1 | Genes used for RT-qPCR analysis.

Gene	Symbol	TaqMan assay ID
Glyceraldehyde 3-phosphate dehydrogenase	GAPDH	Rn01775763_g1
SRY (sex determining region Y)-box 9	SOX9	Rn01751069_mH
Collagen type II	COL2A1	Rn01751069_mH
Aggrecan	ACAN	Rn00573424_m1
Collagen type I	COL1A1	Rn01463848_m1
Runt-related transcription factor 2	RUNX2	Rn01512298_m1
Bone gamma-carboxyglutamate protein	BGLAP	Rn00566386_g1
Secreted phosphoprotein 1	SPP1	Rn01449972_m1
Integrin-binding sialoprotein	IBSP	Rn00561414_m1

Statistical Analyses

SPSS 21.0 (IBM, Armonk, NY, USA) was used for constructing standard box plots for outlier elimination. For statistical inference in Sections "Mechanical Testing" and "Porosity Measurement", a single factor analysis of variance (ANOVA) was performed with SPSS, followed by a Tukey's honestly significant difference *post hoc* test when significance was detected below the $p = 0.05$ value. In Sections "Biochemical Analyses" and "Gene Expression Analyses", the statistical inference was performed using a two-factor ANOVA followed by a Tukey's honestly significant difference *post hoc* test when significance was detected below the $p = 0.05$ value. The model included the two factors (scaffold type and time) and the possible interactions between them. All quantitative results (numerical values and representative diagrams) are expressed as the average ± SD.

Results

Scanning Electron Microscopy

Figures 1 and **2** represent the scanning electron micrographs of all four types of scaffolds. **Figure 1** demonstrates that the fabricated microspheres were uniform in size (Figure S1 in Supplementary Material) and also illustrates the overall porous nature of microsphere-based scaffolds with interconnected pores. Additionally, it highlights the differences in microsphere morphology among the various scaffold groups. The microspheres in PLGA-only scaffolds (**Figure 1A**) were smooth with surface film layers being formed as a result of plasticization of PLGA with ethanol-acetone (Singh et al., 2008). The microspheres in CS scaffolds (**Figures 1B,D**) had minute pores on their surface while the microspheres in TCP scaffolds had a rougher appearance (**Figures 1C,E**) than microspheres in the PLGA-only group. The GRADIENT scaffold image (**Figure 1F**) shows fusion between porous (CS) and rough (TCP) microspheres at the transition region of the scaffold. Apart from the differences in microsphere structure, variations were also observed in the cellular morphology of the cell-seeded constructs (**Figure 2**). At Day 10 (week 1.5), very few cells were observed in the PLGA-only scaffolds residing in pores between the adjacent microspheres, and these cells possessed a rounded morphology (**Figure 2A**). By contrast, a far greater number of cells could be seen in the other three groups with differences appearing in the cellular morphologies. Cells covered the surface of the microspheres almost completely in the CS scaffolds and appeared to be flat with cell–cell connections being evident at the sintering junctions between the adjacent microspheres (**Figure 2B**). Cells

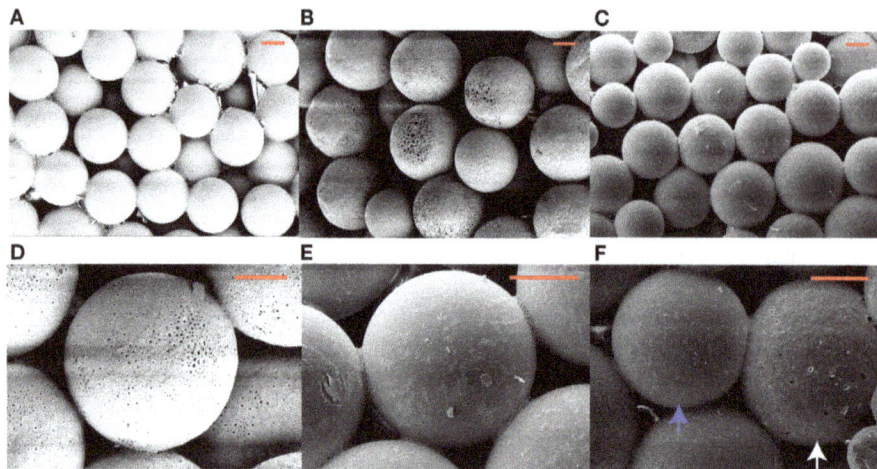

FIGURE 1 | Scanning electron micrographs of acellular microsphere-based scaffolds. The images reveal the distinct morphological features of the microspheres in different scaffold groups: **(A)** PLGA, **(B,D)** CS, **(C,E)** TCP, and **(F)** GRADIENT at the CS (white arrow)-TCP (blue arrow) transition region. Scale bar: 100 μm.

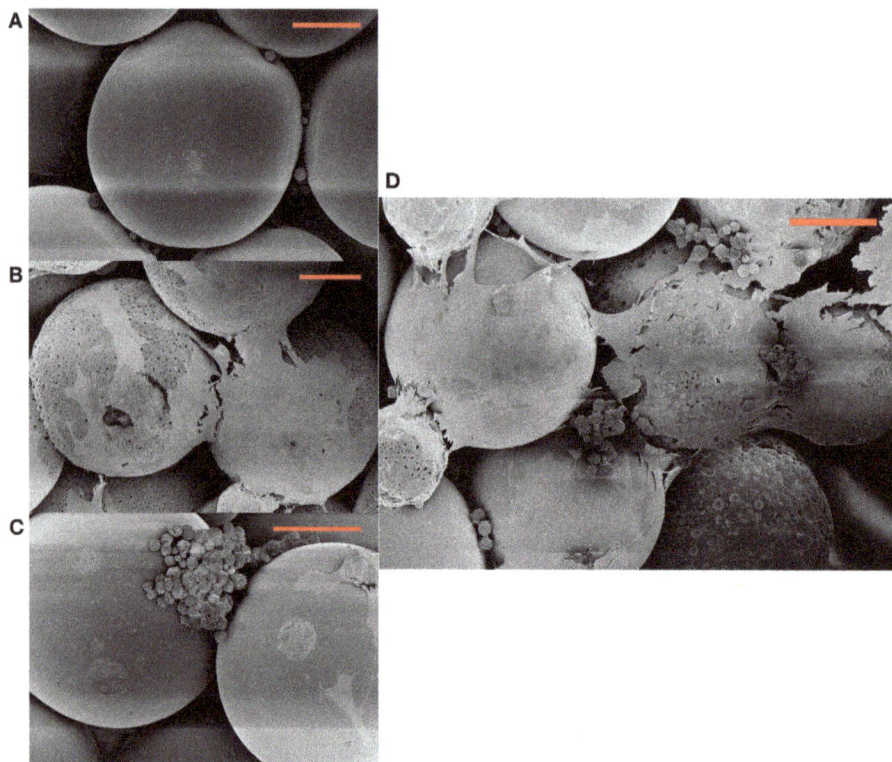

FIGURE 2 | Cellular morphology of rBMSCs at day 10 (week 1.5) on different scaffold groups: (A) PLGA, (B) CS, (C) TCP, and (D) GRADIENT as depicted by the scanning electron micrographs. Scale bar: 100 μm.

in the TCP scaffolds had a round appearance, and were clustered around the microsphere sintering junctions (**Figure 2C**). Both cell types with round (in clusters) and flat morphologies were present in the GRADIENT group (**Figure 2D**). However, no apparent morphological differences were observed in cells from distinct regions of the GRADIENT scaffold.

Mechanical Testing

Tricalcium phosphate acellular scaffolds had an average elastic modulus of 194 ± 16 kPa at week 0 that was 4- ($p < 0.05$), 4.8- ($p < 0.05$), and 2.8-fold ($p < 0.05$) higher than the moduli of PLGA, CS, and GRADIENT scaffolds, respectively (**Figure 3A**). Additionally, among the cell-seeded scaffolds, TCP constructs at week 6 had an average modulus of 0.84 ± 0.55 MPa that was 208.8-fold ($p < 0.05$) higher than the modulus of the CS group (**Figure 3B**). Surprisingly, it was observed that the PLGA constructs at week 6 had an average modulus of 11.4 ± 6.6 MPa (not shown in the figure) that was orders of magnitude higher than the moduli of the other three groups at that time. No significant differences were observed between the elastic moduli of CS and GRADIENT groups at week 6.

Porosity Measurement

The average porosity of CS group was $49.6 \pm 4.4\%$ that was 2.4-fold ($p < 0.05$) higher than the porosity of the PLGA group (**Table 2**). Moreover, the porosities of the scaffolds in the CS group were also statistically significantly higher than the porosities of their counterparts in the TCP and GRADIENT groups. No significant differences in porosities were observed among any other groups.

Biochemical Analysis
DNA Content

The DNA content results (**Figure 4**) revealed no significant differences in the amount of DNA present in the four distinct

types of scaffolds at weeks 0 and 3. At week 6, the DNA content in CS scaffolds was 31.7-fold ($p < 0.05$) higher than the DNA content in the PLGA group. The TCP and GRADIENT groups also outperformed the PLGA control at week 6, with 15- ($p < 0.05$) and 18-fold ($p < 0.05$) higher DNA contents, respectively. Moreover, the DNA content in the CS group at week 6 was statistically significantly higher than the DNA contents in the TCP and GRADIENT groups at that time. Additionally, the CS, TCP, and GRADIENT groups were observed to have statistically significantly higher DNA content at week 6 than their corresponding values at weeks 0 and 3; however, no significant differences in the DNA content over time were observed in the PLGA group.

GAG Content

A trend similar to DNA content was observed in the GAG content (**Figure 5A**), where no significant differences appeared among groups at weeks 0 and 3. At week 6, the net GAG content of the CS scaffolds was 5.5-fold ($p < 0.05$) higher than the GAG content of the PLGA group. Moreover, the GAG content in the CS group at week 6 was also statistically significantly higher than the GAG contents in the TCP and GRADIENT groups. No significant differences in the GAG content were observed among the other three groups week 6, meaning that the CS group was the only group to statistically significantly outperform the PLGA control at that time. The GAG content in the CS scaffolds (22.2 ± 7.5 µg) at week 6 was found to be statistically significantly higher than its corresponding

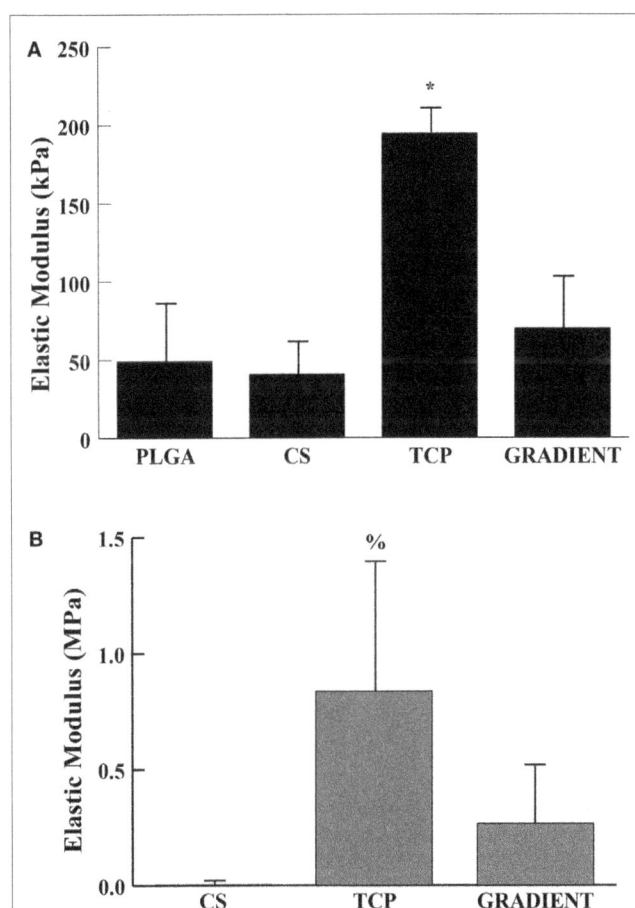

FIGURE 3 | Elastic modulus. (A) Acellular constructs at week 0. (B) Cellular constructs at week 6. All values are expressed as the average ± SD ($n = 3$–5), $p < 0.05$ *Statistically significant change over the other three groups, %statistically significant change over the CS group. PLGA constructs at week 6 are not shown in the figure.

TABLE 2 | Average porosities of different scaffold groups.

Group	Average Porosity (%)
PLGA	21.0 ± 6.8
CS	$49.6 \pm 4.4^*$
TCP	21.6 ± 6.8
GRADIENT	18.4 ± 4.6

*Statistically significantly higher than the other three groups.

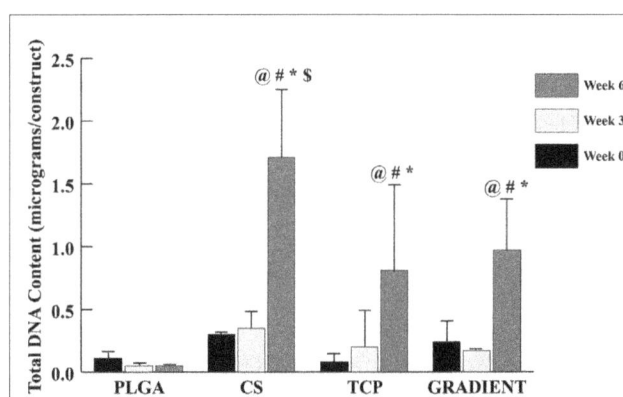

FIGURE 4 | Total DNA content as measured in the microsphere-based scaffolds over weeks 0, 3, and 6. All values are expressed as the average ± SD ($n = 3$–5), $p < 0.05$. @Statistically significant change over week 0 value, #statistically significant change over its value at previous time point, *statistically significant change over the PLGA group at same time point, and $statistically significant change over the TCP and GRADIENT groups at same time point.

values at weeks 0 and 3. The TCP and the GRADIENT groups had significantly higher GAG content at week 6 than their respective values at week 0. Furthermore, the PLGA and TCP groups at week 3 had significantly higher GAG content when it was normalized to the DNA content than the normalized GAG content of the CS and GRADIENT groups at that time (**Figure 5B**). However, at week 6, only the TCP group statistically significantly differed from the PLGA group in the normalized GAG content. It must be noted that the values of GAG content obtained from the biochemical analysis represent both the GAGs present in the ECM secreted by the cells and the CS released by the scaffold and then entrapped within the ECM. The values *do not* represent the CS left entrapped within the polymer matrix, as the GAG content of acellular controls was subtracted at each time point.

HYP Content

At week 0, only the GRADIENT group outperformed the PLGA group in HYP content with 2.6-fold ($p < 0.05$) higher HYP content (**Figure 6A**). Moreover, the HYP content in the GRADIENT group at week 0 was statistically significantly higher than the HYP contents in the CS and TCP groups. Week 3 HYP content results showed that the CS and GRADIENT groups had 1.9- ($p < 0.05$) and 2.9-fold higher HYP content than the PLGA group, respectively. Also, the GRADIENT group at week 3 had statistically significantly higher HYP content than the CS and TCP groups. At week 6, both the CS and the GRADIENT groups outperformed the PLGA control, with HYP contents that were 2.2- ($p < 0.05$) and 2.1-fold ($p < 0.05$) higher, respectively. Additionally, the CS and GRADIENT groups had statistically significant higher HYP contents than the TCP group at week 6. The CS and GRADIENT groups were the only groups that showed statistically significant increases in HYP content over time. The HYP content in the CS group at week 6 was significantly higher than its corresponding values at weeks 0 and 3, whereas the HYP content in the GRADIENT group at week 3 was significantly higher than its HYP content at week 0. In the normalized HYP (per DNA) content, the PLGA, CS, and the GRADIENT groups were statistically significantly higher than the CS group at week 3 (**Figure 6B**), with no significant differences occurring in the normalized HYP content among the PLGA, CS, and GRADIENT groups. The PLGA and TCP groups at week 3 had statistically significantly higher normalized HYP content than their values at week 0 and 6, respectively. No significant differences were observed in the CS and GRADIENT groups over time in the normalized HYP content.

Calcium Content

The calcium content analysis revealed no significant differences between the PLGA and CS groups at week 0 (**Figure 7A**). The calcium contents of TCP and GRADIENT scaffolds at week 0 are not reported because of insufficient sample size ($n < 3$), as some of the samples were lost during processing. At week 3, the calcium content in the PLGA group was statistically significantly greater than the calcium contents in the CS, TCP, and GRADIENT groups. Also, the calcium contents in the CS and TCP groups at week 3 were statistically significantly higher than the calcium content in the GRADIENT group. At week 6, the calcium contents in the CS and GRADIENT groups were

3.4- ($p < 0.05$) and 2.3-fold ($p < 0.05$) greater than the calcium content of the PLGA group. Moreover, the CS group calcium content at week 6 was observed to be statistically significantly higher than the calcium contents of the TCP and GRADIENT groups, and the GRADIENT group was found to be significantly higher than the TCP group in calcium content at week 6. No significant differences were observed in the calcium contents of the PLGA and TCP groups at that time, meaning that only the CS and GRADIENT groups outperformed the PLGA control in calcium content at week 6. The calcium content of the PLGA group increased statistically significantly at week 3 from its week 0 value, followed by a decrease at week 6 that was not statistically significant. The CS group had significantly higher calcium content at week 6 than at weeks 0 and 3. In addition, the GRADIENT group had significantly more calcium at week 6 than at week 3. No significant differences in calcium content of the TCP group were observed over time. The normalized calcium

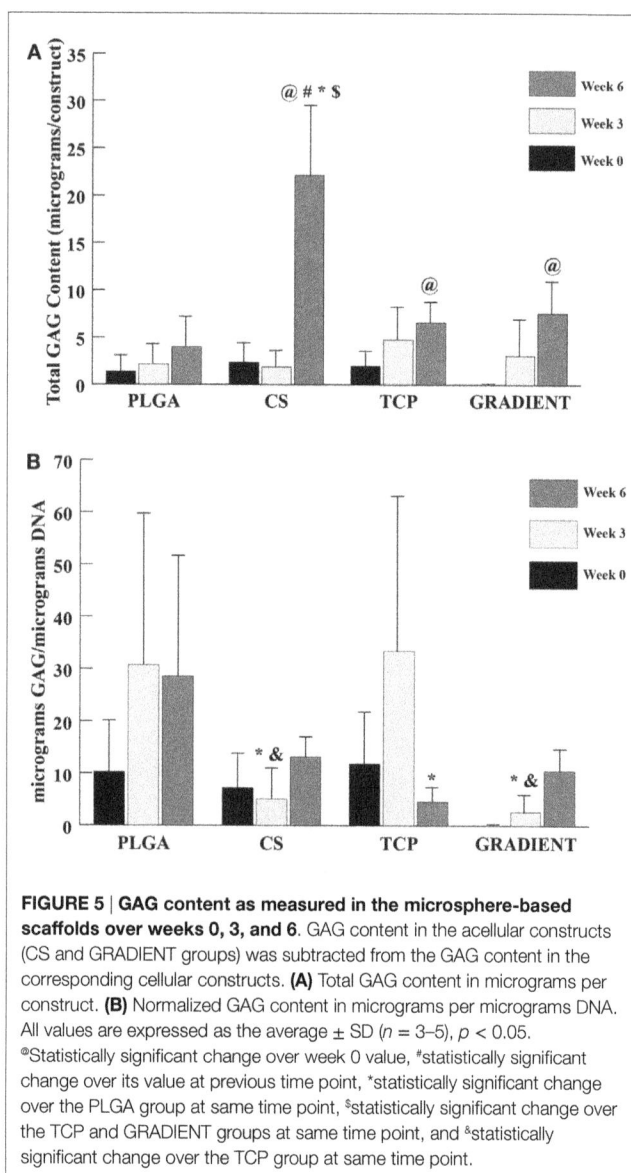

FIGURE 5 | GAG content as measured in the microsphere-based scaffolds over weeks 0, 3, and 6. GAG content in the acellular constructs (CS and GRADIENT groups) was subtracted from the GAG content in the corresponding cellular constructs. **(A)** Total GAG content in micrograms per construct. **(B)** Normalized GAG content in micrograms per micrograms DNA. All values are expressed as the average ± SD ($n = 3–5$), $p < 0.05$. @Statistically significant change over week 0 value, #statistically significant change over its value at previous time point, *statistically significant change over the PLGA group at same time point, $statistically significant change over the TCP and GRADIENT groups at same time point, and &statistically significant change over the TCP group at same time point.

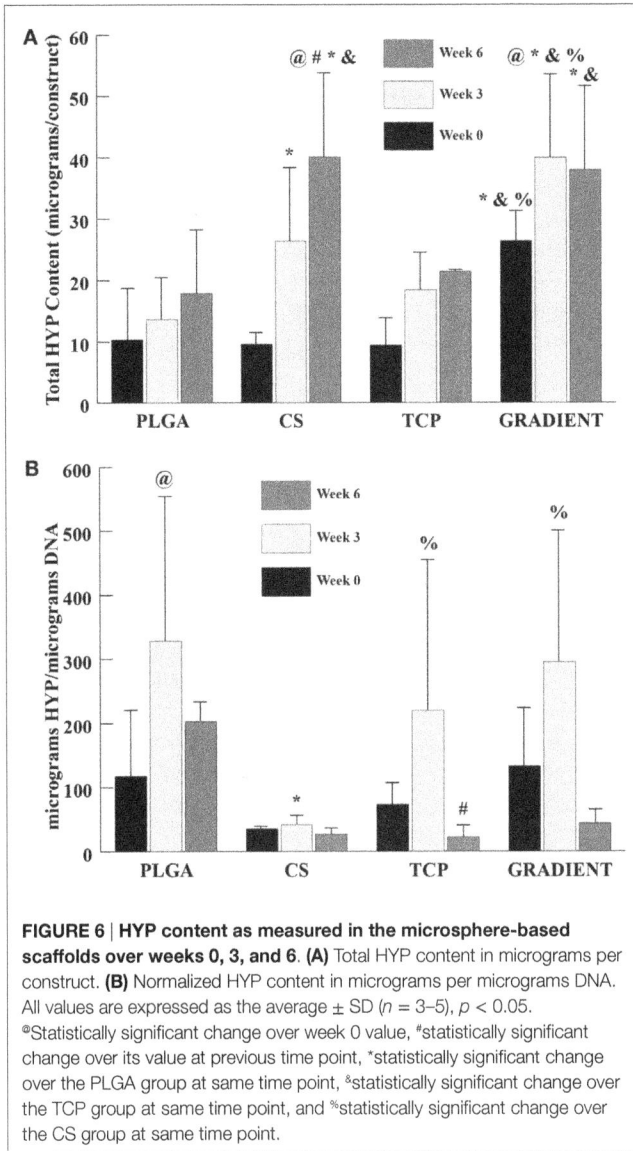

FIGURE 6 | HYP content as measured in the microsphere-based scaffolds over weeks 0, 3, and 6. (A) Total HYP content in micrograms per construct. **(B)** Normalized HYP content in micrograms per micrograms DNA. All values are expressed as the average ± SD ($n = 3–5$), $p < 0.05$. @Statistically significant change over week 0 value, #statistically significant change over its value at previous time point, *statistically significant change over the PLGA group at same time point, &statistically significant change over the TCP group at same time point, and %statistically significant change over the CS group at same time point.

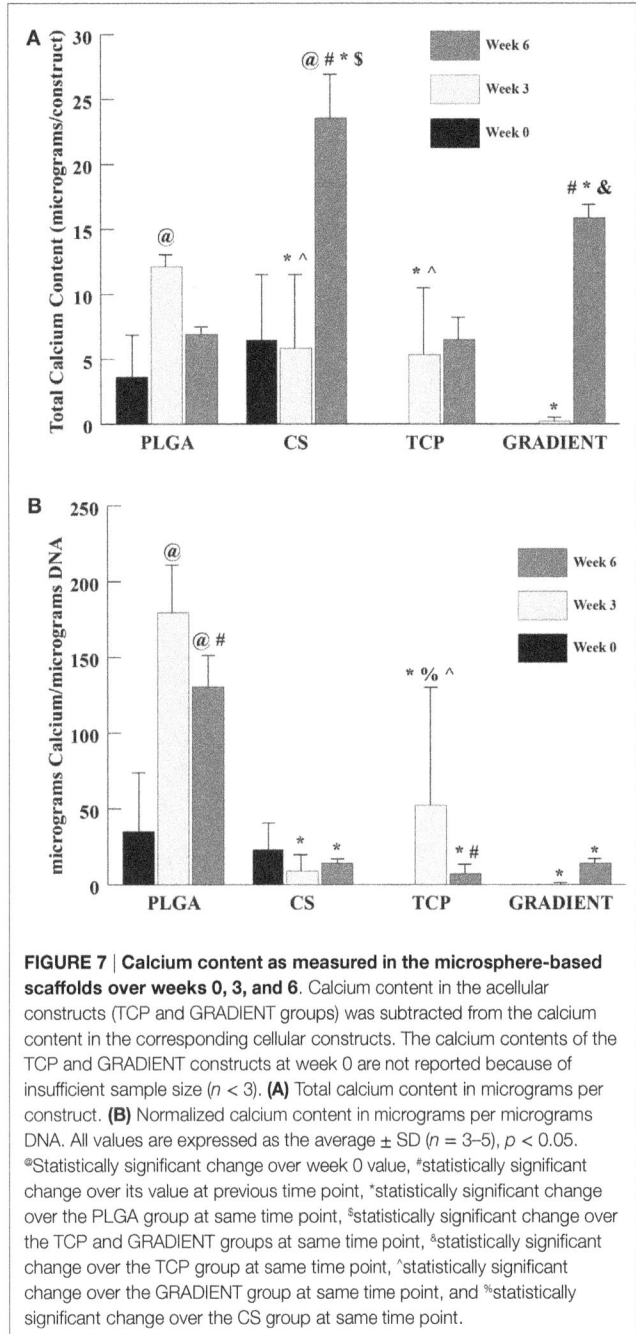

FIGURE 7 | Calcium content as measured in the microsphere-based scaffolds over weeks 0, 3, and 6. Calcium content in the acellular constructs (TCP and GRADIENT groups) was subtracted from the calcium content in the corresponding cellular constructs. The calcium contents of the TCP and GRADIENT constructs at week 0 are not reported because of insufficient sample size ($n < 3$). **(A)** Total calcium content in micrograms per construct. **(B)** Normalized calcium content in micrograms per micrograms DNA. All values are expressed as the average ± SD ($n = 3–5$), $p < 0.05$. @Statistically significant change over week 0 value, #statistically significant change over its value at previous time point, *statistically significant change over the PLGA group at same time point, $statistically significant change over the TCP and GRADIENT groups at same time point, &statistically significant change over the TCP group at same time point, ^statistically significant change over the GRADIENT group at same time point, and %statistically significant change over the CS group at same time point.

content (**Figure 7B**) of PLGA scaffolds at week 3 was statistically significantly higher than the normalized calcium contents in the CS, TCP, and GRADIENT groups. Additionally, the normalized calcium content in the TCP group at week 3 was statistically significantly higher than the normalized calcium contents of the CS and GRADIENT groups. Furthermore, at week 6, the PLGA group's normalized calcium content was significantly higher than the normalized calcium content in the CS, TCP, and GRADIENT groups. The normalized calcium contents in the PLGA group at weeks 3 and 6 were statistically significantly higher than its corresponding value at week 0. However, the normalized calcium contents in the PLGA and TCP groups at week 6 were statistically significantly lower than their corresponding values at week 3. Again, it is to be emphasized that the values of calcium content are intended to represent the calcium present in the ECM secreted by the cells, and the calcium released from the microspheres and retained by the construct, and not the calcium still entrapped within the polymeric matrix.

ALP Activity

At week 0, the ALP activities in the TCP and GRADIENT groups were 2.2- ($p < 0.05$) and 2.5-fold ($p < 0.05$) higher than the ALP activity in the PLGA group (**Figure 8**). Moreover, the ALP activities in the TCP and GRADIENT groups at week 0 were statistically significantly higher than the ALP activity in the CS group. No significant differences were observed in the ALP activities of PLGA and CS groups at week 0, meaning that only the TCP and GRADIENT groups outperformed the PLGA control in ALP activity at that time point. No significant differences in ALP activity were observed over time in the PLGA and CS groups. However, it

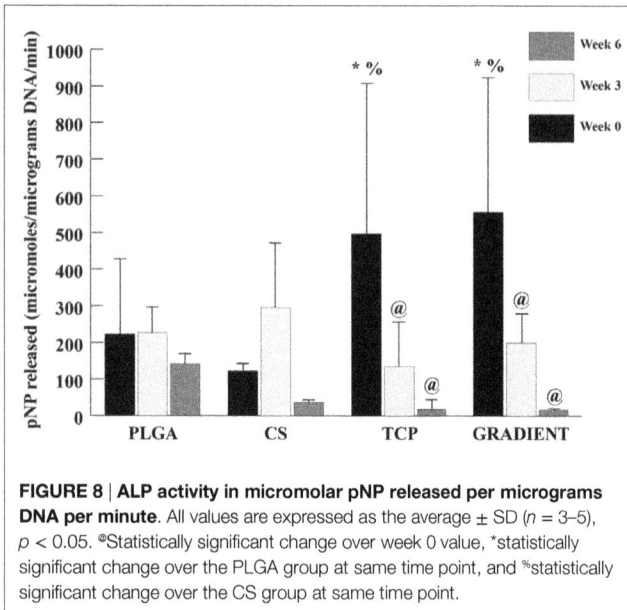

FIGURE 8 | ALP activity in micromolar pNP released per micrograms DNA per minute. All values are expressed as the average ± SD ($n = 3$–5), $p < 0.05$. @Statistically significant change over week 0 value, *statistically significant change over the PLGA group at same time point, and %statistically significant change over the CS group at same time point.

was observed that the ALP activities of the TCP and GRADIENT groups at week 0 were statistically significantly higher than their corresponding values at weeks 3 and 6.

Gene Expression
SOX9 and COL2A1

Relative SOX9 expression (**Figure 9A**) showed no significant differences among groups at week 0 and also no significant differences among the CS, TCP, and GRADIENT groups at week 1.5. The SOX9 expression for PLGA group is not reported at week 1.5 due to insufficient sample size ($n < 3$ as some of the samples were lost during processing). The SOX9 expression for the PLGA group at week 3 was statistically significantly higher than the SOX9 expression of the CS, TCP, and GRADIENT groups. No significant differences among groups were observed in the SOX9 expression at week 6. The PLGA group was found to have statistically significantly higher SOX9 expression at week 3 than at weeks 0 and 6. No significant differences over time were observed in SOX9 expression within any of the other three groups.

The COL2A1 (collagen II) expression (**Figure 9B**) in the PLGA group followed a trend similar to SOX9 expression. No significant differences were observed in COL2A1 expression among the PLGA, CS, and GRADIENT groups at week 0 (the TCP group collagen II expression at week 0 is not reported due to insufficient sample size). The COL2A1 expression of the PLGA group at week 1.5 was statistically significantly higher than the COL2A1 expression of the CS and TCP groups. Additionally, the PLGA group had statistically significantly higher COL2A1 expression than the CS, TCP, and the GRADIENT groups at week 3. The CS group at week 3 had significantly higher COL2A1 expression than the TCP and GRADIENT groups. No significant differences in COL2A1 expression between the other two groups were observed at week 3. The CS group at week 6 outperformed the PLGA group in COL2A1 expression with 2.7-fold ($p < 0.05$)

higher expression. Moreover, the CS group was statistically significantly higher in COL2A1 expression than the TCP and GRADIENT groups. No significant differences were observed in COL2A1 expression among the other three groups at that time, meaning that only the CS group outperformed the PLGA control group in COL2A1 expression at week 6. The COL2A1 expression in the PLGA and CS groups peaked at week 3 with statistically significant higher expression at week 3 than their respective values at earlier time points of weeks 0 and 1.5; however, the expression values in these groups decreased significantly at week 6 compared to their week 3 COL2A1 expression values. No significant differences over time were observed within the other two groups.

ACAN and COL1A1

No significant differences among groups were observed in the ACAN (aggrecan) expression at week 0 (**Figure 9C**). At week 1.5, the ACAN expression in the GRADIENT group was 11.8-fold ($p < 0.05$) higher than the PLGA group. Moreover, the ACAN expression in the GRADIENT group at week 1.5 was statistically significantly higher than the CS and TCP groups. No significant differences among other three groups were observed in the ACAN expression at that time, meaning that only the GRADIENT group outperformed the PLGA control group in ACAN expression at week 1.5. The ACAN expression of the CS group at week 3 was 10.5-fold ($p < 0.05$) higher than the PLGA group. In addition, the ACAN expression in the CS group at week 1.5 was significantly higher than the expression levels in the TCP and GRADIENT groups. Only the CS group outperformed the PLGA group in ACAN expression at week 3, as no significant differences were observed in ACAN expression among the other three groups. At week 6, the TCP group alone outperformed the PLGA group in ACAN expression with a 3.3-fold ($p < 0.05$) higher expression. Moreover, the TCP group also had statistically significantly higher expression than the CS and GRADIENT groups at week 6. No significant differences were observed in ACAN expression over time in the PLGA group. The ACAN expression in the CS group at week 3 was statistically significantly higher than the ACAN expression at the other three time points in the group. The TCP group had statistically significantly higher ACAN expression at week 6 than at weeks 0, 1.5, and 3. Lastly, the GRADIENT group had statistically significantly higher ACAN expression at week 1.5 than ACAN expression at the other 3 weeks.

The COL1A1 (collagen I) expression (**Figure 9D**) of the GRADIENT at week 1.5 was 97-fold ($p < 0.05$) higher than the COL1A1 expression of the PLGA group, which was one of the only instances where a test group outperformed the PLGA control. In addition, the COL1A1 expression of the GRADIENT group was statistically significantly higher than the COL1A1 expression levels of the CS and TCP groups. No significant differences were observed in COL1A1 expression among groups at weeks 0, 3, and 6. Additionally, the week 1.5 COL1A1 expression of the GRADIENT group was statistically significantly higher than its COL1A1 expression at any other time point. No significant differences were observed over time in any other group in the COL1A1 expression.

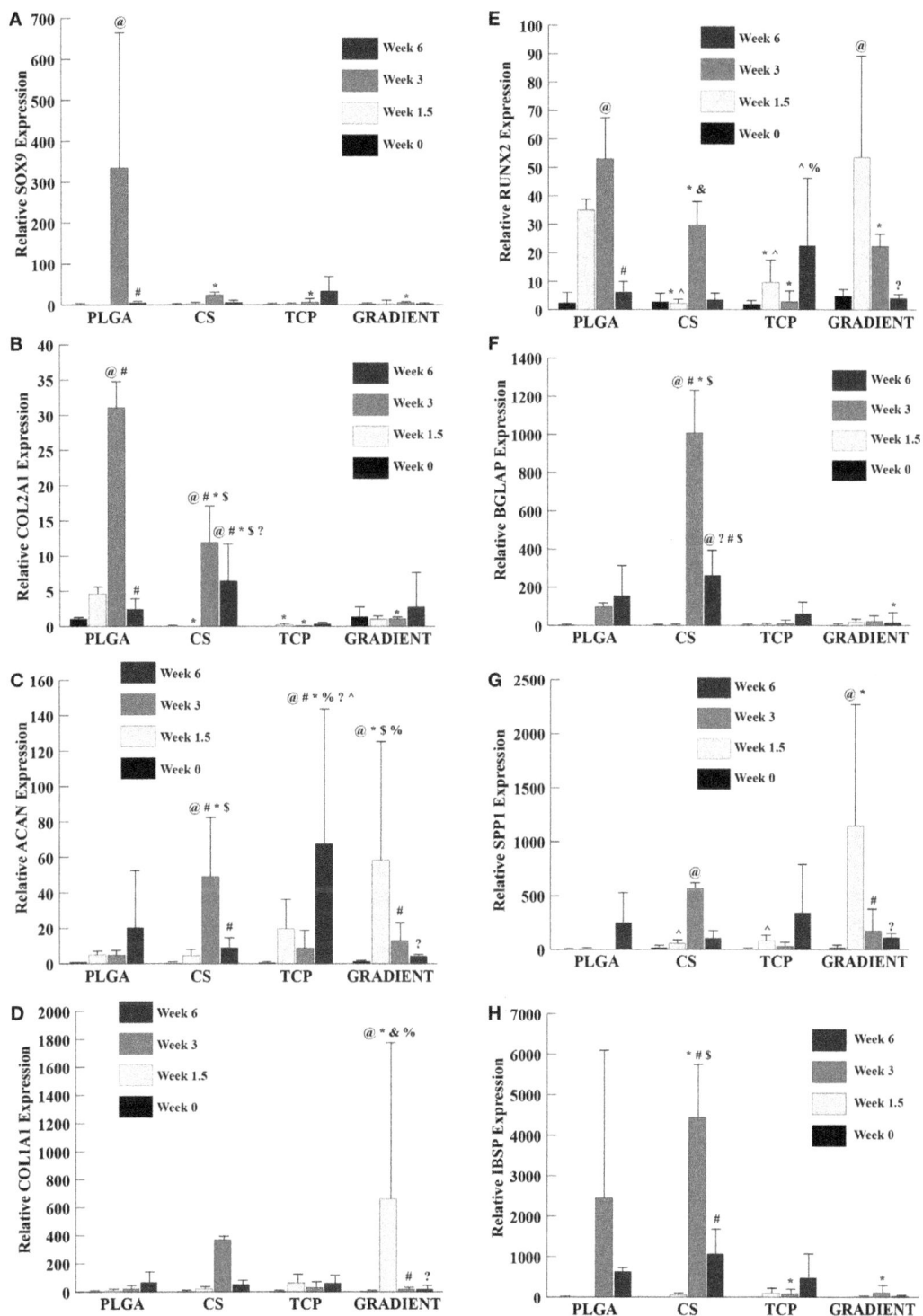

FIGURE 9 | Relative gene expression. All values are expressed as the average ± SD (n = 3–5). **(A)** SOX9 expression: the PLGA group at week 1.5 is not reported because of insufficient sample size (n < 3). **(B)** COL2A1 expression: the TCP group at week 0 is not reported because of insufficient sample size (n < 3). **(C)** ACAN expression. **(D)** COL1A1 expression. **(E)** RUNX2 expression. **(F)** BGLAP expression: the PLGA value at week 1.5 is not reported because of insufficient sample size (n < 3). **(G)** SPP1 expression. **(H)** IBSP expression: the PLGA group at week 1.5 is not reported because of insufficient

sample size (n < 3), p < 0.05. @Statistically significant change over week 0 value, #statistically significant change over its value at previous time point, *statistically significant change over the PLGA group at same time point, $statistically significant change over the TCP and GRADIENT groups at same time point, ?statistically significant change over week 1.5 value, %statistically significant change over the CS group at same time point, &statistically significant change over the TCP group at same time point, and ^statistically significant change over the GRADIENT group at same time point.

RUNX2 and BGLAP

RUNX2 expression (**Figure 9E**) showed no significant differences among groups at week 0. However, at week 1.5, the PLGA and GRADIENT groups had statistically significantly higher RUNX2 expression than the expression levels of the CS and TCP groups, but were not significantly different from each other. At week 3, the PLGA group had statistically significantly higher RUNX2 expression than the other three groups. Moreover, the CS group at week 3 had significantly higher RUNX2 expression than the TCP group. Week 6 expression levels indicated that the TCP group had significantly higher RUNX2 expression than the CS and GRADIENT groups. The PLGA RUNX2 expression at week 3 was found to be statistically significantly higher than its corresponding values at week 0 and week 6, but was not significantly different from its week 1.5 value. The GRADIENT group RUNX2 expression at week 1.5 was statistically significantly higher than at its values at weeks 0 and 6, but did not differ significantly from its value at week 3. No significant differences over time were observed in the RUNX2 expression levels of the CS and TCP groups.

BGLAP expression (**Figure 9F**) showed no significant differences among groups at week 0 and no significant differences among the CS, TCP, and GRADIENT groups at week 1.5 (PLGA value at week 1.5 is not reported because of insufficient sample size). At week 3, the CS group had 10.4-fold ($p < 0.05$) higher BGLAP expression than the PLGA group. Moreover, the CS group had statistically significantly higher BGLAP expression than the TCP and GRADIENT groups. At week 6, the PLGA group had statistically significantly higher BGLAP expression than the GRADIENT group. In addition, the CS group expression level was significantly higher than the expression levels of the TCP and GRADIENT groups. The CS group BGLAP expression at week 3 was statistically significantly higher than its values at weeks 0, 1.5, and 6, respectively. In addition, the CS group BGLAP expression at week 6 was statistically significantly higher than its values at weeks 0 and 1.5, but was significantly lower than its week 3 value. No significant differences over time were observed in the BGLAP expression within any other group.

SPP1 and IBSP

The SPP1 (osteopontin) expression (**Figure 9G**) showed no significant differences among groups at week 0. At week 1.5, the GRADIENT scaffolds had 248-fold ($p < 0.05$) higher SPP1 expression than the PLGA group, another example of gene expression in a test group outperforming the PLGA control. Moreover, the SPP1 expression in the GRADIENT group was statistically significantly higher than the CS and TCP groups. No significant differences among the CS, TCP, and GRADIENT groups were observed in the SPP1 expression levels at week 3 (the PLGA group expression at week 3 is not reported due to insufficient sample size). Again, no significant differences among groups were observed at week 6. The CS group expression at week 3 was statistically significantly higher than at week 0. The GRADIENT group expression at week 1.5 was significantly higher than at weeks 0, 3, and 6. No significant differences over time were observed within any of the remaining two groups.

IBSP expression (**Figure 9H**) showed no significant differences among the CS, TCP, and GRADIENT groups at week 1.5 (the values for CS, TCP, and GRADIENT groups at week 0; and the PLGA group at week 1.5 are not reported because of insufficient sample size). At week 3, the IBSP expression of the CS group was 1.8-fold ($p < 0.05$) higher than the PLGA group. In addition, the CS group IBSP expression at week 3 was statistically significantly higher than the TCP and GRADIENT groups. The PLGA group at week 3 also had significantly higher expression than the TCP and GRADIENT groups. No significant differences among groups were observed at week 6. The CS group IBSP expression at week 3 was statistically significantly higher than at weeks 1.5 and 6. No significant differences were observed over time within any of the other groups.

Discussion

The current study for the first time demonstrated the feasibility of raw material encapsulation in high molecular weight PLGA microsphere-based scaffolds that could potentially be used in large animal models or human patients. This work builds on our previous efforts that spoke of the advantages of raw material encapsulation (in conjunction with growth factors) toward creating a new tissue-specific ECM in low molecular weight PLGA scaffolds (Mohan et al., 2013). Furthermore, employing opposing gradients of CS and TCP to provide bioactive cues and building blocks for simultaneous chondrogenic and osteogenic differentiation of cells is a promising approach for osteochondral interfacial tissue engineering. Additionally, to the best of our knowledge, we are the first group to encapsulate TCP in microsphere-based scaffolds for the bone part of our scaffolds. Most of the other groups utilizing microsphere-based scaffolds have relied on other calcium phosphates and minerals for engineering the bone tissue (Cushnie et al., 2008; Lv et al., 2009; Tahriri and Moztarzadeh, 2014; Xu et al., 2014).

The scanning electron microscopy (SEM) images, depicting the overall porous nature of microsphere-based scaffolds with interconnections among the pores, were in agreement with our previous findings with these scaffolds fabricated with low molecular weight PLGA (Singh et al., 2008). Moreover, raw material encapsulation did not affect the spherical nature of the microspheres; however, it was found to have altered the microstructure of the microspheres. Specifically, the CS microspheres had a porous surface that could be attributed to the solvent removal process during the microsphere fabrication step, as we have also observed previously (Mohan et al., 2013). The presence of sub-micron pores on the CS microspheres contributed toward higher average porosity in these scaffolds compared to the other three groups. The TCP encapsulating microspheres, on the other hand, did not possess pores on their surfaces, but had a rough surface instead. The surface roughness of these microspheres, specifically the presence of ridge-like features, may have resulted from the partitioning of TCP particles on the surface of the microspheres. These surface characteristics of raw material encapsulating microspheres may have great implications in cell attachment or anchorage and also in diffusion of nutrients and wastes in and out of the scaffolds (Persson et al., 2014; Wu et al., 2014). Furthermore, raw material encapsulation impacted the cellular morphology of the seeded rBMSCs. Flat cells with significant cell spreading were observed in the CS and GRADIENT groups while cluster forming round cells could be seen in the TCP and GRAIDENT groups. Though the GRADIENT group contained both flat and round cells, no differences in cell morphologies were observed in cells from distinct regions of the scaffold. The different cell morphologies on microsphere-based scaffolds might suggest that cells responded favorably to the encapsulated raw materials, at least initially, which may have influenced their differentiation along discrete pathways. This initial cellular response to encapsulated raw materials could have pivotal significance in regenerating interfacial tissues that require differentiation of cells from a single source along multiple pathways.

Mechanical testing results demonstrated the compressive moduli of microsphere-based scaffolds to be in the range of articular cartilage (0.1–0.9 MPa) and within an order of magnitude of the moduli for cancellous bone (0.01–2 GPa) (Keaveny and Hayes, 1993; Mansour, 2003; Williams et al., 2003). Moreover, the elastic modulus of TCP scaffolds at week 0 was found to be at least three times as large as any other group, thereby conforming to the observations of Lv et al. demonstrating that calcium phosphates enhance the mechanical properties of polymeric scaffolds (Lv et al., 2009). However, at week 6, the cell seeded TCP constructs had significantly higher modulus than the CS group alone. All the other groups, except for the CS group, had an increase in their elastic moduli from week 0. Differences among groups in degradation rates of the scaffolds, cell proliferation within the scaffolds, and ECM deposition could have all contributed to the increase in moduli. PLGA microspheres are known to degrade via bulk erosion where the rate-limiting step is the diffusion of water molecules into the microsphere core. CS microspheres because of their porous nature may have allowed faster diffusion of the water molecules into their core, thereby initiating the polymer degradation more quickly than in the other three groups. Higher glycolic acid content in PLGA (PLGA50:50) of CS microspheres may have further accelerated polymer degradation in the CS group (Alexis, 2004). Additionally, swelling (Table S3 in Supplementary Material) caused by penetration of water inside of the microspheres may have also played a part in the drop in elastic modulus of CS scaffolds (Mohan et al., 2013). On the other hand, swelling was absent (PLGA and TCP groups) or less pronounced (GRADIENT group) in the other three groups compared to the CS group, which may have prevented the drop in elastic moduli of scaffolds from the PLGA, TCP, and GRADIENT groups at week 6. Moreover, polymer composition (PLGA75:25) and microsphere morphology (absence of minute pores on surface) may have allowed the PLGA, TCP, and GRADIENT scaffolds to further retain their mechanical properties. Surprisingly, the PLGA scaffolds had a tremendous increase in modulus from week 0 to week 6, translating to an elastic modulus orders of magnitude higher than the moduli of the other three groups at week 6. We previously observed a similar trend in elastic moduli in raw material encapsulating low molecular weight PLGA scaffolds where deviations from the overall scaffold structure at week 6 led to a significant increase in elastic modulus (Mohan et al., 2013). Additionally, the elastic moduli of high molecular weight PLGA acellular scaffolds at week 6 (unpublished data) also hinted toward a similar phenomenon.

Therefore, it is speculated that cellular contributions, in conjunction with polymer degradation, led to microscopic changes in the scaffold morphology (closure of pores) that caused the elastic moduli of PLGA constructs to jump at week 6. However, further investigation is needed to better understand the degradation in these high molecular weight PLGA scaffolds and the mechanism of increase in their compressive moduli with time. Altogether, results from the mechanical testing provided information that would be valuable in designing microsphere-based scaffolds for future *in vitro* and *in vivo* studies in rabbits, sheep, etc.

The biochemical content results were found to be consistent with the SEM observations. A small number of cells were observed on the PLGA scaffolds at Day 10, which agreed with the DNA content analysis that revealed low quantities of DNA on these scaffolds throughout the 6-week culture period. By contrast, the DNA contents of all the raw material encapsulating groups increased over time with significant differences appearing at week 6. Our DNA results on microsphere-based scaffolds suggest that raw material encapsulation encouraged rBMSC proliferation on these scaffolds, thus agreeing with the findings of some other groups showing that the raw materials such as CS and β-TCP could cast a positive influence on the proliferative capacity of rBMSCs (Takahashi et al., 2005; Uygun et al., 2009; Todo and Arahira, 2013; Kim et al., 2014). GAG data showed that the CS group had at least a threefold higher GAG content than the rest of the groups at week 6. Since the GAG content of acellular constructs (Table S1 in Supplementary Material) was subtracted at each time point, it is to be stressed that the data primarily represented GAG secreted by the cells and also released CS entrapped within the newly synthesized ECM. A trend similar to GAG content was seen in the HYP content of CS scaffolds suggesting that the encapsulated CS played a significant role in enhancing the cellular GAG and collagen secretion, thus having a modulatory effect on the seeded rBMSCs. However, observance of lower normalized GAG and HYP content in the CS group than the PLGA group suggest that the bioactive effects seen due to CS encapsulation may have been primarily due to the improvement in cellularity without sacrificing biosynthesis on a per cell basis. Calcium content analysis revealed some unanticipated results. The CS group had significantly higher net calcium content than the other groups at week 6, and the PLGA group was higher in calcium per DNA content compared to rest of the groups at that time. The counter-intuitive phenomenon of high calcium (or calcium per DNA) contents in the CS and PLGA groups could be attributed to culture medium components, such as DEX, β-GP, and IGF-I. DEX is a glucocorticoid, which is used extensively *in vitro* as an osteogenic factor. β-GP is the common source for MSCs to form CaP deposits *in vitro* (Shi et al., 2010; Fiorentini et al., 2011). IGF-I is an anabolic signal that does not necessarily influence the proliferation and differentiation of MSCs toward osteoblasts on its own, but it is an important molecule directing the differentiation of already osteogenically committed cells (Hayrapetyan et al., 2014). Thus, the presence of these components likely influenced the commitment of rBMSCs on the microsphere-based scaffolds toward osteogenesis. Furthermore, the ALP activities of the TCP and GRADIENT groups at week 0 were higher than their activities at week 6. The elevated ALP activities in these constructs at earlier time points may have been due to the medium components.

However, failure to observe a similar effect in the other two groups hint that TCP encapsulation might have influenced their behavior initially as seen with the SEM micrographs as well. Lastly, higher normalized HYP and calcium contents in the TCP encapsulating scaffold groups than the CS group at later time points suggest that TCP encapsulation may have improved rBMSC performance by promoting their differentiation in addition to enhancing their proliferation (as seen with DNA content results).

Gene expression results were in agreement with the other results of the study. Relatively higher expressions of SOX9, COL2A1, and RUNX2 by the cells in the PLGA group at week 3 followed by higher mineral content at week 6 (as indicated by the biochemical data) suggest that the DEX in culture the medium may have caused the rBMSCs in the PLGA scaffolds to go down the osteogenic pathway via a cartilage-like intermediate. Higher expression levels of chondrogenic markers (collagen II and aggrecan), in conjunction with up regulation of osteogenic markers (BGLAP and IBSP) by the cells in the CS group at week 3 than compared to the initial time points, suggest a similar phenomenon as observed in the PLGA group. Lower expression of BGLAP and IBSP in the TCP group than the CS group suggests that TCP presence inhibited expression of osteogenic markers by creating a substrate environment that was already high in mineral content, a phenomenon previously observed with hydroxyapatite encapsulating low molecular weight PLGA microsphere-based scaffolds (Dormer et al., 2012a). The cells in the GRADIENT group showed relatively higher expression of ACAN and SPP1 (along with higher expression of RUNX2 by the cells in the group than at week 0) than the cells in the PLGA control group at week 1.5. The higher expression of some chondrogenic and osteogenic markers in the GRADIENT group at earlier time points may be due to faster maturation of rBMSCs toward cartilage- and bone-like cells in this group; however, more evidence is needed to reinforce this speculation.

Overall, the results of the current study indicate that raw material encapsulation into microsphere-based scaffolds influenced the behavior of the seeded rBMSCs. Differences in the cell morphologies and greater cell numbers in the raw material groups leading to enhanced matrix synthesis in these groups demonstrates that the raw materials provide a head start in the (re)generation of tissues. It is of interest to infer the amount of matrix synthesized by cells in the scaffolds beyond the exogenously included amounts. Therefore, the biochemical content (CS and calcium) for the acellular constructs was subtracted from the content of the cell seeded constructs, assuming that the acellular scaffolds degrade and release encapsulated molecules at the same rate as their cellular counterparts. However, we acknowledge that this assumption is weak as cells synthesizing new matrix, and perhaps altering the surrounding pH, etc., will influence the polymer degradation rate, but with the higher molecular weight PLGA, it should be a reasonable approximation that allows us to better evaluate differences among groups due to cellular contribution. In addition, static seeding approach employed in this study has limitations associated with it due to the manual- and operator-dependent nature of the process. However, we followed a uniform manual seeding procedure, and we think that the differences observed in the DNA content at week 0 (24 h post seeding) among various scaffold type might have resulted more from the differences in cell attachment arising due

to differences in scaffold composition than arising from variations in cell seeding. Moreover, we did not specifically explore the dosing effect of CS and TCP, but our group has demonstrated in the past that the concentration of the raw materials can have a significant effect on the differentiation of the cells (Dormer et al., 2012a). Additionally, higher cell number, greater biochemical content, and relatively higher expression of some osteogenic and chondrogenic markers in the GRADIENT group accentuated the advantages of using gradient-based strategies for engineering the osteochondral interface. However, we recognize that these scaffolds not being amenable to histology due to the stiffness of the polymer constructs, given the high molecular weight and slow degradation of the PLGA, was a limitation of the study that would have further elaborated the differences among groups based on their regional material composition, but we have substantiated previously both *in vitro* and *in vivo* that regionalized tissue formation occurs in raw material gradient microsphere-based engineered constructs (Mohan et al., 2011, 2013). Furthermore, the initial effects of raw material encapsulation on a per-cell basis might have been obscured by the culture medium components that appeared to favor osteogenesis. However, it is to be noted that *in vitro* advancements observed initially with raw material encapsulation could translate *in vivo* to a more favorable interaction with infiltrating MSCs, and perhaps facilitate differentiation in a native environment rather than in a medium-governed environment. Lastly, an important consideration in designing scaffolds for clinical use is determining the mechanical integrity. We have shown in our prior work that microsphere-based scaffolds possess adequate mechanical properties for the regeneration of osteochondral tissues and the encapsulation of raw materials may impact those properties (Dormer et al., 2010, 2012a; Mohan et al., 2013). Our mechanical testing results in the current study also agreed with our previous findings; additionally, the results also suggested that the mechanical properties of microsphere-based scaffolds can be impacted by scaffold degradation and cellular matrix synthesized by the seeded cells. Additional cyclic testing in the future may yield interesting information about degree of hysteresis and narrower strain ranges about a fixed strain point (e.g., 5%), with a frequency sweep could yield interesting tan delta profiles as well, which we will consider for future studies.

Altogether, the overall findings emphasize the need to further refine the technology, perhaps by adjusting raw material concentration or by altering PLGA degradation rate. The degradation of the polymer will play a key role in tissue regeneration *in vivo*, where premature failure in scaffold mechanical properties can have a deleterious effect on the regenerating tissue, and extended degradation by contrast could become an obstacle to tissue regeneration. Therefore, it is important to identify a polymer with a biodegradation rate comparable to the neo-tissue formation rate. Additionally, identifying raw material concentrations that are most efficacious in promoting osteogenesis and chondrogenesis would yield valuable information, which could then be leveraged for tailoring scaffold degradation in future sheep or any other large animal model studies. Nevertheless, the current study highlights several benefits of raw material microsphere gradient scaffold technology. The raw material encapsulating microsphere-based scaffolds attempt to regenerate both cartilage and bone simultaneously, thus stressing on the importance of growing cartilage and bone within the physical proximity of each other; many signaling pathways and endogenous proteins responsible for progenitor cell commitment to the osteoblast or chondrocyte lineages have a high degree of interrelatedness (Gordeladze et al., 2009). The raw materials apart from being conductive to tissue (re) generation can also provide inductive signals to the surrounding cells guiding their differentiation. In addition, the raw materials provide clinical significance to microsphere gradient scaffolds, as these scaffolds may be tactically placed for swifter and less costly regulatory approval.

Conclusion

The present study assessed the *in vitro* response of microsphere-based scaffolds with clinical relevance fabricated using a raw material approach. Overall, the results demonstrated that the primary improvements observed with the raw materials-CS and TCP were more due to greater initial interaction with cells and greater cellularity with comparable performance on a per-cell basis rather than on specifically driving differentiation. Moreover, the medium-governed environment that seemed to favor osteogenesis concealed the initial *in vitro* advancements observed with raw material encapsulation. Additionally, there was also evidence of

faster maturation of rBMSCs in the raw material GRADIENT constructs that can be leveraged further to engineer the complex osteochondral interface. Therefore, a strategy combining the "building block" side of the raw material philosophy (as we have done here) with the "signaling" side, for example, by including hydroxyapatite with the TCP, or maybe TGF-β with CS, or by altering the dose of CS (without TGF-β); in a scaffold with a bio-degradation rate comparable to the neo-tissue formation rate, we may be able to achieve the differentiation profiles we seek *in vitro*.

Acknowledgments

This publication was supported by the National Institute of Arthritis and Musculoskeletal and Skin Diseases of the National Institutes of Health under Award Number R01 AR056347. The content is solely the responsibility of the authors and does not necessarily represent the official views of the National Institutes of Health. We would also like to acknowledge support from the Kansas Bioscience Authority Rising Star Award.

References

Alexis, F. (2004). Factors affecting the degradation and drug-release mechanism of poly(lactic acid) and poly[(lactic acid)-co-(glycolic acid)]. *Polym. Int.* 54, 36–46. doi:10.1002/pi.1697

Berkland, C., Kim, K., and Pack, D. W. (2001). Fabrication of PLG microspheres with precisely controlled and monodisperse size distributions. *J. Control. Release* 73, 59–74. doi:10.1016/S0168-3659(01)00289-9

Boyan, B. D., Schwartz, Z., Bonewald, L., and Swain, L. (1989). Localization of 1, 25-(OH) 2D3-responsive alkaline phosphatase in osteoblast-like cells (ROS 17/2.8, MG 63, and MC 3T3) and growth cartilage cells in culture. *J. Biol. Chem.* 264, 11879–11886.

Chen, W.-C., Wei, Y.-H., Chu, I. M., and Yao, C.-L. (2013). Effect of chondroitin sulphate C on the in vitro and in vivo chondrogenesis of mesenchymal stem cells in crosslinked type II collagen scaffolds. *J. Tissue Eng. Regen. Med.* 7, 665–672. doi:10.1002/term.1463

Cushnie, E. K., Khan, Y. M., and Laurencin, C. T. (2008). Amorphous hydroxy-apatite-sintered polymeric scaffolds for bone tissue regeneration: physical characterization studies. *J. Biomed. Mater. Res. A.* 84, 54–62. doi:10.1002/jbm.a.31380

Detamore, M. S., and Athanasiou, K. A. (2003). Tensile properties of the porcine temporomandibular joint disc. *J. Biomech. Eng.* 125, 558–558. doi:10.1115/1.1589778

Dormer, N. H., Busaidy, K., Berkland, C. J., and Detamore, M. S. (2011). Osteochondral interface regeneration of rabbit mandibular condyle with bioactive signal gradients. *J. Oral Maxillofac. Surg.* 69, e50–e57. doi:10.1016/j.joms.2010.12.049

Dormer, N. H., Qiu, Y., Lydick, A. M., Allen, N. D., Mohan, N., Berkland, C. J., et al. (2012a). Osteogenic differentiation of human bone marrow stromal cells in hydroxyapatite-loaded microsphere-based scaffolds. *Tissue Eng. Part A* 18, 757–767. doi:10.1089/ten.TEA.2011.0176

Dormer, N. H., Singh, M., Zhao, L., Mohan, N., Berkland, C. J., and Detamore, M. S. (2012b). Osteochondral interface regeneration of the rabbit knee with macroscopic gradients of bioactive signals. *J. Biomed. Mater. Res. A.* 100, 162–170. doi:10.1002/jbm.a.33225

Dormer, N. H., Singh, M., Wang, L., Berkland, C. J., and Detamore, M. S. (2010). Osteochondral interface tissue engineering using macroscopic gradients of bioactive signals. *Ann. Biomed. Eng.* 38, 2167–2182. doi:10.1007/s10439-010-0028-0

Fiorentini, E., Granchi, D., Leonardi, E., Baldini, N., and Ciapetti, G. (2011). Effects of osteogenic differentiation inducers on in vitro expanded adult mesenchymal stromal cells. *Int. J. Artif. Organs* 34, 998–1011. doi:10.5301/ijao.5000001

Fonseca, C., Caminal, M., Peris, D., Barrachina, J., Fabregas, P. J., Garcia, F., et al. (2014). An arthroscopic approach for the treatment of osteochondral focal defects with cell-free and cell-loaded PLGA scaffolds in sheep. *Cytotechnology* 66, 345–354. doi:10.1007/s10616-013-9581-3

Gordeladze, J. O., Djouad, F., and Brondello, J. M. (2009). Concerted stimuli reg-ulating osteo-chondral differentiation from stem cells: phenotype acquisition regulated by microRNAs. *Acta Pharmacol. Sin.* 30, 1369–1384. doi:10.1038/aps.2009.143

Hayrapetyan, A., Jansen, J. A., and Van Den Beucken, J. J. J. P. (2014). Signaling pathways involved in osteogenesis and their application for bone regenerative medicine. *Tissue Eng. Part B Rev.* 21, 75–87. doi:10.1089/ten.TEB.2014.0119

Jeon, J. H., Bhamidipati, M., Sridharan, B., Scurto, A. M., Berkland, C. J., and Detamore, M. S. (2013). Tailoring of processing parameters for sintering microsphere-based scaffolds with dense-phase carbon dioxide. *J. Biomed. Mater. Res. B Appl. Biomater.* 101, 330–337. doi:10.1002/jbm.b.32843

Keaveny, T. M., and Hayes, W. C. (1993). Mechanical properties of cortical and trabecular bone. *Bone* 7, 285–344.

Kim, H. D., Heo, J., Hwang, Y., Kwak, S.-Y., Park, O. K., Kim, H., et al. (2014). Extracellular-matrix-based and Arg-Gly-Asp-modified photopolymerizing hydro-gels for cartilage tissue engineering. *Tissue Eng. Part A* 21, 757–766. doi:10.1089/ten.TEA.2014.0233

Liao, H.-T., Lee, M.-Y., Tsai, W.-W., Wang, H.-C., and Lu, W.-C. (2013). Osteogenesis of adipose-derived stem cells on polycaprolactone-β-tricalcium phosphate scaffold fabricated via selective laser sintering and surface coating with collagen type I. *J. Tissue Eng. Regen. Med.* doi:10.1002/term.1811

Lv, Q., Nair, L., and Laurencin, C. T. (2009). Fabrication, characterization, and in vitro evaluation of poly(lactic acid glycolic acid)/nano-hydroxyapatite composite microsphere-based scaffolds for bone tissue engineering in rotating bioreactors. *J. Biomed. Mater. Res. A.* 91, 679–691. doi:10.1002/jbm.a.32302

Mansour, J. M. (2003). "Biomechanics of cartilage," in *Kinesiology: the Mechanics and Pathomechanics of Human Movement*, ed. C. A. Oatis (Philadelphia: Lippincott Williams and Wilkins), 66–79.

Mohan, N., Dormer, N. H., Caldwell, K. L., Key, V. H., Berkland, C. J., and Detamore, M. S. (2011). Continuous gradients of material composition and growth factors for effective regeneration of the osteochondral interface. *Tissue Eng. Part A* 17, 2845–2855. doi:10.1089/ten.tea.2011.0135

Mohan, N., Gupta, V., Sridharan, B., Sutherland, A., and Detamore, M. S. (2013). The potential of encapsulating "raw materials" in 3D osteochondral gradient scaffolds. *Biotechnol. Bioeng.* 111, 829–841. doi:10.1002/bit.25145

Pearce, A., Richards, R., Milz, S., Schneider, E., and Pearce, S. (2007). Animal models for implant biomaterial research in bone: a review. *Eur. Cell. Mater.* 13, 1–10.

Persson, M., Lorite, G. S., Kokkonen, H. E., Cho, S.-W., Lehenkari, P. P., Skrifvars, M., et al. (2014). Effect of bioactive extruded PLA/HA composite films on focal adhesion formation of preosteoblastic cells. *Colloids Surf. B Biointerfaces* 121, 409–416. doi:10.1016/j.colsurfb.2014.06.029

Shi, X., Wang, Y., Varshney, R. R., Ren, L., Gong, Y., and Wang, D.-A. (2010). Microsphere-based drug releasing scaffolds for inducing osteogenesis of human mesenchymal stem cells in vitro. *Eur. J. Pharm. Sci.* 39, 59–67. doi:10.1016/j.ejps.2009.10.012

Singh, M. (2008). Tensile properties of the mandibular condylar cartilage. *J. Biomech. Eng.* 130, 011009. doi:10.1115/1.2838062

Singh, M., Morris, C. P., Ellis, R. J., Detamore, M. S., and Berkland, C. (2008). Microsphere-based seamless scaffolds containing macroscopic gradients of encapsulated factors for tissue engineering. *Tissue Eng. Part C Methods* 14, 299–309. doi:10.1089/ten.tec.2008.0167

Tahriri, M., and Moztarzadeh, F. (2014). Preparation, characterization, and in vitro biological evaluation of PLGA/nano-fluorohydroxyapatite (FHA) microsphere-sintered scaffolds for biomedical applications. *Appl. Biochem. Biotechnol.* 172, 2465–2479. doi:10.1007/s12010-013-0696-y

Takahashi, Y., Yamamoto, M., and Tabata, Y. (2005). Osteogenic differentiation of mesenchymal stem cells in biodegradable sponges composed of gelatin and β-tricalcium phosphate. *Biomaterials* 26, 3587–3596. doi:10.1016/j.biomaterials.2004.09.046

Todo, M., and Arahira, T. (2013). In vitro bone formation by mesenchymal stem cells with 3D collagen/β-TCP composite scaffold. *Conf. Proc. IEEE Eng. Med. Biol. Soc.* 2013, 409–412. doi:10.1109/EMBC.2013.6609523

Tracy, M. (1999). Factors affecting the degradation rate of poly(lactide-co-glycolide) microspheres in vivo and in vitro. *Biomaterials* 20, 1057–1062. doi:10.1016/S0142-9612(99)00002-2

Uygun, B. E., Stojsih, S. E., and Matthew, H. W. T. (2009). Effects of immobilized glycosaminoglycans on the proliferation and differentiation of mesenchymal stem cells. *Tissue Eng. Part A* 15, 3499–3512. doi:10.1089/ten.TEA.2008.0405

Williams, S. K., Amiel, D., Ball, S. T., Allen, R. T., Wong, V. W., Chen, A. C., et al. (2003). Prolonged storage effects on the articular cartilage of fresh human osteochondral allografts. *J. Bone Joint Surg. Am.* 85, 2111–2120.

Wu, S. D., Zhang, H., Dong, X. D., Ning, C. Y., and Fok, A. (2014). Physicochemical properties and in vitro cytocompatibility of modified titanium surfaces prepared via micro-arc oxidation with different calcium concentrations. *Appl. Surf.* 329, 347–355. doi:10.1016/j.apsusc.2014.12.039

Xu, W., Wang, L., Ling, Y., Wei, K., and Zhong, S. (2014). Enhancement of compressive strength and cytocompatibility using apatite coated hexagonal mesoporous silica/poly(lactic acid-glycolic acid) microsphere scaffolds for bone tissue engineering. *RSC Adv.* 4, 13495. doi:10.1039/c4ra00626g

Conflict of Interest Statement: The authors declare that the research was conducted in the absence of any commercial or financial relationships that could be construed as a potential conflict of interest.

12

Sensing the difference: the influence of anisotropic cues on cell behavior

José Ballester-Beltrán [1], Manus J. P. Biggs [2], Matthew J. Dalby [3], Manuel Salmerón-Sánchez [1] and Aldo Leal-Egaña [2]*

[1] Division of Biomedical Engineering, School of Engineering, University of Glasgow, Glasgow, UK, [2] Network of Excellence for Functional Biomaterials, National University of Ireland, Galway, Ireland, [3] Institute of Molecular, Cell and Systems Biology, University of Glasgow, Glasgow, UK

From tissue morphogenesis to homeostasis, cells continuously experience and respond to physical, chemical, and biological cues commonly presented in gradients. In this article, we focus our discussion on the importance of nano/micro topographic cues on cell activity, and the role of anisotropic milieus play on cell behavior, mostly adhesion and migration. We present the need to study physiological gradients *in vitro*. To do this, we review different cell migration mechanisms and how adherent cells react to the presence of complex tissue-like environments and cell-surface stimulation in 2D and 3D (e.g., ventral/dorsal anisotropy).

Keywords: surface topography, anisotropic materials, cell–biomaterial interface, cell–matrix anchorage, topographical cues

Edited by:
Elena Martinez,
Institute for Bioengineering of
Catalonia, Spain

Reviewed by:
Dimitrios I. Zeugolis,
National University of Ireland, Ireland
Justin Lee Brown,
Pennsylvania State University, USA

*Correspondence:
Aldo Leal-Egaña,
Center for Cell Engineering, Institute
of Molecular, Cell and Systems
Biology, University of Glasgow,
CMVLS, Joseph Black Building,
Glasgow G12 8QQ, UK
aldo.leal-egana@glasgow.ac.uk

Introduction

When considering cell response to topographical cues, we initially think on classical contact guidance to grooves. This was first reported in 1911, when Harrison observed cells aligning to spider silk (Harrison, 1911). In the 1950s, Weiss and Garber termed this phenomenon contact guidance (Weiss and Garber, 1952). The field was popularized in the 1980s through a collaboration between a cell biologist, Adam Curtis, and an electronic engineer interested in miniaturization, Curtis and Wilkinson (1997), who observed that surface topography gradients can be sensed by adherent cells at the microscale and later, the nanoscale.

In this article, we will focus on the design of novel anisotropic polymeric surfaces and how different parameters influence cell fate. Then, we will review cell migration mechanisms in different environments and the influence that bi-phasic (ventral/dorsal) gradients play on cell activity in *in vivo*-like milieus.

Anisotropic Topography and Cellular Function

Anisotropic Biomaterials

The interplay between heterogeneity and anisotropy persists as the predominat strategy adapted by nature to optimize the function of biological materials. The former relates to the spatial variation (point to point) of the material properties, whereas the latter closely relates to the directional dependence (Ranganathan et al., 2011). Material topography, and in particular micro and nanoscale anisotropic structures, can affect cellular morphology as well as cellular behavior (**Table 1**) (Losert et al., 2013; Cassidy et al., 2014; Londono et al., 2014; Azeem et al., 2015). It is thus necessary to develop a fundamental understanding on the mechanistic processes induced by anisotropic structures in cell biology, in order to gain further insights into the design of biological materials.

TABLE 1 | Topographic characteristic of several of anisotropic polymer scaffolds and their influence on cellular differentiation.

Height/depth	Width	Pitch	Cell type	Differential function	Reference
650 nm	500 nm	3.0 μm	Upregulation of neuronal markers β-Tubulin III and NeuN	Upregulation of neuronal markers β-Tubulin III	Marino et al. (2013)
4.0 μm	2.0 μm	4.0 μm	Primary murine neural progenitor cells	Upregulation of neuronal marker TUJ1	Wang et al. (2012) and Chua et al. (2014)
250 nm	250 nm	500 nm	Human embryonic stem cell line, H1	Upregulation of neuronal markers MAP2	Ankam et al. (2015)
2.0 μm	2.0 μm	4.0 μm	Murine neural progenitor cells	Upregulation of neuronal markers TH, MAP2, and PITX3	Tan et al. (2015)
625 nm	1500 nm	3 μm	Human neural stem cells	Upregulation of neuronal Tuj1 and MAP2 and glial markers GFAP, O4, and Olig2	Yang et al. (2014)
150 nm	250 nm	500 nm	Human MSC	Upregulation of fibro/superficial zone cartilage formation markers PRG4 and COL1	Wu et al. (2014)
200 nm	415 nm	830 nm	Human MSC	No upregulation in the osteospecific marker ALP	Janson et al. (2014)

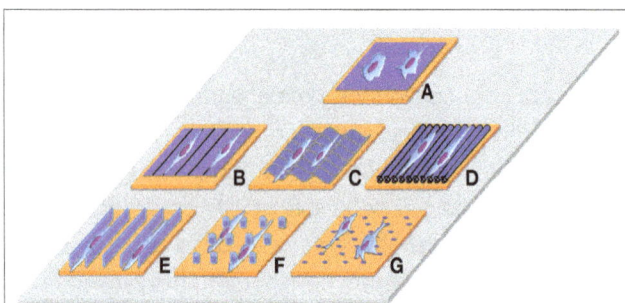

FIGURE 1 | Traditional surfaces used to culture cells on 2D without/with nano/micro topographic cues. (A) Flat surface, **(B)** contact guidance lines, **(C)** grooves, **(D)** aligned fibers, **(E)** 2D confined environments, **(F)** nano/micro pillars **(G)** nano/micro pits.

Novel techniques of nanofabrication and material processing, such as lithographic (Diehl et al., 2005; Zhu et al., 2005; Dalby et al., 2006; Smith et al., 2014) self-assembly (Tsai et al., 2014), electrospinning (Gaharwar et al., 2014), and scratching techniques (Peng et al., 2010; Wang et al., 2013a), offer the ability to create *anisotropic substrates* with feature widths and depths ranging from the macroscale to the microscale down to features sizes as small as 5 nm, facilitating the aquisition of information to help understand this field (Peng et al., 2010; Wang et al., 2013a) (**Figure 1**). These techniques are particularly suited for the generation of anisotropic micro-nanofeatures in polymeric formulations and in particular in thermoplastics. However, with specific reference to load-bearing biomaterials, the topographical modification of metals and their alloys has received much attention recently and several novel techniques including electrical anodization (Xie et al., 2011), acid etching (Att et al., 2009), and femtosecond laser processing (Tavangar et al., 2013) have recently been described.

Both micro (Itala et al., 2003; Germanier et al., 2006; Herrero-Climent et al., 2013) and nanoscale (Biggs et al., 2008; Cassidy et al., 2014; Azeem et al., 2015) groove/ridge topographies are well documented as powerful modulators of contact guidance, being relevant in tissue engineering and biomaterials manufacture. A principal design tenet of anisotropic grating substrates is that of biomimetic extracellular matrix (ECM) design, attempting to mimic the topographical structures imparted by several fibrous components of the ECM. Collagen, being the most abundant protein in the body, encompasses individual fibril elements (e.g., with dimensions of 20–30 nm) to fibril bundles (e.g., from 15–400 μm in diameter). Key to this is that nanogroove surfaces may promote cellular polarization as well as promote aligned self-assembly of ECM components with motifs critical in cell adhesion such as fibronectin and vitronectin. Indeed, the elongated cellular morphology and alignment induced by grooved substrates may resemble the natural state of tissue resident cell populations *in vivo*, and studies indicate that most, if not all, cells, notably fibroblasts (Dalby et al., 2003; Garland et al., 2014), osteoblasts (Lenhert et al., 2005; Wu and Wang, 2013), neurons (Yim et al., 2007; Tonazzini et al., 2014), and MSCs (Dalby et al., 2006; McMurray et al., 2013), undergo significant morphological and functional responses to anisotropic topographies.

The extent to which groove geometry and order can influence cell function is an often overlooked consideration in designing next generation biomaterials. Studies by Tonazzini et al. (2013) show that the loss of neurite guidance is not linear with noise on microgrooved topographies, but is a threshold effect, correlating with changes in focal adhesion (FA) maturation and spatial organization. Here, the authors found that nanogratings with a controlled amount of random nanotopographical noise – or defects – influenced neurite contact guidance at a threshold noise level of aproximately 40 to 50%. Interestingly, a further study by Gamboa and colleagues have identified that the groove orientation does not have to be linear; rather, cell can gain spatial information from anisotropic features. Indeed, cells can cross over individual grooves when they arranged in a waveform pattern, residing both inside and outside of each wave pattern, yet aligning linearly along the long axis of the pattern (Gamboa et al., 2013).

Anisotropic Topography on Cell Adhesion

Critically, nanogroove features seem to directly influence the formation and orientation of FA *in vitro* (Teixeira et al., 2004), probably due to the guiding of ECM proteins. A nice example has been described in the case of fibronectin, a protein which has been shown to selectively adsorb onto the ridge/groove boundaries (De Luca et al., 2015). At present, no clear conclusions have been reached regarding the absolute dimensions required for cellular and FA alignment; rather, this process is cell-specific and density dependent (Clark et al., 1990). It is probable, however, that an interplay between groove width and depth regulates cellular alignment, and a recent study by Crouch et al. (2009) indicated that a grating aspect ratio (depth to width) of 0.16 was required for 95% cellular alignment. Additionally, anisotropic topographies can induce alignment of sub-cellular structures including filopodia (Fujita et al., 2009), nuclei (McKee et al., 2011), and neurite extensions (Tonazzini et al., 2013).

Recent studies indicate that FA alignment is generally more pronounced on patterns with ridge widths between 1 and 5 μm than on grooves and ridged topographies with larger lateral dimensions (Biggs et al., 2008; Yang et al., 2010). Moreover, cells cultured on grooves with nanoscale widths produce FA that are non-polarized (Kim et al., 2013) or almost exclusively oriented obliquely to the topographic patterns (Teixeira et al., 2006). This occurs predominantly on topographical ridges as opposed to grooves, effectively limiting the length of FA formed perpendicular to the groove orientation. Thus, it arises that grooved nanoscale topographies can influence both the adhesion direction as well as adhesion reinforcement (Biggs et al., 2010).

Anisotropic Topography and Cellular Function

The mechanisms by which anisotropic topography and ordered protein deposition influence cellular proliferation and differentiation require more research. Anisotropic arrays of topographical micro and nanoscale gratings have been shown to be potent tools in maintaining the phenotype of primary cells (Zhu et al., 2010) and in differentiating stem cells toward expressing osteogenic (Dalby et al., 2007; Biggs et al., 2009a; Watari et al., 2012), tenogenic (Wojciak et al., 1995), neurogenic (Jeon et al., 2014), adipogenic (Wang et al., 2012), and myogenic (Wang et al., 2013b) transcripts and proteins. The processes that mediate the cellular reaction to anisotropic surface structures, however, are not well understood and may be direct (Cassidy et al., 2014) or indirect (where the surface structure has affected the composition, orientation, or conformation of the adsorbed ECM components)(Perez-Garnes et al., 2011; Ballester-Beltran et al., 2012a).

Multiple studies with mesenchymal stem cell populations point toward the negative effects of micronscale grooves and pronounced cell polarization on osteospecific differentiation (Biggs et al., 2008; Watari et al., 2012), a process appearing to be more influenced by sub 500 nm topographies. Conversely, more adipospecific (Wang et al., 2012) and myogenic (Wang et al., 2013b) differentiation is demonstrated to be enhanced by polarization through micronscale grooved topographies. Periodicity has also been shown to be important in modulating differential function in pluripotent cells. In particular, if mesenchymal stem cells are cultured on grooves with a short feature pitch and become highly aligned, this reduces osteogenesis. However, if the pitch is increased so the grooves are more step cues (around 50 μm pitch), then osteogenesis is achieved with great efficiency (Biggs et al., 2009b).

The mechanism by which anisotropic grating surfaces influence cell function, however, is still being resolved; multiple studies suggest that cells cultured on topographical gratings modulate transcriptional events through adhesion-dependent phosphorylation of downstream signaling molecules (e.g., mediated FA kinases, FAK) (**Figure 2A**). FA pathway signaling has been shown to control essential cellular processes such as growth, survival, migration, and differentiation. Interestingly, extensive evidence has also been generated on the involvement of extracellular signal-related kinase (ERK) 1/2 down-regulation following integrin-mediated FAK activation, in response to grooved substrates (Biggs et al., 2009b; Cassidy et al., 2014).

A Case of Study: Anisotropic Surfaces and Immune Activation

Besides analyzing the influence of anisotropic features in adherent cells, it seems that these surfaces can also induce a significant response in several *non-adherent* cell types (Kwon et al., 2012) (e.g., cells belonging to the immune system).

Several studies have reported on the effects of nanotopographical structures on immune cell motility (Song et al., 2012) and actin rich structures (e.g., lamella and filopodia) are reported to play a significant role in this process (Song et al., 2014). Emerging data suggest that the proteins involved in adhesive processes in cells of the immune system are analogous to those found in FA in adherent cells (Hocde et al., 2009), and that leukocyte binding to ECM components and adsorbed complement proteins can induce FAK-mediated immune cell activation (Bhattacharyya et al., 1999), phagocytosis (Kasorn et al., 2009), and chemokine-mediated migration (Cohen-Hillel et al., 2009). Similarly, Bartneck and colleagues reported that a microstructured topography of regular grooves induced a pro-inflammatory phenotype in macrophages, which was not accompanied by release of pro-inflammatory mediators (Bartneck et al., 2010).

Although the immune response is tightly regulated by the complex interplay of events and interactions between its constituent cells, preliminary studies suggest that anisotropic topographies may be employed to induce cell activation and as in adherent cell types, this may be through FAK-mediated activation of critical signaling pathways.

Perspectives on Cell–Material Interactions

The interactions between cellular populations and engineered substrates are bidirectional; e.g., a mechanical cellular mediated deformation of the scaffold modulates the physical environmental properties. Consequently, in order to better understand the dynamic nature of topographical mediated direction of cellular function stimuli, responsive or "smart" materials are increasingly being employed in cell studies. New reports demonstrate that mechanically active anisotropic topographies can yield critical insight into the role of groove dimension on cellular function through dynamic modulation of the feature dimensions.

Shape memory polymers have recently been employed for this purpose and can be designed with a physiological transition temperature to provide an alternate morphology or topography when subjected to physiological temperatures (e.g., between 32 and 37°C), providing dynamic mechanical cues or anti-adhesive surfaces (Ebara et al., 2014). A study by Gong et al. investigated microgroove surface patterns formed on a cross-linked poly(ε-caprolactone) substrate. Here, a dynamic response to cyclic temperature (e.g., between 32 and 41°C) resulted in the modulation

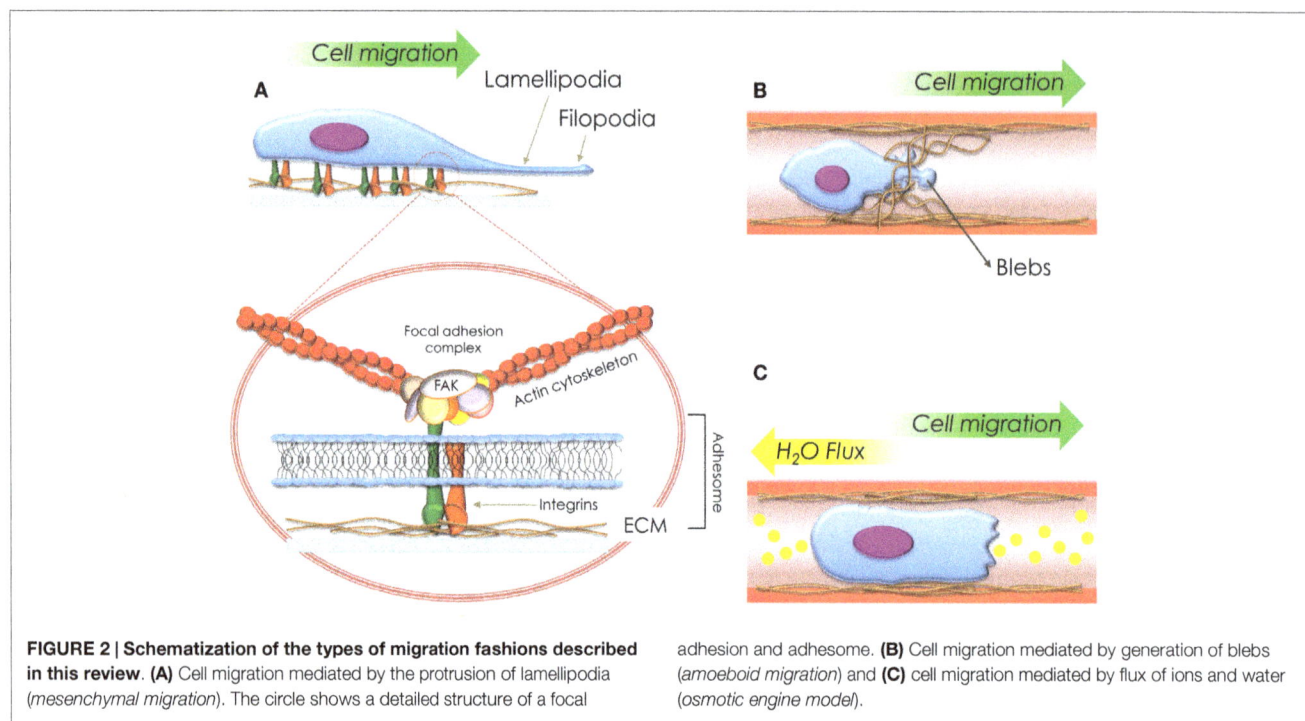

FIGURE 2 | Schematization of the types of migration fashions described in this review. (A) Cell migration mediated by the protrusion of lamellipodia (*mesenchymal migration*). The circle shows a detailed structure of a focal adhesion and adhesome. **(B)** Cell migration mediated by generation of blebs (*amoeboid migration*) and **(C)** cell migration mediated by flux of ions and water (*osmotic engine model*).

of the microgroove dimensions, influencing cell shape and the cytoskeletal arrangement of adherent bone marrow stem cells, which upregulated myospecific genes and proteins (Gong et al., 2014).

Although a large number of studies have reported the effects of nanotopographical structures on modulations to cell function *in vitro* (Dalby et al., 2007; Biggs et al., 2009b), a limited number of studies *in vivo* have been conducted (Fernandez-Yague et al., 2014), particularly in osteointegration and *de novo* bone formation (Xia et al., 2012b; Svensson et al., 2013). A recent study by Yin et al. demonstrated the significant effects of anisotropy in a rat Achilles tendon repair model. Here, anisotropic scaffolds and enhanced alignment resulted in tendon regeneration, while randomly ordered isotropic scaffolds induced ectopic bone formation. Interestingly, the influence of anisotropic micro and nanotopography on osteospecific function seems to be most effectively translated to an *in vivo* response when applied in combination with microscale grating features, indicating a possible synergy between the cellular (micro) and subcellular (nano) in directing regeneration (Kim et al., 2014a).

Considering these indications, it appears logical to expect significant efforts to translate findings from model (e.g., polymer) surfaces into orthopedic materials such as ceramics and metals. However, these materials are hard to manufacture due to the hardness of the materials and the brittle nature of ceramics. Also, while structural orthopedic ceramics, such alumina/zirconia, tend to be highly bio-inert, metals such as titanium and its alloys are highly adhesive to cells due to their reactive oxide layers and both these low and high adhesion environments can mask topographical effects. However, recent advancements in pre-sintering embossing of green ceramics have illustrated that groove patterns in alumina with different widths can be used to influence fibrous tissue (narrow width, 20 μm pitch) and hard tissue (150 μm pitch

with 100 μm groove/50 μm ridge) growth from human osteoprogenitor cells (Nadeem et al., 2013), similarly to results observed on polymers (Biggs et al., 2008).

For metals, there is plenty of literature showing potential effects on more random topographies from etching, blasting, and anodizing (Anselme et al., 2000; McNamara et al., 2011; Sjöström et al., 2012, 2013; Olivares-Navarrete et al., 2015) due to the need for fast fabrication protocols. However, Anselme et al. have indicated potential positive effects for grooves in metals (Anselme et al., 2004). We further note that other cell types have been shown to be responsive to topographies in metals – again though, roughened rather than grooved (Lee et al., 2014; Kim et al., 2015).

As we can observe, anisotropic surfaces can stimulate *in vitro* and *in vivo* cell activity. However, it is still unclear how cell adhesion can be affected by topographic cues. In the next section of this review, we will consider the best understood mechanisms for cell adhesion and migration, focusing further discussions on the influence of ventral and dorsal stimulation on adherent cells.

Cell Motility

During the last years, it has been demonstrated that cell anchorage and motility play important roles in a wide spectrum of biological processes, such as mechano and chemotaxis (Andreas et al., 2014; Charras and Sahai, 2014), as well as wound healing and tissue repair (Gattazzo et al., 2014). Furthermore, similar to tissue repair, several diseases (e.g., cancer) have evolved to use adhesion and migration as part of their pathogenic strategy (Farahani et al., 2014), making research on cell migration an extremely relevant field and showing the necessity to study this process in detail.

Since anisotropic surfaces play a potent role on cell migration, in the next section we will briefly describe different mechanisms used by migrating cells to displace into complex environments, putting into context topographic cues detected on 2D surfaces or 3D milieus.

Cell Migration on 2D: Following the Front
Cell Migration Mediated by the Protrusion of Lamellipodia

One of the most researched migration mechanisms on flat surfaces, at the single-cell scale, corresponds to *mesenchymal migration*.

Mesenchymal migration is recognized by the presence, adhesion, and protrusion of lamellipodium. From the molecular point of view, this type of migration requires cell-matrix adhesion structures (e.g., protein clusters) named *adhesomes*, which are composed by intra-, trans-, and extra- cellular proteins (**Figure 2A**).

The most important mediator between cells and their milieu are heterodimer transmembrane proteins known as integrins. Integrins comprises α- and β- chains. β-subunits interconnect ECM proteins (e.g., collagen, fibronectin, elastin, etc.) with the cytoskeleton (e.g., actin stress fibers), allowing the sensing of elastic and topographical properties of the milieus where they are anchored through the exertion of traction forces (**Figure 2A**). Cell-matrix adhesion and mechanosensing are mediated by non-receptor tyrosine kinases, the most notable of which is FAK, a molecule constitutively associated with the β-integrin subunit. FAK is localized at adhesion structures. It promotes talin recruitment to modulate adhesion reinforcement, and further unraveling of these stimuli by intracellular kinases (e.g., FAK) bound to transmembrane integrins and linking proteins (e.g., vinculin and paxillin) (Ridley et al., 2003; Vicente-Manzanares and Horwitz, 2011; Leal-Egaña et al., 2013).

Adhesion Structures and Cell Polarization

Mesenchymal migration is a cyclic process defined by cell polarization (Ridley et al., 2003). The first step consists in the protrusion of the membrane in the direction of migration. Two different types of protrusion have been identified: lamellipodia (large and broad) and filopodia (spike-like). In both cases, they are driven by actin polymerization and stabilized by their adherence to ECM proteins.

Differences in function have been observed between these protrusions: while filopodia are constituted by parallel actin fibers and are well designed to serve as "sensors" and explore the environment, lamellipodia are constituted by branched actin capable of supporting traction forces involved in cell displacement.

After generation of mature adhesions at the lamellipodia in the cell edge, traction forces generated by the actomyosin network pull the cell body in the direction of the lamellipodia, producing the unidirectional displacement of the cell. During this process, the Arp 2/3 complex plays a preponderant role, inducing actin polymerization at the lamellipodia and generating dendritic actin networks (branches) with pre-existing filaments at the cell front. This polarization defines the final direction of the migration. Simultaneously, during the translocation of the cell body, the Arp 2/3 complex is inhibited at the trailing edge of the cells, inducing detachment of adhesomes and release of the rear part of the cells from the substrate (Vicente-Manzanares and Horwitz, 2011; Hanein and Horwitz, 2012).

Adhesomes attachment/detachment and cell polarization are regulated by two families of GTPases with antagonistic activity and localization in the cell: Rho and Rac. While Rho proteins activate actin polymerization, promote cell adhesion, and generate a leading edge due to their interaction with the Arp 2/3 complex; Rac GTPases produce the disassembly of the actin fibers and the detaching of integrins from ECM proteins, as observed at the trailing edge (Vicente-Manzanares and Horwitz, 2011; Petrie and Yamada, 2012).

Finally, it is important to indicate that, even though it seems that the biological machinery involved in cell migration could also be related to the sense of topographic cues, there is not clear information about the mechanisms by which cells can sense differences in structure and geometrical organization of 2D milieus during their displacement.

Cell Motility Within Complex 3D Milieus

During recent years, several biophysical mechanisms used for cells during migration have been studied, which are described in the next section of this review. These migration mechanisms, mostly observed in migrating cells within complex environments (e.g., micro-channels, filamentous 3D milieus), can give us clues about the way cells could interact with topographic cues found in 3D milieu.

Cell Migration Mediated by the Protrusion of Lobopodia

When cells migrate within 3D elastic environments, a special type of protrusion, named lobopodia, can be observed. Lobopodia are mostly represented as non-sharp cylindrical protrusions that might be driven by intracellular pressure rather than actin polymerization (Petrie and Yamada, 2012). Moreover, and although it has been shown that lobopodia contraction is mediated by RhoA-ROCK-myosin II signaling, this type of migration still remains less understood and poorly characterized (Petrie et al., 2014).

With respect to lobopodia, there is little information about structure and composition, although it has been proposed that the myosin IIa acts through vimentin filaments (polarized to the anterior of lobopodial cells and anchored to the nucleus, likely by nesprin-3) easing cell migration (DeSimone and Horwitz, 2014). Particularly, Petrie et al. (2014) suggests that the nucleus physically divides the cell in two compartments, maintaining differences in hydrostatic pressure between the leading and the rear parts of the cell.

Cell Migration Mediated by Generation of Blebs

Displacement through plasma membrane blebbing is one of the simplest biological mechanisms used by migrating cells (Charras and Paluch, 2008; Fackler and Grosse, 2008). Traditionally named *amoeboid* migration, this process is characterized by the formation of spherical membrane protrusions (e.g., blebs) (**Figure 2B**), produced by contraction of the actomyosin cortex. This phenomena is dependant on cortical tension and the integrity of actin cortex (Charras and Paluch, 2008).

From the molecular point of view, *amoeboid* migration is dependent on the activity of Rho GTPase and actomyosin contractility. However, it is noteworthy to remark that, differently to *mesenchymal* migration, the blebbing mechanism generates low traction forces since the Arp 2/3 complex is not required (Bergert et al., 2012). As bleb motility requires less energy than *mesenchymal* cell translocation, this mechanism has been mostly studied on metastatic cells, due to their capacity to escape from anti-tumor treatments based on protease inhibitors, or during their speedy migration onto low adherent surfaces and/or confined environments.

It is important to indicate that, although several cancers exhibit only one migration style, several cancer lines can easily switch from *mesenchymal* to *amoeboid* displacement when they are embedded within three-dimensional (3D) matrices (Bergert et al., 2012; Paluch and Raz, 2013). Moreover, Bergert and colleagues demonstrated that when the Arp 2/3 complex is inhibited (e.g., by using the compound CK-666 in Walker cells cultured on 2D surfaces), lamellipodia are replaced by bleb formation, probably by controlling the actin cortex and/or cortical tension (Bergert et al., 2012).

However, it is important to indicate that even though current research has demonstrated the use of blebs as a mechanism for cell migration, there is a lack of information concerning the mechanisms involved in translocation and forces implied in cell movement (Charras and Paluch, 2008; Paluch and Raz, 2013). Then, and although it is still unclear, the mechanisms by which cells translocate themselves using blebs appear related to periodicity in the formation of protrusions and the regular generation of small pseudopodia on the leading edge allowing the translocation of the cytosol and intracellular organelles through them (Charras and Paluch, 2008; Paluch and Raz, 2013).

It is important to indicate that, although migration mediated by blebs have been mostly studied on scaffolds exhibiting topographic cues (e.g., micro channels, fibrous matrices), there is no information regarding the influence that these topographic cues play on cell migration. However, and as was previously noted, first attempts to solve this question have been focused on immune-cells exhibiting an amoeboid migration fashion.

Cell Migration Mediated by Flux of Ions and Water

Recently, Stroka and colleagues demonstrated *in vitro* that neoplastic cells migrating in confined 3D matrices use an actin/myosin-independent mechanism based on the permeation of ions and water through trans-membrane channels (**Figure 2C**). This new translocation strategy, named the *osmotic engine model* (Papadopoulos and Saadoun, 2014; Stroka et al., 2014a), can explain cell displacement within 3D environments (e.g., 3 μm-wide channels) in the presence of myosin, Rho/Rock kinase, and/or $\beta1$ integrin inhibitors (Balzer et al., 2012; Stroka et al., 2014b).

Although this process is currently under study, mathematical and biochemical analysis have revealed that this type of migration requires the coordinated activity of polarized ion channels and aquaporins, which modulate fluxes of ions and water from the leading (flux in) to the trailing edge (flux out), where the sodium hydrogen exchanger-1 (NHE-1) and aquaporin 5 (AQP5) –recruited by cortical actin polymerization – seem to play a preponderant role on cell motility and regulation of intracellular pH (Stroka et al., 2014a,b).

Role of the Nucleus on Cell Migration Within 3D Milieus

The nucleus is the largest and stiffest organelle in cells. Since cell migration within 3D matrices is restricted by the pore cut-off/size distribution, cells need to squeeze the nucleus through via myosin-II mediated contraction (Friedl et al., 2011).

During the lobopodia-based migration, via the actomyosin contractility, the nucleus acts as a piston pressurizing the leading compartment. This results in bleb formation, lobopodia formation, and protrusion, and finally cell migration. Recently, Petri and colleagues compared the intracellular hydrostatic pressure in front of the nucleus, for cells cultured on/in 2D and 3D environments, finding differences of approximately 10-fold between these two systems (from approximately 300 to 700 Pa in lamellipodia compared to approximately 2200 Pa in lobopodia). According to the authors, when cells are confined within defined 3D micro channels (approximately 20 μm diameter), the nucleus compartmentalize the intracellular volume, this then acts as a piston, which enhances the hydrostatic pressures at the frontal edge of the cell with respect to the rear edge (approximately 2400 vs. 900 Pa). This results in bleb formation, lobopodia formation, and protrusion, and finally cell migration. Molecularly, the actomyosin-vimentin-nesprin-3 complex (e.g., intermediate filaments) seems to be responsible for pulling the nuclei to the front of the cell, and its influence on the cell displacement within 3D channels (Petrie et al., 2014).

Cell Migration on Nano/Micro Topographic Designed Environments

It is known that cells can switch spontaneously between different migration mechanisms after remodeling cytoskeleton arrangement depending on their environment. Thus, *in vitro* and *in vivo* gradients may lead to changes in cell migration among other important cellular processes. In almost all cases, the migration fashion will be dependent on the balance between actin polymerization, rear contractility, and adhesion. First attempts to explain this behavior have been done in 3D micro-channels after analysis of actin organization at the leading edge. According to the authors, there are two different F-actin networks involved in cell sensing and migration: one polymerizing at the cell-matrix interface (Wilson et al., 2013) and a "free" fragment growing on the leading edge. Both structures can communicate and interact mechanically (Wilson et al., 2013), suggesting that cytoskeleton, compartmentalization, and hydrostatic pressures produced by the nucleus as well as sensing of topographic characteristics of the cell milieu by migrating cells are intimately related. However, as was previously discussed, the biological mechanism by which cells recognize topographic cues, and their influence on cell migration, is still far away for being explained.

Physiological Gradients and Bi-Phasic Biophysical Stimulation

Traditionally, cell culture has been performed on 2D substrates where cells sense and respond to ventral stimulation (e.g., topographical cues). However, standard flat surfaces differ from *in vivo* milieus, where cells are subjected to complex 3D gradients,

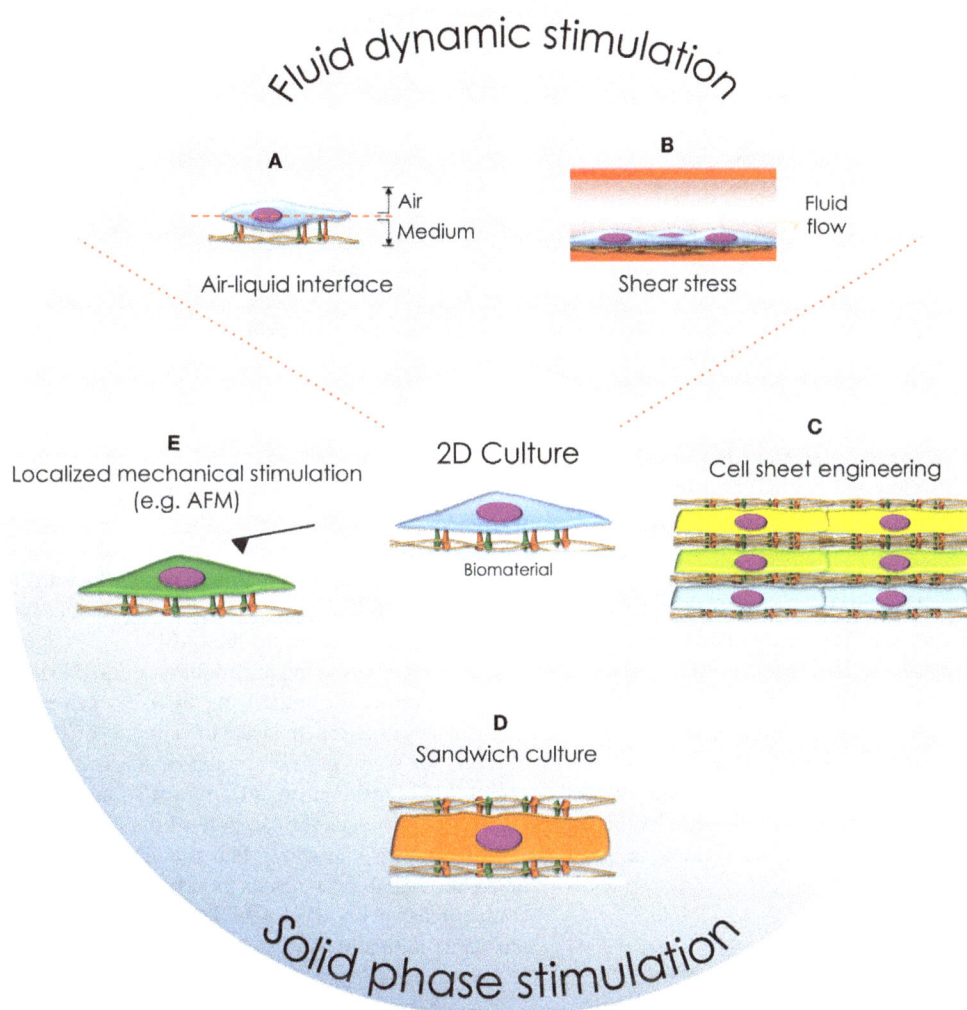

FIGURE 3 | Cell culture systems developed to mimic the physiological environment *in vitro*. (A) Air-liquid interface culture and **(B)** cell culture under fluid flow conditions. **(C)** Cell-sheet engineering, **(D)** sandwich culture, and **(E)** localized dorsal stimulation using an AFM cantilever.

such as differential ventral/dorsal exposure to liquid-gas phases (e.g., lungs), shear stress produced by fluid flow (e.g., endothelial tissues), or surrounded by an ECM (e.g., parenchymal tissues) (**Figure 3**).

These complex environmental stimuli have been reconstituted *in vitro*, with the purpose to study cell behavior in physiological-like conditions. Here, we will focus on the simultaneous ventral/dorsal stimulation of cells, seeking to recapitulate the physiological cell behavior.

Fluid Dynamic Stimulation
This type of stimulation can be divided in two groups, according to the physical sub-phase involved in cellular stimulation:

Liquid-Gas Phase Stimulation
The epithelium is a polarized tissue where cells are ventrally anchored to the ECM and dorsally contacting a gas phase. Thus, fully immersed epithelial cells cultures (e.g., traditional culture strategy on 2D substrates) differ from the physiological

environment. Consequently, alternative methods allowing dorsal contact to a gas phase have been developed (e.g., roller bottles, rocking platforms, and inverted cultures) (Voisin et al., 1977).

Nowadays, the use of the air-liquid interface culture (ALI, **Figure 3A**) has become a traditional system used to cultivate epithelial cells because it resembles the physiological condition (Voisin et al., 1977; Zamora et al., 1983, 1986; De Borja Callejas et al., 2014) and thus makes possible to perform drug testing, among other analysis, in physiologically relevant environments (Kooter et al., 2013; Kim et al., 2014b; Ashraf et al., 2015).

Dynamic Fluid Flow Stimulation
Blood vessels are internally covered by endothelial cells, exposing their ventral surfaces to parenquimal tissues (e.g., ECM), and dorsally to the lumen of the vessels: being stimulated by forces produced by fluid displacement (e.g., shear stress). Therefore, new *in vitro* culture systems providing constant flow or even pulsatile stress have been performed (**Table 2**; **Figure 3B**).

TABLE 2 | Effect of fluid flow on different cell lineages.

Cell type	Effect of fluid flow	Reference
Endothelial cells	Cell alignment Release of vaso-active substances (e.g., endothelin-1) and nitric oxide synthase	Ishibazawa et al. (2011) and Vozzi et al. (2014)
Vascular smooth muscle cells	Decrease cell proliferation Increase NO production Increase of fibroblast growth factor (FGF)-2 production	Papadaki et al. (1998) and Lindner et al. (1991)
Osteoblast cells	Induction of NO and prostaglandin E2 production Activation of growth factor signaling pathways Alteration in the Wnt/β-catenin and bone formation signaling pathway	Smalt et al. (1997) and Jia et al. (2014)
Stem cells	Cell alignment Increase in the angiogenic and vasculogenic potential of endothelial cells derived from human embryonic stem cells (hESC) Positive modulation of the stem cell proliferation and differentiation	Metallo et al. (2008), Huang et al. (2005), Lim et al. (2013), and Potter et al. (2014)

It is now well characterized that the excitation of the dorsal receptors stimulates protein kinase C (PKC) and the mitogen-activated protein (MAP) kinase pathways, resulting in gene transcription modulation and control of e.g., endothelial growth and vaso-active substances secretion such as endothelin-1 and endothelial nitric oxide synthase-3 (Vozzi et al., 2014).

The influence of shear stress has also been studied on additional cell lineages, such as vascular smooth muscle cells, since these can be encounter in endothelium-desquamated injuries and are therefore involved in the response to vascular wounds. Furthermore, the effect on osteocytes has been studied, since the fluid flow over the osteocyte network has been suggested to be the main cellular signal-generating factor (e.g., as a result of mechanical loading of bone) (Piekarski and Munro, 1977; Cowin and Weinbaum, 1998; Knothe Tate et al., 1998, 2000) (**Table 2**).

Solid Phase Stimulation

Cells embed within 3D milieus are subjected to physical (e.g., stiffness and pores), chemical (e.g., cytokines and growth factors), and biological (e.g., cell-cell contact and cell-ECM adhesion) gradients during tissue morphogenesis and homeostasis. Among the strategies developed to recreate this environment, hydrogels represent a convenient and well-studied system due to their structural and compositional similarities to natural ECM and the advances in material chemistry that allow tunable physical, chemical, and functional properties (Sant et al., 2010; Pedron et al., 2015).

Here, we will focus on cell culture systems that trigger bi-phasic adhesion signaling such as, sandwich culture, cell sheet engineering, and dorsal stimulation [e.g., by atomic force microscopy (AFM)] (**Figures 3C–E**, respectively) (Takahashi et al., 2013). In these systems, even if cells are not completely embedded within a 3D matrix, the stimulation of dorsal cell receptors triggers cell adhesion and specific signaling pathways that determine cell fate as a balance between ventral and dorsal stimulation.

Sandwich cultures involve confining cells within two substrates – dorsally and ventrally – with the same or different properties. One of the best known examples are collagen constructs, used preferentially in culture of hepatocytes since these cells lose their metabolic functions when attached to 2D substrates. However, the use of sandwich cultures made of ECM proteins (e.g., collagen on the top and the bottom), allow hepatocytes to maintain their polarization and metabolic activity (e.g., albumin, urea, transferrin, fibrinogen, and bile salt secretion, as well as cytochrome activity (P450 activity) restored (Swift et al., 2010 and Dunn et al., 1992, respectively). Furthermore, this type of culture allows hepatocytes to generate bile canalicular networks (Bi et al., 2006). Thus, this system is a very straightforward tool to study *in vitro* hepatocellular function, such as protein synthesis and/or drug metabolism (Xia et al., 2009, 2012a).

Cell-sheet engineering techniques are based in stacking 2D cell layers, including the underlying ECM, to generate a 3D tissue that consists of alternate layers of cells and ECM. The technique enables the study of more complex environments, mimicking the multidimensional organization of some tissues and organs. This system stresses the key role of dorsal stimulation for hepatocyte cultures and shows that the 3D coculture of hepatocyte and endothelial cells results in a powerful tool to gain more comprehensive knowledge of liver metabolism, detoxification, and signaling pathways *in vitro* (Harimoto et al., 2002; Kim and Rajagopalan, 2010).

We, among others, have been involved in the research of new alternatives for sandwich cultures, such as the use of ventral and dorsal surfaces with different properties/characteristics (e.g., stiffness and/or topological patterns) (Ballester-Beltrán et al., 2015). This system has shown cell morphology to be related to substrate rigidity and the ability of cells to reorganize ECM proteins adsorbed to these surfaces (Beningo et al., 2004; Ballester-Beltran et al., 2012b; Ballester-Beltrán et al., 2014). Furthermore, it has been shown that sandwich-like cultures can modify cell spreading/elongation and migration rates depending on the substrates properties, resulting in closer 3D environment behaviors (Beningo et al., 2004; Ballester-Beltrán et al., 2015).

Cells cultured within these bi-phasic systems adhere to the ventral and dorsal substrates, exerting tensional forces on each surface (e.g., spatially tunable mechanotransduction). This was first observed when osteosarcoma U2OS cells were ventrally attached to 2D fibronectin-coated glass. In this configuration, cells were dorsally stimulated by AFM using a fibronectin-coated cantilever (**Figure 3E**). In response to this stimulus, cells adhered and spread on the cantilever forming new fibrillar actin fibers connecting both surfaces, which enabled the cells to contract and pull the cantilever (Chaudhuri et al., 2009). Hence, cell interaction mediated by dorsal stimulation triggers changes in the cytoskeleton arrangement and generates new adhesion structures. This might link ventral and dorsal sides, allowing a complex response to bi-phasic stimuli, such as the fact that dorsal stimulation induces modification of ventral adhesions (Fuentes et al., 2011; Ballester-Beltrán et al., 2015), indicating the existence of a clear balance between ventral and dorsal stimulation.

When aligned electrospun fibers are used to stimulate dorsal cell adhesion, cells elongate and align in the direction of the fibers. Interestingly, when sandwich-like cultures consist of aligned fibers contacting cells ventrally, and a flat surface stimulating cells dorsally, cells remain aligned to ventral fibers. These results suggest that the topographical cues play a major role irrespective of which surface they are presented to (Ballester-Beltran et al., 2013). As expected, this alignment is depending on the cell adhesion to fibers, since cells were not able to align when they were coated with non-adhesive proteins (e.g., albumin).

Outlook and Conclusion

In this review, we have shown the important role gradients have *in vivo* and different methods to recapitulate them *in vitro*. We had special attention to the study of topographical cues since its ability to mimic the fibrillar structure of the ECM is key to unravel cell biology *in vivo*.

Novel methodologies would allow studying these surface gradients in closer 3D physiological environments. For example, here we have shown those offering a bi-phasic stimulation (adhesion-gas, adhesion-fluid flow, and adhesion-adhesion). These technical strategies could be combined with 2D gradients on both dorsal and ventral sides, in order to investigate 3D environments-like e.g., topographical gradients on a 2D ventral substrate and fluid flow through the z axis. These studies would set up the basis to answer complex biological questions as well as new methods to mimic the micro/nano pathological surroundings and drug assessment.

Acknowledgments

This work was supported by MRC grant MR/L022710/1 "synergistic microenvironments for non-union bone defects."

References

Andreas, K., Sittinger, M., and Ringe, J. (2014). Toward *in situ* tissue engineering: chemokine-guided stem cell recruitment. *Trends Biotechnol.* 32, 483–492. doi:10.1089/scd.2005.14.329

Ankam, S., Lim, C. K., and Yim, E. K. (2015). Actomyosin contractility plays a role in MAP2 expression during nanotopography-directed neuronal differentiation of human embryonic stem cells. *Biomaterials* 47C, 20–28. doi:10.1016/j.biomaterials.2015.01.003

Anselme, K., Bigerelle, M., Loison, I., Noël, B., and Hardouin, P. (2004). Kinetic study of the expression of beta-catenin, actin and vinculin during osteoblastic adhesion on grooved titanium substrates. *Biomed. Mater. Eng.* 14, 545–556.

Anselme, K., Linez, P., Bigerelle, M., Le Maguer, D., Le Maguer, A., Hardouin, P., et al. (2000). The relative influence of the topography and chemistry of TiAl6V4 surfaces on osteoblastic cell behaviour. *Biomaterials* 21, 1567–1577. doi:10.1016/S0142-9612(00)00042-9

Ashraf, S., Brockman-Schneider, R., Gern, J.E. (2015). Propagation of rhinovirus-C strains in human airway epithelial cells differentiated at air-liquid interface. *Methods Mol Biol* 1221, 63–70. doi:10.1007/978-1-4939-1571-2_6

Att, W., Yamada, M., and Ogawa, T. (2009). Effect of titanium surface characteristics on the behavior and function of oral fibroblasts. *Int. J. Oral Maxillofac. Implants* 24, 419–431. doi:10.1016/S0022-3913(10)60106-0

Azeem, A., English, A., Kumar, P., Satyam, A., Biggs, M., Jones, E., et al. (2015). The influence of anisotropic nano- to micro-topography on in vitro and in vivo osteogenesis. *Nanomedicine* 5, 693–711. doi:10.2217/nnm.14.218

Ballester-Beltran, J., Cantini, M., Lebourg, M., Rico, P., Moratal, D., Garcia, A. J., et al. (2012a). Effect of topological cues on material-driven fibronectin fibrillogenesis and cell differentiation. *J. Mater. Sci. Mater. Med.* 23, 195–204. doi:10.1007/s10856-011-4532-z

Ballester-Beltran, J., Lebourg, M., Rico, P., and Salmeron-Sanchez, M. (2012b). Dorsal and ventral stimuli in cell-material interactions: effect on cell morphology. *Biointerphases* 7, 39. doi:10.1007/s13758-012-0039-5

Ballester-Beltrán, J., Lebourg, M., Rico, P., and Salmerón-Sánchez, M. (2015). Cell migration within confined sandwich-like nanoenvironments. *Nanomedicine* 10, 815–828. doi:10.2217/nnm.14.217

Ballester-Beltran, J., Lebourg, M., and Salmeron-Sanchez, M. (2013). Dorsal and ventral stimuli in sandwich-like microenvironments. Effect on cell differentiation. *Biotechnol. Bioeng.* 110, 3048–3058. doi:10.1002/bit.24972

Ballester-Beltrán, J., Moratal, D., Lebourg, M., and Salmerón-Sánchez, M. (2014). Fibronectin-matrix sandwich-like microenvironments to manipulate cell fate. *Biomater. Sci.* 2, 381–389. doi:10.1039/C3BM60248F

Balzer, E., Tong, Z., Paul, C., Hung, W. C., Stroka, K., Boggs, A., et al. (2012). Physical confinement alters tumor cell adhesion and migration phenotypes. *FASEB J.* 26, 4045–4056. doi:10.1096/fj.12-211441

Bartneck, M., Schulte, V. A., Paul, N. E., Diez, M., Lensen, M. C., and Zwadlo-Klarwasser, G. (2010). Induction of specific macrophage subtypes by defined micro-patterned structures. *Acta Biomater.* 6, 3864–3872. doi:10.1016/j.actbio.2010.04.025

Beningo, K. A., Dembo, M., and Wang, Y. L. (2004). Responses of fibroblasts to anchorage of dorsal extracellular matrix receptors. *Proc. Natl. Acad. Sci. U.S.A.* 101, 18024–18029. doi:10.1073/pnas.0405747102

Bergert, M., Chandradoss, S., Desai, R., and Paluch, E. (2012). Cell mechanics control rapid transitions between blebs and lamellipodia during migration. *Proc. Natl. Acad. Sci. U.S.A.* 109, 14434–14439. doi:10.1073/pnas.1207968109

Bhattacharyya, S. P., Mekori, Y. A., Hoh, D., Paolini, R., Metcalfe, D. D., and Bianchine, P. J. (1999). Both adhesion to immobilized vitronectin and Fcepsilon-RI cross-linking cause enhanced focal adhesion kinase phosphorylation in murine mast cells. *Immunology* 98, 357–362. doi:10.1046/j.1365-2567.1999.00883.x

Bi, Y. A., Kazolias, D., and Duignan, D. B. (2006). Use of cryopreserved human hepatocytes in sandwich culture to measure hepatobiliary transport. *Drug Metab. Dispos.* 34, 1658–1665. doi:10.1124/dmd.105.009118

Biggs, M. J., Richards, R., Gadegaard, N., McMurray, R., Affrossman, S., Wilkinson, C., et al. (2009a). Interactions with nanoscale topography: adhesion quantification and signal transduction in cells of osteogenic and multipotent lineage. *J. Biomed. Mater. Res. A* 91, 195–208. doi:10.1002/jbm.a.32196

Biggs, M. J., Richards, R. G., Gadegaard, N., Wilkinson, C. D. W., Oreffo, R. O. C., and Dalby, M. J. (2009b). The use of nanoscale topography to modulate the dynamics of adhesion formation in primary osteoblasts and ERK/MAPK signalling in STRO-1+ enriched skeletal stem cells. *Biomaterials* 30, 5094–5103. doi:10.1016/j.biomaterials.2009.05.049

Biggs, M. J., Richards, R. G., and Dalby, M. J. (2010). Nanotopographical modification: a regulator of cellular function through focal adhesions. *Nanomedicine* 6, 619–633. doi:10.1016/j.nano.2010.01.009

Biggs, M. J., Richards, R. G., McFarlane, S., Wilkinson, C. D., Oreffo, R. O., and Dalby, M. J. (2008). Adhesion formation of primary human osteoblasts and the functional response of mesenchymal stem cells to 330nm deep microgrooves. *J. R. Soc. Interface* 5, 1231–1242. doi:10.1002/jbm.a.32196

Cassidy, J. W., Roberts, J. N., Smith, C. A., Robertson, M., White, K., Biggs, M. J., et al. (2014). Osteogenic lineage restriction by osteoprogenitors cultured on nanometric grooved surfaces: the role of focal adhesion maturation. *Acta Biomater.* 10, 651–660. doi:10.1016/j.actbio.2013.11.008

Charras, G., and Paluch, E. (2008). Blebs lead the way: how to migrate without lamellipodia. *Nature* 9, 730–736. doi:10.1038/nrm2453

Charras, G., and Sahai, E. (2014). Physical influence of the extracellular environment on cell migration. *Nat. Rev.* 15, 813–824. doi:10.1038/nrm3897

Chaudhuri, O., Parekh, S. H., Lam, W. A., and Fletcher, D. A. (2009). Combined atomic force microscopy and side-view optical imaging for mechanical studies of cells. *Nat. Methods* 6, 383–387. doi:10.1038/nmeth.1320

Chua, J. S., Chng, C. P., Moe, A. A., Tann, J. Y., Goh, E. L., Chiam, K. H., et al. (2014). Extending neurites sense the depth of the underlying topography during neuronal differentiation and contact guidance. *Biomaterials* 35, 7750–7761. doi:10.1016/j.biomaterials.2014.06.008

Clark, P., Connolly, P., Curtis, A. S., Dow, J. A., and Wilkinson, C. D. (1990). Topographical control of cell behaviour: II. Multiple grooved substrata. *Development* 108, 635–644.

Cohen-Hillel, E., Mintz, R., Meshel, T., Garty, B. Z., and Ben-Baruch, A. (2009). Cell migration to the chemokine CXCL8: paxillin is activated and regulates adhesion and cell motility. *Cell. Mol. Life Sci.* 66, 884–899. doi:10.1007/s00018-009-8447-5

Cowin, S. C., and Weinbaum, S. (1998). Strain amplification in the bone mechanosensory system. *Am. J. Med. Sci.* 316, 184–188. doi:10.1097/00000441-199809000-00006

Crouch, A. S., Miller, D., Luebke, K. J., and Hu, W. (2009). Correlation of anisotropic cell behaviors with topographic aspect ratio. *Biomaterials* 30, 1560–1567. doi:10.1016/j.biomaterials.2008.11.041

Curtis, A., and Wilkinson, C. (1997). Topographical control of cells. *Biomaterials* 18, 1573–1583. doi:10.1016/S0142-9612(97)00144-0

Dalby, M. J., Gadegaard, N., Tare, R., Andar, A., Riehle, M., Herzyk, P., et al. (2007). The control of human mesenchymal cell differentiation using nanoscale symmetry and disorder. *Nat. Mater.* 6, 997–1003. doi:10.1038/nmat2013

Dalby, M. J., McCloy, D., Robertson, M., Wilkinson, C. D., and Oreffo, R. O. (2006). Osteoprogenitor response to defined topographies with nanoscale depths. *Biomaterials* 27, 1306–1315. doi:10.1016/j.biomaterials.2005.08.028

Dalby, M. J., Riehle, M. O., Yarwood, S. J., Wilkinson, C. D., and Curtis, A. S. (2003). Nucleus alignment and cell signaling in fibroblasts: response to a micro-grooved topography. *Exp. Cell Res.* 284, 274–282. doi:10.1016/S0014-4827(02)00053-8

De Borja Callejas, F., Martinez-Anton, A., Alobid, I., Fuentes, M., Cortijo, J., Picado, C., et al. (2014). Reconstituted human upper airway epithelium as 3-d *in vitro* model for nasal polyposis. *PLoS ONE* 9:e100537. doi:10.1371/journal.pone.0100537

De Luca, A. C., Zink, M., Weidt, A., Mayr, S. G., and Markaki, A. E. (2015). Effect of microgrooved surface topography on osteoblast maturation and protein adsorption. *J. Biomed. Mater. Res. A.* doi:10.1002/jbm.a.35407

DeSimone, D. W., and Horwitz, A. R. (2014). Many modes of motility. *Science* 345, 1002–1003. doi:10.1126/science.1259176

Diehl, K. A., Foley, J. D., Nealey, P. F., and Murphy, C. J. (2005). Nanoscale topography modulates corneal epithelial cell migration. *J. Biomed. Mater. Res. A* 75, 603–611. doi:10.1002/jbm.a.30467

Dunn, J. C., Tompkins, R. G., and Yarmush, M. L. (1992). Hepatocytes in collagen sandwich: evidence for transcriptional and translational regulation. *J. Cell Biol.* 116, 1043–1053. doi:10.1083/jcb.116.4.1043

Ebara, M., Uto, K., Idota, N., Hoffman, J. M., and Aoyagi, T. (2014). The taming of the cell: shape-memory nanopatterns direct cell orientation. *Int. J. Nanomedicine* 9(Suppl. 1), 117–126. doi:10.2147/IJN.S50677

Fackler, O., and Grosse, R. (2008). Cell motility through plasma membrane blebbing. *J. Cell Biol.* 181, 879–884. doi:10.1083/jcb.200802081

Farahani, E., Patra, H. K., Jangamreddy, J. R., Rashedi, I., Kawalec, M., Rao Pariti, R. K., et al. (2014). Cell adhesion molecules and their relation to (cancer) cell stemness. *Carcinogenesis* 35, 747–759. doi:10.1093/carcin/bgu045

Fernandez-Yague, M. A., Abbah, S. A., McNamara, L., Zeugolis, D. I., Pandit, A., and Biggs, M. J. (2014). Biomimetic approaches in bone tissue engineering: integrating biological and physicomechanical strategies. *Adv. Drug Deliv. Rev.* doi:10.1016/j.addr.2014.09.005

Friedl, P., Wolf, K., and Lammerding, J. (2011). Nuclear mechanics during cell migration. *Curr. Opin. Cell Biol.* 23, 55–64. doi:10.1016/j.ceb.2010.10.015

Fuentes, D. E., Bae, C., and Butler, P. J. (2011). Focal adhesion induction at the tip of a functionalized nanoelectrode. *Cell. Mol. Bioeng.* 4, 616–626. doi:10.1007/s12195-011-0214-7

Fujita, S., Ohshima, M., and Iwata, H. (2009). Time-lapse observation of cell alignment on nanogrooved patterns. *J. R. Soc. Interface* 6(Suppl. 3), S269–S277. doi:10.1098/rsif.2008.0428.focus

Gaharwar, A. K., Nikkhah, M., Sant, S., and Khademhosseini, A. (2014). Anisotropic poly (glycerol sebacate)-poly (ε-caprolactone) electrospun fibers promote endothelial cell guidance. *Biofabrication* 7, 015001. doi:10.1088/1758-5090/7/1/015001

Gamboa, J. R., Mohandes, S., Tran, P. L., Slepian, M. J., and Yoon, J. Y. (2013). Linear fibroblast alignment on sinusoidal wave micropatterns. *Colloids Surf. B Biointerfaces* 104, 318–325. doi:10.1016/j.colsurfb.2012.11.035

Garland, S. P., McKee, C. T., Chang, Y. R., Raghunathan, V. K., Russell, P., and Murphy, C. J. (2014). A cell culture substrate with biologically relevant size-scale topography and compliance of the basement membrane. *Langmuir* 30, 2101–2108. doi:10.1021/la403590v

Gattazzo, F., Urciuolo, A., and Bonaldo, P. (2014). Extracellular matrix: a dynamic microenvironment for stem cell niche. *Biochim. Biophys. Acta* 1840, 2506–2519. doi:10.1016/j.bbagen.2014.01.010

Germanier, Y., Tosatti, S., Broggini, N., Textor, M., and Buser, D. (2006). Enhanced bone apposition around biofunctionalized sandblasted and acid-etched titanium implant surfaces – a histomorphometric study in miniature pigs. *Clin. Oral Implants Res.* 17, 251–257. doi:10.1111/j.1600-0501.2005.01222.x

Gong, T., Zhao, K., Yang, G., Li, J., Chen, H., Chen, Y., et al. (2014). The control of mesenchymal stem cell differentiation using dynamically tunable surface microgrooves. *Adv. Healthc. Mater.* 3, 1608–1619. doi:10.1002/adhm.201300692

Hanein, D., and Horwitz, A. (2012). The structure of cell-matrix adhesions: the new frontier. *Curr. Opin. Cell Biol.* 24, 134–140. doi:10.1016/j.ceb.2011.12.001

Harimoto, M., Yamato, M., Hirose, M., Takahashi, C., Isoi, Y., Kikuchi, A., et al. (2002). Novel approach for achieving double-layered cell sheets co-culture: overlaying endothelial cell sheets onto monolayer hepatocytes utilizing temperature-responsive culture dishes. *J Biomed Mater Res* 62, 464–470. doi:10.1002/jbm.10228

Harrison, R. (1911). On the stereotropism of embryonic cells. *Science* 34, 279–281. doi:10.1126/science.34.870.279

Herrero-Climent, M., Lazaro, P., Rios, J. V., Lluch, S., Marques, M., Guillem-Marti, J., et al. (2013). Influence of acid-etching after grit-blasted on osseointegration of titanium dental implants: *in vitro* and *in vivo* studies. *J. Mater. Sci. Mater. Med.* 24, 2047–2055. doi:10.1007/s10856-013-4935-0

Hocde, S. A., Hyrien, O., and Waugh, R. E. (2009). Cell adhesion molecule distribution relative to neutrophil surface topography assessed by TIRFM. *Biophys. J.* 97, 379–387. doi:10.1016/j.bpj.2009.04.035

Huang, H., Nakayama, Y., Qin, K., Yamamoto, K., Ando, J., Yamashita, J., et al. (2005). Differentiation from embryonic stem cells to vascular wall cells under *in vitro* pulsatile flow loading. *J. Artif. Organs* 8, 110–118. doi:10.1007/s10047-005-0291-2

Ishibazawa, A., Nagaoka, T., Takahashi, T., Yamamoto, K., Kamiya, A., Ando, J., et al. (2011). Effects of shear stress on the gene expressions of endothelial nitric oxide synthase, endothelin-1, and thrombomodulin in human retinal microvascular endothelial cells. *Invest. Ophthalmol. Vis. Sci.* 52, 8496–8504. doi:10.1167/iovs.11-7686

Itala, A., Koort, J., Ylanen, H. O., Hupa, M., and Aro, H. T. (2003). Biologic significance of surface microroughing in bone incorporation or porous bioactive glass implants. *J. Biomed. Mater. Res. A* 67A, 496–503. doi:10.1002/jbm.a.10501

Janson, I. A., Kong, Y. P., and Putnam, A. J. (2014). Nanotopographic substrates of poly (methyl methacrylate) do not strongly influence the osteogenic phenotype of mesenchymal stem cells *in vitro*. *PLoS ONE* 9:e90719. doi:10.1371/journal.pone.0090719

Jeon, K. J., Park, S. H., Shin, J. W., Kang, Y. G., Hyun, J. S., Oh, M. J., et al. (2014). Combined effects of flow-induced shear stress and micropatterned surface morphology on neuronal differentiation of human mesenchymal stem cells. *J. Biosci. Bioeng.* 117, 242–247. doi:10.1016/j.jbiosc.2013.08.002

Jia, Y. Y., Li, F., Geng, N., Gong, P., Huang, S. J., Meng, L. X., et al. (2014). Fluid flow modulates the expression of genes involved in the Wnt signaling pathway in osteoblasts in 3D culture conditions. *Int. J. Mol. Med.* 33, 1282–1288. doi:10.3892/ijmm.2014.1694

Kasorn, A., Alcaide, P., Jia, Y., Subramanian, K. K., Sarraj, B., Li, Y., et al. (2009). Focal adhesion kinase regulates pathogen-killing capability and life span of neutrophils via mediating both adhesion-dependent and -independent cellular signals. *J. Immunol.* 183, 1032–1043. doi:10.4049/jimmunol.0802984

Kim, J., Bae, W. G., Choung, H. W., Lim, K. T., Seonwoo, H., Jeong, H. E., et al. (2014a). Multiscale patterned transplantable stem cell patches for bone tissue regeneration. *Biomaterials* 35, 9058–9067. doi:10.1016/j.biomaterials.2014.07.036

Kim, J. S., Klosener, J., Flor, S., Peters, T. M., Ludewig, G., Thorne, P. S., et al. (2014b). Toxicity assessment of air-delivered particle-bound polybrominated diphenyl ethers. *Toxicology* 317, 31–39. doi:10.1016/j.tox.2014.01.005

Kim, J., Kim, H. N., Lim, K. T., Kim, Y., Seonwoo, H., Park, S. H., et al. (2013). Designing nanotopographical density of extracellular matrix for controlled morphology and function of human mesenchymal stem cells. *Sci. Rep.* 3, 3552. doi:10.1038/srep03552

Kim, S. S., Wen, W., Prowse, P., and Hamilton, D. W. (2015). Regulation of matrix remodelling phenotype in gingival fibroblasts by substratum topography. *J. Cell. Mol. Med.* doi:10.1111/jcmm.12451

Kim, Y., and Rajagopalan, P. (2010). 3D hepatic cultures simultaneously maintain primary hepatocyte and liver sinusoidal endothelial cell phenotypes. *PLoS ONE* 5:e15456. doi:10.1371/journal.pone.0015456

Knothe Tate, M. L., Knothe, U., and Niederer, P. (1998). Experimental elucidation of mechanical load-induced fluid flow and its potential role in bone metabolism and functional adaptation. *Am. J. Med. Sci.* 316, 189–195. doi:10.1097/00000441-199809000-00007

Knothe Tate, M. L., Steck, R., Forwood, M. R., and Niederer, P. (2000). In vivo demonstration of load-induced fluid flow in the rat tibia and its potential implications for processes associated with functional adaptation. *J. Exp. Biol.* 203, 2737–2745.

Kooter, I.M., Alblas, M.J., Jedynska, A.D., Steenhof, M., Houtzager, M.M., Van Ras, M. (2013). Alveolar epithelial cells (A549) exposed at the air-liquid interface to diesel exhaust: First study in TNO's powertrain test center. *Toxicol In Vitro* 27, 2342–2349. doi:10.1016/j.tiv.2013.10.007

Kwon, K. W., Park, H., Song, K. H., Choi, J. C., Ahn, H., Park, M. J., et al. (2012). Nanotopography-guided migration of T cells. *J. Immunol.* 189, 2266–2273. doi:10.4049/jimmunol.1102273

Leal-Egaña, A., Díaz-Cuenca, A., and Boccaccini, A. (2013). Tuning of cell-biomaterial anchorage for tissue regeneration. *Adv. Mater. Weinheim* 25, 4049–4057. doi:10.1002/adma.201301227

Lee, V. K., Lanzi, A. M., Haygan, N., Yoo, S. S., Vincent, P. A., and Dai, G. (2014). Generation of multi-scale vascular network system within 3D hydrogel using 3D bio-printing technology. *Cell. Mol. Bioeng.* 7, 460–472. doi:10.1007/s12195-014-0340-0

Lenhert, S., Meier, M. B., Meyer, U., Chi, L., and Wiesmann, H. P. (2005). Osteoblast alignment, elongation and migration on grooved polystyrene surfaces patterned by Langmuir-Blodgett lithography. *Biomaterials* 26, 563–570. doi:10.1016/j.biomaterials.2004.02.068

Lim, K. T., Kim, J., Seonwoo, H., Chang, J. U., Choi, H., Hexiu, J., et al. (2013). Enhanced osteogenesis of human alveolar bone-derived mesenchymal stem cells for tooth tissue engineering using fluid shear stress in a rocking culture method. *Tissue Eng. Part C Methods* 19, 128–145. doi:10.1089/ten.tec.2012.0017

Lindner, V., Lappi, D. A., Baird, A., Majack, R. A., and Reidy, M. A. (1991). Role of basic fibroblast growth factor in vascular lesion formation. *Circ. Res.* 68, 106–113. doi:10.1161/01.RES.68.1.106

Londono, C., Loureiro, M. J., Slater, B., Lucker, P. B., Soleas, J., Sathananthan, S., et al. (2014). Nonautonomous contact guidance signaling during collective cell migration. *Proc. Natl. Acad. Sci. U.S.A.* 111, 1807–1812. doi:10.1073/pnas.1321852111

Losert, W., Driscoll, M., Guven, C., Sun, X. Y., and Fourkas, J. (2013). Cellular contact guidance through dynamic sensing of surface topography. *Biophys. J.* 104, 148A–148A. doi:10.1016/j.bpj.2012.11.840

Marino, A., Ciofani, G., Filippeschi, C., Pellegrino, M., Pellegrini, M., Orsini, P., et al. (2013). Two-photon polymerization of sub-micrometric patterned surfaces: investigation of cell-substrate interactions and improved differentiation of neuron-like cells. *ACS Appl. Mater. Interfaces* 5, 13012–13021. doi:10.1021/am403895k

McKee, C. T., Raghunathan, V. K., Nealey, P. F., Russell, P., and Murphy, C. J. (2011). Topographic modulation of the orientation and shape of cell nuclei and their influence on the measured elastic modulus of epithelial cells. *Biophys. J.* 101, 2139–2146. doi:10.1016/j.bpj.2011.09.042

McMurray, R. J., Wann, A. K. T., Thompson, C. L., Connelly, J. T., and Knight, M. M. (2013). Surface topography regulates wnt signaling through control of primary cilia structure in mesenchymal stem cells. *Sci. Rep.* 3, 3545. doi:10.1038/srep03545

McNamara, L. E., Sjöström, T., Burgess, K. E., Kim, J. J., Liu, E., Gordonov, S., et al. (2011). Skeletal stem cell physiology on functionally distinct titania nanotopographies. *Biomaterials* 32, 7403–7410. doi:10.1016/j.biomaterials.2011.06.063

Metallo, C. M., Vodyanik, M. A., de Pablo, J. J., Slukvin, I. I., and Palecek, S. P. (2008). The response of human embryonic stem cell-derived endothelial cells to shear stress. *Biotechnol. Bioeng.* 100, 830–837. doi:10.1002/bit.21809

Nadeem, D., Sjostrom, T., Wilkinson, A., Smith, C. A., Oreffo, R. O., Dalby, M. J., et al. (2013). Embossing of micropatterned ceramics and their cellular response. *J. Biomed. Mater. Res. A* 101, 3247–3255. doi:10.1002/jbm.a.34622

Olivares-Navarrete, R., Hyzy, S. L., Haithcock, D. A., Cundiff, C. A., Schwartz, Z., and Boyan, B. D. (2015). Coordinated regulation of mesenchymal stem cell differentiation on microstructured titanium surfaces by endogenous bone morphogenetic proteins. *Bone* 73, 208–216. doi:10.1016/j.bone.2014.12.057

Paluch, E., and Raz, E. (2013). The role and regulation of blebs in cell migration. *Curr. Opin. Cell Biol.* 25, 582–590. doi:10.1016/j.ceb.2013.05.005

Papadaki, M., Tilton, R. G., Eskin, S. G., and McIntire, L. V. (1998). Nitric oxide production by cultured human aortic smooth muscle cells: stimulation by fluid flow. *Am. J. Physiol.* 274, H616–H626.

Papadopoulos, M., and Saadoun, S. (2014). Key roles of aquaporins in tumor biology. *Biochim. Biophys. Acta.* doi:10.1016/j.bbamem.2014.09.001

Pedron, S., Becka, E., and Harley, B. A. (2015). Spatially gradated hydrogel platform as a 3D engineered tumor microenvironment. *Adv. Mater.* 27, 1567–1572. doi:10.1002/adma.201404896

Peng, P., Shi, T., Liao, G., and Tang, Z. (2010). Combined AFM nano-machining and reactive ion etching to fabricate high aspect ratio structures. *J. Nanosci. Nanotechnol.* 10, 7287–7290. doi:10.1166/jnn.2010.2858

Perez-Garnes, M., Gonzalez-Garcia, C., Moratal, D., Rico, P., and Salmeron-Sanchez, M. (2011). Fibronectin distribution on demixed nanoscale topographies. *Int. J. Artif. Organs* 34, 54–63. doi:10.5301/IJAO.2011.6316

Petrie, R., Koo, H., and Yamada, K. (2014). Generation of compartmentalized pressure by a nuclear piston governs cell motility in a 3D matrix. *Science* 345, 1062–1065. doi:10.1126/science.1256965

Petrie, R., and Yamada, K. (2012). At the leading edge of three-dimensional cell migration. *J. Cell Sci.* 125, 5917–5926. doi:10.1242/jcs.093732

Piekarski, K., and Munro, M. (1977). Transport mechanism operating between blood supply and osteocytes in long bones. *Nature* 269, 80–82. doi:10.1038/269080a0

Potter, C. M., Lao, K. H., Zeng, L., and Xu, Q. (2014). Role of biomechanical forces in stem cell vascular lineage differentiation. *Arterioscler. Thromb. Vasc. Biol.* 34, 2184–2190. doi:10.1161/ATVBAHA.114.303423

Ranganathan, S. I., Ostoja-Starzewski, M., and Ferrari, M. (2011). Quantifying the anisotropy in biological materials. *J. Appl. Mech. Trans. ASME* 78, 064501-1–064501-4. doi:10.1115/1.4004553

Ridley, A., Schwartz, M., Burridge, K., Firtel, R., Ginsberg, M., Borisy, G., et al. (2003). Cell migration: integrating signals from front to back. *Science* 302, 1704–1709. doi:10.1126/science.1092053

Sant, S., Hancock, M. J., Donnelly, J. P., Iyer, D., and Khademhosseini, A. (2010). Biomimetic gradient hydrogels for tissue engineering. *Can. J. Chem. Eng.* 88, 899–911. doi:10.1002/cjce.20411

Sjöström, T., McNamara, L. E., Meek, R. M., Dalby, M. J., and Su, B. (2013). 2D and 3D nanopatterning of titanium for enhancing osteoinduction of stem cells at implant surfaces. *Adv. Healthc. Mater.* 2, 1285–1293. doi:10.1002/adhm.201200353

Sjöström, T., McNamara, L. E., Yang, L., Dalby, M. J., and Su, B. (2012). Novel anodization technique using a block copolymer template for nanopatterning of titanium implant surfaces. *ACS Appl. Mater. Interfaces* 4, 6354–6361. doi:10.1021/am301987e

Smalt, R., Mitchell, F. T., Howard, R. L., and Chambers, T. J. (1997). Induction of NO and prostaglandin E2 in osteoblasts by wall-shear stress but not mechanical strain. *Am. J. Physiol.* 273, E751–E758.

Smith, C. L. C., Thilsted, A. H., Garcia-Ortiz, C. E., Radko, I. P., Marie, R., Jeppesen, C., et al. (2014). Efficient excitation of channel plasmons in tailored, UV-lithography-defined V-grooves. *Nano Lett.* 14, 1659–1664. doi:10.1021/nl5002058

Song, K. H., Kwon, K. W., Choi, J. C., Jung, J., Park, Y., Suh, K. Y., et al. (2014). T cells sense biophysical cues using lamellipodia and filopodia to optimize intraluminal path finding. *Integr. Biol. (Camb.)* 6, 450–459. doi:10.1039/c4ib00021h

Song, K. H., Kwon, K. W., Song, S., Suh, K. Y., and Doh, J. (2012). Dynamics of T cells on endothelial layers aligned by nanostructured surfaces. *Biomaterials* 33, 2007–2015. doi:10.1016/j.biomaterials.2011.12.002

Stroka, K., Jiang, H., Gu, Z., Sun, S., and Konstantopoulos, K. (2014a). Bioengineering paradigms for cell migration in confined microenvironments. *Curr. Opin. Cell Biol.* 30, 41–51. doi:10.1016/j.ceb.2014.06.001

Stroka, K., Jiang, H., Chen, S. H., Tong, Z., Wirtz, D., Sun, S., et al. (2014b). Water permeation drives tumor cell migration in confined microenvironments. *Cell* 157, 611–623. doi:10.1016/j.cell.2014.02.052

Svensson, S., Suska, F., Emanuelsson, L., Palmquist, A., Norlindh, B., Trobos, M., et al. (2013). Osseointegration of titanium with an antimicrobial nanostructured noble metal coating. *Nanomedicine* 9, 1048–1056. doi:10.1016/j.nano.2013.04.009

Swift, B., Pfeifer, N. D., and Brouwer, K. L. (2010). Sandwich-cultured hepatocytes: an *in vitro* model to evaluate hepatobiliary transporter-based drug interactions and hepatotoxicity. *Drug Metab. Rev.* 42, 446–471. doi:10.3109/03602530903491881

Takahashi, H., Shimizu, T., Nakayama, M., Yamato, M., and Okano, T. (2013). The use of anisotropic cell sheets to control orientation during the self-organization of 3D muscle tissue. *Biomaterials* 34, 7372–7380. doi:10.1016/j.biomaterials.2013.06.033

Tan, K., Tann, J., Sathe, S. R., Goh, S., Ma, D., Goh, E., et al. (2015). Enhanced differentiation of neural progenitor cells into neurons of the mesencephalic dopaminergic subtype on topographical patterns. *Biomaterials* 43, 32–43. doi:10.1016/j.biomaterials.2014.11.036

Tavangar, A., Tan, B., and Venkatakrishnan, K. (2013). The influence of laser-induced 3-D titania nanofibrous platforms on cell behavior. *J. Biomed. Nanotechnol.* 9, 1837–1846. doi:10.1166/jbn.2013.1679

Teixeira, A. I., McKie, G. A., Foley, J. D., Bertics, P. J., Nealey, P. F., and Murphy, C. J. (2006). The effect of environmental factors on the response of human corneal epithelial cells to nanoscale substrate topography. *Biomaterials* 27, 3945–3954. doi:10.1016/j.biomaterials.2006.01.044

Teixeira, A. I., Nealey, P. F., and Murphy, C. J. (2004). Responses of human keratocytes to micro- and nanostructured substrates. *J. Biomed. Mater. Res. A* 71, 369–376. doi:10.1002/jbm.a.30089

Tonazzini, I., Cecchini, A., Elgersma, Y., and Cecchini, M. (2014). Interaction of SH-SY5Y cells with nanogratings during neuronal differentiation: comparison with primary neurons. *Adv. Healthc. Mater.* 3, 581–587. doi:10.1002/adhm.201300216

Tonazzini, I., Meucci, S., Faraci, P., Beltram, F., and Cecchini, M. (2013). Neuronal differentiation on anisotropic substrates and the influence of nanotopographical noise on neurite contact guidance. *Biomaterials* 34, 6027–6036. doi:10.1016/j.biomaterials.2013.04.039

Tsai, H. Y., Pitera, J. W., Miyazoe, H., Bangsaruntip, S., Engelmann, S. U., Liu, C. C., et al. (2014). Two-dimensional pattern formation using graphoepitaxy of PS-b-PMMA block copolymers for advanced FinFET device and circuit fabrication. *ACS Nano* 8, 5227–5232. doi:10.1021/nn501300b

Vicente-Manzanares, M., and Horwitz, A. (2011). Adhesion dynamics at a glance. *J. Cell Sci.* 124, 3923–3927. doi:10.1242/jcs.095653

Voisin, C., Aerts, C., Jakubczk, E., and Tonnel, A. B. (1977). [La culture cellulaire en phase gazeuse. Un nouveau modele experimental d'etude *in vitro* des activites des macrophages alveolaires]. *Bull. Eur. Physiopathol. Respir.* 13, 69–82.

Vozzi, F., Bianchi, F., Ahluwalia, A., and Domenici, C. (2014). Hydrostatic pressure and shear stress affect endothelin-1 and nitric oxide release by endothelial cells in bioreactors. *Biotechnol. J.* 9, 146–154. doi:10.1002/biot.201300016

Wang, P. Y., Li, W. T., Yu, J., and Tsai, W. B. (2012). Modulation of osteogenic, adipogenic and myogenic differentiation of mesenchymal stem cells by submicron grooved topography. *J. Mater. Sci. Mater. Med.* 23, 3015–3028. doi:10.1007/s10856-012-4748-6

Wang, Y., Jiang, S., Shi, H., Zhang, W., Qiao, J., Wu, M., et al. (2013a). Heteroepitaxy of anisotropic polycaprolactone films for the guidance of smooth muscle cell growth. *Chem. Commun.* 49, 10421–10423. doi:10.1039/C3CC46359A

Wang, Z. Y., Teo, E. Y., Chong, M. S., Zhang, Q. Y., Lim, J., Zhang, Z. Y., et al. (2013b). Biomimetic three-dimensional anisotropic geometries by uniaxial stretch of poly(ε-caprolactone) films for mesenchymal stem cell proliferation, alignment, and myogenic differentiation. *Tissue Eng. Part C Methods* 19, 538–549. doi:10.1089/ten.tec.2012.0472

Watari, S., Hayashi, K., Wood, J., Russell, P., Nealey, P., Murphy, C., et al. (2012). Modulation of osteogenic differentiation in hMSCs cells by submicron topographically-patterned ridges and grooves. *Biomaterials* 33, 128–136. doi:10.1016/j.biomaterials.2011.09.058

Weiss, P., and Garber, B. (1952). Shape and movement of mesenchyme cells as functions of the physical structure of the medium. *Proc. Natl. Acad. Sci. U.S.A.* 38, 264–280. doi:10.1073/pnas.38.3.264

Wilson, K., Lewalle, A., Fritzsche, M., Thorogate, R., Duke, T., and Charras, G. (2013). Mechanisms of leading edge protrusion in interstitial migration. *Nat. Commun.* 4, 289. doi:10.1038/ncomms3896

Wojciak, B., Crossan, J., Curtis, A., and Wilkinson, C. (1995). Grooved substrata facilitate *in vitro* healing of completely divided flexor tendons. *J. Mater. Sci. Mater. Med.* 6, 266–271. doi:10.1007/BF00120269

Wu, X., and Wang, S. (2013). Biomimetic calcium carbonate concentric microgrooves with tunable widths for promoting MC3T3-E1 cell functions. *Adv. Healthc. Mater.* 2, 326–333. doi:10.1002/adhm.201200205

Wu, Y. N., Law, J. B. K., He, A. Y., Low, H. Y., Hui, J. H. P., Lim, C. T., et al. (2014). Substrate topography determines the fate of chondrogenesis from human mesenchymal stem cells resulting in specific cartilage phenotype formation. *Nanomedicine* 10, 1507–1516. doi:10.1016/j.nano.2014.04.002

Xia, L., Arooz, T., Zhang, S., Tuo, X., Xiao, G., Susanto, T. A., et al. (2012a). Hepatocyte function within a stacked double sandwich culture plate cylindrical bioreactor for bioartificial liver system. *Biomaterials* 33, 7925–7932. doi:10.1016/j.biomaterials.2012.06.078

Xia, L., Feng, B., Wang, P., Ding, S., Liu, Z., Zhou, J., et al. (2012b). *In vitro* and *in vivo* studies of surface-structured implants for bone formation. *Int. J. Nanomedicine* 7, 4873–4881. doi:10.2147/IJN.S29496

Xia, L., Ng, S., Han, R., Tuo, X., Xiao, G., Leo, H. L., et al. (2009). Laminar-flow immediate-overlay hepatocyte sandwich perfusion system for drug hepatotoxicity testing. *Biomaterials* 30, 5927–5936. doi:10.1016/j.biomaterials.2009.07.022

Xie, L., Liao, X., Yin, G., Huang, Z., Yan, D., Yao, Y., et al. (2011). Preparation, characterization, *in vitro* bioactivity, and osteoblast adhesion of multi-level porous titania layer on titanium by two-step anodization treatment. *J. Biomed. Mater. Res. A* 98, 312–320. doi:10.1002/jbm.a.33120

Yang, K., Jung, H., Lee, H. R., Lee, J. S., Kim, S. R., Song, K. Y., et al. (2014). Multiscale, hierarchically patterned topography for directing human neural stem cells into functional neurons. *ACS Nano* 8, 7809–7822. doi:10.1021/Nn501182f

Yang, Y., Kusano, K., Frei, H., Rossi, F., Brunette, D. M., and Putnins, E. E. (2010). Microtopographical regulation of adult bone marrow progenitor cells chondrogenic and osteogenic gene and protein expressions. *J. Biomed. Mater. Res. A* 95, 294–304. doi:10.1002/jbm.a.32838

Yim, E. K., Pang, S. W., and Leong, K. W. (2007). Synthetic nanostructures inducing differentiation of human mesenchymal stem cells into neuronal lineage. *Exp. Cell Res.* 313, 1820–1829. doi:10.1016/j.yexcr.2007.02.031

Zamora, P.O., Benson, J.M., Li, A.P., Brooks, A.L. (1983). Evaluation of an exposure system using cells grown on collagen gels for detecting highly volatile mutagens in the CHO/HGPRT mutation assay. *Environ Mutagen* 5, 795–801.

Zamora, P.O., Gregory, R.E., Li, A.P., Brooks, A.L. (1986). An in vitro model for the exposure of lung alveolar epithelial cells to toxic gases. *J Environ Pathol Toxicol Oncol* 7, 159–168.

Zhu, B., Lu, Q., Yin, J., Hu, J., and Wang, Z. (2005). Alignment of osteoblast-like cells and cell-produced collagen matrix induced by nanogrooves. *Tissue Eng.* 11, 825–834. doi:10.1089/ten.2005.11.825

Zhu, J., Li, J., Wang, B., Zhang, W. J., Zhou, G., Cao, Y., et al. (2010). The regulation of phenotype of cultured tenocytes by microgrooved surface structure. *Biomaterials* 31, 6952–6958. doi:10.1016/j.biomaterials.2010.05.058

Conflict of Interest Statement: The authors declare that the research was conducted in the absence of any commercial or financial relationships that could be construed as a potential conflict of interest. The Review Editor Dimitrios I. Zeugolis declares that, despite being affiliated to the same institution as author Manus J. P. Biggs, the review process was handled objectively and no conflict of interest exists.

13

Bioceramics and Scaffolds: A Winning Combination for Tissue Engineering

Francesco Baino*, Giorgia Novajra and Chiara Vitale-Brovarone

Department of Applied Science and Technology, Institute of Materials Physics and Engineering, Politecnico di Torino, Turin, Italy

Edited by:
Malcolm Xing,
University of Manitoba, Canada

Reviewed by:
Gwendolen Clair Reilly,
University of Sheffield, UK
Qiang Chen,
Southeast University, China

*Correspondence:
Francesco Baino
francesco.baino@polito.it

In the last few decades, we have assisted to a general increase of elder population worldwide associated with age-related pathologies. Therefore, there is the need for new biomaterials that can substitute damaged tissues, stimulate the body's own regenerative mechanisms, and promote tissue healing. Porous templates referred to as "scaffolds" are thought to be required for three-dimensional tissue growth. Bioceramics, a special set of fully, partially, or non-crystalline ceramics (e.g., calcium phosphates, bioactive glasses, and glass–ceramics) that are designed for the repair and reconstruction of diseased parts of the body, have high potential as scaffold materials. Traditionally, bioceramics have been used to fill and restore bone and dental defects (repair of hard tissues). More recently, this category of biomaterials has also revealed promising applications in the field of soft-tissue engineering. Starting with an overview of the fundamental requirements for tissue engineering scaffolds, this article provides a detailed picture on recent developments of porous bioceramics and composites, including a summary of common fabrication technologies and a critical analysis of structure–property and structure–function relationships. Areas of future research are highlighted at the end of this review, with special attention to the development of multifunctional scaffolds exploiting therapeutic ion/drug release and emerging applications beyond hard tissue repair.

Keywords: hydroxyapatite, calcium phosphate, bioglass, glass–ceramic, composite, bioactivity, porosity

INTRODUCTION

The term "tissue engineering" was up to the mid 1980s loosely applied in the literature in cases of surgical manipulation of tissues and organs or in a broader sense when prosthetic devices or biomaterials were used. A clear definition was given by Langer and Vacanti (1993) as follows:

> Tissue engineering is an interdisciplinary field that applies the principles of engineering and life science toward the development of biological substitutes that restore, maintain, or improve the tissue function.

Without a doubt, tissue engineering aims to provide a permanent solution to the replacement of tissues that are either defective or have been lost due to different pathological conditions, and it has emerged as a promising alternative to tissue or organ transplantation. This approach uses interdisciplinary tools to produce devices that have the potential to integrate and regenerate a specific functional tissue upon implantation. A key component of this strategy is a synthetic framework referred to as scaffold, which serves as a guiding two- or three-dimensional (2- or 3-D) structure for both hard- and soft-tissue development both *in vitro* and *in vivo*. Due to its open system of interconnected pores, the scaffold provides a mechanically stable environment that can host the required cells and biological components (seeded in the laboratory prior to implantation), allow cell migration, adhesion and growth, and support the organization of the growing tissue when implanted *in vivo* (Nerem, 1991). This is further enhanced by the use of "signaling," which is another building block of tissue engineering. Signaling involves biochemical and biomechanical signals (delivered by the scaffold), which activate *in vivo* mechanisms of tissue regeneration, coaxing the cells into creating viable tissues and, thus, determining whether the scaffold turns into integrated tissue (Rutenberg et al., 2004; Johnson et al., 2007).

Many different materials have been investigated and engineered (natural and synthetic, bioresorbable, and permanent) to construct scaffolds. Among these, bioceramics have been extensively considered since these materials generally show better tissue responses compared to polymers and metals (Hench, 1998). Some bioceramics, such as hydroxyapatite (HA) and alumina, are intended to be permanent devices, thus they do not release their components into the human body and are expected to generate no foreign body reactions. On the other hand, if designed as resorbable biomaterials (e.g., most bioactive glasses) with various resorption kinetics (from days to months), their ion dissolution products (typically Ca, Si, Na, and phosphate ions) can be usually processed via normal metabolism (Habibovic and Barralet, 2011) or even exploited to exert a desired therapeutic effect, such as promotion of angiogenesis and antibacterial properties (Gerhardt et al., 2011; Hoppe et al., 2011; Mourino et al., 2012; Vargas et al., 2013).

Given the inorganic nature and mechanical rigidity of bioceramics, their traditional fields of application have been related to hard tissue repair, such as bone and teeth. However, several studies have also demonstrated the potential of bioceramics as an innovative route to regenerate various types of damaged soft tissues (Baino et al., 2016b; Miguez-Pacheco et al., 2015a).

This article will look at bioceramic materials used as scaffolds for hard- and soft-tissue engineering. First, basic scaffold requirements are examined and an overview of bioceramics used to produce a variety of scaffolds is given. Then, the main fabrication technologies used for making scaffolds are presented discussing both advantages and limitations. Further directions for the research are finally discussed, highlighting the promise of multifunctional engineered systems that combine the "conventional" proprieties of bioceramics and new, smart added values for improved therapeutic action (e.g., ion release and drug delivery).

SCAFFOLD REQUIREMENTS AND CRITICAL ISSUES

Tissue engineering scaffolds have been widely studied with the hope of designing implantable biomaterials that can produce the most appropriate host response in which the clinical situation

demands while supporting the growth and regeneration of complex 3-D tissues. There are several widely accepted requirements that should characterize an ideal scaffold (Hutmacher, 2000; Jones et al., 2007; Gerhardt and Boccaccini, 2010; Baino and Vitale-Brovarone, 2011), as summarized in **Table 1**.

A major difficulty in the design of scaffolds is to simultaneously tailor these requirements due to their competing nature in fulfilling host tissue demands, namely, if a specific requisite is accomplished, another one might in turn be negatively affected.

A crucial aspect for the successful outcome of scaffolds for load-bearing applications (e.g., bone tissue repair) is the need to balance the porosity of a scaffold with its mechanical proprieties (Vitale-Brovarone et al., 2009). As described in **Table 1**, a highly interconnected porous structure (typically a pore content above 50 vol.%) is essential to enable full integration of the scaffold once it is implanted. However, porosity affects the mechanical

TABLE 1 | Design criteria for tissue engineering scaffolds.

Requirements	Description
(i) Geometry	It must initially fill complex 3-D defects, subsequently guiding the tissue to match the original 3-D anatomy
(ii) Bioactivity	Stimulation of rapid tissue attachment to the implant surface (without formation of scar/fibrous tissue) and creation of a stable long-term bonding that prevents micromotion at the interface and the onset of an inflammatory response
(iii) Biocompatibility	Ability to support normal cellular activity including molecular signaling systems without any local and/or systemic toxic effects to the host tissue
(iv) Chemical and biological stability/ biodegradability	Depending on the specific application; if the scaffold must remain *in situ* indefinitely, materials with high stability must be selected; conversely, if it is intended to be a temporary device, the scaffold must degrade gradually over a predetermined period of time and be replaced by the natural host tissue
(v) Porous structure	The scaffold must possess an interconnected porous structure with a large surface-to-volume ratio and pore size of at least 100 μm in diameter (ideal for bone repair) to allow cell penetration, tissue in-growth, facilitate vascularization of the construct, and nutrient transport
(vi) Mechanical competence/ compliance	The mechanical performance of the scaffold, which is determined by both the properties of the biomaterial and the porous structure, must be sufficient to withstand implantation handling and support the loads and stresses that the new tissue will ultimately bear. Adequate elastic compliance (low stiffness) with soft tissue is required for non-osseous applications
(vii) Biological properties	Special properties, such as the promotion of angiogenesis, stimulation of cell differentiation, and antibacterial effect, can be achieved by the release of appropriate ions from the scaffold material. These added values are typically imparted to bioactive glass scaffolds by carefully designing the glass composition
(viii) Fabrication	The scaffold should be easily tailored in size and shape to the diseased or injured area that the new tissue will replace
(ix) Commercialization potential	The scaffold should be produced with an automated technique in a reproducible manner; it should be fabricated and sterilized according to international standards for commercial production and clinical use

competence of the component, as strength and stiffness progressively diminish when the volume fraction of porosity is increased (Gibson, 1989).

If the scaffold is intended to be bioresorbable, the achievement of mechanical competence becomes a further hurdle since degradable materials tend to be mechanically more and more fragile over time. Additional complications in the development of bioresorbable scaffolds are (i) the maintenance of strength and stability of the interface during the degradation period and replacement by the natural host tissue and (ii) matching the rate of resorption with that of the expected specific tissue regeneration. It is also important that the breakdown products of the biomaterial can be readily metabolized without causing any local or systemic adverse reaction (Hoppe et al., 2011).

Another aspect that is worth mentioning concerns the limitation of elastic modulus mismatch, which is crucial for the long-term success of implant bonding to both hard and soft tissues. Several studies demonstrated that the discontinuous change in elastic properties at the tissue–implant interface results in large stress gradients to the host tissue ultimately leading to failure of the implanted material (Hench and Greenspan, 2013).

Optimization of all the physicochemical parameters summarized in **Table 1** is an extremely difficult task due to their complex and still partially unexplained interlocking. The rate and quality of tissue integration have been related to a dependence on scaffold pore size, porosity volume fraction, and pore interconnection (Karageorgiu and Kaplan, 2005). Moreover, the role of strut microstructure and pore geometry has to be considered with respect to their influence on entrapment and recruitment of growth factors in addition to their influence on scaffold mechanics. Deconvoluting the relative effects of these parameters is complicated by the bioactivity of many bioceramics, which is mediated through two principal mechanisms: (i) directly through dissolution and release of ionic products *in vitro* and *in vivo*, elevating local concentrations of soluble species that interact directly with local cells or influence cell behavior by their effect on local pH and (ii) indirectly through the influence that surface chemistry will have on protein adsorption, growth factor entrapment, and subsequent cell attachment and function. A valuable picture on these important issues in view of optimizing scaffold design and fabrication has been recently given by Hing (2005).

A highly challenging field of research concerns the strategies for imparting special "biological" properties to tissue engineering scaffolds, with particular reference to the use of bioactive glasses. It has been demonstrated that key mechanisms leading to enhanced new bone growth are related to the controlled release of ionic dissolution products (e.g., soluble silica and calcium ions) from the degrading bioactive glass (Hench, 2009). Specifically, a series of studies have shown that bioactive silicate glasses and their ionic dissolution products enhance osteogenesis by regulating osteoblast proliferation, differentiation, and gene expression (Xynos et al., 2000, 2001; Jell and Stevens, 2006; Jell et al., 2008). Sun et al. (2007) showed that 45S5 Bioglass® promotes human osteoblast proliferation: in the presence of critical concentrations of Si and Ca ions, within 48 h osteoblasts that are capable of differentiating into a mature osteocyte phenotype begin to proliferate and regenerate new bone and, at the same time, osteoblasts that

are not in the correct phase of the cell cycle and unable to proceed toward differentiation are switched into apoptosis by the ionic dissolution products.

The relative contribution of specific ion dissolution products from bioactive glasses or Si-substituted calcium phosphates to osteogenesis have been controversially debated in the literature (Bohner, 2009; Hoppe et al., 2011). It has been hypothesized that the high Si concentration from bioactive glass could be a major factor in stimulating osteoblasts to grow quickly, which might be effective for melt-derived bioactive glasses (Xynos et al., 2001; Sun et al., 2007). However, Bielby et al. (2004) found no significant differences in the proliferation of human primary osteoblasts grown in conditioned cell culture media containing similar Ca, P, and Na ions but different Si ion concentrations released from a sol–gel bioactive glass. Therefore, further studies are required to gain quantitative knowledge and to confirm the mechanisms by which ion dissolution products from bioactive glass may affect gene expression in bone cells.

Recent findings also indicate that controlled release of low concentrations of ionic dissolution products from bioactive glasses can induce angiogenesis that plays a key role in the regeneration process of both hard and soft tissue (Gerhardt et al., 2011; Vargas et al., 2013). The role of angiogenic and osteogenic factors in the adaptive response and interaction of osteoblasts and endothelial cells during the processes of bone development and bone repair has been reviewed in detail by Kanczler and Oreffo (2008).

Early studies suggesting that the ability of bioactive glasses to induce differentiation of non-osseous cells (e.g., muscle precursor cells exposed to phosphate glasses) have been recently reported (Ahmed et al., 2004).

BIOCERAMICS: A SHORT OVERVIEW

Bioceramics is a large class of specially designed ceramics for the repair and reconstruction of diseased or damaged parts of the body. Current forms of application in clinical use include solid pieces (used, for instance, in the reconstruction of middle ear ossicles or as load-bearing components of joint prostheses), powders and granules for bone filling, coatings on metal joint prostheses, injectable formulations (bone cement), and porous scaffolds (**Figure 1**). Based on their tissue response, bioceramics can be classified into three major families: nearly inert (e.g., alumina and zirconia), bioactive (e.g., bioactive glass), and resorbable ceramics [e.g., β- and α-tricalcium phosphate (TCP)] (Hench, 1996). Nearly, inert ceramics are generally used as femoral heads and acetabular cups for hip replacement as well as to fabricate dental implants; however, usually these materials are not used as scaffolds due to their inertness that triggers the formation of a 1- to 3-μm thick "protective" fibrous capsule on the surface of the implant. Even if there is no aggressive foreign body response, there is no bond between the implant and the host tissue (Hench, 1996).

The ability of creating a stable bond with the host tissue is of primary importance in the selection of bioceramics for making scaffolds. In this regard, bioactive as well as bioresorbable ceramics represent a valuable solution. Furthermore, the latter ones exhibit the added value of degrading gradually over a period of

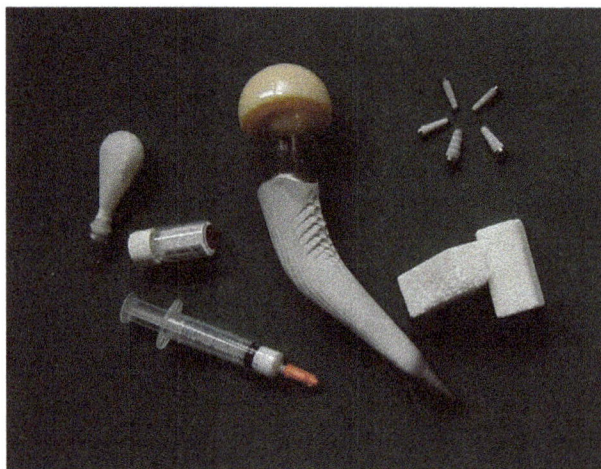

FIGURE 1 | Examples of commercial bioceramics for medical applications: powders and granules for use as bone fillers (typically calcium phosphates or bioactive glass), hemispherical acetabular cup (alumina) for hip joint prosthesis, hydroxyapatite coating on femoral metal stem, porous scaffolds (usually calcium phosphates or bioactive glass/glass–ceramic). Image reproduced from © Dorozhkin (2010a).

time while being replaced by the natural host tissue and, therefore, disappear once their task of acting as templates for new tissue has been completed (Baino and Vitale-Brovarone, 2011; Fu et al., 2011a,b).

The following sections focus on the main types of bioceramics that are currently used to fabricate scaffolds by schematically grouping the materials in their specific class from a microstructural viewpoint: crystalline ceramics, bioactive glasses, glass–ceramics, and composites. Applications and clinical developments are also shortly discussed.

Crystalline Ceramics

The major representatives of this class are calcium phosphates that are among the most widely used crystalline ceramics for bone tissue regeneration. This is due to their exceptional properties that include (i) similarity, in terms of structure and chemical composition, to the mineral phase of bone, and (ii) osteoconductivity, i.e., the ability of providing a biocompatible interface along with bone migrates, and thus bonds to the host tissue without the formation of scar tissue (Cao and Hench, 1996; LeGeros, 2002).

Synthetic HA ($Ca_{10}(PO_4)_6(OH)_2$) has a stoichiometric calcium-to-phosphate ratio of 1:67 and, from a crystallographic point of view, is the calcium phosphate phase most similar to natural bone apatite. Because of its excellent biocompatibility and osteoconductivity, HA is successfully used as bone filler in the form of cement or granules and in the form of coatings on metallic joint prostheses. However, its use as a scaffold material is limited because of its low mechanical properties and extremely slow resorption rate (Barrere et al., 2006).

It is partly for this reason that other calcium phosphates have emerged with different degrees of solubility depending mainly

on the calcium-to-phosphorous ratio (the rate of dissolution increases with decreasing Ca/P ratio) as well as on the crystallographic structure (Hench, 1996; Dorozhkin, 2007, 2010a,b). The interested reader is addressed to specific publications dealing with calcium phosphate bioceramics (Legeros et al., 2003; Dorozhkin, 2012).

A common drawback to all calcium phosphate bioceramics produced in a porous form is their low mechanical properties (brittleness, low fatigue strength) that largely limit their clinical use to non-major load-bearing parts of the skeleton. We have to consider that calcium phosphate scaffolds are often consolidated by sintering that, however, does not occur under a viscous flow regime, and thus may not lead to full densification of scaffold struts. Other materials, such as a few bioactive glass–ceramics and composites, seem to be more suitable for fabricating high-strength, tough scaffolds (Baino and Vitale-Brovarone, 2011; Fu et al., 2011a,b).

Besides calcium phosphates, alumina is another well-known example of crystalline ceramic that has been widely used for decades to fabricate components of hip and knee joint prostheses (femur head, acetabular cup, and tibial plate) primarily due to its high-strength suitable for load-bearing applications, excellent wear resistance, and bioinertness (associated with maintenance of the desired physico-chemical and mechanical properties over time) (Rahaman et al., 2007). Porous alumina is clinically used only in the fabrication of orbital implants (spherical porous scaffolds) for enucleation that should allow fibrovascular ingrowth through the pore network and remain in the patient's anophthalmic socket indefinitely without undergoing degradation (Baino et al., 2014; Baino and Vitale-Brovarone, 2015a).

Bioactive Glasses

It has been extensively proved that bioactive glasses are able to strongly bond to living tissues (primarily bone) creating a stable interface and to trigger a range of biological responses, such as tissue regeneration and angiogenesis while degrading over time (Hench, 2006; Jones, 2013).

These properties of bioactive glasses arise from a time-dependent modification of their surface that occurs on exposure to physiological environment. The glass surface forms a biologically active layer of HA that provides the bonding interface with host tissues, while the dissolution products (Si, Na, Ca, phosphate ions, etc.) stimulate the cells to produce new tissue (Cao and Hench, 1996).

The first bioactive glass, belonging to the $45SiO_2–24.5Na_2O–24.5CaO–6P_2O_5$ (wt.%) system (45S5 Bioglass®), was developed by Prof. Larry Hench and coworkers in the late 1960s (Hench et al., 1971) and is in clinical use since 1985. Over the years, many other silicate, borate, and phosphate glasses have been proposed for biomedical applications, as reviewed elsewhere (Baino and Vitale-Brovarone, 2011; Rahaman et al., 2011).

Bioactive glasses are commonly produced by traditional melting-quenching routes or the sol–gel technique. Melt-derived glasses can be poured into molds to produce rods and bars or cast as components of various sizes and shapes. The melt can also be quenched in cold water to obtain a "frit," i.e., granules and pieces of different sizes that can be easily powdered and further processed to fabricate porous scaffolds (Baino and Vitale-Brovarone, 2011). Finally, the glasses can be also spun to fabricate glass fibers that in the last decade have attracted increasing interest for application in soft-tissue engineering, especially the phosphate ones, as guides for muscle or nerve repair (Vitale-Brovarone et al., 2012a) as well as for the fabrication of glassy bone scaffolds (Gu et al., 2013). For melt-derived silicate glasses, the silica content should be <60 mol.% to allow the glass to bond with bone (Wilson et al., 1981). However, HA layer formation and bone bonding can be also achieved with glasses with up to 90 mol.% silica if the glass is obtained by a sol–gel process (Li et al., 1991). In general, sol–gel glasses were found to form a nanocrystalline HA surface layer more rapidly than melt-derived glasses due to the higher surface area available for ion-exchange phenomena (tens vs. few meter square per gram).

In the last decade, the advent of mesoporous bioactive glasses (MBGs) allowed combining superior bioactive properties (formation of a surface HA layer within few hours from contact with biological fluids) and drug uptake/release abilities in a single, multifunctional biomaterial (Arcos and Vallet-Regí, 2013).

Glass–Ceramics

Glass can be converted by heating into a partially crystalline material containing various kinds of crystalline phases with controlled size and content depending on the thermal treatment parameters. Generally, the resulting glass–ceramic material exhibits superior mechanical properties with respect to its parent glass, specifically higher elastic modulus, hardness, failure strength, and wear resistance. Scaffolds are often produced by sintering, which requires glasses to be heated above their glass transition temperature in order to initiate localized flow. Many bioactive glasses, including 45S5 Bioglass®, crystallize immediately above their glass transition temperature; therefore, sintered bioactive glass scaffolds are often glass–ceramic scaffolds (Gerhardt and Boccaccini, 2010; Baino and Vitale-Brovarone, 2011).

45S5 Bioglass®-derived scaffolds suffer from some drawbacks as the base glass tends to crystallize before full densification is achieved (sintering end), thereby originating extremely brittle glass–ceramic porous products; furthermore, scaffold bioactivity seems to be partially suppressed by the development of a sodium–calcium–silicate crystalline phase (Chen et al., 2006). In the attempt to overcome these drawbacks, interesting results have been obtained by various research groups that proposed alternative glass–ceramics. For instance, Vitale-Brovarone et al. (2007) used the bioactive glass CEL2 ($45SiO_2$–$26CaO$–$15Na_2O$–$3P_2O_5$–$4K_2O$–$7MgO$ mol.%) to fabricate foam-like glass–ceramic scaffolds exhibiting compressive strength up to 1 MPa (porosity 70 vol.%) and an excellent biological compatibility with osteoblasts; more recently, the same research group successfully optimized the process parameters to obtain scaffolds with higher strength (5–6 MPa) within the typical range of cancellous bone (2–12 MPa) (Vitale-Brovarone et al., 2009; Baino et al., 2013). Glass–ceramic bone-like scaffolds based on the experimental glass SCNA ($57SiO_2$–$34CaO$–$6Na_2O$–$3Al_2O_3$ mol.%) can reach a compressive strength of 15 MPa (porosity around 65 vol.%), which makes them suitable for load-bearing applications but

retain an extremely moderate bioactivity (Vitale-Brovarone et al., 2012b; Baino and Vitale-Brovarone, 2014).

Composites

A crucial aspect for the success of scaffolds in tissue engineering and regeneration of tissues is that the structure and properties of the scaffolds must be pertinent to the tissue concerned and the mechanical loads that it will experience *in vivo*. Like most ceramic materials, bioceramics have the disadvantage of exhibiting low fracture toughness (i.e., brittleness) and this could limit their use in load-bearing applications. Furthermore, their high stiffness may restrict the use of bioceramics in non-osseous applications, where adequate compliance with soft tissues is necessary (Miguez-Pacheco et al., 2015a).

One approach that aims to overcome these problems is the combination of bioceramics with polymers to produce a composite scaffold, which makes the most of both materials. Typically, bioceramics are added as fillers or coatings to the polymer matrix to improve its mechanical proprieties, i.e., to increase strength and stiffness as well as to effectively induce enhanced bioactivity (Mohamad Yunos et al., 2008).

Following an alternative strategy, Bretcanu et al. (2007) fabricated porous composites by using a bioceramic scaffold (45S5 Bioglass®) as a porous inorganic matrix and by coating it with poly(3-hydroxybutyrate) (P3HB). The polymer was specifically introduced to strengthen the 45S5 Bioglass® scaffold structure, in fact, the P3HB layer acted as a glue, thereby holding the inorganic particles together when the scaffold struts started to fail. The compressive strength of such a composite scaffold (up to 1.5 MPa) was twice than that of bare 45S5 Bioglass® scaffolds (up to 0.4 MPa) (Chen et al., 2006).

Added values, such as drug uptake/release, are also provided to the composite if mesoporous glass particles are used as a second phase (Arcos and Vallet-Regí, 2013).

Both non-degradable and degradable polymers have been used in the fabrication of composite scaffolds; however, stable polymers often have low biocompatibility as they tend to become surrounded by a fibrous capsule once implanted. Therefore, there have been several attempts to create composites based on the combination of biodegradable polymers and bioceramics. The first composites investigated were comprised of HA or TCP used as inorganic phases while poly(L-lactic acid) (PLLA), poly(D/L-lactic acid) (PDLLA), poly(glycolic acid) (PGA), and their copolymers (PLGA) as organic ones (Ambrosio et al., 2001; Deng et al., 2001; Kasaga et al., 2001; Xu et al., 2004). HA/polyethylene porous composites, marketed under the commercial name "Hapex," are currently used in the clinical practice for the repair of orbital floor fractures (Tanner, 2010).

More recently, attention has moved toward nano-bioceramic/polymer composites, which have the potential to improve interaction with the host tissue/cells (Erol-Taygun et al., 2013). In this regard, one of the most fascinating challenges is to develop smart composite biomaterials with nanoscale interaction between the bioactive inorganic phase and the organic one, so that the scaffold could degrade as a single material rather than having mismatched degradation rates of glass and polymer phase. As recently underlined by Jones (2009), this intimate interaction should allow cells to come into contact with both phases at one time, and the scaffold should degrade at a single rate.

A special mention should be devoted to the so-called "star gels," which are a particular type of organically modified silicates ("ormosils") having an organic core surrounded by flexible arms that are terminated in alkoxysilane groups able to form a silica-like network during the sol–gel process (Vallet-Regí et al., 2006). These hybrid materials show bioactive properties and have fracture toughness higher than that of sol–gel glasses and comparable to that of cancellous bone, thus having promise for tissue engineering applications that require good long-term fatigue behavior (Manzano et al., 2006).

Fabrication of bioceramic/metal composites has been also reported where the ceramic phase is applied in the form of a coating. Metallic materials, such as stainless steel, titanium, and Co–Cr–Mo alloy, have become the materials of choice for load-bearing prostheses due to high-strength, good fatigue resistance, and favorable machining properties. Some metallic materials, however, may produce adverse effects such as the release of significant amounts of metal ions into the tissues, which may result in complications, such as inflammatory and immune reactions (Alvarez and Nakajima, 2009). Thus, there is a need to further improve the biocompatibility between metallic materials and host tissue (primarily bone). Wang et al. (2009) prepared porous TiNbZr alloy scaffold coated with calcium phosphate to improve osteoconductivity. Cell culture experiments showed that the surface-modified TiNbZr scaffolds were more favorable for the adhesion and proliferation of osteoblast-like cells compared to bare metal scaffolds.

FABRICATION TECHNOLOGIES OF BIOCERAMIC SCAFFOLDS

A wide range of processing routes has been proposed for the production of bioceramic porous scaffolds for tissue engineering. These include techniques developed *ad hoc* or often adapted from other contexts, such as foaming, solid freeform fabrication (SFF), starch consolidation, organic phase burning-out, and sponge replication.

These various methods provide a mean to control the 3-D structure of tissue engineering constructs, and processing can strongly influence various characteristics of the scaffold. Each method, in fact, is best suited for producing a specific range of pore size and distribution, interconnectivity and overall porosity in addition to strut thickness and orientation. Thus, the most appropriate technique must be accurately selected to meet the demands of the specific type of tissue (Colombo, 2006).

Moreover, each fabrication method differs in terms of overall cost, making some of them attractive for a large-scale production, while others are more appropriate for the development of value-added products.

The following sections examine the main available techniques to fabricate bioceramic scaffolds, highlighting time by time the merits and drawbacks of each method. A comparison of these techniques is given in **Table 2**. An overview of the main methods used to fabricate bioceramic containing composite scaffolds is also provided.

Foaming Methods

Highly porous ceramics can be produced by dispersing a gas in the form of bubbles into a ceramic suspension or colloidal sols, followed by solidification, to obtain pores in the range of 20 µm up to 1–2 mm (Jones and Hench, 2003). The various foaming techniques developed in the literature are based on two approaches: (i) incorporating an external gas by mechanical frothing, injection of a stream of gas, or introduction of an aerosol propellant and (ii) evolution of a gas *in situ*. The decisive step in direct foaming methods is the stabilization and setting of the wet foams. These, in fact, need to be set in order to maintain their porous morphology before heating at high temperature for sintering/ceramization. Furthermore, several transformations in the bubble structure might occur within the interval between foam generation and foam solidification. For instance, the gas bubbles initially have a spherical shape (nucleation phase) and later grow as polyhedral cells (Colombo, 2006). In order to retain the cellular morphology and prevent the collapse of the foamed structure, surfactants are generally used to stabilize the bubbles formed in the liquid phase as they reduce the surface tension of the gas–liquid interfaces. Surfactants stabilize the system for a limited period of time; hence, a further mechanism is then required to provide a more permanent form of stabilization (Sepulveda and Binner, 1999).

The incorporation of bubbles can be brought about by a variety of processing routes.

H_2O_2 foaming involves mixing ceramic powder with an aqueous solution of H_2O_2 as a foaming agent; then, the resulting mixture is cast into molds and stored into an oven at 60°C. At this temperature, H_2O_2 decomposes and the oxygen released tends to form bubbles in the slurry and, thus, gives rise to the foaming process. The sample is then sintered to obtain crystalline ceramics, bioactive glass, and calcium phosphate scaffolds depending on the initial powders (Navarro et al., 2004). By varying the amount of H_2O_2 incorporated and the thermal treatment, the percentage of porosity and pore size can be modulated. However, an intrinsic shortcoming of this foaming method is that pores are interconnected only in a laminar manner, resulting in poor interconnection in the direction perpendicular to the laminae (Li et al., 2002).

An alternative to H_2O_2 foaming is *in situ* polymerization of an organic monomer (or gel-cast foaming). A high-solid-load aqueous ceramic suspension is prepared that also incorporates an organic monomer, which must be soluble in water (e.g., acrylates) together with an initiator and a catalyst to provide *in situ* polymerization (Ortega et al., 2002; Wu et al., 2011b). The two latter ingredients are necessary to control the actual beginning of the polymerization reaction (i.e., the induction time – period of inactivity between the addition of reagents and the polymerization reaction onset), which, in the processing of porous ceramics, must take place during casting. After the addition of a foaming agent (surfactant), the suspension is mechanically agitated to obtain a wet ceramic foam. The foam is cast into the appropriate mold and, after polymerization is complete, the green body is strong enough to be removed from the mold and

TABLE 2 | Comparison of different techniques (listed in alphabetical order) for the fabrication of bioceramic scaffolds (non-composite) on the basis of their advantages and disadvantages.

Technique	Advantages	Disadvantages	Reference
Foaming methods (general)	Allows manufacturing of both closed and open-cell foams; good versatility of final part shapes, as the solution can be cast in molds without additional machining	Difficulty in achieving high interconnectivity; non-porous external surface	Jones and Hench (2003) and Colombo (2006)
H_2O_2 foaming	Simple	Low porosity control laminar pore structure with poor 3-D interconnection	Li et al. (2002) and Navarro et al. (2004)
Sol–gel foaming	Hierarchical structure can be obtained (macroporous scaffold combined with ordered mesoporous texture)	Need for a high degree of control of the foam	Akkus et al. (2002) and Jones and Hench (2004)
In situ polymerization of organic monomer (gel-cast foaming)	Highly porous ceramic; high-strength properties due to the less flawed structure and dense struts and walls produced	Low pore interconnectivity	Sepulveda and Binner (1999), Ortega et al. (2002), Ramay and Zhang (2003), and Wu et al. (2011b)
Organic phase burning-out/space holder	High mechanical strength	Difficult to obtain a homogeneous distribution of pores; poor interconnectivity	Baino et al. (2009) and Wu et al. (2009)
Solid freeform fabrication (SFF) (general)	Customized objects; reproducible	Costly; resolution needs to be improved to the micro-scale	Hollister (2005)
SLA	Complex internal features can be obtained	Only applicable using ceramic/photopolymer blends	Levy et al. (1997), Tesavibul et al. (2012), Scalera et al. (2014), and Sabree et al. (2015)
SLS	High accuracy; good mechanical strength; a broad range of materials can be processed	High temperatures during process; trapped powder is difficult to remove	Hutmacher et al. (2004)
3-D printing	Fast processing; no toxic components; water used as a binder; tunable mechanical properties	Trapped powder issue	Yun et al. (2007), Fu et al. (2011a,b), Garcia et al. (2011), Wu et al. (2011a), Bose et al. (2013), and Liu et al. (2013)
Sponge replication	Reticulated open-cell material; applicable to any ceramic material that can be dispersed into a suspension; no toxic chemicals needed	Mechanical properties might be poor	Chen et al. (2006), Zhu et al. (2008), Vitale-Brovarone et al. (2009), Zhu and Kaskel (2009), Wu et al. (2010), Baino et al. (2013), and Baino and Vitale-Brovarone (2014)
Starch consolidation	Environment-friendly; low-cost	Pores might be poorly interconnected	Lyckfeldt and Ferreira (1998) and Vitale-Brovarone et al. (2004, 2005)
Thermal bonding of short glass fibers	Simple; no need for any additional material except fibers and mold; glassy scaffolds can be obtained	Mechanical properties might be poor	Pirhonen et al. (2003), Moimas et al. (2006), Gu et al. (2013), and Tirkkonen et al. (2013)

transferred to an oven for drying, burning-out of the polymer, and sintering of ceramic particles. The resulting ceramic foam exhibits higher strength magnitudes compared to other conventional methods due to the less flawed structure (low amount and size of the defects) and dense struts and walls produced. However, the porous structure results poorly interconnected and non-homogeneous (Sepulveda and Binner, 1999). The final cell size distribution and strut thickness can be engineered during processing by controlling enlargement of bubbles and thinning of lamellas (cell walls) upon the induction period. This can be efficiently done by altering the concentration of the initiator and the catalyst; however, other parameters such as temperature and pH have also been found to play a significant role (Sepulveda and Binner, 1999). Another advantage of this technique is the ability to produce porous scaffolds with a high degree of complexity. The casting process, in fact, allows shaping forms/profiles without the need of machining. Additionally, if further details are required, the dried green foams are strong enough to withstand machining (Colombo, 2006). Gel-cast foaming has also been combined with the foam replica method (the latter described in Section "Sponge

Replica Method") to produce HA scaffolds with interconnected pores (Ramay and Zhang, 2003). Gel-cast foaming can also involve the use of gelling polymers (e.g., gelatin) with no need for initiator and catalyst (e.g., gelation can take place with a decrease in temperature); in this case, a supplementary freeze–drying step before sintering is necessary (Novajra et al., 2015a,b). The structure of a scaffold produced by gel-cast foaming is shown in **Figure 2**.

A third option is sol–gel foaming, a process that combines sol–gel technology – a chemical-based wet synthesis route, which involves the conversion of a solution containing ceramic precursors (sol) into a network of covalently bonded silica via inorganic polymerization reactions – and mechanical frothing (Akkus et al., 2002). After heat treatment, a glass or glass–ceramic construct can be obtained exhibiting a hierarchical structure with interconnected macropores for tissue ingrowth (10–500 µm) and a mesoporous texture (channels in the 2–50 nm range) that promotes cell adhesion and adsorption of biological metabolites while intensifying the rate of surface reactions *in vitro* and *in vivo* (especially the formation of surface HA layer) (Jones and Hench,

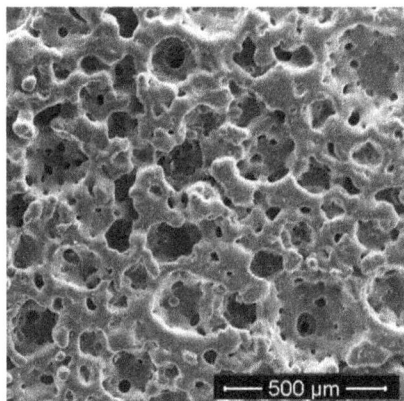

FIGURE 2 | Bioactive glass–ceramic scaffold obtained by gel-cast foaming followed by a freeze–drying step before sintering (courtesy of Giorgia Novajra).

2004). The latter feature is tuned by including in the sol a surfactant that acts as a template for supramolecular self-assembly; this process is also referred to as evaporation-induced self-assembly (EISA) (Brinker et al., 1999). The steps involved in the process are (1) preparation of a sol from a mixture of distilled water, appropriate precursors (metal alkoxides, such as tetraethylorthosilicate and triethylphosphate), salts ($CaNO_3$), and a hydrolysis catalyst (dilute acid), (2) foaming by vigorous agitation with the addition of a gelling agent, a surfactant, and distilled water, (3) casting of foamed mixture into molds, (4) aging to achieve gelation of the sol, (5) removal of the solvent by drying at low temperature, and (6) sintering to obtain porous components. Highly bioactive bone-like 3-D scaffolds can be successfully obtained by this method (Jones and Hench, 2004); an unavoidable limitation is the intrinsic brittleness of the porous product due to the nanoporous texture, which poses critical issues in view of the safe implantation of the device (too low mechanical properties) (Baino and Vitale-Brovarone, 2011).

Starch Consolidation

This method uses corn-, rice-, or potato-derived starch granules both as a pore former and a binder to fabricate porous ceramics. The main advantages of this processing technique are its low cost and its environment-friendly nature.

The process involves mixing of starch granules, ceramic powder, and distilled water to obtain a suspension that is continuously stirred and maintained at 60–80°C. In this temperature range, starch undergoes swelling due to water absorption, leading to a gel-like material that, after consolidation, is thermally treated to burn-out the organic phase and to sinter the ceramic matrix. Low dimensional changes occur during consolidation and drying, which ease the control of the ultimate dimensions of the component after sintering (Lyckfeldt and Ferreira, 1998).

Historically, this method was one of the first used to process bioactive glasses in a porous form (Vitale-Brovarone et al., 2004, 2005); albeit the mechanical properties of the resulting glass–ceramic scaffolds (compressive strength about 6 MPa) were

comparable to those of cancellous bone (2–12 MPa), the porosity was too low (40 vol.%) and poorly interconnected for deeming an eventual clinical application. Therefore, other polymer phases (apart from starch) have been experimented as a pore former for tissue engineering bioactive glass scaffolds.

Organic Phase Burning-Out

The organic phase burning-out (or space-holder method) is another strategy for producing porous scaffolds. In this method, ceramic powders are mixed together with a solid polymeric phase of synthetic [e.g., poly(methyl methacrylate) or polyethylene microbeads] (Baino et al., 2009) or natural origin (e.g., rice husk) (Wu et al., 2009). Afterwards, the blend is pressed to obtain a "green body" and thermally treated at high temperature. Upon heating, the polymeric particles that fill in the space within the volume of the component decompose, whereas the inorganic particles sinter, leading to a porous body displaying a negative replica of the original sacrificial template (Colombo, 2006; Baino and Vitale-Brovarone, 2011). Since sintering requires higher temperatures than pyrolysis, the ceramic matrix has to be partially consolidated before removal of the sacrificial material, so that the porous structure does not collapse during the polymer removal step; therefore, binders are generally incorporated in the mixture (Studart et al., 2006).

Both closed and open cell ceramic foams can be obtained, depending on the volume fraction and nature (significantly affecting the amount of gas developed during burning-out) of the sacrificial polymer. Nevertheless, pore interconnectivity is generally low due to the difficulty in maintaining a homogeneous distribution of the polymer spheres (Baino et al., 2009; Wu et al., 2009). Due to the presence of thick, dense struts, scaffolds produced by this method can exhibit high mechanical strength, even comparable to that of cortical bone (Baino et al., 2009).

In order to attain a highly porous structure, a large proportion of the polymeric phase in the starting mixture is necessary. This typically causes the development of a large amount of gas during heating that can cause the formation of cracks in the ceramic body (Bretcanu et al., 2014). Thus, the process needs to be attentively controlled to avoid the formation of defects in the final component.

Sponge Replica Method

The sponge replication method was patented by Schwartzwalder and Somers (1963) and, since then, it has become the most popular and effective method of producing foam-like ceramic scaffolds for tissue engineering. This success is primarily attributed to the simplicity and flexibility of the method, as it is applicable to any ceramic material that can be appropriately dispersed into a suspension. It has been observed that the reticulated open-cell structure (i.e., consisting of interconnected voids surrounded by a web of ceramic ligaments, the struts) that can be obtained using the foam replica method is the most suitable for bone tissue engineering scaffolds (**Table 1**) as it closely mimics the 3-D trabecular architecture of cancellous bone (**Figure 3**). Another key strength of this method is that the starting sponge can be easily cut and conformed to match the size and shape of the tissue defect, so that – at least ideally – personalized scaffolds

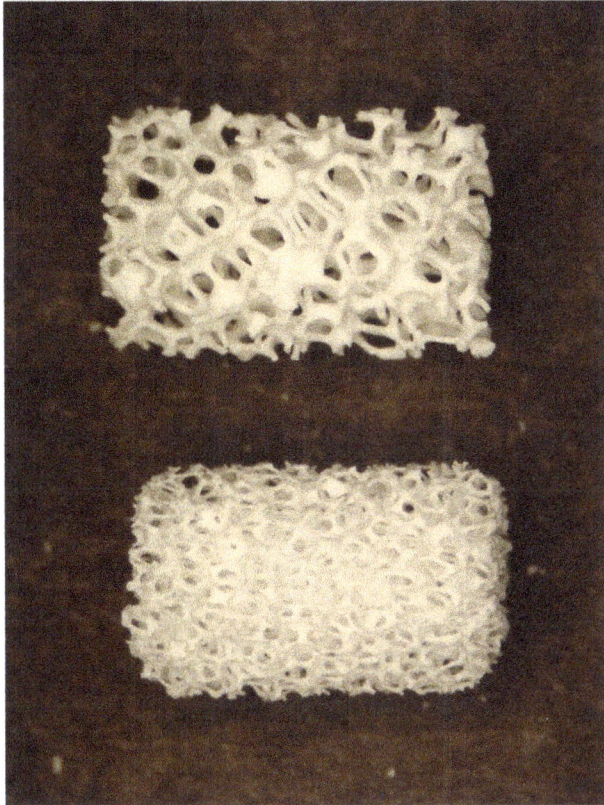

FIGURE 3 | Photographs of two commercially available hydroxyapatite cylindrical scaffolds with different porosity produced by sponge replica method. The length of the scaffolds is about 15 mm. Image adapted from © Dorozhkin (2010a).

could be fabricated according to the patient's clinical needs (Vitale-Brovarone et al., 2009).

This process involves the impregnation of an open-cell porous template of synthetic (typically a polyurethane sponge) or natural material (e.g., marine sponge) with a slurry of finely divided ceramic powder and a binding agent [e.g., poly(vinyl alcohol), colloidal silica]. The sponge is then squeezed to remove the excess slurry and enable the coating of the sponge struts with a thin layer of the slurry. After drying, the coated template is pyrolyzed while the remaining ceramic coating is sintered at higher temperatures to obtain a porous ceramic exhibiting the same architecture as the sacrificial template (positive replica). Therefore, the morphological characteristics of the ceramic foam are directly related to those of the polymeric template used (Schwartzwalder and Somers, 1963).

The most crucial step in the process is the production of a uniform coating on the polymeric structure. In more detail, the affecting factors are (1) the rheology of the impregnating suspension and (2) its adhesion on the struts of the polymeric sponge. The suspension should be sufficiently fluid to allow penetration into the cells of the sponge upon compression and expansion, but viscous enough to avoid drainage of the remaining coating. It is also worth mentioning that incomplete removal of the excess

slurry leads to a structure with a certain degree of closed porosity (Schwartzwalder and Somers, 1963; Colombo, 2006).

The sponge replica method has been recently applied in combination with EISA method to produce hierarchical porous bioactive glass scaffolds, where a polyurethane foam and a surfactant were used as co-templates for scaffold macropores and mesopores, respectively (Zhu et al., 2008; Zhu and Kaskel, 2009). These scaffolds are highly bioactive but exhibit dramatic brittleness due to the presence of the mesoporous texture. Wu et al. (2010) tried to improve the mechanical properties of these hierarchical porous constructs by depositing a silk coating on the strut, but their compressive strength still remained too low (few hundreds of kilopascal) for deeming a safe clinical application.

Solid Freeform Fabrication

Solid freeform fabrication, also referred to as rapid prototyping, denotes a set of emerging moldless techniques that use layer-wise manufacturing strategies to create scaffolds with customized external shape and pre-designed internal architecture (strut features, pore arrangement, size, and distribution) directly from a computer-generated 3-D model. This model is a 3-D reconstruction of the patient-specific tissue defect, which can be acquired from patient's computed tomography data or magnetic resonance imaging. Further details regarding the micro-environment can be developed by making use of computer-aided design (CAD). One of the main advantages of SFF technology is the ability to fabricate components with highly reproducible architecture and compositional variation (Hutmacher et al., 2004). This set of techniques is particularly valuable to produce functionally graded bioceramic and composites (Miao and Sun, 2010).

A number of SFF strategies have been adopted to manufacture scaffolds for tissue engineering applications (Hollister, 2005).

Stereolitography (SLA) uses a blend of ceramic powders and a photocurable monomer. A UV laser beam, which cures the monomer, is selectively scanned over the surface of the blend following the cross-sectional profiles of the CAD model; subsequent layers are built directly on top of previously cured layers with new layers of blend being deposited. After this step, the material not cured by the laser can be drained away and sintering is performed to produce the final object (Levy et al., 1997; Hutmacher et al., 2004). Fabrication of HA and amorphous calcium phosphate scaffolds for hard tissue repair using SLA has been extensively reported in the literature (Hollister, 2005; Scalera et al., 2014). Recently, Tesavibul et al. (2012) proposed the use of a lithographic method to fabricate 45S5 Bioglass®-derived scaffolds with highly ordered pore arrangement. Stereolitographic fabrication of wollastonite containing glass–ceramic scaffolds with high-strength properties was also reported by Sabree et al. (2015) (**Figure 4**).

Selective laser sintering (SLS) is a technique that employs a CO_2 laser beam to sinter thin layers of powdered ceramic materials to form 3-D objects. The laser beam is scanned over the powder bed following CAD data, thus raising the temperature of powders only in selected areas. In this way, particles fuse together and subsequent layers can be built directly on the top of the previously sintered material. Scaffolds from nano-HA and β-TCP as well as ceramic/polymer composites have been prepared using SLS technology (Hutmacher et al., 2004). Gao et al. (2014)

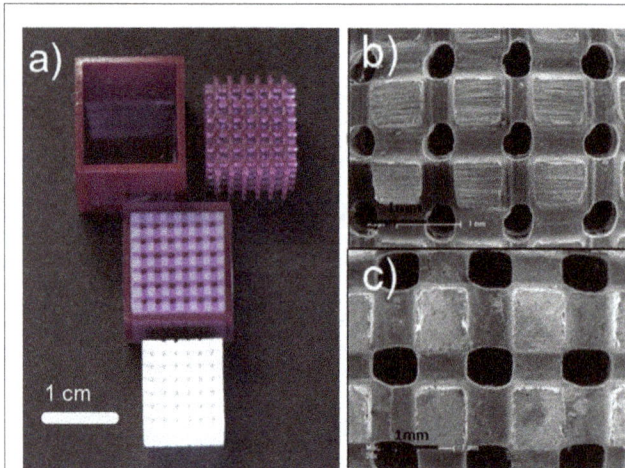

FIGURE 4 | Wollastonite containing glass–ceramic scaffolds produced by stereolithography: (A) original mold fabricated by stereolithography, filled mold and final sintered scaffold structure showing shrinkage after sintering (1200°C); (B,C) SEM images showing a general view of the scaffold structure and morphology (nominal pore size of 400 and 500 μm, respectively). Images adapted from © Sabree et al. (2015).

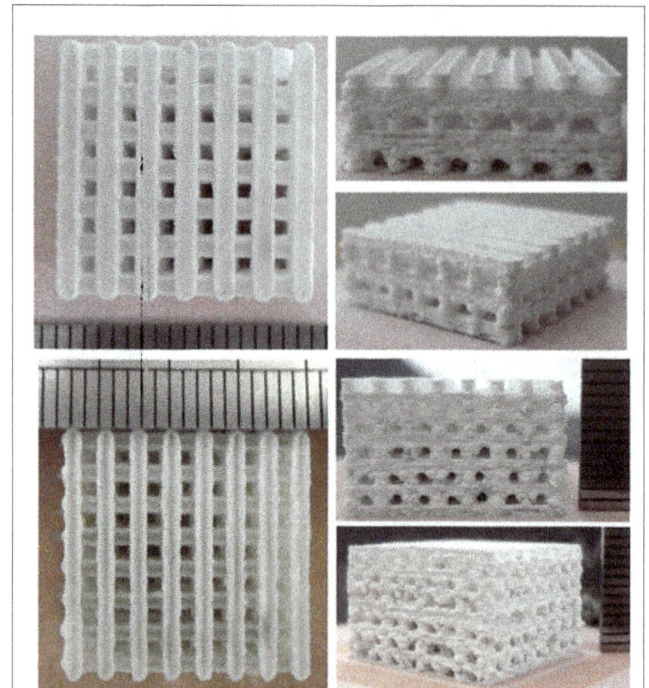

FIGURE 5 | Calcium phosphate (HA/β-TCP = 60/40 wt.%/wt.%) scaffolds fabricated by selective laser sintering: the scaffold architecture in 3-D is built up layer by layer. Images adapted from © Gao et al. (2014).

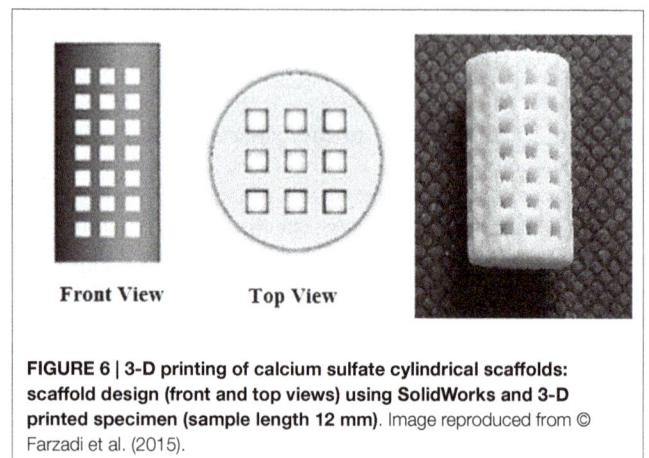

Front View   **Top View**

FIGURE 6 | 3-D printing of calcium sulfate cylindrical scaffolds: scaffold design (front and top views) using SolidWorks and 3-D printed specimen (sample length 12 mm). Image reproduced from © Farzadi et al. (2015).

recently reported the fabrication of biphasic calcium phosphate scaffolds by SLS, too (**Figure 5**).

A third very valuable option to produce porous ceramic scaffolds is 3-D printing (3DP), developed in the early 1990s at MIT. 3DP is a powder-based technology that employs a printer head – which moves in accordance to the object profile being generated by a computer system – to eject and deposit binder onto the powder surface and bonds the granules in the selected regions. Subsequently, a fresh layer of powder is laid down by a set of rollers. The cycle continues until the whole object is completed and at this point an airflow is used to remove unbound powder. The objects are sintered at high temperatures to achieve sufficient strength of the bodies and to remove the binder safely. Binders can be either organic (e.g., starch based) or water based. A wide variety of ceramic materials for tissue engineering have been processed using 3DP, such as HA, calcium phosphates, calcium sulfate, bioactive glasses, and ceramic composites, with a regular 3-D architecture and pore arrangement (**Figure 6**); however, extensive optimization is needed to process good quality parts with 3DP for any new material/composition, which is – together with the quite high cost of instrumentation – the major drawback of this approach (Bose et al., 2013).

Methods referred to as robocasting and direct ink-write assembling belong to the broad class of 3DP techniques. In this regard, bioactive glass scaffolds with a regular arrangement of pores in 3-D and extraordinarily high mechanical performances in compression and flexure were proposed for possible application in the substitution of cortical bone and load-bearing segments of the skeleton (Fu et al., 2011a,b; Liu et al., 2013).

3-D printing has also been applied to fabricate MBG scaffolds. Yun et al. (2007) and Garcia et al. (2011) prepared hierarchical 3-D porous MBG scaffolds using a combination of double polymer

template and rapid prototyping techniques. In their study, they mixed MBG gel with methylcellulose and then printed, sintered at 500–700°C to remove polymer templates and obtained MBG scaffolds. Although the obtained MBG scaffolds have uniform pore structure, their mechanical strength is compromised because of the incorporation of methylcellulose, which results in some micropores. Recently, Wu et al. (2011a) reported a new facile method to prepare hierarchical and multi-functional MBG scaffolds with controllable pore architecture, excellent mechanical strength, and mineralization ability for bone regeneration by a modified 3DP technique using poly(vinyl alcohol) as a binder. The obtained 3DP MBG scaffolds possess a compressive mechanical strength (16 MPa), which is about 200 times that of the MBG scaffolds prepared using a traditional polyurethane foam as a template.

Thermal Bonding of Short Glass Fibers

Porous 3-D scaffolds can also be obtained using glass fibers as a starting material. The fibers, with diameters typically ranging from tens to few hundreds of micrometers, are cut and disposed into a mold in a random arrangement with porosity originating from the free space between them. Then, a thermal treatment allows this porous structure to be stabilized by thermally bonding (sintering) the glass fibers in order to obtain glass scaffolds. The scaffolds produced by this method show a high degree of pore interconnectivity and the final scaffold structure can be tailored acting on the fiber size, the sintering time, and temperature (Pirhonen et al., 2003; Moimas et al., 2006).

Since 45S5 Bioglass® is not easy to draw into fibers without devitrification due to its narrow working range, other glass formulations that can be easily spun have been proposed in the literature for fibrous scaffold production, in particular, silicate (e.g., 13–93, 9–93) and borate bioactive glasses (e.g., 13–99B3) as well as mixtures of them (Gu et al., 2013). A porous scaffold made of glass fibers with nominal composition $11.1–12.0\ Na_2O$, $15.0–17.1\ K_2\cdot O$, $2.8–3.3\ MgO$, $12.7–15.2\ CaO$, $2.7–3.8\ P_2O_5$, $1.0–1.4\ B_2O_3$, $0.0–0.6\ TiO_2$, and $48.5–52.0\ SiO_2$ wt.% (Tirkkonen et al., 2013) is currently available on the market (Inion BioRestore™, Inion Oy, Tampere, Finland) as a graft material (porous morsels) for bone defect restoration. Research studies on thermally bonded phosphate glass fibrous scaffolds are currently ongoing (**Figure 7**).

Processing Technologies for Bioceramic Containing Composite Scaffolds

Numerous fabrication techniques have been described to produce 3-D porous bioceramic/polymer composite scaffolds, including space-holder, gas foaming, thermally induced phase separation

(TIPS), and SFF. These methods have been extensively reviewed in the literature (Rezwan et al., 2006; Mohamad Yunos et al., 2008). Among all, TIPS can be considered the technique of choice if scaffolds with highly oriented porosity need to be prepared. This pore structure differs considerably from the isotropic structure and equiaxed pores that are typically obtained by the "conventional" methods. The TIPS process has been widely used to produce composite scaffolds based on PLGA and PDLLA foams containing 45S5 Bioglass® particles as bioactive inclusions (Maquet et al., 2003, 2004; Verrier et al., 2004; Blacher et al., 2005).

Polymer-coated bioceramic scaffolds can be produced by a dipping method that involves the dipping of a bioceramic scaffold in a polymer solution followed by drying in air (Bretcanu et al., 2007); the polymer coating is useful to improve the mechanical properties of the scaffold, especially the fracture toughness (Rehorek et al., 2013).

A dip-coating approach has been also reported to apply a biomimetic calcium phosphate layer on metal scaffolds (TiNbZr alloy) to improve their biocompatibility (Wang et al., 2009).

A highly versatile and promising approach to produce bioceramic scaffolds coated with different materials (polymers, other ceramic phases) is the electrophoretic deposition (EPD), which uses the electrophoresis mechanism for the movement of charged particles suspended in a solution under an electric field, in order to deposit them in an ordered manner on a substrate to develop thin and thick films and coatings (Boccaccini et al., 2010). Fiorilli et al. (2015) reported the successful EPD of MBG onto a strong, nearly inert glass–ceramic scaffold to obtain a bioactive high-strength construct for load-bearing applications in bone tissue engineering. The use of EPD to produce carbon nanotube (CNT) coatings for smart applications in tissue engineering has been also investigated, for example, Meng et al. (2011) incorporated CNTs into 45S5 Bioglass®-derived glass–ceramic scaffolds by EPD and cultured mesenchymal stem cells on the constructs with and without electrical stimulation, and they observed that the electrical conductivity associated with the CNTs can promote the proliferation and differentiation of the cells attached onto the scaffold.

CLINICAL APPLICATIONS OF BIOCERAMIC SCAFFOLDS: PRESENT AND FUTURE

An overview of the applications of bioceramic scaffolds in medicine is summarized in **Table 3**. As a result of biomechanical limitations, bioactive glasses, glass–ceramics, and calcium phosphates are mainly used in low-/non-load-bearing applications or compressive load situations in solid or powder form, such as bone restoration and augmentation, middle ear repair, vertebral, and iliac crest replacements (Hench, 1998; Dorozhkin, 2010a). Thermal-sprayed HA coatings on metal joint prostheses are also used in the clinical practice by surgeons (Sun et al., 2001). Bioactive glass–ceramic porous coatings on alumina acetabular cups have been recently proposed to improve osteointegration of prosthetic devices (Vitale-Brovarone et al., 2012b; Baino et al., 2015, 2016a).

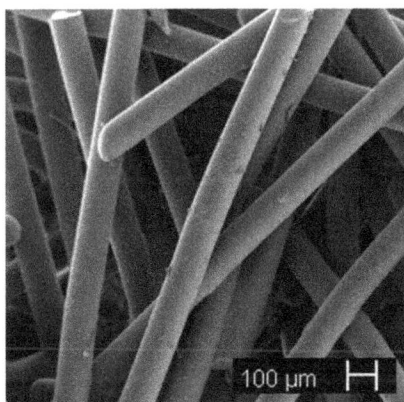

FIGURE 7 | Resorbable glass fibrous scaffold obtained by thermal bonding of short glass fibers (courtesy of Giorgia Novajra).

TABLE 3 | Applications of bioceramic scaffolds in tissue engineering.

Field of application	Material/scaffold involved	Recipient	Stage of use/research	Reference
Bone defect repair	Porous scaffolds made of HA, biphasic calcium phosphates, bioactive glasses (e.g., 45S5 Bioglass®, 13–93)	H	Clinical use (the products are FDA approved)	Hench (1998) and Dorozhkin (2010a, 2012)
Joint prosthesis	Bioactive glass–ceramic coating with trabecular architecture on bioceramic acetabular cup	–	Promising experimental results achieved in the framework of the EC-funded project "MATCh." Neither *in vitro* nor *in vivo* tests are currently available in the literature	Vitale-Brovarone et al. (2012a,b) and Baino et al. (2015, 2016a,b)
Orbital implant	Porous spheres made of alumina (the so-called "Bioceramic implant"), HA (examples of commercial products: coralline HA – Bioeye®, synthetic HA – FCI3, bovine HA – Molteno M-sphere) or 45S5 Bioglass®/polyethylene composite (Medpor-Plus)	H	HA and alumina implants, being FDA approved since many years, are routinely used in the clinical practice Early uses of 45S5 Bioglass®/polyethylene composite spheres in the clinical practice	Naik et al. (2007) and Baino et al. (2014)
Wound healing	45S5 Bioglass®/polymer composite meshes	AS	No study involving human patients available	Day et al. (2004) and Rai et al. (2010)
Skin tissue engineering	Fibrous constructs comprising MBG fibers as such or in combination with a polymer	–	No biological study available	Hong et al. (2010) and Jia et al. (2011)
Lung tissue engineering	Sol–gel glass foams or PDLLA/45S5 Bioglass® porous composites	IV	No *in vivo* study available	Tan et al. (2002) and Verrier et al. (2004)
Muscle tissue engineering	Phophate glass fibrous constructs	–	No *in vivo* study available	Ahmed et al. (2004), Shah et al. (2014), and Shah et al. (2015)
Peripheral nerve repair	Bioactive glass fibrous constructs	AS	No study involving human patients available	Vitale-Brovarone et al. (2012a) and Kim et al. (2015)

H, humans; AS, animal study; IV, in vitro tests with cells.

All the applications of bioactive ceramics take the advantage of bioactivity and minimize mechanical-property requirements, which may be an issue in the case of highly porous implants. Stock porous blocks of various size made of HA, (biphasic) calcium phosphate, and a few bioactive glasses (**Table 3**) are currently marketed worldwide and clinically implanted in humans for the repair of small bone defects; these implants can be contoured intraoperatively by the surgeon to match the size/shape of the defect. SFF-derived custom-made HA porous scaffolds are produced if a high accuracy on the size or complex shapes are needed, such as implants for orbital floor repair (Levy et al., 1997). Trabecular bone – which can be actually considered a natural bioceramic-based composite – from bone banks is also used as a restorative material (Schlickewei and Schlickewei, 2007).

A special non-osseous application where (porous) bioceramics are widely used is the fabrication of orbital implants for enucleated patients. Porous spherical implants (scaffolds) made of bovine, coralline, and synthetic HA as well as alumina are routinely implanted upon anophthalmic socket surgery as they are biocompatible and allow fibrovascularization within their pore network (Baino et al., 2014). Early human trials with 45S5 Bioglass®/polyethylene composite porous orbital implants showed promising results, including an enhanced implant fibrovascularization compared to other available devices (Naik et al., 2007), which can be due to the angiogenic effect of bioactive glass.

In recent years, the use of bioceramic and composite scaffolds – usually comprising bioactive glass as an inorganic phase – has also been proposed for some emerging applications in contact with soft tissues. In this regard, the angiogenic potential of bioactive glasses has opened new perspectives in skin tissue engineering. Day et al. (2004) first showed *in vitro* (using fibroblasts) and *in vivo* (in rats) the ability of 45S5 Bioglass® incorporated into PGA meshes to increase scaffold neovascularization, which would be highly beneficial during the engineering of larger soft tissue constructs. Nano-sized 45S5 Bioglass® particles were also used by Rai et al. (2010) in the fabrication of a novel poly(3-hydroxyoctanoate)-based composite scaffold for wound dressing: the incorporation of bioactive glass nanoparticles accelerated blood clotting time and enhanced the wettability, surface roughness, and overall biocompatibility of the scaffold.

Hong et al. (2010) investigated the use of ultrathin MBG hollow fibers (diameter around 600 nm), fabricated by electrospinning combined with a phase-separation inducing agent [poly(ethylene oxide)], as a multifunctional system for skin tissue engineering (support to the regenerated tissue and release of anti-inflammatory drugs) when organized in the form of 3-D macroporous membranes. MBGs were also mixed with chitosan to produce composite films by freeze–drying for possible use as hemostatic membranes for skin repair (Jia et al., 2011).

Bioactive glass scaffolds have been also proposed for lung tissue engineering applications. In a study by Tan et al. (2002), sol–gel-derived bioactive glass foams with surface modifications to include amine or mercaptan groups and/or coated with laminin were manufactured and placed in culture with murine lung epithelial cells to determine the best conditions to promote cell growth and proliferation. Based on histological examination of the cell cultures, there was full colonization of the foams by the lung cells and it was shown that the laminin-coated, amine-modified foams were most effective in promoting cell growth and attachment.

In another study, Verrier et al. (2004) proposed the use of PDLLA/45S5 Bioglass® porous composites for lung tissue engineering performing *in vitro* biocompatibility assays with a human lung carcinoma A549 cell line. Two hours after cell seeding, a general increase of cell adhesion according to the increased content of Bioglass® (0, 5, and 40 wt.%) in the PDLLA foams was observed, but cell proliferation studies over a period of 4 weeks revealed a better aptitude of A549 cells to proliferate on scaffolds containing only 5 wt.% of glass. These results seem to indicate the possibility of using bioactive glasses in lung tissue engineering approaches, although a lot of future work, including testing with the different cell types found in this complex tissue, is necessary for further advancements.

The results reported by Verrier et al. (2004) demonstrate that the concentration of bioactive glass in tissue engineering polymer-based constructs should be always optimized depending on the considered tissues that we want to regenerate. This dose-dependent effect was also observed in another study by the same research group, in which PLGA/45S5 Bioglass® composite tubular foam scaffolds (porosity about 93 vol.%, size of interconnected macropores in the 50–300 μm range, wall thickness within 1.5–3.0 mm) were fabricated via TIPS (Boccaccini et al., 2005); the authors proposed the use of the produced constructs for the regeneration of tissues requiring a tubular shape scaffold, such as blood vessels and trachea.

The research group led by Prof. Jonathan Knowles also carried out a few studies with phosphate glasses for applications in muscle regeneration. Ahmed et al. (2004) found that CaO–Na₂O–Fe₂O₃–P₂O₅ glass fibers allowed attachment, proliferation, and differentiation of conditionally immortal muscle precursor cell line with the formation of myotubes along the axis of the fibers. Shah et al. (2005) found that human masseter-derived cells seeded on a 3-D mesh construct not only attached and proliferated but also migrated along the fibers forming multinucleated myotubes. It was also found that 3-D aligned fiber scaffolds were able to support unidirectional cell alignment and caused an up-regulation of genes encoding for myogenic regulatory factors (Shah et al., 2014), even when the glass fibers were embedded into a collagen gel to form a composite scaffold (Shah et al., 2015). Glass fibers were also found to support and direct axonal regeneration both *in vitro* and *in vivo* (Vitale-Brovarone et al., 2012a; Kim et al., 2015).

Because of their ability to bond to soft tissues and to elicit desirable biological responses, such as angiogenesis, bioactive glasses have been recently proposed in a non-porous form for some other interesting non-osseous applications. A few examples concern the use of bioactive glass particulate for the treatment of gastric ulcers, injectable radioactive glasses for killing cancer cells in liver tumor, glass/polymer composites for cardiac tissue engineering, and glass/polymer tubes for peripheral nerve regeneration. These applications, not restricted to porous scaffolds, have been recently reviewed by some leading scientists in the field (Baino et al., 2016b; Miguez-Pacheco et al., 2015a,b).

SUMMARY AND OUTLOOK

Progress in tissue engineering has led to the development of porous materials designed and manufactured to act as a scaffold for the growth of new tissue in order to restore the natural state and function of diseased parts of the body. Bioceramics have demonstrated to be highly suitable materials for tissue engineering scaffolds and developments in processing methods have provided a mean to control the 3-D architecture of such scaffolds. In spite of remarkable advances, bioceramics have not yet reached their full potential but research is ongoing.

Besides "traditional" use for osseous defect repair, a variety of innovative applications are emerging; for instance, recent studies have interestingly highlighted the suitability of bioactive glasses and glass–ceramics for wound healing applications and soft-tissue engineering (Baino et al., 2016b; Miguez-Pacheco et al., 2015a). For these applications, where softer and more flexible materials are needed, inorganic–organic hybrids could be an even better solution. These materials are interpenetrating networks of inorganic and organic components that interact at a molecular level; they behave as a single phase and, thus, degrade as one material (overcoming the main drawback related to composite biomaterials). Their mechanical properties as well as bioactivity can be tailored by varying the constituents and synthesis/processing parameters (Jones, 2009, 2013).

The use of porous bioceramics as parts of a complex prosthetic devices and not only as a bone-filling material for the restoration of osseous defects but also as a "warm" challenge that has recently arisen. In this regard, a fascinating approach that has been put forward is the use of glass-derived scaffolds as osteointegrative trabecular coatings on ceramic acetabular cup of hip joint prosthesis. These coatings are expected to induce biological fixation of the prosthesis while eliminating the need for invasive screws, cements, or threading to fix implants in place (Vitale-Brovarone et al., 2012b; Baino and Vitale-Brovarone, 2015b; Baino et al., 2015, 2016a).

The development of multifunctional bioceramics that combine the "conventional" properties of 3-D porous bioactive scaffolds and the added value of therapeutic ion release also has great potential. In this regard, bioactive glasses can be doped with various trace elements to provide a smart strategy for the controlled delivery of ions *in situ*, such as Sr, Cu, Zn, Ga, or Co, which may lead to therapeutic effects upon their release into the cellular environment (e.g., promotion of angiogenesis, antibacterial action) (Hoppe et al., 2011; Mourino et al., 2012).

Fabrication of bioceramic components with hierarchical porosity has also recently attracted the interest of biomaterials scientists (Colombo et al., 2010). The use of MBGs either in the form of macro-/mesoporous scaffolds or as coatings can add valuable extra-functionalities to the (base) scaffold. The mesoporous texture and high surface area of these glasses intensify the rate of surface reactions, leading to a faster release of ionic species upon glass dissolution. Therefore, not only the classical bioactivity mechanism is speeded up (fast formation of a surface layer of HA that allows strong bone bonding *in vivo*) but also therapeutic metal ions, previously incorporated within the glass network, can be quickly released upon contact with biological fluids (Wu and Chang, 2014). The solubility rate of MBGs can be tailored by controlling the textural parameters (e.g., mesopore structure and size) and by changing the glass composition so that they dissolve at controlled rates matching those of the tissue growth. A further added value is using MBGs as carriers for the controlled delivery of drug molecules that can be incorporated in the material mesopores (Arcos and Vallet-Regí, 2013), thereby creating a multifunctional tissue engineering implantable device.

New strategies for scaffold fabrication are also emerging both to improve the scaffold performance and to develop ever more sustainable processing routes. For instance, highly porous bioactive glass scaffolds were successfully produced by an innovative method based on preceramic polymers containing micro- and nano-sized fillers (Fiocco et al., 2014). Silica from the decomposition of the silicone resins reacted with the oxides deriving from the fillers, yielding glass–ceramic components after heating at 1000°C. Despite the limited mechanical strength, the obtained samples possessed suitable porous architecture and promising biocompatibility and bioactivity, as testified by preliminary *in vitro* tests. This method has also been very recently applied to fabricate wollastonite/diopside composite foams for bone tissue engineering applications (Fiocco et al., 2015).

If an oriented pore microstructure and high mechanical properties are required, freezing of ceramic slurries can represent a valuable, relatively simple strategy to this aim (Liu et al., 2012).

In summary, new, continuous advances in scaffold processing technologies and novel emerging applications of porous scaffolds in both hard- and soft-tissue engineering bring further honor to the long history of ceramics in medicine. We forecast a bright future for bioceramics, which will indeed provide an ever increasing contribution in improving the quality of life of mankind.

AUTHOR CONTRIBUTIONS

FB conceived the study, performed literature search and wrote the paper. GN performed literature search and wrote the paper. CV-B wrote the paper. All authors critically revised the manuscript.

FUNDING

The research leading to these results has received funding from the EU Seventh Framework Programme (FP7/2007-2013) under grant agreements no. 286548 (MATCh), no. 280575 (Restoration) and no. 264526 (GlaCERCo).

REFERENCES

Ahmed, I., Collins, C. A., Lewis, M. P., Olsen, I., and Knowles, J. C. (2004). Processing, characterisation and biocompatibility of iron-phosphate glass fibres for tissue engineering. *Biomaterials* 25, 3223–3232. doi:10.1016/j.biomaterials.2003.10.013

Akkus, O., Pujol, J., and Qi, G. (2002). Bioactive sol-gel foams for tissue repair. *J. Biomed. Mater. Res.* 59, 340–348. doi:10.1002/jbm.1250

Alvarez, K., and Nakajima, H. (2009). Metallic scaffolds for bone regeneration. *Materials* 2, 790–832. doi:10.3390/ma2030790

Ambrosio, A. M. A., Sahota, J. S., Khan, Y., and Laurencin, C. T. (2001). A novel amorphous calcium phosphate polymer ceramic for bone repair: I. Synthesis and characterization. *J. Biomed. Mater. Res.* 58, 295–301. doi:10.1002/1097-4636(2001)58:3<295::AID-JBM1020>3.0.CO;2-8

Arcos, D., and Vallet-Regí, M. (2013). Bioceramics for drug delivery. *Acta Mater.* 61, 890–911. doi:10.1016/j.actamat.2012.10.039

Baino, F., Ferraris, M., Bretcanu, O., Verné, E., and Vitale-Brovarone, C. (2013). Optimization of composition, structure and mechanical strength of bioactive 3-D glass-ceramic scaffolds for bone substitution. *J. Biomater. Appl.* 27, 872–890. doi:10.1177/0885328211429193

Baino, F., Marshall, M., Kirk, N., and Vitale-Brovarone, C. (2016a). Design, selection and characterization of novel glasses and glass-ceramics for use in prosthetic applications. *Ceram. Int.* 42, 1482–1491. doi:10.1016/j.ceramint.2015.09.094

Baino, F., Novajra, G., Miguez-Pacheco, V., Boccaccini, A. R., and Vitale-Brovarone, C. (2016b). Bioactive glasses: special applications outside the skeletal system. *J. Non Cryst. Solids* 432, 15–30. doi:10.1016/j.jnoncrysol.2015.02.015

Baino, F., Perero, S., Ferraris, S., Miola, M., Balagna, C., Verné, E., et al. (2014). Biomaterials for orbital implants and ocular prostheses: overview and future prospects. *Acta Biomater.* 10, 1064–1087. doi:10.1016/j.actbio.2013.12.014

Baino, F., Tallia, F., Novajra, G., Minguella, J., Montealegre, M. A., Korkusuz, F., et al. (2015). Novel bone-like porous glass coatings on Al₂O₃ prosthetic substrates. *Key Eng. Mater.* 631, 236–240. doi:10.4028/www.scientific.net/KEM.631.236

Baino, F., Verné, E., and Vitale-Brovarone, C. (2009). 3-D high strength glass-ceramic scaffolds containing fluoroapatite for load-bearing bone portions replacement. *Mater. Sci. Eng. C* 29, 2055–2062. doi:10.1016/j.msec.2009.04.002

Baino, F., and Vitale-Brovarone, C. (2011). Three-dimensional glass-derived scaffolds for bone tissue engineering: current trends and forecasts for the future. *J. Biomed. Mater. Res. A* 97, 514–535. doi:10.1002/jbm.a.33072

Baino, F., and Vitale-Brovarone, C. (2014). Mechanical properties and reliability of glass-ceramic foam scaffolds for bone repair. *Mater. Lett.* 118, 27–30. doi:10.1016/j.matlet.2013.12.037

Baino, F., and Vitale-Brovarone, C. (2015a). Ceramics for oculo-orbital surgery. *Ceram. Int.* 41, 5213–5231. doi:10.1016/j.ceramint.2014.12.086

Baino, F., and Vitale-Brovarone, C. (2015b). Trabecular coating on curved alumina substrates using a novel bioactive and strong glass-ceramic. *Biomed. Glasses* 1, 31–40. doi:10.1515/bglass-2015-0003

Barrere, F., Van Blitterswijk, C. A., and De Groot, K. (2006). Bone regeneration: molecular and cellular interactions with calcium phosphate ceramics. *Int. J. Nanomed.* 1, 317–332.

Bielby, R. C., Christodoulou, I. S., Pryce, R. S., Radford, W. J., Hench, L. L., and Polak, J. M. (2004). Time- and concentration-dependent effects of dissolution products of 58S sol-gel bioactive glass on proliferation and differentiation of murine and human osteoblasts. *Tissue Eng.* 10, 1018–1026. doi:10.1089/ten.2004.10.1018

Blacher, S., Maquet, V., Jerome, R., Pirard, J. P., and Boccaccini, A. R. (2005). Study of the connectivity properties of bioglass®-filled polylactide foam scaffolds by image analysis and impedance spectroscopy. *Acta Biomater.* 1, 565–574. doi:10.1016/j.actbio.2005.06.003

Boccaccini, A. R., Blaker, J. J., Maquet, V., Day, R. M., and Jerome, R. (2005). Preparation and characterisation of poly(lactide-co-glycolide) (PLGA) and PLGA/bioglass® composite tubular foam scaffolds for tissue engineering applications. *Mater. Sci. Eng. C* 25, 23–31. doi:10.1016/j.msec.2004.03.002

Boccaccini, A. R., Keim, S., Ma, R., Li, Y., and Zhitomirsky, I. (2010). Electrophoretic deposition of biomaterials. *J. R. Soc. Interface* 7, S581–S613. doi:10.1098/rsif.2010.0156.focus

Bohner, M. (2009). Silicon-substituted calcium phosphates – a critical view. *Biomaterials* 30, 6403–6406. doi:10.1016/j.biomaterials.2009.08.007

Bose, S., Vahabzadeh, S., and Bandyopadhyay, A. (2013). Bone tissue engineering using 3D printing. *Mater. Today* 16, 496–504. doi:10.1016/j.mattod.2013.11.017

Bretcanu, O., Baino, F., Verné, E., and Vitale-Brovarone, C. (2014). Novel resorbable glass-ceramic scaffolds for hard tissue engineering: from the parent phosphate glass to its bone-like macroporous derivatives. *J. Biomater. Appl.* 28, 1287–1303. doi:10.1177/0885328213506759

Bretcanu, O., Chen, Q., Misra, S. K., Boccaccini, A. R., Verné, E., and Vitale-Brovarone, C. (2007). Biodegradable polymer coated 45S5 bioglass-derived glass-ceramic scaffolds for bone tissue engineering. *Glass. Tech. Eur. J. Glass. Sci. Tech. A* 48, 227–234.

Brinker, C. J., Lu, Y., Sellinger, A., and Fan, H. (1999). Evaporation-induced self-assembly: nanostructures made easy. *Adv. Mater.* 11, 579–585. doi:10.1002/(SICI)1521-4095(199905)11:7<579::AID-ADMA579>3.0.CO;2-R

Cao, W., and Hench, L. L. (1996). Bioactive materials. *Ceram. Int.* 22, 493–507. doi:10.1016/0272-8842(95)00126-3

Chen, Q. Z., Thompson, I. D., and Boccaccini, A. R. (2006). 45S5 bioglass®-derived glass-ceramic scaffolds for bone tissue engineering. *Biomaterials* 27, 2414–2425. doi:10.1016/j.biomaterials.2005.11.025

Colombo, P. (2006). Conventional and novel processing methods for cellular ceramics. *Philos. Trans. A Math. Phys. Eng. Sci.* 364, 109–124. doi:10.1098/rsta.2005.1683

Colombo, P., Vakifahmetoglu, C., and Costacurta, S. (2010). Fabrication of ceramic components with hierarchical porosity. *J. Mater. Sci.* 45, 5425–5455. doi:10.1007/s10853-010-4708-9

Day, R. M., Boccaccini, A. R., Shurey, S., Roether, J. A., Forbes, A., Hench, L. L., et al. (2004). Assessment of polyglycolic acid mesh and bioactive glass for soft-tissue engineering scaffolds. *Biomaterials* 25, 5857–5866. doi:10.1016/j.biomaterials.2004.01.043

Deng, X., Hao, J., and Wang, C. (2001). Preparation and mechanical properties of nanocomposites of poly(D,L lactide) with Ca-deficient hydroxyapatite nanocrystals. *Biomaterials* 22, 2867–2873. doi:10.1016/S0142-9612(01)00031-X

Dorozhkin, S. V. (2007). Calcium orthophosphates. *J. Mater. Sci.* 42, 1061–1095. doi:10.1007/s10853-006-1467-8

Dorozhkin, S. V. (2010a). Calcium orthophosphates as bioceramics: state of the art. *J. Funct. Mater.* 1, 22–107. doi:10.3390/jfb1010022

Dorozhkin, S. V. (2010b). Amorphous calcium (ortho)phosphates. *Acta Biomater.* 6, 4457–4475. doi:10.1016/j.actbio.2010.06.031

Dorozhkin, S. V. (2012). Biphasic, triphasic and multiphasic calcium orthophosphates. *Acta Biomater.* 8, 963–977. doi:10.1016/j.actbio.2011.09.003

Erol-Taygun, M., Zheng, K., and Boccaccini, A. R. (2013). Nanoscale bioactive glasses in medical applications. *Int. J. Appl. Glass Sci.* 4, 136–148. doi:10.1111/ijag.12029

Farzadi, A., Waran, V., Solati-Hashjin, M., Rahman, Z. A. A., Asadi, M., and Osman, N. A. A. (2015). Effect of layer printing delay on mechanical properties and dimensional accuracy of 3D printed porous prototypes in bone tissue engineering. *Ceram. Int.* 41, 8320–8330. doi:10.1016/j.ceramint.2015.03.004

Fiocco, L., Bernardo, E., Colombo, P., Cacciotti, I., Bianco, A., Bellucci, D., et al. (2014). Novel processing of bioglass ceramics from silicone resins containing micro- and nano-sized oxide particle fillers. *J. Biomed. Mater. Res. A* 102, 2502–2510. doi:10.1002/jbm.a.34918

Fiocco, L., Elsayed, H., Ferroni, L., Gardin, C., Zavan, B., and Bernardo, E. (2015). Bioactive wollastonite-diopside foams from preceramic polymers and reactive oxide fillers. *Materials* 8, 2480–2494. doi:10.3390/ma8052480

Fiorilli, S., Baino, F., Cauda, V., Crepaldi, M., Vitale-Brovarone, C., Demarchi, D., et al. (2015). Electrophoretic deposition of mesoporous bioactive glass on glass-ceramic foam scaffolds for bone tissue engineering. *J. Mater. Sci.: Mater. Med.* 26, 1–12. doi:10.1007/s10856-014-5346-6

Fu, Q., Saiz, E., Rahaman, M. N., and Tomsia, A. P. (2011a). Bioactive glass scaffolds for bone tissue engineering: state of the art and future perspectives. *Mater. Sci. Eng. C* 31, 1245–1256. doi:10.1016/j.msec.2011.04.022

Fu, Q., Saiz, E., and Tomsia, A. P. (2011b). Bioinspired strong and highly porous glass scaffolds. *Adv. Funct. Mater.* 21, 1058–1063. doi:10.1002/adfm.201002030

Gao, C., Deng, Y., Feng, P., Mao, Z., Li, P., Yang, B., et al. (2014). Current progress in bioactive ceramic scaffolds for bone repair and regeneration. *Int. J. Mol. Sci.* 15, 4714–4732. doi:10.3390/ijms15034714

Garcia, A., Izquierdo-Barba, I., Colilla, M., De Laorden, C. L., and Vallet-Regí, M. (2011). Preparation of 3-D scaffolds in the SiO_2-P_2O_5 system with tailored hierarchical mesomacroporosity. *Acta Biomater.* 7, 1265–1273. doi:10.1016/j.actbio.2010.10.006

Gerhardt, L. C., and Boccaccini, A. R. (2010). Bioactive glass and glass-ceramic scaffolds for bone tissue engineering. *Materials* 3, 3867–3910. doi:10.3390/ma3073867

Gerhardt, L. C., Widdows, K. L., Erol, M. M., Burch, C. W., Sanz-Herrera, J. A., Ochoa, I., et al. (2011). The pro-angiogenic properties of multi-functional bioactive glass composite scaffolds. *Biomaterials* 32, 4096–4108. doi:10.1016/j.biomaterials.2011.02.032

Gibson, L. J. (1989). Modelling the mechanical behaviour of cellular materials. *Mater. Sci. Eng. A* 110, 1–36. doi:10.1016/0921-5093(89)90154-8

Gu, Y., Huang, W., Rahaman, M. N., and Day, D. E. (2013). Bone regeneration in rat calvarial defects implanted with fibrous scaffolds composed of a mixture of silicate and borate bioactive glasses. *Acta Biomater.* 9, 9126–9136. doi:10.1016/j.actbio.2013.06.039

Habibovic, P., and Barralet, J. E. (2011). Bioinorganics and biomaterials: bone repair. *Acta Biomater.* 7, 3013–3026. doi:10.1016/j.actbio.2011.03.027

Hench, L. L. (1996). "Ceramics, glasses, and glass-ceramics," in *Biomaterials Science: An Introduction to Materials in Medicine*, eds Ratner B. D., Hoffman A. S., Schoen F. J., and Lemons J. E. (San Diego, CA: Academic Press), 73–84.

Hench, L. L. (1998). Bioceramics. *J. Am. Ceram. Soc.* 81, 1705–1728. doi:10.1111/j.1151-2916.1998.tb02540.x

Hench, L. L. (2006). The story of bioglass®. *J. Mater. Sci.: Mater. Med.* 17, 967–978. doi:10.1007/s10856-006-0432-z

Hench, L. L. (2009). Genetic design of bioactive glass. *J. Eur. Ceram. Soc.* 29, 1257–1265. doi:10.1016/j.jeurceramsoc.2008.08.002

Hench, L. L., and Greenspan, D. (2013). Interactions between bioactive glass and collagen: a review and new perspectives. *J. Aust. Ceram. Soc.* 49, 1–40.

Hench, L. L., Splinter, R. J., Allen, W. C., and Greenlee, T. K. (1971). Bonding mechanisms at the interface of ceramic prosthetic materials. *J. Biomed. Mater. Res.* 5, 117–141. doi:10.1002/jbm.820050611

Hing, K. A. (2005). Bioceramic bone graft substitutes: influence of porosity and chemistry. *Int. J. Appl. Ceram. Technol.* 2, 184–199. doi:10.1111/j.1744-7402.2005.02020.x

Hollister, S. J. (2005). Porous scaffold design for tissue engineering. *Nat. Mater.* 4, 518–524. doi:10.1038/nmat1421

Hong, Y., Chen, X., Jing, X., Fan, H., Gu, Z., and Zhang, X. (2010). Fabrication and drug delivery of ultrathin mesoporous bioactive glass hollow fibers. *Adv. Funct. Mater.* 20, 1503–1510. doi:10.1002/adfm.200901627

Hoppe, A., Guldal, N., and Boccaccini, A. R. (2011). Biological response to ionic dissolution products from bioactive glass and glass-ceramics in the context of bone tissue engineering. *Biomaterials* 32, 2757–2774. doi:10.1016/j.biomaterials.2011.01.004

Hutmacher, D. W. (2000). Scaffolds in tissue engineering bone and cartilage. *Biomaterials* 21, 2529–2543. doi:10.1016/S0142-9612(00)00121-6

Hutmacher, D. W., Sittinger, M., and Risbud, M. V. (2004). Scaffold-based tissue engineering: rationale for computer-aided design and solid freeform fabrication systems. *Trends Biotechnol.* 22, 354–362. doi:10.1016/j.tibtech.2004.05.005

Jell, G., Notingher, I., Tsigkou, O., Notingher, P., Polak, J. M., Hench, L. L., et al. (2008). Bioactive glass-induced osteoblast differentiation: a noninvasive spectroscopic study. *J. Biomed. Mater. Res. A* 86, 31–40. doi:10.1002/jbm.a.31542

Jell, G., and Stevens, M. M. (2006). Gene activation by bioactive glasses. *J. Mater. Sci. Mater. Med.* 17, 997–1002. doi:10.1007/s10856-006-0435-9

Jia, T. B., Chen, J. Y., Feng, X. X., and Chang, J. (2011). Fabrication and characterization of chitosan/mesoporous bioactive glasses porous films. *J. Clin. Rehabil. Tissue Eng. Res.* 15, 7877–7880.

Johnson, P. C., Mikos, A. G., Fisher, J. P., and Jansen, J. A. (2007). Strategic directions in tissue engineering. *Tissue Eng.* 13, 2827–2837. doi:10.1089/ten.2007.0335

Jones, J. R. (2009). New trends in bioactive scaffolds: the importance of nanostructure. *J. Eur. Ceram. Soc.* 29, 1275–1281. doi:10.1016/j.jeurceramsoc.2008.08.003

Jones, J. R. (2013). Review of bioactive glass: from Hench to hybrids. *Acta Biomater.* 9, 4457–4486. doi:10.1016/j.actbio.2012.08.023

Jones, J. R., Gentleman, E., and Polak, J. (2007). Bioactive glass scaffolds for bone regeneration. *Elements* 3, 393–399. doi:10.2113/GSELEMENTS.3.6.393

Jones, J. R., and Hench, L. L. (2003). Regeneration of trabecular bone using porous ceramics. *Curr. Opin. Solid State Mater. Sci.* 7, 301–307. doi:10.1016/j.cossms.2003.09.012

Jones, J. R., and Hench, L. L. (2004). Factors affecting the structure and properties of bioactive foam scaffolds for tissue engineering. *J. Biomed. Mater. Res. B* 68, 36–44. doi:10.1002/jbm.b.10071

Kanczler, J. M., and Oreffo, R. O. (2008). Osteogenesis and angiogenesis: the potential for engineering bone. *Eur. Cells Mater. J.* 15, 100–114.

Karageorgiu, V., and Kaplan, D. (2005). Porosity of 3D biomaterial scaffolds and osteogenesis. *Biomaterials* 26, 5474–5491. doi:10.1016/j.biomaterials.2005.02.002

Kasuga, T., Ota, Y., Nogami, M., and Abe, Y. (2000). Preparation and mechanical properties of polylactide acid composites containing hydroxyapatite fibres. *Biomaterials* 22, 9–23. doi:10.1016/S0142-9612(00)00091-0

Kim, Y. P., Lee, G. S., Kim, J. W., Kim, M. S., Ahn, H. S., Lim, J. Y., et al. (2015). Phosphate glass fibres promote neurite outgrowth and early regeneration in a peripheral nerve injury model. *J. Tissue Eng. Regen. Med.* 9, 236–246. doi:10.1002/term.1626

Langer, R., and Vacanti, J. P. (1993). Tissue engineering. *Science* 260, 920–926. doi:10.1126/science.8493529

LeGeros, R. Z. (2002). Properties of osteoconductive biomaterials: calcium phosphates. *Clin. Orthop. Relat. Res.* 395, 81–98. doi:10.1097/00003086-200202000-00009

Legeros, R. Z., Lin, S., Rohanizadeh, R., Mijares, D., and LeGeros, J. P. (2003). Biphasic calcium phosphate bioceramics: preparation, properties and applications. *J. Mater. Sci.: Mater. Med.* 14, 201–220.

Levy, R. A., Chu, T. G., Halloran, J. W., Feinberg, S. E., and Hollister, S. (1997). CT-generated porous hydroxyapatite orbital floor prosthesis as a prototype bioimplant. *AJNR Am. J. Neuroradiol.* 18, 1522–1525.

Li, R., Clark, A. E., and Hench, L. L. (1991). An investigation of bioactive glass powders by sol-gel processing. *J. Appl. Biomater.* 2, 231–239. doi:10.1002/jab.770020403

Li, S. H., De Wijn, J. R., Layrolle, P., and De Groot, K. (2002). Synthesis of macroporous hydroxyapatite scaffolds for bone tissue engineering. *J. Biomed. Mater. Res.* 61, 109–120. doi:10.1002/jbm.10163.abs

Liu, X., Rahaman, M. N., Fu, Q., and Tomsia, A. P. (2012). Porous and strong bioactive glass (13-93) scaffolds prepared by unidirectional freezing of camphene-based suspensions. *Acta Biomater.* 8, 415–423. doi:10.1016/j.actbio.2011.07.034

Liu, X., Rahaman, M. N., Hilmas, G. E., and Bal, B. S. (2013). Mechanical properties of bioactive glass (13-93) scaffolds fabricated by robotic deposition for structural bone repair. *Acta Biomater.* 9, 7025–7034. doi:10.1016/j.actbio.2013.02.026

Lyckfeldt, O., and Ferreira, J. M. F. (1998). Processing of porous ceramics by starch consolidation. *J. Eur. Ceram. Soc.* 18, 131–140. doi:10.1016/S0955-2219(97)00101-5

Manzano, M., Arcos, D., Delgado, M. R., Ruiz, E., Gil, F. J., and Vallet-Regí, M. (2006). Bioactive star gels. *Chem. Mater.* 18, 5696–5703. doi:10.1021/cm0615370

Maquet, V., Boccaccini, A. R., Pravata, L., Notingher, I., and Jerome, R. (2003). Preparation, characterization, and in vitro degradation of bioresorbable and bioactive composites based on bioglass®-filled polylactide foams. *J. Biomed. Mater. Res. A* 66, 335–346. doi:10.1002/jbm.a.10587

Maquet, V., Boccaccini, A. R., Pravata, L., Notingher, I., and Jerome, R. (2004). Porous poly([alpha]-hydroxyacid)/bioglass(R) composite scaffolds for bone tissue engineering. I: preparation and in vitro characterisation. *Biomaterials* 25, 4185–4894. doi:10.1016/j.biomaterials.2003.10.082

Meng, D., Narayan Rath, S., Mordan, N., Salih, V., Kneser, U., and Boccaccini, A. R. (2011). In vitro evaluation of 45S5 bioglass®-derived glass-ceramic scaffolds coated with carbon nanotubes. *J. Biomed. Mater. Res. A* 99, 435–444. doi:10.1002/jbm.a.33185

Miao, X., and Sun, D. (2010). Graded/gradient porous biomaterials. *Materials* 3, 26–47. doi:10.3390/ma3010026

Miguez-Pacheco, V., Hench, L. L., and Boccaccini, A. R. (2015a). Bioactive glasses beyond bone and teeth: emerging applications in contact with soft tissues. *Acta Biomater.* 13, 1–15. doi:10.1016/j.actbio.2014.11.004

Miguez-Pacheco, V., Greenspan, D., Hench, L. L., and Boccaccini, A. R. (2015b). Bioactive glasses in soft tissue repair. *Am. Ceram. Soc. Bull.* 94, 27–31.

Mohamad Yunos, D., Bretcanu, O., and Boccaccini, A. R. (2008). Polymer-bioceramic composites for tissue engineering scaffolds. *J. Mater. Sci.* 43, 4433–4442. doi:10.1007/s10853-008-2552-y

Moimas, L., Biasotto, M., Di Lenarda, R., Olivo, A., and Schmid, C. (2006). Rabbit pilot study on the resorbability of three-dimensional bioactive glass fibre scaffolds. *Acta Biomater.* 2, 191–199. doi:10.1016/j.actbio.2005.09.006

Mourino, V., Cattalini, J. P., and Boccaccini, A. R. (2012). Metallic ions as therapeutic agents in tissue engineering scaffolds: an overview of their biological applications and strategies for new developments. *J. R. Soc. Interface* 9, 401–419. doi:10.1098/rsif.2011.0611

Naik, M. N., Murthy, R. K., and Honavar, S. G. (2007). Comparison of vascularization of Medpor and Medpor-plus orbital implants: a prospective, randomized study. *Ophthal. Plast. Reconstr. Surg.* 23, 463–467. doi:10.1097/IOP.0b013e318158ec8e

Navarro, M., Del Valle, S., Martínez, S., Zeppetelli, S., Ambrosio, L., Planell, J. A., et al. (2004). New macroporous calcium phosphate glass ceramic for guided bone regeneration. *Biomaterials* 25, 4233–4241. doi:10.1016/j.biomaterials.2003.11.012

Nerem, R. M. (1991). Cellular engineering. *Ann. Biomed. Eng.* 19, 529–545. doi:10.1007/BF02367396

Novajra, G., Perdika, P., Pisano, R., Baino, F., Jones, J. R., Boccaccini, A. R., et al. (2015a). Tailoring of bone scaffold properties using silicate/phosphate glass mixtures. *Key Eng. Mater.* 631, 283–288. doi:10.4028/www.scientific.net/KEM.631.283

Novajra, G., Perdika, P., Pisano, R., Miola, M., Bari, A., Jones, J. R., et al. (2015b). Structure optimisation and biological evaluation of bone scaffolds prepared by co-sintering of silicate and phosphate glasses. *Adv. Appl. Ceram.* 114, S48–S55. doi:10.1179/1743676115Y.0000000035

Ortega, F. S., Sepulveda, P., and Pandolfelli, V. C. (2002). Monomer systems for the gelcasting of foams. *J. Eur. Ceram. Soc.* 22, 1395–1401. doi:10.1016/S0955-2219(01)00486-1

Pirhonen, E., Moimas, L., and Haapanen, J. (2003). Porous bioactive 3-D glass fiber scaffolds for tissue engineering applications manufactured by sintering technique. *Key Eng. Mater.* 240-242, 237–240. doi:10.4028/www.scientific.net/KEM.240-242.237

Rahaman, M. N., Day, D. E., Bal, B. S., Fu, Q., Jung, S. B., Bonewald, L. F., et al. (2011). Bioactive glass in tissue engineering. *Acta Biomater.* 7, 2355–2373. doi:10.1016/j.actbio.2011.03.016

Rahaman, M. N., Yao, A., Sonny Bal, B., Garino, J. P., and Ries, M. D. (2007). Ceramics for prosthetic hip and knee joint replacement. *J. Am. Ceram. Soc.* 90, 1965–1988. doi:10.1111/j.1551-2916.2007.01725.x

Rai, R., Boccaccini, A. R., Knowles, J. C., Locke, I. C., Gordge, M. P., McCormick, A., et al. (2010). Fabrication of a novel poly(3-hydroxyoctanoate)/nanoscale bioactive glass composite film with potential as a multifunctional wound dressing. *AIP Conf. Proc.* 1255, 126–128. doi:10.1063/1.3455552

Ramay, H. R., and Zhang, M. (2003). Preparation of porous hydroxyapatite scaffolds by combination of the gel-casting and polymer sponge methods. *Biomaterials* 24, 3293–3302.

Rehorek, L., Chlup, Z., Meng, D., Yunos, D. M., Boccaccini, A. R., and Dlouhy, I. (2013). Response of 45S5 bioglass® foams to tensile loading. *Ceram. Int.* 39, 8015–8020. doi:10.1016/j.ceramint.2013.03.070

Rezwan, K., Chen, Q. Z., Blaker, J. J., and Boccaccini, A. R. (2006). Biodegradable and bioactive porous polymer/inorganic composite scaffolds for bone tissue engineering. *Biomaterials* 27, 3413–3431. doi:10.1016/j.biomaterials.2006.01.039

Rutenberg, M. S., Hamazaki, T., Singh, A. M., and Terada, N. (2004). Stem cell plasticity: beyond alchemy. *Int. J. Hematol.* 79, 15–21. doi:10.1007/BF02983528

Sabree, I., Gough, J. E., and Derby, B. (2015). Mechanical properties of porous ceramic scaffolds: influence of internal dimensions. *Ceram. Int.* 41, 8425–8432. doi:10.1016/j.ceramint.2015.03.044

Scalera, F., Esposito Corcione, C., Montagna, F., Sannino, A., and Maffezzoli, A. (2014). Development and characterization of UV curable epoxy/hydroxyapatite suspensions for stereolithography applied to bone tissue engineering. *Ceram. Int.* 40, 15455–15462. doi:10.1016/j.ceramint.2014.06.117

Schlickewei, W., and Schlickewei, C. (2007). The use of bone substitutes in the treatment of bone defects-the clinical view and history. *Macromol. Symp.* 253, 10–23. doi:10.1002/masy.200750702

Schwartzwalder, K., and Somers, A. V. (1963). *Method of Making a Porous Shape of Sintered Refractory Ceramic Articles.* U.S. Patent No. 3090094.

Sepulveda, P., and Binner, J. G. P. (1999). Processing of cellular ceramics by foaming and in situ polymerisation of organic monomers. *J. Eur. Ceram. Soc.* 19, 2059–2066. doi:10.1016/S0955-2219(99)00024-2

Shah, R., Knowles, J. C., Hunt, N. P., and Lewis, M. P. (2015). Development of a novel smart scaffold for human skeletal muscle. *J. Tissue Eng. Regen. Med.* doi:10.1002/term.1780

Shah, R., Ready, D., Knowles, J. C., Hunt, N. P., and Lewis, M. P. (2014). Sequential identification of a degradable phosphate glass scaffold for skeletal muscle regeneration. *J. Tissue Eng. Regen. Med.* 8, 801–810. doi:10.1002/term.1581

Shah, R., Sinanan, A. C. M., Knowles, J. C., Hunt, N. P., and Lewis, M. P. (2005). Craniofacial muscle engineering using a 3-dimensional phosphate glass fibre construct. *Biomaterials* 26, 1497–1505. doi:10.1016/j.biomaterials.2004.04.049

Studart, A. R., Gonzenbach, U. T., Tervoort, E., and Gauckler, L. J. (2006). Processing routes to macroporous ceramics: a review. *J. Am. Ceram. Soc.* 89, 1771–1789. doi:10.1111/j.1551-2916.2006.01044.x

Sun, J. Y., Yang, Y. S., Zhong, J. P., and Greenspan, D. C. (2007). The effect of the ionic products of bioglass® dissolution on human osteoblasts growth cycle *in vitro*. *J. Tissue Eng. Regen. Med.* 1, 281–286. doi:10.1002/term.34

Sun, L., Berndt, C. C., Gross, K. A., and Kucuk, A. (2001). Material fundamentals and clinical performance of plasma-sprayed hydroxyapatite coatings: a review. *J. Biomed. Mater. Res.* 58, 570–592. doi:10.1002/jbm.1056.abs

Tan, A., Romanska, H. M., Lenza, R., Jones, J. R., Hench, L. L., Polak, J. M., et al. (2002). The effect of 58S bioactive sol-gel derived foams on the growth of murine lung epithelial cells. *Key Eng. Mater.* 240-242, 719–724. doi:10.4028/www.scientific.net/KEM.240-242.719

Tanner, K. E. (2010). Bioactive ceramic-reinforced composites for bone augmentation. *J. R. Soc. Interface* 7, S541–S557. doi:10.1098/rsif.2010.0229.focus

Tesavibul, P., Felzmann, R., Gruber, S., Liska, R., Thompson, I., Boccaccini, A. R., et al. (2012). Processing of 45S5 bioglass® by lithography-based additive manufacturing. *Mater. Lett.* 41, 81–84. doi:10.1016/j.matlet.2012.01.019

Tirkkonen, L., Haimi, S., Huttunen, S., Wolff, J., Pirhonen, E., Sandor, G. K., et al. (2013). Osteogenic medium is superior to growth factors in differentiation of human adipose stem cells towards bone-forming cells in 3D culture. *Eur. Cell. Mater.* 25, 144–158.

Vallet-Regí, M., Salinas, A. J., and Arcos, D. (2006). From the bioactive glasses to the star gels. *J. Mater. Sci.: Mater. Med.* 17, 1011–1017. doi:10.1007/s10857-006--0437-7

Vargas, G. E., Haro Durand, L. A., Cadena, V., Romero, M., Mesones, R. V., Mackovic, M., et al. (2013). Effect of nano-sized bioactive glass particles on the angiogenic properties of collagen based composites. *J. Mater. Sci. Mater. Med.* 24, 1261–1269. doi:10.1007/s10856-013-4892-7

Verrier, S., Blaker, J. J., Maquet, V., Hench, L. L., and Boccaccini, A. R. (2004). PDLLA/bioglass® composites for soft-tissue and hard-tissue engineering: an in vitro cell biology assessment. *Biomaterials* 25, 3013–3021. doi:10.1016/j.biomaterials.2003.09.081

Vitale-Brovarone, C., Baino, F., and Verné, E. (2009). High strength bioactive glass-ceramic scaffolds for bone regeneration. *J. Mater. Sci. Mater. Med.* 20, 643–653. doi:10.1007/s10856-008-3605-0

Vitale-Brovarone, C., Di Nunzio, S., Bretcanu, O., and Verné, E. (2004). Macroporous glass-ceramic materials with bioactive properties. *J. Mater. Sci.: Mater. Med.* 15, 209–217.

Vitale-Brovarone, C., Novajra, G., Lousteau, J., Milanese, D., Raimondo, S., and Fornaro, M. (2012a). Phosphate glass fibres and their role in neuronal polarization and axonal growth direction. *Acta Biomater.* 8, 1125–1136. doi:10.1016/j.actbio.2011.11.018

Vitale-Brovarone, C., Baino, F., Tallia, F., Gervasio, C., and Verné, E. (2012b). Bioactive glass-derived trabecular coating: a smart solution for enhancing osteointegration of prosthetic elements. *J. Mater. Sci.: Mater. Med.* 23, 2369–2380. doi:10.1007/s10856-012-4643-1

Vitale-Brovarone, C., Verné, E., Bosetti, M., Appendino, P., and Cannas, M. (2005). Microstructural and in vitro characterization of SiO_2-Na_2O-CaO-MgO glass-ceramic bioactive scaffolds for bone substitutes. *J. Mater. Sci.: Mater. Med.* 16, 909–917.

Vitale-Brovarone, C., Verné, E., Robiglio, L., Appendino, P., Bassi, F., Martinasso, G., et al. (2007). Development of glass-ceramic scaffolds for bone tissue engineering: characterisation, proliferation of human osteoblasts and nodule formation. *Acta Biomater.* 3, 199–208. doi:10.1016/j.actbio.2006.07.012

Wang, X., Li, Y., Hodgson, P. D., and Wen, C. E. (2009). Biomimetic modification of porous TiNbZr alloy scaffold for bone tissue engineering. *Tissue Eng. Part A* 16, 309–316. doi:10.1089/ten.tea.2009.0074

Wilson, J., Pigott, G. H., Schoen, F. J., and Hench, L. L. (1981). Toxicology and biocompatibility of bioglasses. *J. Biomed. Mater. Res.* 15, 805–817. doi:10.1002/jbm.820150605

Wu, C., and Chang, J. (2014). Multifunctional mesoporous bioactive glasses for effective delivery of therapeutic ions and drug/growth factors. *J. Control. Release* 193, 282–295. doi:10.1016/j.jconrel.2014.04.026

Wu, C., Luo, Y., Cuniberti, G., Xiao, Y., and Gelinsky, M. (2011a). Three-dimensional printing of hierarchical and tough mesoporous bioactive glass scaffolds with a controllable pore architecture, excellent mechanical strength and mineralization ability. *Acta Biomater.* 7, 2644–2650. doi:10.1016/j.actbio.2011.03.009

Wu, Z. Y., Hill, R. G., Yue, S., Nightingale, D., Lee, P. D., and Jones, J. R. (2011b). Melt-derived bioactive glass scaffolds produced by a gel-cast foaming technique. *Acta Biomater.* 7, 1807–1816. doi:10.1016/j.actbio.2010.11.041

Wu, C., Zhang, Y., Zhu, Y., Friis, T., and Xiao, Y. (2010). Structure-property relationships of silk-modified mesoporous bioglass scaffolds. *Biomaterials* 31, 3429–3438. doi:10.1016/j.biomaterials.2010.01.061

Wu, S. C., Hsu, H. C., Hsiao, S. H., and Ho, W. F. (2009). Preparation of porous 45S5 bioglass®-derived glass-ceramic scaffolds by using rice husk as a porogen additive. *J. Mater. Sci. Mater. Med.* 20, 1229–1236. doi:10.1007/s10856-009-3690-8

Xu, H. H. K., Quinn, J. B., Takagi, S., and Chow, L. C. (2004). Synergistic reinforcement of in situ hardening calcium phosphate composite scaffold for bone tissue engineering. *Biomaterials* 25, 1029–1037. doi:10.1016/S0142-9612(03)00608-2

Xynos, I. D., Edgar, A. J., Buttery, L. D. K., Hench, L. L., and Polak, J. M. (2001). Gene-expression profiling of human osteoblasts following treatment with the ionic products of bioglass® 45S5 dissolution. *J. Biomed. Mater. Res.* 55, 151–157. doi:10.1002/1097-4636(200105)55:2<151::AID-JBM1001>3.3.CO;2-4

Xynos, I. D., Hukkanen, M. V. J., Batten, J. J., Buttery, L. D., Hench, L. L., and Polak, J. M. (2000). Bioglass® 45S5 stimulates osteoblast turnover and enhances bone formation *in vitro*: implications and applications for bone tissue engineering. *Calcif. Tissue Int.* 67, 321–329. doi:10.1007/s002230001134

Yun, H. S., Kim, S. E., and Hyeon, Y. T. (2007). Design and preparation of bioactive glasses with hierarchical pore network. *Chem. Commun. (Camb.)* 2139–2141. doi:10.1039/b702103h

Zhu, Y., and Kaskel, S. (2009). Comparison of the in vitro bioactivity and drug release property of mesoporous bioactive glasses (MBGs) and bioactive glasses (BGs) scaffolds. *Microporous Mesoporous Mater.* 118, 176–182. doi:10.1016/j.micromeso.2008.08.046

Zhu, Y., Wu, C., Ramaswamy, Y., Kockrick, E., Simon, P., Kaskel, S., et al. (2008). Preparation, characterization and in vitro bioactivity of mesoporous bioactive glasses (MBGs) scaffolds for bone tissue engineering. *Microporous Mesoporous Mater.* 112, 494–503. doi:10.1016/j.micromeso.2007.10.029

Conflict of Interest Statement: The authors declare that the research was conducted in the absence of any commercial or financial relationships that could be construed as a potential conflict of interest.

14

Development of Magnesium and Siloxane-Containing Vaterite and Its Composite Materials for Bone Regeneration

Shinya Yamada[1], Akiko Obata[1]*, Hirotaka Maeda[1], Yoshio Ota[2] and Toshihiro Kasuga[1]*

[1] Department of Frontier Materials, Graduate School of Engineering, Nagoya Institute of Technology, Nagoya, Japan,
[2] Yabashi Industries Co., Ltd., Ogaki, Japan

Development of novel biomaterials with Mg^{2+}, Ca^{2+}, and silicate ions releasability for bone regeneration is now in progress. Several inorganic ions have been reported to stimulate bone-forming cells. We featured Ca^{2+}, silicate, and especially, Mg^{2+} ions as growth factors for osteoblasts. Various biomaterials, such as ceramic powders and organic–inorganic composites, that release the ions, have been developed and investigated for their cytocompatibilities in our previous work. Through the investigation, providing the three ions was found to be effective to activate osteogenic cells. Magnesium and siloxane-containing vaterite was prepared by a carbonation process as an inorganic particle that can has the ability to simultaneously release Ca^{2+}, silicate, and Mg^{2+} ions to biodegradable polymers. Poly (L-lactic acid) (PLLA)- and bioactive PLLA-based composites containing vaterite coatings were discussed regarding their degradability and cytocompatibility using a metallic Mg substrate as Mg^{2+} ion source. PLLA/SiV composite film, which has a releasability of silicate ions besides Ca^{2+} ion, was coated on a pure Mg substrate to be compared with the PLLA/V coating. The degradability and releasability of inorganic ions were morphologically and quantitatively monitored in a cell culture medium. The bonding strength between the coatings and Mg substrates was one of the key factors to control Mg^{2+} ion release from the substrates. The cell culture tests were conducted using mouse osteoblast-like cells (MC3T3-E1 cells); cellular morphology, proliferation, and differentiation on the materials were evaluated. The PLLA/V and PLLA/SiV coatings on Mg substrates were found to enhance the proliferation, especially the PLLA/SiV coating possessed a higher ability to induce the osteogenic differentiation of the cells.

Keywords: bioceramics, magnesium, calcium, silicate, bone regeneration

Edited by:
Aldo R. Boccaccini,
University of Erlangen-Nuremberg,
Germany

Reviewed by:
Steve Meikle,
University of Brighton, UK
Alexander Hoppea,
Johnson Matthey, Netherlands

*Correspondence:
Akiko Obata
obata.akiko@nitech.ac.jp;
Toshihiro Kasuga
kasuga.toshihiro@nitech.ac.jp

INTRODUCTION

Various types of bioactive ceramics and glasses have been investigated for application in bone regeneration (Jarcho, 1981; Winter et al., 1981; LeGeros, 2002). Calcium phosphate and calcium silicate glasses, such as Bioglass® 45S5, are well known to have excellent bioactivity and promote new bone formation *in vivo*. Recently, several ions released from these materials have been found to influence cell functions and some of the ions can accelerate osteogenesis, angiogenesis, and antibacterial activity (Hoppe et al., 2011). Calcium (Ca^{2+}) ions released from composite materials, consisting of a type II collagen gel and hydroxyapatite (HA), have been demonstrated to have a stimulatory effect on the activation of mouse primary osteoblasts (Maeno et al., 2005). Ca^{2+} ion concentrations of 2–4 mM are reported to be suitable for enhancing the proliferation and survival of osteoblasts, whereas concentrations of 6–8 mM favor their differentiation and biomineralization of extracellular matrix (ECM). Ca^{2+} ion concentrations >10 mM were found to be cytotoxic for cells.

Stimulatory effects for the enhancement of bone formation were found for the soluble silica species and Ca^{2+} ions that were released from Bioglass® 45S5 (Xynos et al., 2000a). The cellular numbers of human osteoblasts (HOBs) cultured in the ionic products of Bioglass® 45S5, obtained by its dissolution in Dulbecco's modified eagle medium (DMEM), increased by 155.1 ± 6.5% compared with normal DMEM after 4 days of culture. HOBs cultured on the Bioglass® 45S5 disk exhibited higher alkaline phosphatase (ALP) activity, which is known to be associated with osteoblastic differentiation of HOBs, compared with those grown on a bioinert (plastic) substrate, after 6 days of culture (Xynos et al., 2000b). Trace amounts of Ca^{2+} and silicate ions are believed to be beneficial for the promotion of bone formation.

Additionally, magnesium (Mg^{2+}) ions have been reported to enhance cell adhesion to materials, along with the differentiation and biomineralization of osteoblasts. The expression of various integrin family members, which are a class of adhesion proteins, was increased on Mg^{2+}-modified alumina compared with Mg^{2+}-free controls (Zreiqat et al., 2002). The stimulatory effects of Mg^{2+} ions on early bone cell differentiation have also been reported, whereby osteoblasts cultured on bioactive SiO_2–CaO–P_2O_5–MgO glass exhibited a high ALP activity (Saboori et al., 2009). Moreover, the effects of Mg^{2+} ions on angiogenic function have been clarified by Maier et al. (2004). Mg^{2+} ions stimulate the proliferation of human umbilical vein endothelial cells (HUVECs) and enhance the mitogenic response to angiogenic factors. These stimulatory effects of the released inorganic ions on cellular activities should be beneficial to the design of new biomaterials for bone regeneration.

Magnesium- and siloxane-containing vaterite (MgSiV) has been developed as a material that provides Mg^{2+}, Ca^{2+}, and silicate ions upon degradation in our previous work (Yamada et al., 2014a). Of the calcium carbonates, vaterite, calcite, and aragonite, vaterite is the most thermodynamically unstable polymorph. The chemical structure and their degradation behavior in physical condition were examined. From cell culture tests, mouse osteoblast-like cells had an improved proliferation, differentiation, and mineralization in the extract of the MgSiV and the dependence on the ion-type contained in the extract; these cell functions were significantly enhanced when all of the ions, Mg^{2+}, Ca^{2+}, and silicate ions, were simultaneously provided to the cells.

The improved functions of the cells were also observed in the results of the cell culture tests for metallic magnesium (Mg) substrates coated with a siloxane-containing vaterite (SiV) and poly (L-lactic acid) (PLLA) composite layer (Yamada et al., 2013, 2014b). The metallic Mg substrate coated with the composite layer releases the three kinds of ions at the same time; Ca^{2+} and silicate ions are supplied by SiV, and Mg^{2+} ions are from the metallic Mg substrates. The cell proliferation and differentiation were accelerated on the metallic Mg substrate coated with the composite layer in comparison with those on the sample releasing only Ca^{2+} and Mg^{2+} ions or no ions.

The up-regulation effects by the three kinds of ions on the cells were found to be similar even though the providing process was different between the MgSiV and the Mg substrate coated with the composite layer. These findings imply that biomaterials providing the three kinds of ions would be good for achievement of the rapid mineralization of osteogenic cells. In addition, such inorganic ions supplied by bioceramics can be regarded to be one of the important factors for promoting bone formation in vivo.

In this review, we provide an overview of materials providing Mg^{2+}, Ca^{2+}, and silicate ions, i.e., the MgSiV and the Mg substrates coated with PLLA/SiV composite layer, and osteoblast-like cell reactions to the materials. In addition, new composite materials that possess an excellent 3D structure (cotton wool-like structure), flexibility, and a providing ability of Ca^{2+} and silicate ions are introduced as well. They have been expected to be good candidates for bone fillers.

MAGNESIUM- AND SILOXANE-CONTAINING VATERITE

The development of SiV (Nakamura et al., 2013) and its composites with biodegradable polymer, such as PLLA or poly(lactic-co-glycolic acid) (PLGA), as materials providing Ca^{2+} and silicate ions has been published in our previous work (Obata et al., 2009, 2010; Wakita et al., 2010; Fujikura et al., 2013). Electrospun fibre-mats consisting of the PLLA/SiV composites possessed excellent cell compatibility in vitro and a formation of mineralized tissue in vivo. Especially, in the results of cell culture tests, the PLLA/SiV composites accelerated the proliferation and the differentiation of mouse osteoblast-like cells in comparison with a composite consisting of vaterite and PLLA (Obata et al., 2009). This implies that the ions released from the PLLA/SiV composites, particularly silicate ions, must contribute to the enhanced cell functions. Many reports demonstrated that such ions are able to enhance osteogenic cell functions, proliferation, differentiation, and mineralization, and regarded to be one of the important factors for bone formation in the body (Hoppe et al., 2011). Thus, the SiV-containing composites are expected to be some of the good candidates for new biomaterials promoting bone formation.

In contrast, the ions released from the SiV and its composites are believed to have no up-regulation effect on cell adhesion. Cell adhesion is a significant process of progressing proliferation for adherent cells, such as osteoblasts and fibroblasts. To improve cell adhesion should be useful to improve proliferation and following biological reactions of these cells. Mg^{2+} ions have been found to improve cell adhesion to substrate surfaces (Zreiqat et al., 2002). Thus, to incorporate magnesium to the SiV was expected to achieve new biomaterials having higher cell compatibility, along with enhanced cell adhesion, proliferation, differentiation, and mineralization. In addition, MgSiV is expected to possess buffering action in aqueous solution since it releases carbonate ions as well, while most of silica-based bioactive glasses, such as 45S5-type bioactive glass, increase its surrounding pH. This might be good for cells cultured on the material surfaces. The preparation of MgSiV powders has been reported in our previous work (Yamada et al., 2014a). In the present short review, some of their significant results are introduced briefly.

Preparation

Magnesium and siloxane-containing vaterite powders were synthesized by a carbonation process in methanol using calcium hydroxide, 3-aminopropyltriethoxysilane (APTES), and magnesium hydroxide as calcium, silicate, and magnesium sources, respectively (Yamada et al., 2014a). All the chemicals were mixed into the slurry under carbon dioxide gas flow, resulting in the formation of a precursor gel. The obtained gel was aged for 12 h at room temperature, dried at 110°C for 24 h, and then grounded to form particles. The obtained MgSiV contained 2.0 wt% of magnesium and 2.8 wt% of silicon. SiV powders were also prepared by the same method without adding magnesium source.

Structure

The prepared MgSiV samples exhibit flat-spherical morphology, around 1.3 μm in diameter and 0.6 μm in thickness (**Figure 1**). They consist of primary particles with several being 10 nm in size. On the other hand, the SiV have a spherical morphology, ~1.4 μm in diameter. The reason why the morphologies are different between the two samples is that it is expected that the orientation of the vaterite phase in MgSiV might be varied by Mg^{2+} ions. Vaterite is known to have a characteristic symmetry and orientation of carbonate ions in its crystalline structure. The orientation is parallel to the c-axis (Wang and Becker, 2009). The siloxane derived from APTES is believed to contribute to the stabilization of the c-face (Nakamura et al., 2013). The Mg^{2+} ions in the MgSiV might influence the orientation, resulting in the formation of the flat-spherical particles. The surface areas of the two samples are also different; they were 103 and 34 m^2/g for the MgSiV and SiV, respectively, from the results of BET–nitrogen adsorption.

The crystalline phase of MgSiV consists predominantly of vaterite one and contains small amounts of calcite and calcium magnesium carbonate. X-ray diffraction (XRD) pattern of the MgSiV demonstrates that the peaks corresponding to the c-axis-dependent plane of vaterite shifted to a higher angle (**Figure 2**). By

contrast, the ab plane shows no shift. Mg might be incorporated into the vaterite crystalline structure and substitute for some of the Ca-sites in vaterite, since the lattice spacing for the vaterite (004) plane changed from 0.426 to 0.421 nm by adding Mg to SiV. The MgSiV and SiV were found to also contain the amorphous calcium carbonate (ACC) phase in their structures from the results of Fourier transform infrared spectroscopy (FTIR) analysis (data not shown here).

Ion Release

The MgSiV powders release Mg^{2+}, Ca^{2+}, and silicate ions through their crystalline transformation from vaterite to aragonite phase in aqueous solution. They were immersed in the Tris–HCl buffer solution (pH 7.4) for 7 days, and the amount of the released ions was measured by inductively coupled plasma atomic emission spectroscopy (ICP-AES) (**Figure 3**). Their crystalline phases at each time point during the immersion were characterized by XRD (**Figure 4**). The crystalline phase of the MgSiV transformed from vaterite into aragonite in 12 h after the immersion and simultaneously released 60% of the total Mg and 80% of the total Si. The release of the two ions continued until day 7, while the release rate decreased after 12 h. A total amount of 83% of the total Mg and almost all Si in the MgSiV were released in the 7 days. On the other hand, the Ca-release behavior was different from those of Mg and Si. The amount of the released Ca was maximum after 12 h and then continued to decline until day 7. The increase in the Ca amount in 12 h after the immersion is believed to originate from the dissolution of ACC. On the other hand, the decline in the amount is due to the formation of precipitates at the bottom of the containers used.

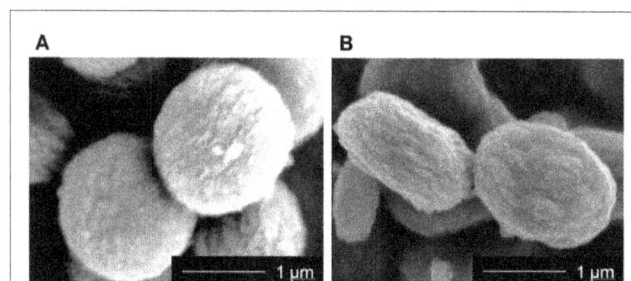

FIGURE 1 | SEM images of (A) SiV and (B) MgSiV. Reprinted with permission from Yamada et al. (2014a).

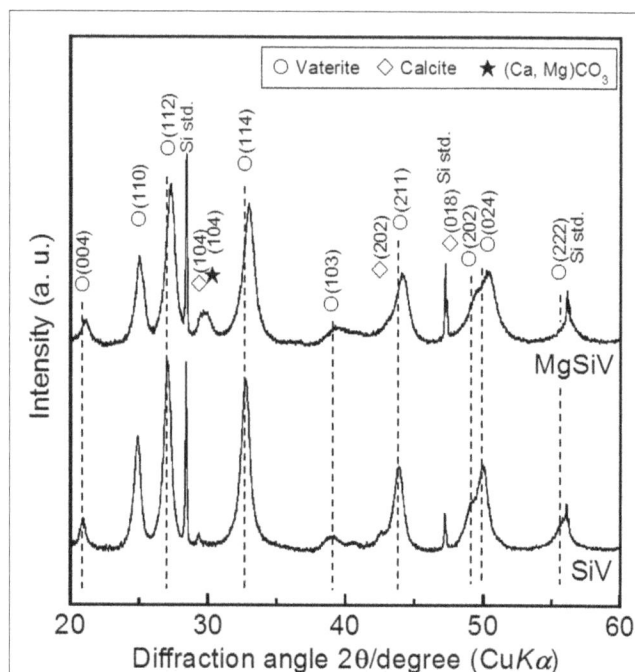

FIGURE 2 | XRD patterns of SiV and MgSiV. Reprinted with permission from Yamada et al. (2014a).

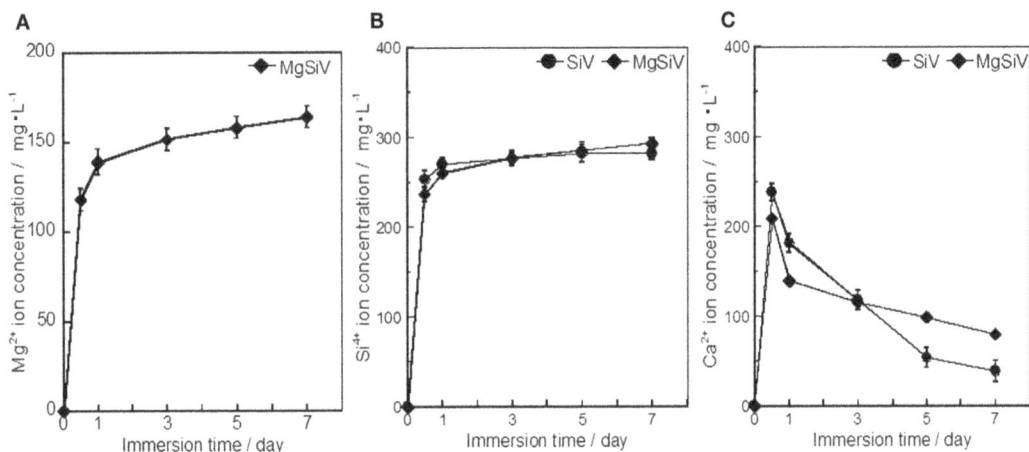

FIGURE 3 | Amounts of (A) Mg, (B) Si, and (C) Ca elements dissolved from SiV and MgSiV. Reprinted with permission from Yamada et al. (2014a).

The SiV powders possess ion-release behavior similar to the MgSiV. The transformation of the crystal phase of the SiV is, however, different from the MgSiV; its phase changed from vaterite to calcite in 12 h after the immersion. This is because aragonite phase precipitates more easily in an aqueous solution containing a large amount of Mg^{2+} ions (Kitano, 1962; Bischoff, 1968; Sawada et al., 1990; Böttcher et al., 1997; Morse et al., 1997; Kitamura, 2001; Zhang et al., 2012). No Mg^{2+} ion is incorporated in the lattice of aragonite because it has a tightly bound hydration shell (Falini et al., 1996, 2009). After 12 h, small peaks corresponding to vaterite phase are still seen for the MgSiV, while the crystal phase of SiV completely transformed to calcite. Mg must be incorporated into the vaterite crystalline structure in the MgSiV, since the peaks corresponding to vaterite in the MgSiV shifted compared with those of the SiV. The Mg incorporated into the vaterite dissolved from the MgSiV in 12 h, because the peaks revert to the original positions of the SiV. Vaterite disappeared and the predominant crystalline phase was aragonite after 7 days. The particle shape of the MgSiV varied after the immersion; no original MgSiV particles were found, but needle-like ones, which is a typical shape of aragonite, were newly observed in the samples after 7 days of immersion.

PLLA/SiV COMPOSITE COATING ON A METALLIC MAGNESIUM SUBSTRATE

Metallic Mg and its alloys possess biodegradability and proper mechanical properties and are regarded to be good candidates for metallic biomaterials (Staiger et al., 2006; Witte et al., 2008; Witte, 2010). They have the suitable properties for being used as vascular stents or orthopedic implants; they possess high reactivity with water and dissolve in body fluid through corrosion, which would contribute to the avoidance of secondary surgery after healing and achieve a complete replacement of bone tissue. In addition, they have the similar Yong's modulus (41–45 GPa) to that of human cortical bone, which might contribute to the decrease of bone resorption around the implants. The modulus is lower

than that of any other metallic biomaterials, such as titanium alloys (Staiger et al., 2006).

On the other hand, there are concerns that metallic Mg rapidly degrades and produces corrosion, hydroxyl ions, and bubbles of hydrogen gas around the surrounding tissues (Witte et al., 2005). This induces an extremely high local alkali concentration (pH > 9.0) on the metallic Mg surface, which is harmful for cells (Shen et al., 2012). The bubbles of hydrogen gas formed in 1 week after implantation, which induced vacant spaces around the metallic Mg. This is attributed to poor integration of the metallic Mg implanted into body tissue (Witte et al., 2005). To solve these problems, the metallic Mg surfaces were coated with biodegradable polymer, such as poly(ε-caprolactone) (PCL) and PLLA (Wong et al., 2010; Xu and Yamamoto, 2012). The cytocompatibility of the metallic Mg was improved by the polymer coatings.

Bioactive coatings consisting of PLLA-based composites containing SiV or vaterite (V) powders have been developed in our previous work, since Mg^{2+}, Ca^{2+}, and silicate ions must be provided from the metallic Mg, vaterite phase, and siloxane in the SiV, respectively, which were expected to enhance osteogenic cell activities. The adhesion, proliferation, and differentiation of MC3T3-E1 cells cultured on the prepared samples were estimated to clarify the effects of the each ion released from the samples on the cell functions (Yamada et al., 2013, 2014b).

Preparation
The SiV and V powders were prepared by a carbonation method aforementioned. The composites of PLLA and SiV or V were prepared by a melt-blending method, dissolved in chloroform, and then coated on surfaces of a commercially available pure metallic Mg with a spin coater. The amount of SiV or V in the composites was set to be 60 wt% (~47 vol%).

Morphology, Bonding Strength, and Degradation
The surface morphology of the coatings on the metallic Mg was different among the PLLA/SiV, PLLA/V, and pure PLLA

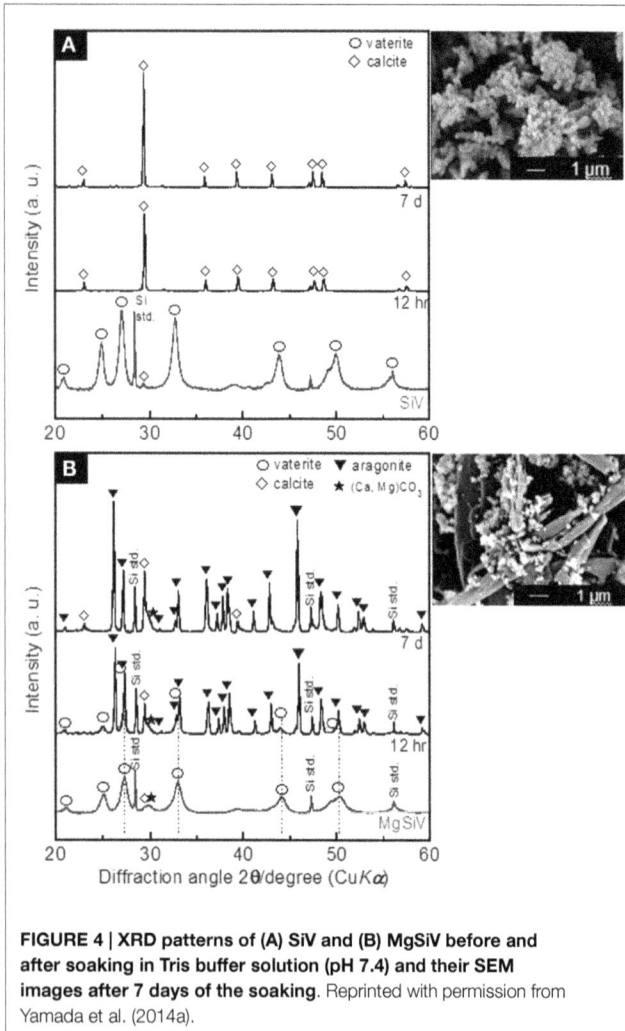

FIGURE 4 | XRD patterns of (A) SiV and (B) MgSiV before and after soaking in Tris buffer solution (pH 7.4) and their SEM images after 7 days of the soaking. Reprinted with permission from Yamada et al. (2014a).

(**Figures 5A–C**), since the diameters of the powders are different; it is ~1.5 μm for SiV and 0.5 μm for V. The thickness also varied among them; it was 5.3 ± 0.4, 3.0 ± 0.1, and 1.8 ± 0.2 μm for PLLA/SiV, PLLA/V, and pure PLLA. Roughnesses of the coatings were 0.40 ± 0.00, 0.19 ± 0.01, and 0.08 ± 0.01 μm for the PLLA/SiV, PLLA/V, and pure PLLA, respectively. This might be due to the difference in the viscosity of the composite or pure PLLA solution. The layer prepared using a spin-coating method depends on the concentration and viscosity of polymer solutions (Schubert and Dunkel, 2003).

Tensile bonding strength tests for the three types of coating demonstrated that the PLLA/SiV coating possesses the highest strength; the rank order of the strength was the PLLA/SiV > PLLA/V > pure PLLA. The difference in the bonding strength would be due to the changes in the molecular weight of PLLA in the coatings by adding the powders. The bonding mechanism was reported to be influenced by molecular weight of polymer in coatings (Xu and Yamamoto, 2012). More free ends of the polymer chains are in the polymers with a lower molecular weight in comparison with those with a higher molecular weight. In the case of the PLLA composite coatings, a larger number of

free carboxyl groups for electrostatic intermolecular interaction between polymer chain and the metallic Mg surface is supposed to be contained in PLLA/SiV, based on the results of the tensile bonding tests. The molecular weights are, however, 82 kDa for PLLA/SiV, 46 kDa for PLLA/V, and 90 kDa for pure PLLA. The varied coating thicknesses of the coatings between them might contribute to the differences in the bonding strength.

All the coated samples release a trace amount of Mg^{2+} ions in α-MEM, while no detachment of the coating layer from the metallic Mg substrates was happened for them. The amount of the ions significantly decreases by the coatings compared with the uncoated (pure) metallic Mg, except the PLLA/V coating (**Figure 6**). Up to 30 μg/mL of the ions were released from the uncoated Mg for 7 days of culturing. On the other hand, the PLLA/SiV and PLLA-coated samples released only 11 and 5 μg/mL of the ions, respectively. The PLLA/V-coated sample possessed a completely different releasing behavior from those of the other two samples; the value of the released ions was the same level of the uncoated Mg at day 3 (16 μg/mL) and then reached about 1.4 times as large as that at day 7 (43 μg/mL). This might be because a large amount of pores formed on the surface of the PLLA/V coating, while no pore or tiny one were done on the surfaces of the other two samples (**Figures 5D–F**). The pores on the PLLA/V coating were generated through the detachment of V powders and the degradation of the PLLA matrix. The Ca^{2+} ions released from the PLLA/V coating might accelerate the corrosion of the metallic Mg, resulting in the enhanced release of Mg^{2+} ion. Thus, the chemical component of the filler in coatings is important for achievement of suppressing the corrosion of the metallic Mg and the rapid release of Mg^{2+} ions from the substrates.

Cytocompatibility

The proliferation of MC3T3-E1 cells on the three types of coated samples and the uncoated one was evaluated by counting live cells after 1, 3, and 7 days of culturing (**Figure 7A**). Results represent the mean values of the experiments in triplicate. Statistical analysis was performed using Student's t-test and single-factor ANOVA (SPSS 21 software; IBM, USA) followed by Tukey's multiple comparison test. Values of $p < 0.05$ were considered to be significant. Although almost no proliferation ability was found for the cells cultured on the metallic Mg, the cells proliferated on the coated samples, especially the proliferation on the PLLA/SiV- and PLLA/V-coated samples was excellent. The uncoated sample should degrade rapidly and generate extremely high alkali condition surrounding its surface after seeding the cells, resulting in the poor cell activity. The polymer coatings suppress such harmful influence on the seeded cells by the metallic Mg, which improves the cell activity. The surface morphology and roughness of the coatings might relate to the cell proliferation ability. However, although the PLLA/SiV coating possess much rougher surface than the PLLA/V one, the proliferation ability of the cells was the similar between the two samples. The crystallinity of polymer was also reported to influence cell proliferation (Park and Cima, 1996; Iafisco et al., 2012). The crystallinities of PLLAs in the PLLA/SiV, PLLA/V, and pure PLLA coatings were 12, 9, and 14%, respectively. Thus, the cells on the samples can be regarded to proliferate independently of the crystallinity of the coatings. The Ca^{2+} and Mg^{2+} ions released

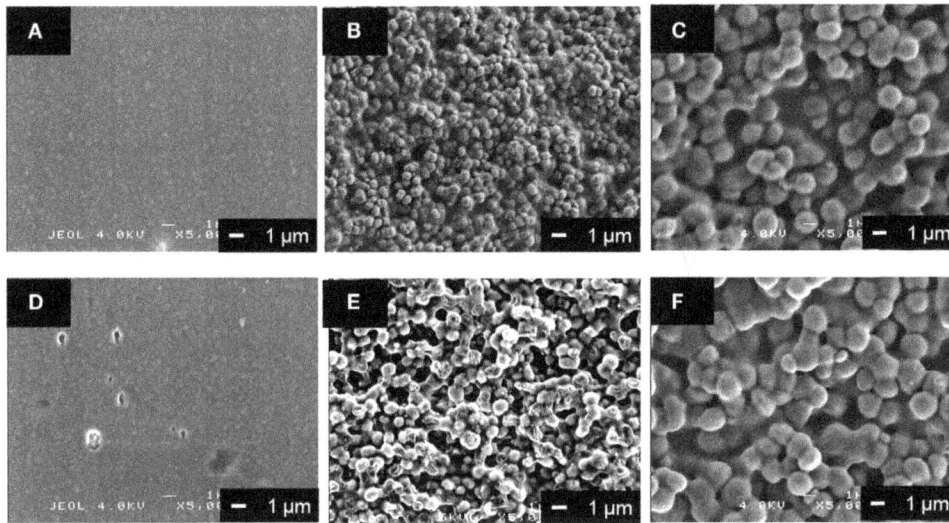

FIGURE 5 | SEM images of (A,D) PLLA coating, (B,E) PLLA/V coating, and (C,F) PLLA/SiV coating (A–C) before and (D–F) after soaking in α-MEM at 37°C for 7 days. Reprinted with permission from Yamada et al. (2013).

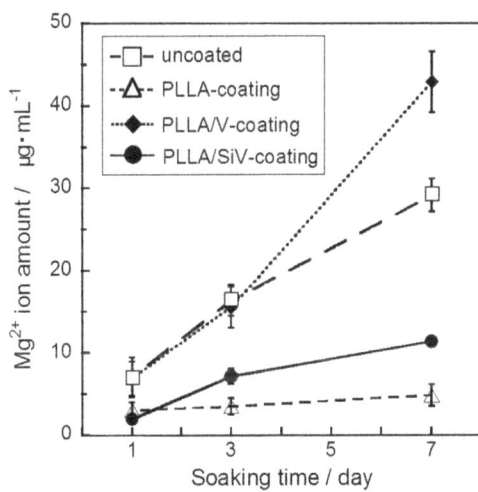

FIGURE 6 | Mg^{2+} ion concentrations dissolved from uncoated, PLLA coating, PLLA/V coating, and PLLA/SiV coating. Reprinted with permission from Yamada et al. (2013).

from the PLLA/SiV- and PLLA/V-coated samples may influence the cell proliferation, since the two ions have been reported to influence osteoblast functions (Diba et al., 2012).

Although there was no significant difference in the proliferation between the PLLA/SiV and PLLA/V coatings, adhering and spreading of the cells varied between the two. The morphology of the cells cultured on the two samples was observed after staining with a Giemsa's solution (**Figure 7C**). The cells exhibit spindle-like shape on the PLLA/SiV coating, while they did circular and a less-spread shape on the PLLA/V one. The aspect ratios of the cells varied between the two samples; the ratio of PLLA/SiV samples

was higher than that of the PLLA/V ones. The proliferation is comparable between the two samples; nevertheless, the instability of the PLLA/V coatings as shown in **Figure 5E** might inhibit the cell spreading.

The osteogenic differentiation of the cells varied on the three types of coated samples. The rank order of the ALP activity was the PLLA/SiV > PLLA/V > pure PLLA ≈ the uncoated Mg substrate after 21 days of culturing (**Figure 7B**). There are two possible reasons why the differentiation varied among the samples, the shape of adhesive cells, and the ions released from the samples. Cell morphologies influence gene expression (Lavenus et al., 2011). As aforementioned, the cells showed a good spreading on the PLLA/SiV coating in comparison with those on the PLLA/V ones. The good spreading should be good for exhibiting their high performances. On the other hand, the ions, especially silicate ions, are known to accelerate osteogenic cell differentiation (Xynos et al., 2001). In addition, MgSiV is expected to possess buffering action in aqueous solution since it releases carbonate ions as well, while most of silica-based bioactive glasses, such as 45S5-type bioactive glass, increase its surrounding pH. This might be good for cells cultured on the material surfaces. Thus, the PLLA/SiV coating is useful for improving the cytocompatibility of the metallic Mg because of its strong bonding with the Mg surface, the stability in an aqueous solution, and the ability of providing three kinds of ions, Mg^{2+}, Ca^{2+}, and silicate ions, which enhance osteogenic cell functions.

BONE-VOID FILLERS WITH COTTON WOOL-LIKE STRUCTURE AND ION-PROVIDING ABILITY

Bone-void filler is one of the most common biomaterials for bone reconstruction. Materials for the bone-void fillers are required to

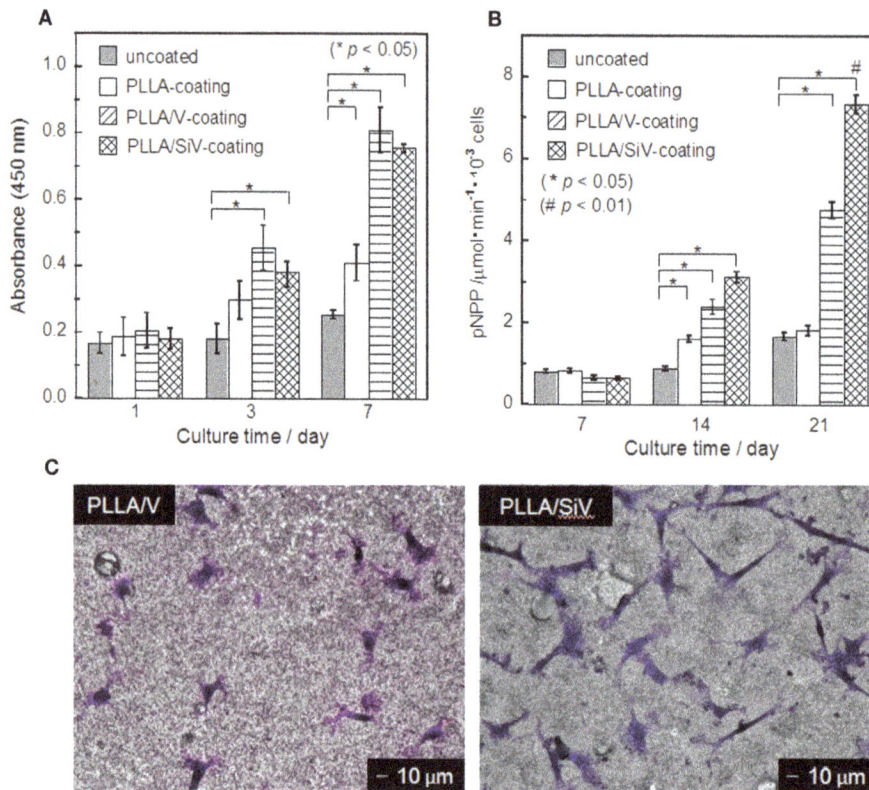

FIGURE 7 | (A) Cell number (mean ± SEM; *$p < 0.05$ as compared to uncoated by t-test), **(B)** ALP activity (mean ± SEM; *$p < 0.05$ as compared to uncoated by t-test, #$p < 0.05$ as compared to other three samples by Tukey's multiple comparison test), and **(C)** morphology of MC3T3-E1 cells cultured on samples. **(C)** After 3 days of culturing. Reprinted with permission from Yamada et al. (2013).

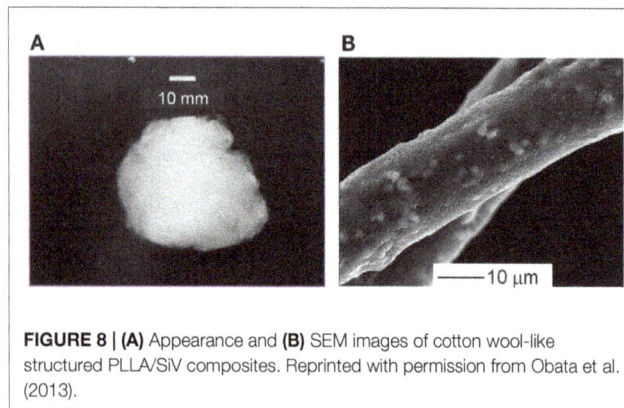

FIGURE 8 | (A) Appearance and **(B)** SEM images of cotton wool-like structured PLLA/SiV composites. Reprinted with permission from Obata et al. (2013).

have bioactivity and porous structure for achieving excellent cell integration and rapid bone regeneration in body. Electrospun fibremats have been widely investigated for the use in bone tissue engineering because of their flexibility and high interconnected porosity (Li et al., 2002; Sill and von Recum, 2008). A conventional electrospinning system consists of a syringe pomp, a power supply, and a metallic plate (collector). A polymer-based solution is put in a syringe set in the syringe pomp and then electrically charged with the power supply. The electrically charged solution is sprayed onto the earthed collector. Electrospun fibers

tightly overlap one another on the collector, resulting in the fabrication of fibremats. However, fabricating thick fibremats, e.g., several millimeter in thickness, had been regarded to be difficult with the conventional electrospinning system, because electrospun fibers hardly sprayed onto a collector when thickness of fibremats formed reaches several hundred micrometer (Pham et al., 2006). Pore sizes of electrospun fibremats are not enough big to induce tissue ingrowth. PLLA/SiV composites having a cotton wool-like structure have been developed with two-types of our original electrospinning systems (Kasuga et al., 2012; Obata et al., 2013). The obtained samples were evaluated in their mechanical properties, ion-releasing ability, and cell compatibility.

Preparation

Two different systems for electrospinnig were used to fabricate a cotton wool-like structure. One is the system having a vessel (100 mm in diameter) filled with ethanol as a collector (Kasuga et al., 2012). Electrospun fibers are collected in the ethanol, which avoids adhesion between the fibers. In addition, electrical charges on electrospun fibers are expected to be neutralized instantly after entering the ethanol. The electrospun fibers contain large gaps between them, resulting in the formation of 3D structure. Another one is the system having a metallic plate collector (like a conventional system) and a fan which blows air against electrospun fibers (Obata et al., 2013). The air can immediately evaporate the solvent in the electrospun fibers (chloroform) in between a tip of syringe and the collector and prevent the fiber sticking to each other.

Structure, Ions-Releasing Ability, and Mechanical Properties

The PLLA composite containing 10, 20, or 30 wt% of SiV with a cotton wool-like structure has been successfully fabricated. The fibers are 10–20 μm in diameter and have pores with ~1 μm in diameter on their surfaces. The SiV powders disperse inside of the fibers and some of them are observed on the fiber surfaces (**Figure 8**). The pores might be formed due to the evaporation of chloroform in the fibers during the electrospinning (Huang et al., 2003; Kim et al., 2005). The pores are expected to play a role in the achievement of ion releasing from the fibers in an aqueous solution. An aqueous solution must penetrate inside the fibers through the pores, and the SiV powders can be exposed to the solution even at central parts of the fibers. In fact, Ca^{2+} and silicate ions gradually release from the fibers and their amounts depend on the contents of SiV in the composite fibers. Thus, the amounts of the ions released are controllable by changing the content of SiV. When the samples are used as bone-void fillers, they would be tightly packed into irregularly shaped bone defects. Mechanical elasticities of the prepared samples are almost the same as that of the pure PLLA sample. That is, they are able to be packed into such defects without collapse. In addition, handling of the samples during operation must be improved.

Cell Compatibility

The cotton wool-like structured samples are required to have the ability of cell penetration to achieve rapid bone regeneration inside of them in body. Although the pore size of the samples can be easily varied by mechanically pressing, when their porosity is set to 90 and 96%, the pore sizes in the samples are enough to induce the cell penetration. Results of culture tests using MC3T3-E1 cells for the samples with 90 and 96% in porosity demonstrated that cells successfully migrate into the cotton wool-like structures and proliferate inside of them. In addition, the live cell numbers in the cotton wool-like structures were significantly higher than those on the fibremats. This implies that the cotton wool-like structure can provide a large space allowing the cells to adhere and proliferate.

SUMMARY

Since inorganic ions were found to stimulate osteogenic cells to proliferate, differentiate, and mineralize, several types of biomaterials releasing such ions have been developed. In this review, we focused on materials releasing three types of ions, Ca^{2+}, Mg^{2+}, and silicate ions, and their cytocompatibility with osteoblast-like cells. The materials possessed the controlled release of the ions in the culture media. Providing several types of the ions simultaneously was important for achieving enhanced cell functions. Especially, the materials releasing all the three types of ions exhibited higher properties than the others in the results of cell culture tests. Combinatorial effects of inorganic ions provided on cells might exist and are expected to be minutely clarified in the future.

REFERENCES

Bischoff, J. L. (1968). Kinetics of calcite nucleation: magnesium ion inhibition and ionic strength catalysis. *J. Geophys. Res.* 73, 3315–3322. doi:10.1029/JB073i010p03315

Böttcher, M. E., Gehlken, P.-L., and Steele, D. F. (1997). Characterization of inorganic and biogenic magnesium calcites by Fourier transform infrared spectroscopy. *Solid State Ionics.* 101–103, 1379–1385. doi:10.1016/S0167-2738(97)00235-X

Diba, M., Tapia, F., Boccaccini, A. R., and Strobel, L. A. (2012). Magnesium-containing bioactive glasses for biomedical applications. *Int. J. Appl. Glass Sci.* 3, 221–253. doi:10.1111/j.2041-1294.2012.00095.x

Falini, G., Fermani, S., Tosi, G., and Dinelli, E. (2009). Calcium carbonate morphology and structure in the presence of seawater ions and humic acids. *Cryst. Growth Des.* 9, 2065–2072. doi:10.1021/cg8002959

Falini, G., Gazzano, M., and Ripamonti, A. (1996). Magnesium calcite crystallizatin from water-alcohol mixtures. *Chem. Commun.* 9, 1037–1038. doi:10.1039/cc9960001037

Fujikura, K., Lin, S., Nakamura, J., Obata, A., and Kasuga, T. (2013). Preparation of electrospun fiber mats using siloxane-containing vaterite and biodegradable polymer hybrids for bone regeneration. *J. Biomed. Mater. Res. B Appl. Biomater.* 101, 1350–1358. doi:10.1002/jbm.b.32952

Hoppe, A., Güldal, N. S., and Boccaccini, A. R. (2011). A review of the biological response to ionic dissolution products from bioactive glasses and glass-ceramics. *Biomaterials* 32, 2757–2774. doi:10.1016/j.biomaterials.2011.01.004

Huang, Z.-M., Zhang, Y.-Z., Kotaki, M., and Ramakrishna, S. (2003). A review on polymer nanofibers by electrospinning and their applications in nanocomposites. *Compos. Sci. Technol.* 63, 2223–2253. doi:10.1016/S0266-3538(03)00178-7

Iafisco, M., Palazzo, B., Ito, T., Otsuka, M., Senna, M., Delgado-Lopez, J. M., et al. (2012). Preparation of core–shell poly(l-lactic) acid-nanocrystalline apatite hollow microspheres for bone repairing applications. *J. Mater. Sci. Mater. Med.* 23, 2659–2669. doi:10.1007/s10856-012-4732-1

Jarcho, M. (1981). Calcium phosphate ceramics as hard tissue prosthetics. *Clin. Orthop. Relat. Res.* 157, 259–278.

Kasuga, T., Obata, A., Maeda, H., Ota, Y., Yao, X., and Oribe, K. (2012). Siloxane-poly(lactic acid)-vaterite composites with 3D cotton-like structure. *J. Mater. Sci. Mater. Med.* 23, 2349–2357. doi:10.1007/s10856-012-4607-5

Kim, G.-T., Lee, J.-S., Shin, J.-H., Ahn, Y.-C., Hwang, Y.-J., Shin, H.-S., et al. (2005). Investigation of pore formation for polystyrene electrospun fiber: effect of relative humidity. *Korean J. Chem. Eng.* 22, 783–788. doi:10.1007/BF02705799

Kitamura, M. (2001). Crystallization and transformation mechanism of calcium carbonate polymorphs and the effect of magnesium ion. *J. Colloid Interface Sci.* 236, 318–327. doi:10.1006/jcis.2000.7398

Kitano, Y. (1962). The behavior of various inorganic ions in the separation of calcium carbonate from a bicarbonate solution. *Bull. Chem. Soc. Jpn.* 35, 1973–1980. doi:10.1246/bcsj.35.1973

Lavenus, S., Berreur, M., Trichet, V., Pilet, P., Louarn, G., and Layrolle, P. (2011). Adhesion and osteogenic differentiation of human mesenchymal stem cells on titanium nanopores. *Eur. Cell. Mater.* 22, 84–96.

LeGeros, R. Z. (2002). Properties of osteoconductive biomaterials: calcium phosphates. *Clin. Orthop. Relat. Res.* 395, 81–98. doi:10.1097/00003086-200202000-00009

Li, W. J., Laurencin, C. T., Caterson, E. J., Tuan, R. S., and Ko, F. K. (2002). Electrospun nanofibrous structure: a novel scaffold for tissue engineering. *J. Biomed. Mater. Res.* 60, 613–621. doi:10.1002/jbm.10167

Maeno, S., Niki, Y., Matsumoto, H., Morioka, H., Yatabe, T., Funayama, A., et al. (2005). The effect of calcium ion concentration on osteoblast viability, proliferation and differentiation in monolayer and 3D culture. *Biomaterials* 26, 4847–4855. doi:10.1016/j.biomaterials.2005.01.006

Maier, J. A., Bernardini, D., Rayssiguier, Y., and Mazur, A. (2004). High concentrations of magnesium modulate vascular endothelial cell behaviour in vitro. *Biochim. Biophys. Acta* 1689, 6–12. doi:10.1016/j.bbadis.2004.02.004

Morse, J. W., Wang, Q., and Tsio, M. Y. (1997). Influences of temperature and Mg:Ca ratio on CaCO3 precipitates from seawater. *Geology* 25, 85–87. doi:10.1 130/0091-7613(1997)025<0085:IOTAMC>2.3.CO;2

Nakamura, J., Poologasundarampillai, G., Jones, J. R., and Kasuga, T. (2013). Tracking the formation of vaterite particles containing aminopropyl-functionalized silsesquioxane and their structure for bone regenerative medicine. *J. Mater. Chem. B* 1, 4446–4454. doi:10.1039/c3tb20589d

Obata, A., Hotta, T., Wakita, T., Ota, Y., and Kasuga, T. (2010). Electrospun microfiber meshes of silicon-doped vaterite/poly(lactic acid) hybrid for guided bone regeneration. *Acta Biomater.* 6, 1248–1257. doi:10.1016/j.actbio.2009.11.013

Obata, A., Ozasa, H., Kasuga, T., and Jones, J. R. (2013). Cotton wool-like poly(lactic acid)/vaterite composite scaffolds releasing soluble silica for bone tissue engineering. *J. Mater. Sci. Mater. Med.* 24, 1649–1658. doi:10.1007/s10856-013-4930-5

Obata, A., Tokuda, S., and Kasuga, T. (2009). Enhanced in vitro cell activity on silicon-doped vaterite/poly(lactic acid) composites. *Acta Biomater.* 5, 57–62. doi:10.1016/j.actbio.2008.08.004

Park, A., and Cima, L. G. (1996). In vitro cell response to differences in poly-L-lactide crystallinity. *J. Biomed. Mater. Res.* 31, 117–130. doi:10.1002/jbm.1996.820310102

Pham, Q. P., Sharma, U., and Mikos, A. G. (2006). Electrospun poly (ε-caprolactone) microfiber and multilayer nanofiber/microfiber scaffolds: characterization of scaffolds and measurement of cellular infiltration. *Biomacromolecules* 7, 2796–2805. doi:10.1021/bm060680j

Saboori, A., Rabiee, M., Moztarzadeh, F., Sheikhi, M., Tahriri, M., and Karimi, M. (2009). Synthesis, characterization and in vitro bioactivity of sol-gel-derived SiO$_2$-CaO-P$_2$O$_5$-MgO bioglass. *Mater. Sci. Eng. C* 29, 335–340. doi:10.1016/j.msec.2008.07.004

Sawada, K., Ogino, T., and Suzuki, T. (1990). The distribution coefficients of Mg^{2+} ion between CaCO$_3$ polymorphs and solution and the effects on the formation and transformation of CaCO$_3$ in water. *J. Cryst. Growth* 106, 393–399. doi:10.1016/0022-0248(90)90084-X

Schubert, D., and Dunkel, T. (2003). Spin coating from a molecular point of view: its concentration regimes, influence of molar mass and distribution. *Mater. Res. Innovat.* 7, 314–321. doi:10.1007/s10019-003-0270-2

Shen, Y., Liu, W., Wen, C., Pan, H., Wang, T., Darvell, B. W., et al. (2012). Bone regeneration: importance of local pH-strontium-doped borosilicate scaffold. *J. Mater. Chem.* 22, 8662–8670. doi:10.1039/c2jm16141a

Sill, T. J., and von Recum, H. A. (2008). Electrospinning: applications in drug delivery and tissue engineering. *Biomaterials* 29, 1989–2006. doi:10.1016/j.biomaterials.2008.01.011

Staiger, M. P., Pietak, A. M., Huadmai, J., and Dias, G. (2006). Magnesium and its alloys as orthopedic biomaterials: a review. *Biomaterials* 27, 1728–1734. doi:10.1016/j.biomaterials.2005.10.003

Wakita, T., Obata, A., Poologasundarampillai, G., Jones, J. R., and Kasuga, T. (2010). Preparation of electrospun siloxane-poly(lactic acid)-vaterite hybrid fibrous membranes for guided bone regeneration. *Compos. Sci. Technol.* 70, 1889–1893. doi:10.1016/j.compscitech.2010.05.014

Wang, J., and Becker, U. (2009). Structure and carbonate orientation of vaterite (CaCO3). *Am. Mineral.* 94, 380–386. doi:10.2138/am.2009.2939

Winter, M., Griss, P., de Groot, K., Tagai, H., Heimke, G., von Dijk, H. J., et al. (1981). Comparative histocompatibility testing of seven calcium phosphate ceramics. *Biomaterials* 2, 159–IN151. doi:10.1016/0142-9612(81)90043-0

Witte, F. (2010). The history of biodegradable magnesium implants: a review. *Acta Biomater.* 6, 1680–1692. doi:10.1016/j.actbio.2010.02.028

Witte, F., Hort, N., Vogt, C., Cohen, S., Ulrich Kainer, K., Willumeit, R., et al. (2008). Degradable biomaterials based on magnesium corrosion. *Curr. Opin. Solid State Mater. Sci.* 12, 63–72. doi:10.1016/j.cossms.2009.04.001

Witte, F., Kaese, V., Haferkamp, H., Switzer, E., Meyer-Lindenberg, A., Wirth, C. J., et al. (2005). In vivo corrosion of four magnesium alloys and the associated bone response. *Biomaterials* 26, 3557–3563. doi:10.1016/j.biomaterials.2004.09.049

Wong, H. M., Yeung, K. W., Lam, K. O., Tam, V., Chu, P. K., Luk, K. D., et al. (2010). A biodegradable polymer-based coating to control the performance of magnesium alloy orthopaedic implants. *Biomaterials* 31, 2084–2096. doi:10.1016/j.biomaterials.2009.11.111

Xu, L., and Yamamoto, A. (2012). Characteristics and cytocompatibility of biodegradable polymer film on magnesium by spin coating. *Colloids Surf. B Biointerfaces* 93, 67–74. doi:10.1016/j.colsurfb.2011.12.009

Xynos, I. D., Edgar, A. J., Buttery, L. D., Hench, L. L., and Polak, J. M. (2000a). Ionic products of bioactive glass dissolution increase proliferation of human osteoblasts and induce insulin-like growth factor II mRNA expression and protein synthesis. *Biochem. Biophys. Res. Commun.* 276, 461–465. doi:10.1006/bbrc.2000.3503

Xynos, I. D., Hukkanen, M. V., Batten, J. J., Buttery, L. D., Hench, L. L., and Polak, J. M. (2000b). Bioglass ®45S5 stimulates osteoblast turnover and enhances bone formation in vitro: implications and applications for bone tissue engineering. *Calcif. Tissue Int.* 67, 321–329. doi:10.1007/s002230001134

Xynos, I. D., Edgar, A. J., Buttery, L. D., Hench, L. L., and Polak, J. M. (2001). Gene-expression profiling of human osteoblasts following treatment with the ionic products of Bioglass® 45S5 dissolution. *J. Biomed. Mater. Res.* 55, 151–157. doi:10.1002/1097-4636(200105)55:2<151::AID-JBM1001>3.0.CO;2-D

Yamada, S., Maeda, H., Obata, A., Lohbauer, U., Yamamoto, A., and Kasuga, T. (2013). Cytocompatibility of siloxane-containing vaterite/poly(L-lactic acid) composite coatings on metallic magnesium. *Materials* 6, 5857. doi:10.3390/ma6125857

Yamada, S., Ota, Y., Nakamura, J., Sakka, Y., and Kasuga, T. (2014a). Preparation of siloxane-containing vaterite doped with magnesium. *J. Ceram. Soc. Jpn.* 122, 1010–1015. doi:10.2109/jcersj2.122.1010

Yamada, S., Yamamoto, A., and Kasuga, T. (2014b). Poly(L-lactic acid)/vaterite composite coatings on metallic magnesium. *J. Mater. Sci. Mater. Med.* 25, 2639–2647. doi:10.1007/s10856-014-5302-5

Zhang, Z., Xie, Y., Xu, X., Pan, H., and Tang, R. (2012). Transformation of amorphous calcium carbonate into aragonite. *J. Cryst. Growth* 343, 62–67. doi:10.1016/j.jcrysgro.2012.01.025

Zreiqat, H., Howlett, C. R., Zannettino, A., Evans, P., Schulze-Tanzil, G., Knabe, C., et al. (2002). Mechanisms of magnesium-stimulated adhesion of osteoblastic cells to commonly used orthopaedic implants. *J. Biomed. Mater. Res.* 62, 175–184. doi:10.1002/jbm.10270

Conflict of Interest Statement: The authors declare that the research was conducted in the absence of any commercial or financial relationships that could be construed as a potential conflict of interest.

15

Adult Stem Cell Therapies for Wound Healing: Biomaterials and Computational Models

Daniele Tartarini[1]* and Elisa Mele[2]*

[1] Department of Mechanical Engineering, Insigneo Institute for in silico Medicine, University of Sheffield, Sheffield, UK,
[2] Department of Materials, Loughborough University, Loughborough, UK

Edited by:
Alessandro Polini,
Radboud University Medical Centre,
Netherlands

Reviewed by:
Mikaël M. Martino,
Osaka University, Japan
Elizabeth R. Balmayor,
Technical University Munich,
Germany

*Correspondence:
Daniele Tartarini
d.tartarini@sheffield.ac.uk;
Elisa Mele
e.mele2@lboro.ac.uk

The increased incidence of diabetes and tumors, associated with global demographic issues (aging and life styles), has pointed out the importance to develop new strategies for the effective management of skin wounds. Individuals affected by these diseases are in fact highly exposed to the risk of delayed healing of the injured tissue that typically leads to a pathological inflammatory state and consequently to chronic wounds. Therapies based on stem cells (SCs) have been proposed for the treatment of these wounds, thanks to the ability of SCs to self-renew and specifically differentiate in response to the target bimolecular environment. Here, we discuss how advanced biomedical devices can be developed by combining SCs with properly engineered biomaterials and computational models. Examples include composite skin substitutes and bioactive dressings with controlled porosity and surface topography for controlling the infiltration and differentiation of the cells. In this scenario, mathematical frameworks for the simulation of cell population growth can provide support for the design of bioconstructs, reducing the need of expensive, time-consuming, and ethically controversial animal experimentation.

Keywords: mesenchymal stem cells, adipose stem cells, wound healing, cell-based modeling approaches, FLAME, Chaste

INTRODUCTION

Human skin is a large and complex organ that is designated to protect the body against environmental insults, and it acts as barrier against chemical, mechanical, and thermal stresses, infections, and dehydration (Martin, 1997). Thanks to the presence of specific receptors and terminations of the peripheral nervous system, the skin exerts also regulatory and sensory functions, including regulation of body temperature, touch, and pain perception (Lumpkin and Caterina, 2007). Injuries, diseases, or surgical procedures can compromise the integrity of this vital organ with the disruption of its physiologic condition and the consequent formation of wounds (Metcalfe and Ferguson, 2007; Shaw and Martin, 2009). Once the skin is wounded, a cascade of biological processes starts in order to restore the normal tissue anatomy and assure wound closure (Bielefeld et al., 2013). If the healing process is delayed or it fails, a state of pathologic inflammation is established, resulting in chronic wounds. Impaired healing is often associated with ischemia, diabetes mellitus, tumor, venous and pressure ulcers, severe infections, and it can be the cause of reduced quality of life, disability, and even death (Gurtner et al., 2008).

In recent years, diverse strategies have been developed to effectively manage and cure chronic wounds (Metcalfe and Ferguson, 2007). Among these, therapies based on stem cells (SCs) are attractive thanks to the unique ability of these cells to self-renew and differentiate into function-specific cellular phenotypes (Wong et al., 2012). In particular, two types of adult SCs are relevant for promoting skin regeneration: mesenchymal stem cells (MSCs) and adipose-derived stromal cells (ASCs). The aim of this review is to provide an overview of the recent advances in the wound management area with emphasis on how biomaterials and SCs (MSCs and ASCs) can be combined to produce advanced wound dressings; how mathematical models and computation frameworks can be advantageously exploited to better understand the mechanisms of tissue regeneration and to design more effective medical devices.

INSTRUCTIVE BIOMATERIAL-BASED SCAFFOLDS

The ultimate aim of bioconstructs for wound healing is to accelerate the skin repair by creating a favorable environment for cell proliferation and differentiation, and mimicking the physicochemical and mechanical properties of the skin (Shevchenko et al., 2010; Yildirimer et al., 2012). Ideal biomedical devices for wound management should be able to reduce inflammation and microbial invasion. They should effectively absorb exudates, promote gas permeability, and deliver functional biomacromolecules to the wound site. Attempts to produce these advanced devices have led to the combination of SCs with properly structured biomaterials. Examples include epidermal, dermal, and dermoepidermal (composite) skin substitutes that encapsulate SCs and bioactive dressings with controlled porosity and surface topography for enhanced cell infiltration and differentiation. As biomaterials, collagen and hyaluronic acid [the major components of the extracellular matrix (ECM)] together with fibrin (abundant in blood clots and naturally involved in wound healing) are widely used for their high biocompatibility, degradability, and ability to promote cell proliferation, migration, and differentiation (Hu et al., 2014). On the other hand, biocompatible and biodegradable synthetic polymers, such as polycaprolactone, polylactic acid, polyglycolic acid, poly(vinyl alcohol), poly(ethylene glycol), and polyurethanes, are of interest in wound care, because they can be easily processed and their properties (mechanical strength and degradation rate) can be controlled and engineered (Moura et al., 2013). Lastly, polysaccharides, such as chitosan and its derivatives, are used for their antimicrobial and homeostatic activity and ability to stimulate fibroblasts proliferation, tissue granulation, reepithelialization, and collagen deposition (Hu et al., 2014).

Mesenchymal Stem Cells

Mesenchymal stem cells are multipotent SCs that can be isolated from bone marrow and other tissues, including adipose and nerve tissue, amniotic fluid, and dermis (Fu and Li, 2009). They are capable to repair not only mesenchymal tissues (bone, cartilage, muscle, marrow, tendon, and ligament) but also liver, heart, nervous tissue, and skin. Furthermore, MSCs exhibit site-specific differentiation, responding to environmental cues and adapting their functions to diverse biomolecular contexts (Jackson et al., 2012). MSCs are involved in nearly all of the wound healing

phases, stimulating angiogenesis, reducing local inflammation, and promoting the formation of the extracellular matrix. MSCs exhibit also antimicrobial activity, through the secretion of antimicrobial proteins or immune-modulating factors (Isakson et al., 2015; Zahorec et al., 2015). Preclinical studies have demonstrated that the local injection of bone marrow-derived MSCs (BM-MSCs) into an incisional full-thickness wound strongly reduces the healing time, promoting angiogenesis, reepithelialization, and granulation (Wu et al., 2007; Chen et al., 2008). Accelerated wound closure of diabetic ulcers has been also shown in preclinical and early human trials when BM-MSCs are used, thanks the production of key cytokines and growth factors, and differentiation in keratinocytes and endothelial cells (Badiavas and Falanga, 2003; Falanga et al., 2007; Jackson et al., 2012; Isakson et al., 2015). However, as the delivery of MSCs through direct injection can induce rapid cell death, novel strategies based on the use of MSC-seeded scaffolding materials have been proposed with the aim to promote cell adhesion, proliferation, and migration.

Cell- and collagen-derived dermal equivalents (DEs) have been produced using human BM-MSCs and MSCs from umbilical cord's Wharton Jelly (UC-MSCs) in coculture with the keratinocyte cell line HaCaT (Schneider et al., 2010). Differently from cell-based DEs (without collagen), the cells were distributed homogenously in the collagen-based DEs, spreading and migrating within the porous structure of the scaffold. Furthermore, ECM proteins and growth factors were highly expressed indicating that collagen-based DEs efficiently directed cell proliferation and ECM remodeling. BM-MSCs and skin-derived (SD) MSCs in combination with collagen-based dermal substitutes (Integra and Pelnac) have been used also for the treatment of full-thickness wounds (Shevchenko et al., 2010; Leonardi et al., 2012; da Silva Jeremias et al., 2014). Studies on a murine model highlighted that Integra was faster colonized in animals receiving MSCs than in control ones (no MSCs) because MSCs promoted cell migration to the wound site and vascularization of the scaffold mainly due to a paracrine mechanism. SD-MSCs well adhered and established cytoplasmic extensions within the matrices, maintaining their phenotypic profile and creating a three-dimensional (3D) cell culture. A recent study has investigated the temporal and spatial migration of MSCs *in vivo* through porous collagen scaffolds loaded with stromal cell-derived factor-1α, demonstrating that the chemotactic cue promoted the recruitment of MSCs to the injured area. Consequently, the enrichment of the wound site with MSCs facilitated the reepithelialization and neovascularization of the tissue (Chen et al., 2015).

Together with DEs, micro- or nanostructured scaffolds for MSC-based therapies have been developed. Composite nanofibrous substrates of collagen and poly(L-lactic acid-co-e-caprolactone) (PLLCL) have been produced by electrospinning and used to direct the epidermal differentiation of human BM-MSCs (Jin et al., 2011). The physical characteristics (size, network organization, and mechanical properties) of the nanofibers and the biochemical cues of collagen were exploited to recreate a fibrillary environment mimicking the native skin. BM-MSCs cultured on the collagen-PLLCL nanofibers exhibited an excellent proliferation rate and their fibroblastic morphology gradually progressed toward that one of epidermal cells. Electrospun nanofibers of collagen and poly (D,L)-lactic-co-glycolic acid (PLGA) containing BM-MSCs were instead proposed for the treatment of full-thickness skin wounds (Ma et al., 2011). The collagen-PLGA scaffolds were implanted *in vivo* and MSCs promoted collagen synthesis and reepithelialization of the insulted skin.

As proved by clinical trials, collagen- and fibrin-based biomedical devices combined with MSCs are particularly promising for non-healing and chronic wounds (Li et al., 2015). A study on 20 patients, whose non-healing wounds (burns, lower extremity ulcers, and decubitus ulcers) were treated with a collagen sponge impregnated with BM-MSCs (Yoshikawa et al., 2008), has showed complete recovery and regeneration of the native tissue for the majority of the cases. In another study, complete or significant closure of diabetic ulcers has been observed using fibrin glue and collagen matrix containing BM-MSCs (Ravari et al., 2011).

Adipose Stem Cells

Multipotent SCs from the adipose tissue are clinically attractive because they can be easily extracted in large amounts and possess high recovery yield (Hassan et al., 2014). It have been demonstrated that ASCs enhance wound healing by differentiating into endogenous skin cells, enhancing epithelial migration and dermal fibroblast proliferation, promoting angiogenesis, secreting cytokines and growth factors (insulin-like growth factor, hepatocyte growth factor, vascular endothelial growth factor), and reducing scar formation.

Similarly to MSCs, ASCs are typically administered by direct injection or topically through gel matrices. However, these approaches are detrimental for cell survival, and hardly provide a microenvironment suitable for cell proliferation and differentiation. In order to achieve therapeutic efficacy, bilayer nanofibrous structures have been proposed for the delivery of ASCs (Pan et al., 2014). Electrospun fibers of poly(e-caprolactone-co-lactide)/poloxamer (PLCL/poloxamer) have been combined with a substrate of dextran and gelatin by mimicking the multilayer structure of the skin. While the electrospun scaffold provided mechanical support and protection of the injured area against external stresses, the hydrogel offered a physiological environment for ASCs proliferation. Nanofibers of polyvinyl alcohol (PVA), gelatin, and azide have been developed for directing the differentiation of ASCs to keratinocytes (Ravichandran et al., 2013). Cells grown on scaffolds functionalized with azine expressed keratin and filaggrin (markers of epidermal differentiation), acquiring the characteristic morphology of keratinocytes. Chitosan-electrospun mats reinforced with cellulose or chitin nanocrystals have been also proposed as highly biocompatible and non-cytotoxic scaffolds for ASCs proliferation (Naseri et al., 2014, 2015).

Together with electrospinning, freeze drying has been used as technology to create 3D porous constructs. Structures of poly(3-hydroxybutyrate-co-hydroxyvalerate) (PHBV) loaded with ASCs have been tested *in vivo*, demonstrating that the mechanical properties of the scaffolds were able to control contraction stresses during tissue repair, whereas ASCs enhanced granulation, reepithelialization, and vascularization (Zonari et al., 2015). Scarring was strongly reduced during healing and, after 28 days of treatment with PHBV/ASCs samples, the new-formed tissue was characterized by a well-organized dermal matrix with sebaceous glands and hair follicles.

Preclinical studies have demonstrated that ASCs combined with engineered scaffolds based on natural biomaterials, such as collagen and cellulose derivatives, have high potential therapeutic effects in wound healing, because they increase the epithelialization rate, granulation, and downregulate the inflammatory response (Hassan et al., 2014; Rodrigues et al., 2014).

COMPUTATIONAL MODELS

The variety and complexity of the biochemical and biophysical processes involved in tissue regeneration alongside their intrinsic multiscale nature highlight the need of computational models both to fully understand cell growth and to design efficient scaffolds and tissue substitutes (Langer and Vacanti, 1993; Hori et al., 2004; Byrne et al., 2007; O'Dea et al., 2012). Aspects to be considered are the timely release of growth factors and therapeutic agents and the controlled degradation of the scaffold during wound healing to allow cells proliferation; especially for *in vivo* tissue regeneration that is more efficient than replacement (Yildirimer et al., 2012; Yildirimer and Seifalian, 2014). Multiphase models have been used to describe these time-dependent processes *in vitro* in a perfusion bioreactor, with particular attention for the interplay between cell growth, access to nutrients, and scaffold degradation (O'Dea et al., 2013). Cell population and culture medium have been modeled as viscous fluids within the porous scaffold, while the scaffold and ECM have been treated as rigid porous materials. The model has predicted that scaffold and ECM heterogeneity impacts on the mechanical properties of the regenerated tissue with effects on the future success of the implant. Further computational methods have modeled cell spreading and tissue regeneration *in vitro* using porous scaffolds by considering transport and consumption of nutrients, ECM deposition, cell population dynamics, cell attachment, migration and intercellular interactions (Sengers et al., 2007; O'Dea et al., 2012; O'Dea et al., 2014; Yildirimer and Seifalian, 2014). The diffusion of nutrients, oxygen, and biochemical signals is mainly accounted in the models as advection–reaction–diffusion equations and depends on the type of bioreactor or scaffold used. Finite element methods (FEM) and computational fluid dynamics (CFD) models have been proposed to understand how the scaffold/bioreactor structure and porosity affect the distribution of nutrients and consequently the cellular growth rate (Olivares and Lacroix, 2013). Although comprehensive computational models specifically conceived for skin regeneration are unavailable to date, most of the already developed methodologies can provide insights in modeling skin and wound healing. In the following, we will focus on the computational models suitable for skin regeneration, in particular for cell population dynamics, human skin homeostasis, and growth factors interactions.

Continuum and Individual-Based Models of Cell Populations

Models for cell population growth are classified by the underlying mathematical approach: continuum, individual-based, and hybrid (O'Dea et al., 2012; Van Liedekerke et al., 2015). The debate on the adoption of a continuum versus an individual-based approach is extensively addressed in O'Dea et al. (2012). Continuum approaches are mainly based on multiphase or mixture theory that describes systems made of several interacting constituents, like a biological tissue (O'Dea et al., 2012): different cell types, ECM, and interstitial fluid. These systems can be represented as a mixture of continua, occupying the same spatial region, whose interactions are described through force balance equations and constitutive relations. Continuum models can be solved efficiently via FEM but cell properties are spatially averaged. On the other hand, individual-based or agent-based models (ABMs) are preferred when the number of initial cells is relatively small, which is the typical scenario for scaffolds seeded with SCs, and when subcellular phenomena need to be addressed, like cell signaling, cell cycle, cell–cell interaction, space occupancy. ABMs allow to explicitly express and study single cell behavior, signaling, proliferation, and movement (Youssef et al., 2007). Cell behavior is modeled through simple rules that take into account the cell cycle, the status of neighbors, and the space occupancy. These models are divided in on-lattice and off-lattice (**Figure 1**), depending on whether the cells are constrained in a lattice or are free to move in the space. Cellular automata (CA) models (**Figure 1A**) represent a cell as a lattice site with a fixed volume; biological and physical interactions are encoded in each cell as rules. Cell division, migration, and death are accounted shifting neighbors within an interaction radius. In Cellular Potts models (CPM), **Figure 1B**, a cell occupies several

contiguous lattice sites (Graner and Glazier, 1992). Migration, growth, and shape change are modeled with a Markov chain Monte Carlo method and only favorable energetic configurations are accounted. In **Figure 1C**, lattice sites are compartments hosting several cells. This approach is similar to CA, but single cell position is not computed.

In off-lattice cell-centered ABM models (**Figure 1D**), cells are free to move in the space (also called lattice-free approach) and are modeled as spheres or ellipsoids. Nevertheless, when it is necessary to account the influence of mechanical forces on the cells (cell–scaffold and cell–ECM interaction), they are modeled as a deformable objects (Byrne and Drasdo, 2009). Off-lattice cell-centered ABM models have been used to model 2D *in vitro* epithelial tissues (Walker et al., 2004; Sun et al., 2007) and skin tissue growth in 3D (Adra et al., 2010); in both cases, the Flexible Large-scale Agent Modeling Environment (FLAME) computational framework for agent-based simulation has been used (Richmond et al., 2010). Further work on the lattice-free cell-centered approach has been done to take into account cell–cell and cell–environment interactions (Meineke et al., 2001; van Leeuwen et al., 2009). The models considered the cells connected through linear over-damped springs, and they have been used to simulate epithelial growth of the intestinal crypt. Voronoi polyhedra have been used (**Figure 1E**) to model a more realistic cell shape and contact surface in dense tissues with many neighboring cells, like in epithelia and skin (Fletcher et al., 2013). These models are implemented in the Cancer, Heart and Soft Tissue Environment

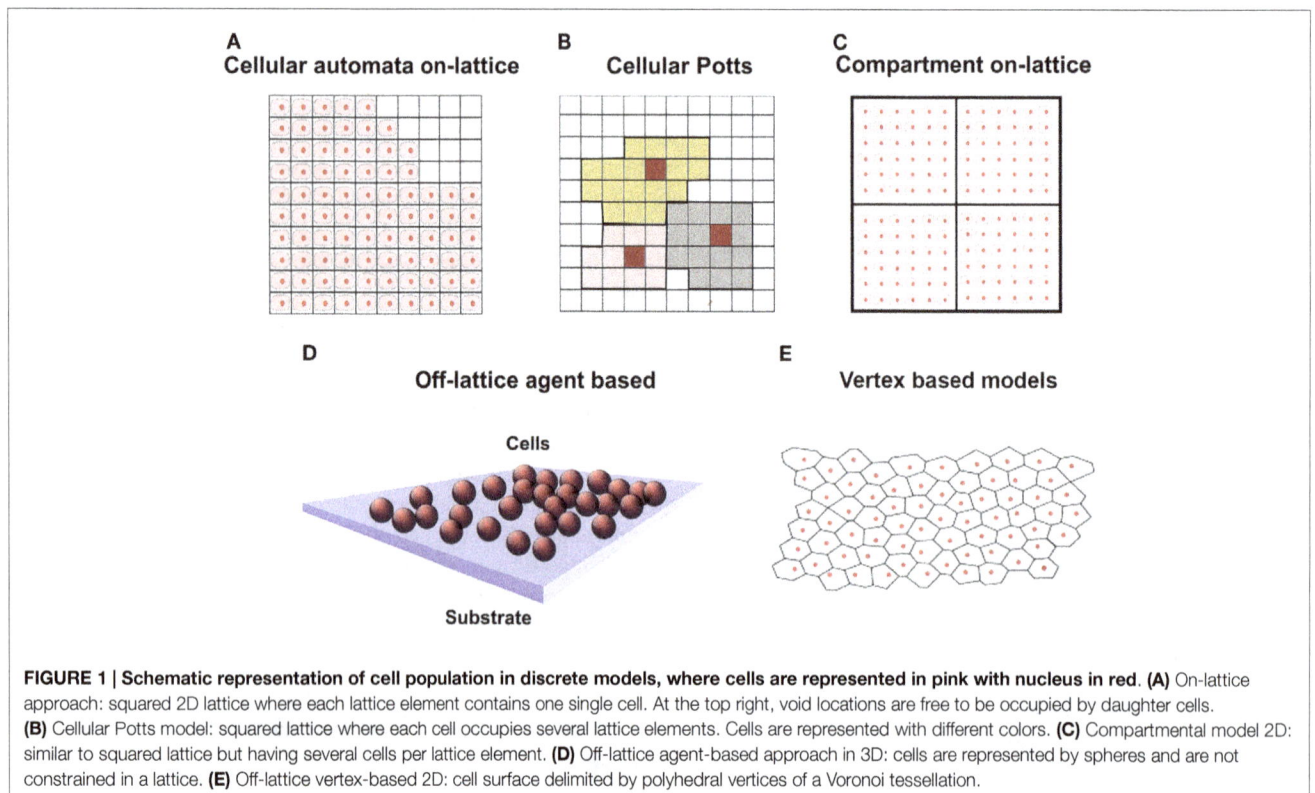

FIGURE 1 | Schematic representation of cell population in discrete models, where cells are represented in pink with nucleus in red. (A) On-lattice approach: squared 2D lattice where each lattice element contains one single cell. At the top right, void locations are free to be occupied by daughter cells. **(B)** Cellular Potts model: squared lattice where each cell occupies several lattice elements. Cells are represented with different colors. **(C)** Compartmental model 2D: similar to squared lattice but having several cells per lattice element. **(D)** Off-lattice agent-based approach in 3D: cells are represented by spheres and are not constrained in a lattice. **(E)** Off-lattice vertex-based 2D: cell surface delimited by polyhedral vertices of a Voronoi tessellation.

TABLE 1 | Comparison of cell population models (Van Liedekerke et al., 2015).

Computational models		
	Characteristics	Limitations
On-lattice models		
• Individual representation of cells		
• Precise cell position		
• Simulation of cell movement, division, and death		
(A) Cellular automata models	• Large-scale simulations	• Inappropriate description of cell mechanics and adhesion
	• Efficient parameter sensitivity	• Fixed cell size
(B) Cell Potts models	• Flexible and extensible framework	• Sensitivity analysis limited by computational complexity
	• High cell density can be simulated	• Physics partially represented
(C) Compartmental models	• Cell position resolved at the lattice compartment level	• Scale linked to lattice size
	• Efficient parameter sensitivity analysis	• Representation of physical interaction with energy function
Off-lattice models		
• Individual representation of cells		
• Physical laws directly represented		
• Variable cell size		
(D) Center-based models (CBM) with spherical cells	• Equation of motion is intuitive and extendable	• Cell–cell forces are pairwise and can generate artifacts
	• Effective code parallelization	• Large simulations (over 10^6 cells) limited by computational time
(E) Vertex-based models	• Suitable for highly packed populations	• Computational complexity limits simulations to thousands of cells
	• Forces and mechanical stresses at subcellular level can be modeled	

(CHASTE) framework. The features and limitations of the computational models described above are summarized in **Table 1**. The computational power required for simulations depends on the model and the number of cells involved and code parallelization improves performances (Richmond et al., 2010; Harvey et al., 2015).

Hybrid cell-center-continuous approaches have also been proposed and implemented (Cheng et al., 2009; Chung et al., 2010). They are based on a CA model for the cell cycle, cell proliferation, migration and collision, and on reaction–diffusion equation for nutrient concentration. These models have been used to investigate a typical condition of bioreactors where tissue regeneration is slowed by nutrient limitations, allowing the identification of more effective seeding strategies.

Computational Models for Human Epidermis

As discussed previously, only few works have reported on computational models for skin and wound healing (*in virtuo* analysis), due to the complexity of this biological process. The epidermis studies available are based on ABM models with an initial population of SCs. Cells are generally approximated with spheres of 10 μm, and their behavioral rules are taken from literature or experimental data. ABMs have been used to investigate the organization and self-regulation of keratinocytes (Sun et al., 2007), the role of growth factors on cell–cell and cell–ECM interaction (Adra et al., 2010), the effect of the presence of fibroblasts on the expansion rate of keratinocyte colony (Sun et al., 2008), the spatio-temporal dynamics of epidermis homeostasis under normal and pathological conditions (Zhang et al., 2014), and the importance of SCs in long-term skin epithelium regeneration and homeostasis (Li et al., 2013). ABMs have been used to study the behavior *in vitro* of normal human keratinocytes under varying extracellular calcium concentrations, observing that the cell–substrate contact is crucial in the self-organization of the colony and that rapid wound closure is promoted in a low calcium media (Sun et al., 2007; Smallwood, 2011). A multiscale integrated model of human epidermis have been developed coupling ABM (through FLAME) with the expression and signaling of growth factors for specific subcellular mechanisms through COmplex PAthway SImulator (COPASI) (Hoops et al., 2006). FLAME has been also used to predict the dynamics of cell colonies over 3 years comparing different hypotheses of SC generation of epithelium (Li et al., 2013). The ABM models allow to explore alternative hypothesis about skin structure and dynamics over different conditions in timeframes longer than those feasible *in vitro* and in different regimes of nutrients or biochemical signals. ABM simulations of epithelial wounds made with FLAME can efficiently exploit parallel computational architectures and using GPUs obtain nearly real-time results (Richmond et al., 2010).

FUTURE DIRECTIONS

Differently from bone tissue engineering where the understanding of bone structure, biomechanics, and tissue formation relies on a highly cross-disciplinary research (biomaterial engineering, biology, and computer science), the current state of the art of skin regeneration for wound healing is still sector-based. On one hand, advanced biomedical dressings have been developed using different classes of biomaterials and SCs; on the other hand, computational modeling has not yet been completely exploited to study skin growth and cell–biomaterial interaction. The complexity of the biological phenomena involved hardly permits the existence of a one-fits-all computational framework. Currently, the most mature frameworks supporting the research in this area (open source and supporting the main operating systems) are CHASTE for multiscale and multiphase problems (Mirams et al., 2013), CompuCell3D for multicellular organisms (morphogenesis) (Izaguirre et al., 2004), and FLAME for generic agent-based systems. Tools based on FEM also exist: FEniCS (Logg et al., 2012),

ANSYS, and Abaqus. Theoretical and computational models can provide detailed information of physical and biological entities within the evolving/healing tissue that are not easily accessible with experimental studies: fluid and mechanical stress, cell density, and nutrient levels. Nevertheless, their prediction power at systems biology level is strictly linked to robust validation against biological models (Smallwood et al., 2004). The use of these technologies to predict the behavior of cells during wound closure and the role played by the dressing is fundamental to progress in this area, allowing the reduction of animal tests.

AUTHOR CONTRIBUTIONS

DT and EM conceived and wrote the main manuscript text, according to their competency.

FUNDING

DT acknowledges the project "Accelerating *in silico* cancer research with graphic processors" of the Engineering and Physical Science Research Council (EPSRC) for the financial support.

REFERENCES

Adra, S., Sun, T., MacNeil, S., Holcombe, M., and Smallwood, R. (2010). Development of a three dimensional multiscale computational model of the human epidermis. *PLoS ONE* 5:e8511. doi:10.1371/journal.pone.0008511

Badiavas, E. V., and Falanga, V. (2003). Treatment of chronic wounds with bone marrow-derived cells. *Arch. Dermatol.* 139, 510–516. doi:10.1001/archderm.139.4.510

Bielefeld, K. A., Amini-Nik, S., and Alman, B. A. (2013). Cutaneous wound healing: recruiting developmental pathways for regeneration. *Cell Mol. Life Sci.* 70, 2059–2081. doi:10.1007/s00018-012-1152-9

Byrne, D. P., Lacroix, D., Planell, J. A., Kelly, D. J., and Prendergast, P. J. (2007). Simulation of tissue differentiation in a scaffold as a function of porosity, Young's modulus and dissolution rate: application of mechanobiological models in tissue engineering. *Biomaterials* 28, 5544–5554. doi:10.1016/j.biomaterials.2007.09.003

Byrne, H., and Drasdo, D. (2009). Individual-based and continuum models of growing cell populations: a comparison. *J. Math. Biol.* 58, 657–687. doi:10.1007/s00285-008-0212-0

Chen, G., Tian, F., Li, C., Zhang, Y., Weng, Z., Zhang, Y., et al. (2015). In vivo real-time visualization of mesenchymal stem cells tropism for cutaneous regeneration using NIR-II fluorescence imaging. *Biomaterials* 53, 265–273. doi:10.1016/j.biomaterials.2015.02.090

Chen, L., Tredget, E. E., Wu, P. Y. G., and Wu, Y. (2008). Paracrine factors of mesenchymal stem cells recruit macrophages and endothelial lineage cells and enhance wound healing. *PLoS ONE* 3:e1886. doi:10.1371/journal.pone.0001886

Cheng, G., Markenscoff, P., and Zygourakis, K. (2009). A 3D hybrid model for tissue growth: the interplay between cell population and mass transport dynamics. *Biophys. J.* 97, 401–414. doi:10.1016/j.bpj.2009.03.067

Chung, C. A., Lin, T.-H., Chen, S.-D., and Huang, H.-I. (2010). Hybrid cellular automaton modeling of nutrient modulated cell growth in tissue engineering constructs. *J. Theor. Biol.* 262, 267–278. doi:10.1016/j.jtbi.2009.09.031

da Silva Jeremias, T., Grecco Machado, R., Coutinho Visoni, S. B., Pereima, M. J., Leonardi, D. F., and Goncalves Trentin, A. (2014). Dermal substitutes support the growth of human skin-derived mesenchymal stromal sells: potential tool for skin regeneration. *PLoS ONE* 9:e89542. doi:10.1371/journal.pone.0089542

Falanga, V., Iwamoto, S., Chartier, M., Yufit, T., Butmarc, J., Kouttab, N., et al. (2007). Autologous bone marrow-derived cultured mesenchymal stem cells delivered in a fibrin spray accelerate healing in murine and human cutaneous wounds. *Tissue Eng.* 13, 1299–1312. doi:10.1089/ten.2006.0278

Fletcher, A. G., Osborne, J. M., Maini, P. K., and Gavaghan, D. J. (2013). Implementing vertex dynamics models of cell populations in biology within a consistent computational framework. *Prog. Biophys Mol. Biol.* 113, 299–326. doi:10.1016/j.pbiomolbio.2013.09.003

Fu, X., and Li, H. (2009). Mesenchymal stem cells and skin wound repair and regeneration: possibilities and questions. *Cell Tissue Res.* 335, 317–321. doi:10.1007/s00441-008-0724-3

Graner, F., and Glazier, J. (1992). Simulation of biological cell sorting using a two-dimensional extended Potts model. *Phys. Rev. Lett.* 69, 2013–2016. doi:10.1103/PhysRevLett.69.2013

Gurtner, G. C., Werner, S., Barrandon, Y., and Longaker, M. T. (2008). Wound repair and regeneration. *Nature* 453, 314–321. doi:10.1038/nature07039

Harvey, D. G., Fletcher, A. G., Osborne, J. M., and Pitt-Francis, J. (2015). A parallel implementation of an off-lattice individual-based model of multicellular populations. *Comput. Phys. Comm.* 192, 130–137. doi:10.1016/j.cpc.2015.03.005

Hassan, W. U., Greiser, U., and Wang, W. (2014). Role of adipose-derived stem cells in wound healing. *Wound Rep. Reg.* 22, 313–325. doi:10.1111/wrr.12173

Hoops, S., Sahle, S., Gauges, R., Lee, C., Pahle, J., Simus, N., et al. (2006). COPASI – a complex pathway simulator. *Bioinformatics* 22, 3067–3074. doi:10.1093/bioinformatics/btl485

Hori, Y., Inoue, S., Hirano, Y., and Tabata, Y. (2004). Effect of culture substrates and fibroblast growth factor addition on the proliferation and differentiation of rat bone marrow stromal cells. *Tissue Eng.* 10, 995–1005. doi:10.1089/ten.2004.10.995

Hu, M. S., Maan, Z. N., Wu, J. C., Rennert, R. C., Hong, W. X., Lai, T. S., et al. (2014). Tissue engineering and regenerative repair in wound healing. *Ann. Biomed. Eng.* 42, 1494–1507. doi:10.1007/s10439-014-1010-z

Isakson, M., de Blacam, C., Whelan, D., McArdle, A., and Clover, A. J. P. (2015). Mesenchymal stem cells and cutaneous wound healing: current evidence and future potential. *Stem Cells Int.* 2015, 831095. doi:10.1155/2015/831095

Izaguirre, J. A., Chaturvedi, R., Huang, C., Cickovski, T., Coffland, J., Thomas, G., et al. (2004). CompuCell, a multi-model framework for simulation of morphogenesis. *Bioinformatics* 20, 1129–1137. doi:10.1093/bioinformatics/bth050

Jackson, W. M., Nesti, L. J., and Tuan, R. S. (2012). Concise review: clinical translation of wound healing therapies based on mesenchymal stem cells. *Stem Cells Transl. Med.* 1, 44–50. doi:10.5966/sctm.2011-0024

Jin, G., Prabhakaran, M. P., and Ramakrishna, S. (2011). Stem cell differentiation to epidermal lineages on electrospun nanofibrous substrates for skin tissue engineering. *Acta Biomater.* 7, 3113–3122. doi:10.1016/j.actbio.2011.04.017

Langer, R., and Vacanti, J. P. (1993). Tissue engineering. *Science* 260, 920–926. doi:10.1126/science.8493529

Leonardi, D., Oberdoerfer, D., Fernandes, M. C., Meurer, R. T., Pereira-Filho, G. A., Cruz, P., et al. (2012). Mesenchymal stem cells combined with an artificial dermal substitute improve repair in full-thickness skin wounds. *Burns* 38, 1143–1150. doi:10.1016/j.burns.2012.07.028

Li, M., Zhao, Y., Hao, H., Han, W., and Fu, X. (2015). Mesenchymal stem cell-based therapy for nonhealing wounds: today and tomorrow. *Wound Rep. Reg.* 23, 465–482. doi:10.1111/wrr.12304

Li, X., Upadhyay, A. K., Bullock, A. J., Dicolandrea, T., Xu, J., Binder, R. L., et al. (2013). Skin stem cell hypotheses and long term clone survival – explored using agent-based modelling. *Sci. Rep.* 3, 1904. doi:10.1038/srep01904

Logg, A., Mardal, K. A., and Wells, G. (2012). *Automated Solution of Differential Equations by the Finite Element Method*, Vol. 84. (Berlin; Heidelberg: Springer).

Lumpkin, E. A., and Caterina, M. J. (2007). Mechanisms of sensory transduction in the skin. *Nature* 445, 858–865. doi:10.1038/nature05662

Ma, K., Liao, S., He, L., Lu, J., Ramakrishna, S., and Chan, C. K. (2011). Effects of nanofiber/stem cell composite on wound healing in acute full-thickness skin wounds. *Tissue Eng. Part A* 17, 1413–1424. doi:10.1089/ten.tea.2010.0373

Martin, P. (1997). Wound healing – aiming for perfect skin regeneration. *Science* 276, 75–81. doi:10.1126/science.276.5309.75

Meineke, F. A., Potten, C. S., and Loeffler, M. (2001). Cell migration and organization in the intestinal crypt using a lattice-free model. *Cell Prolif.* 34, 253–266. doi:10.1046/j.0960-7722.2001.00216.x

Metcalfe, A. D., and Ferguson, M. W. J. (2007). Tissue engineering of replacement skin: the crossroads of biomaterials, wound healing, embryonic development, stem cells and regeneration. *J. R. Soc. Interface* 4, 413–437. doi:10.1098/rsif.2006.0179

Mirams, G. R., Arthurs, C. J., Bernabeu, M. O., Bordas, R., Cooper, J., Corrias, A., et al. (2013). Chaste: an open source C++ library for computational physiology and biology. *PLoS Comput. Biol.* 9:e1002970. doi:10.1371/journal.pcbi.1002970

Moura, L. I., Dias, A. M., Carvalho, E., and de Sousa, H. C. (2013). Recent advances on the development of wound dressings for diabetic foot ulcer treatment – a review. *Acta Biomater.* 9, 7093–7114. doi:10.1016/j.actbio.2013.03.033

Naseri, N., Algan, C., Jacobs, V., John, M., Oksman, K., and Mathew, A. P. (2014). Electrospun chitosan-based nanocomposite mats reinforced with chitin nanocrystals for wound dressing. *Carbohydr. Polym.* 109, 7–15. doi:10.1016/j.carbpol.2014.03.031

Naseri, N., Mathew, A. P., Girandon, L., Frohlich, M., and Oksman, K. (2015). Porous electrospun nanocomposite mats based on chitosan-cellulose nanocrystals for wound dressing: effect of surface characteristics of nanocrystals. *Cellulose* 22, 521–534. doi:10.1007/s10570-014-0493-y

O'Dea, R. D., Byrne, H. M., and Waters, S. L. (2012). "Continuum modelling of in vitro tissue engineering: a review. Studies in mechanobiology, tissue engineering and biomaterials," in *Computational Modeling in Tissue Engineering*, Vol. 10, ed. Liesbet G. (Berlin; Heidelberg: Springer), 229–266.

O'Dea, R. D., Nelson, M. R., El Haj, A. J., Waters, S. L., and Byrne, M. H. (2014). A multiscale analysis of nutrient transport and biological tissue growth in vitro. *Math. Med. Biol.* 32, 345–366. doi:10.1093/imammb/dqu015

O'Dea, R. D., Osborne, J. M., Haj El, A. J., Byrne, H. M., and Waters, S. L. (2013). The interplay between tissue growth and scaffold degradation in engineered tissue constructs. *J. Math. Biol.* 67, 1199–1225. doi:10.1007/s00285-012-0587-9

Olivares, A. L., and Lacroix, D. (2013). "Computational methods in the modeling of scaffolds for tissue engineering," in *Computational Modeling in Tissue Engineering*, ed. Liesbet G. (Berlin; Heidelberg: Springer), 107–126.

Pan, J.-F., Liu, N.-H., Sun, H., and Xu, F. (2014). Preparation and characterization of electrospun PLCL/poloxamer nanofibers and dextran/gelatin hydrogels for skin tissue engineering. *PLoS ONE* 9:e112885. doi:10.1371/journal.pone.0112885

Ravari, H., Hamidi-Almadari, D., Salimifar, M., Bonakdaran, S., Parizadeh, M. R., and Koliakos, G. (2011). Treatment of non-healing wounds with autologous bone marrow cells, platelets, fibrin glue and collagen matrix. *Cytotherapy* 13, 705–711. doi:10.3109/14653249.2011.553594

Ravichandran, R., Venugopal, J. R., Sundarrajan, S., Mukherjee, S., Forsythe, J., and Ramakrishna, S. (2013). Click chemistry approach for fabricating PVA/gelatin nanofibers for the differentiation of ADSCs to keratinocytes. *J. Mater. Sci. Mater. Med.* 24, 2863–2871. doi:10.1007/s10856-013-5031-1

Richmond, P., Walker, D., Coakley, S., and Romano, D. (2010). High performance cellular level agent-based simulation with FLAME for the GPU. *Brief. Bioinform.* 11, 334–347. doi:10.1093/bib/bbp073

Rodrigues, C., de Assis, A., Moura, D., Halmenschlager, G., Saffi, J., Xavier, L. L., et al. (2014). New therapy of skin repair combining adipose-derived mesenchymal stem cells with sodium carboxymethylcellulose scaffold in a pre-clinical rat model. *PLoS ONE* 9:e96241. doi:10.1371/journal.pone.0096241

Schneider, R. K., Anraths, J., Kramann, R., Bornemann, J., Bovi, M., Knüchel, R., et al. (2010). The role of biomaterials in the direction of mesenchymal stem cell properties and extracellular matrix remodelling in dermal tissue engineering. *Biomaterials* 31, 7948–7959. doi:10.1016/j.biomaterials.2010.07.003

Sengers, B. G., Taylor, M., Please, C. P., and Oreffo, R. O. C. (2007). Computational modelling of cell spreading and tissue regeneration in porous scaffolds. *Biomaterials* 28, 1926–1940. doi:10.1016/j.biomaterials.2006.12.008

Shaw, T. J., and Martin, P. (2009). Wound repair at a glance. *J. Cell Sci.* 122, 3209–3213. doi:10.1242/jcs.031187

Shevchenko, R. V., James, S. L., and James, S. E. (2010). A review of tissue-engineered skin bioconstructs available for skin reconstruction. *J. R. Soc. Interface* 7, 229–258. doi:10.1098/rsif.2009.0403

Smallwood, R. (2011). "Cell-centred modeling of tissue behaviour," in *Understanding the Dynamics of Biological Systems*, eds W. Dubitzky, J. Southgate, and H. Fuß (London: Springer), 175–194.

Smallwood, R. H., Holcombe, W. M. L., and Walker, D. C. (2004). Development and validation of computational models of cellular interaction. *J. Mol. Histol.* 35, 659–665. doi:10.1007/s10735-004-2660-1

Sun, T., McMinn, P., Coakley, S., Holcombe, M., Smallwood, R., and MacNeil, S. (2007). An integrated systems biology approach to understanding the rules of keratinocyte colony formation. *J. R. Soc. Interface* 4, 1077–1092. doi:10.1098/rsif.2007.0227

Sun, T., McMinn, P., Holcombe, M., Smallwood, R., and MacNeil, S. (2008). Agent based modelling helps in understanding the rules by which fibroblasts support keratinocyte colony formation. *PLoS ONE* 3:e2129. doi:10.1371/journal.pone.0002129

van Leeuwen, I. M., Mirams, G. R., Walter, A., Fletcher, A., Murray, P., Osborne, J., et al. (2009). An integrative computational model for intestinal tissue renewal. *Cell Prolif.* 42, 617–636. doi:10.1111/j.1365-2184.2009.00627.x

Van Liedekerke, P., Palm, M. M., Jagiella, N., and Drasdo, D. (2015). Simulating tissue mechanics with agent-based models: concepts, perspectives and some novel results. *Comp. Part. Mech.* 2, 401–444. doi:10.1007/s40571-015-0082-3

Walker, D. C., Hill, G., and Wood, S. M. (2004). Agent-based computational modeling of wounded epithelial cell monolayers. *Nanobioscience* 3, 153–163. doi:10.1109/tnb.2004.833680

Wong, V. W., Levi, B., Rajadas, J., Longaker, M. T., and Gurtner, G. C. (2012). Stem cell niches for skin regeneration. *Int. J. Biomater.* 2012, 1–8. doi:10.1155/2012/926059

Wu, Y., Chen, L., Scott, P. G., and Tredget, E. E. (2007). Mesenchymal stem cells enhance wound healing through differentiation and angiogenesis. *Stem Cells* 25, 2648–2659. doi:10.1634/stemcells.2007-0226

Yildirimer, L., and Seifalian, A. M. (2014). Three-dimensional biomaterial degradation – material choice, design and extrinsic factor considerations. *Biotechnol. Adv.* 32, 984–999. doi:10.1016/j.biotechadv.2014.04.014

Yildirimer, L., Thanh, N. T. K., and Seifalian, A. M. (2012). Skin regeneration scaffolds: a multimodal bottom-up approach. *Trends Biotechnol.* 30, 638–648. doi:10.1016/j.tibtech.2012.08.004

Yoshikawa, T., Mitsuno, H., Nonaka, I., Sen, Y., Kawanishi, K., Inada, Y., et al. (2008). Wound therapy by marrow mesenchymal cell transplantation. *Plast. Reconstr. Surg.* 121, 860–877. doi:10.1097/01.prs.0000299922.96006.24

Youssef, B. B., Cheng, G., Zygourakis, K., and Markenscoff, P. (2007). Parallel implementation of a cellular automaton modeling the growth of three-dimensional tissues. *Int. J. High Perform. Comp. App.* 21, 196–209. doi:10.1177/1094342007074873

Zahorec, P., Koller, J., Danisovic, L., and Bohac, M. (2015). Mesenchymal stem cells for chronic wounds therapy. *Cell Tissue Bank.* 16, 19–26. doi:10.1007/s10561-014-9440-2

Zhang, H., Hou, W., Henrot, L., Schnebert, S., Dumas, M., Heusele, C., et al. (2014). Modelling epidermis homoeostasis and psoriasis pathogenesis. *J. R. Soc. Interface* 12, 20141071. doi:10.1098/rsif.2014.1071

Zonari, A., Martins, T. M., Paula, A. C., Boeloni, J. N., Novikoff, S., Marques, A. P., et al. (2015). Polyhydroxybutyrate-co-hydroxyvalerate structures loaded with adipose stem cells promote skin healing with reduced scarring. *Acta Biomater.* 17, 170–181. doi:10.1016/j.actbio.2015.01.043

Conflict of Interest Statement: The authors declare that the research was conducted in the absence of any commercial or financial relationships that could be construed as a potential conflict of interest.

16

Matrix-immobilized BMP-2 on microcontact printed fibronectin as an *in vitro* tool to study BMP-mediated signaling and cell migration

*Kristin Hauff [1,2], Chiara Zambarda [1,3], Miriam Dietrich [1], Maria Halbig [1,3], Anna Luise Grab [1], Rebecca Medda [1,3] and Elisabetta Ada Cavalcanti-Adam [1,3]**

[1] Department of Biophysical Chemistry, Institute of Physical Chemistry, University of Heidelberg, Heidelberg, Germany, [2] Applied Chemistry, University of Reutlingen, Reutlingen, Germany, [3] Department of New Materials and Biosystems, Max Planck Institute for Intelligent Systems, Stuttgart, Germany

Edited by:
Anna Lagunas,
Instituto de Salud Carlos III, Spain

Reviewed by:
Claudio G. Rolli,
Weizmann Institute of Science, Israel
Boaz Mizrahi,
Technion – Israel Institute of
Technology, Israel
Kevin Shakesheff,
University of Nottingham, UK

*Correspondence:
Elisabetta Ada Cavalcanti-Adam,
Institute of Physical Chemistry,
University of Heidelberg, Im
Neuenheimer Feld 253, Heidelberg
69120, Germany
ada.cavalcanti-adam@
urz.uni-heidelberg.de

During development, growth factors (GFs) such as bone morphogenetic proteins (BMPs) exert important functions in several tissues by regulating signaling for cell differentiation and migration. *In vivo*, the extracellular matrix (ECM) not only provides support for adherent cells, but also acts as reservoir of GFs. Several constituents of the ECM provide adhesive cues, which serve as binding sites for cell trans-membrane receptors, such as integrins. In conveying adhesion-mediated signaling to the intracellular compartment, integrins do not function alone but rather crosstalk and cooperate with other receptors, such as GF receptors. Here, we present a strategy for the immobilization of BMP-2 onto cellular fibronectin (cFN), a key protein of the ECM, to investigate GF-mediated signaling and migration. Following biotinylation, BMP-2 was linked to biotinylated cFN using NeutrAvidin as cross-linker. Characterization with quartz crystal microbalance with dissipation monitoring and enzyme-linked immunosorbent assay confirmed the efficient immobilization of BMP-2 on cFN over a period of 24 h. To validate the bioactivity of matrix-immobilized BMP-2 (iBMP-2), we investigated short- and long-term responses of C2C12 myoblasts, which are an established *in vitro* model for BMP-2 signaling, in comparison to soluble BMP-2 (sBMP-2) or in absence of GFs. Similarly to sBMP-2, iBMP-2 triggered Smad 1/5 phosphorylation and translocation of the complex to the nucleus, corresponding to the activation of BMP-mediated Smad-dependent pathway. Additionally, successful suppression of myotube formation was observed after 6 days in sBMP-2 and iBMP-2. We next implemented this approach in the fabrication of cFN micropatterned stripes by soft lithography. These stripes allowed cell-surface interaction only on the patterned cFN, since the surface in between was passivated, thus serving as platform for studies on directed cell migration. During a 10-h observation time, the migratory behavior, especially the cells' net displacement, was increased in presence of BMP-2. As such, this versatile tool retains the bioactivity of GFs and allows the presentation of ECM adhesive cues.

Keywords: BMP-2, fibronectin, microcontact printing, C2C12 myoblasts, BMP/Smad signaling

Introduction

The use of growth factors (GFs), such as bone/body morphogenetic proteins (BMPs), in biomedical applications is gaining importance over the last few years (Crouzier et al., 2011; Kang et al., 2011). The lack of control over the amount and release of GFs often leads to unwanted ectopic side effects (Cheung and Phillips, 2006; Carragee et al., 2011). Especially BMP-2 is already used for clinical applications, however, ectopic bone formation has been observed (Rosen, 2009; Luca et al., 2010). The immobilization of the GFs not only reduces ectopic side effects but also proves to be more cost-efficient, since lower amounts are required to obtain the desired local effect (Igwe et al., 2012), while allowing for sustained presentation. Current challenges in GF immobilization strategies are represented by (i) achieving control over the amount of the immobilized molecule and (ii) avoiding hindrance and interference with GF bioactivity (Almodóvar et al., 2014).

Bone morphogenetic proteins were originally investigated for their ability to regulate the formation of new bone. At the cellular level, BMPs direct and participate in different processes like cell growth, apoptosis, differentiation, and migration (Sotobori et al., 2006). BMPs bind the heteromeric receptor complexes composed of type I and type II trans-membrane serine/threonine kinase receptors (Miyazono et al., 2005; Sieber et al., 2009). The activation of BMP receptors follows two different routes: activation through preformed receptor complexes triggers a Smad-dependent pathway, while complexes formed upon BMP binding, the so-called BMP-induced signaling complexes, initiate the activation of Smad-independent, p38-dependent pathways (Nohe, 2001). The Smad-dependent signaling pathway is mediated by endocytosis through functional clathrin-coated pits, while Smad-independent pathways rely on the association of caveolae with the receptor complexes (Hartung et al., 2006). Nevertheless, recent studies on the covalent immobilization of BMP-2 on surfaces indicated that BMP-2 internalization is not necessary to trigger Smad 1/5 phosphorylation, suggesting that BMP-dependent pathways might be already activated by GF binding to the receptors (Pohl et al., 2012). Concerning the role of BMP in cell migration, Smad-independent pathways have been observed during BMP-2-mediated migratory effects. It has been reported that BMP-2 can activate Cdc42/PAK/LIMK and p38/MK2/Hsp25 pathways independently (Gamell et al., 2008).

The extracellular matrix (ECM) is a meshwork of glycoproteins and glycosaminoglycans, which provide structural and functional integrity to tissues and organs. Amongst them, proteins such as collagens and elastin, and glycoproteins such as fibronectin (FN) are secreted and arranged in a fibrillar network by various cell types, e.g., fibroblasts. FN is an abundant protein that exists in two isoforms derived by alternative splicing: the soluble plasma FN circulating in the blood and the insoluble cellular fibronectin (cFN), which is a component of the ECM. The interactions between cells and FN are mediated by the cell-binding motif RGD (arginine–glycine–aspartate) present in FN (Hynes, 2009).

The ECM not only offers a support for adherent cells and regulates cell migration and differentiation (Yamaguchi et al., 2005),

but also presents a reservoir of GFs, which influence cell behavior (Folkman et al., 1988; Taipale and Keski-Oja, 1997; Hynes, 2009). Proteoglycans, for example, bind fibroblast growth factors (FGFs) and vascular endothelial growth factors (VEGFs) through their heparin chains (Hynes, 2009). ECM proteins that do not contain such a pronounced sugar moiety are also able to interact with GFs. For instance, FN, vitronectin, and collagen type II have been shown to bind insulin-like GF-binding protein 5, hepatocyte GF, and transforming growth factor-β (TGF-β) through specific binding sites, respectively (Xu et al., 2004; Hynes, 2009). How GFs transduce information from the matrix to the cells has not yet been conclusively clarified. Different processes may occur for different GFs. One possibility is that GFs interact with their receptors while they are bound to the matrix and the ECM proteins act like cofactors. The release of GFs upon degradation of the ECM due to injury or proteolytic activity is also possible (Hynes, 2009). This results in the availability of GFs that can interact with their receptors at the cell membrane independent of matrix components. This presentation mode offers a spatially and temporarily defined stimulation with soluble GFs. Among them, it is known that the cells secrete TGF-β as latency-associated peptide and it interacts with fibrillins, incorporating into the ECM. Proteolytic degradation or mechanical stretching by trans-membrane integrins releases active TGF-β molecules that bind to their respective TGF-β receptors (Horiguchi et al., 2012).

Several approaches have been developed to immobilize GFs to ECM components. For the delivery of BMP-2, new ECM biomimetic systems have been reported, like inkjet printing of BMP-2 patterns on fibrin substrates (Phillippi et al., 2008), soft biopolymeric films presenting BMP-2 and hyaluronan hydrogels (Patterson et al., 2010; Crouzier et al., 2011).

Combining the presentation of GFs with adhesive matrix molecules offers the possibility to investigate the signaling and crosstalk of different pathways involved in cell adhesion and migration. An approach to better define, engineer, and analyze cell behavior is the fabrication of micropatterned adhesive substrates, which present spatially defined ECM proteins surrounded by non-adhesive molecules to backfill the area in between (Jackman et al., 1999; Folch and Toner, 2000; Whitesides et al., 2001; Zheng et al., 2012). Additionally, to assess and quantify complex cellular processes such as cell migration, micropatterned stripes serve as excellent substrates to determine migration speed and persistence (Petrie et al., 2009; Vedula et al., 2012; Kasten et al., 2014).

In this study, we use microcontact printing to manufacture FN-coated surfaces (Csucs et al., 2003), which are further functionalized with immobilized BMP-2 (iBMP-2) molecules. We report on the influence of matrix-iBMP-2 on cell behavior. We chose C2C12 myoblasts as in vitro system, since this cell line is an established model for BMP-2 signaling. These cells fuse and form contractile myotubes in the absence of BMP-2, but commit to the osteogenic lineage upon BMP-2 exposure (Katagiri et al., 1994). The phosphorylation and translocation of certain Smad proteins, namely Smad 1/5/8, can be used as short-time read-out signal to determine the bioactivity of BMP-2 (Sieber et al., 2009; Bragdon et al., 2011).

Materials and Methods

Preparation of Protein Solutions

Cellular fibronectin from human foreskin fibroblasts (Sigma-Aldrich, St. Louis, MO, USA) was dissolved in sterile water (1 mg/ml) and dialyzed against PBS overnight using Dispo Biodialyzer (MWCO 5 kDa, Sigma-Aldrich). Recombinant human BMP-2 (rhBMP-2) derived from *E. coli* or *CHO* cells (355-BEC/CF, 355-BM/CF, R&D Systems, Minneapolis, MN, USA) was reconstituted in 1 M NaCl (99.5% p.a. ACS ISO, Carl Roth, Karlsruhe) in PBS to a concentration of 0.1 mg/ml. NeutrAvidin (NA; A2666, Life Technologies, Eugene, OR, USA) was dissolved in PBS (5 mg/ml).

Biotinylation of cFN and BMP-2

For protein biotinylation at free amines on the lysine side chains, EZ-Link® NHS-PEG 12-biotin (Thermo Scientific, Rockford, IL, USA) was dissolved in dry dimethyl sulfoxide (DMSO, Merck, Darmstadt) to a concentration of 25 mM. For labeling cFN, a 100-fold molar excess of the linker was added to the protein. BMP-2 was labeled by adding a molar excess of 40, respectively. Afterwards, the solutions were incubated at room temperature (RT) for 1 h while shaking. Biotinylated cFN (cFN-biotin) or BMP-2 (BMP-2-biotin) was purified overnight by dialysis against PBS or 1 M NaCl in PBS, respectively.

Fluorescent Conjugation of cFN

To visualize the micro patterned structures, cFN was fluorescently labeled. Atto-647N-NHS dye (ATTO-TEC GmbH, Siegen, Germany) was dissolved in dry DMSO (10 mg/ml) and added to the cFN solution at a molar excess of 50. The solution was incubated for 1 h while shaking. To remove unconjugated fluorophores, the mixture was dialyzed overnight against PBS yielding fluorescently labeled cFN (cFN-647).

Photolithography and Microcontact Printing

Photolithography was used to produce the stamp master. Besides the silanization step, all production steps were performed in a clean room. A silicon wafer (Silicon Materials, Kaufering, Germany) with a diameter of 5 cm was spin coated using the negative photoresist SU-8 2002 (Microchem Corp., Newton, MA, USA) according to the manufacturer's instructions, yielding a thickness of 2.7 μm. Then, a soft bake at 65°C for 2 min and at 95°C for another 2 min was performed. Contact exposure through a chrome mask, aligned by a custom-made vacuum mask holder, was achieved with UV light (exposure time 1.9 s). Here, a mask with a line width of 20 μm and spacing of 50 μm was used. Following post-baking at 65°C for 3 min, the resist was developed in mr-DEV 600 developer (micro resist technology GmbH, Berlin) for 75 s. The stamp master was dried in a stream of nitrogen and silanized with 1H1H2H2H-perfluorooctyltrichlorosilane (ABCR GmbH & Co. KG, Karlsruhe, Germany) in a desiccator for 6 h.

Polydimethylsiloxane (PDMS) (Sylgard 184 Silicon Elastomer Kit, Dow Corning, Seneffe, Belgium) was prepared according to the manufacturer's instructions and degassed under vacuum. One milliliter of PDMS was poured into a Petri dish containing the stamp master, degassed in vacuum, and subsequently cured at

65°C overnight. Afterwards, the PDMS was detached from the stamp master, cut into 1 cm² stamps, incubated in *n*-hexane for 30 min, and sonicated in *n*-hexane for 5 min to remove unreacted monomers or crosslinkers.

For microcontact printing, the stamp surface was coated with a mixture of 5 μl of cFN solution and 45 μl of PBS to obtain a final concentration of 0.1 mg/ml. As an alternative to the striped structure, a homogeneous PDMS stamp was applied to produce surfaces homogeneously covered with cFN. The solution was incubated for 40 min, after which the excess cFN was removed. To minimize the amount of labeled cFN, a mixture consisting of a ratio of 9:1 was incubated on the homogenous stamps with an area of 1cm². Glass coverslips (Carl Roth, Karlsruhe, Germany) were cleaned with ethanol in an ultrasonic bath for 15 min. Before use, the glass slides were dried under a stream of nitrogen and treated with oxygen plasma [GigaEtch, PVA TePla, Kirchheim (München), Germany] at 0.4 mbar and 150 W for 10 min. The stamps were washed twice with 100 μl PBS, dried, and immediately placed onto the glass for 30 s. The stamps were carefully removed from the coverslip and rinsed with PBS several times. To prevent unspecific cell adhesion between the stripes, the cFN-patterned surfaces were incubated with 100 μl of 0.1 mg/ml poly-L-lysine-g-poly (ethylene glycol) [PLL (20 kDa)-g(3.5)–PEG (2 kDa), PLL–PEG, Surface Solutions, Switzerland] in HEPES buffer for 30 min (see **Figure 1**). To minimize the amount of PLL–PEG per substrate, a piece of parafilm was used to ensure an even coverage. Samples were then washed with PBS.

For soluble BMP-2 (sBMP-2), cFN and cFN-647 were added in equal amount, while for the iBMP-2, the biotinylated cFN (cFN-biotin) was used. For the immobilization of BMP-2, the cFN-biotin micropatterned surfaces were incubated with NA at a concentration of 0.01 mg/ml in PBS for 30 min followed by washing with PBS. Afterwards, 50 μl of BMP-2-biotin in PBS with a final concentration of 0.01 μg/μl was added for 1 h. Since the stamped surfaces have an area of approximately 1 cm², the maximal possible surface concentration was 0.5 μg/cm². The biotin linker consists of a 56 Å PEG spacer that mediates the immobilization of BMP-2 to NA and at the same time allows for a certain degree of mobility due to its length.

Quartz Crystal Microbalance with Dissipation Monitoring

The interaction between cFN-biotin, NA, and BMP-2-biotin from *E. coli* cells was investigated using a quartz crystal microbalance with dissipation monitoring (QCM-D). All QCM-D experiments were performed in an E4 QCM-D from Q-Sense (Vaestra Froelunda, Sweden) using open modules. The sensing elements were silica-coated QCM-D crystals (QSX 303, Vaestra Froelunda, Sweden) with a fundamental frequency of 4.95 MHz. FN was microcontact printed on the activated sensor using a flat stamp as described in Section "Photolithography and Microcontact Printing." The passivation step was not necessary as only sensors with a homogeneous layer of FN were prepared and the surfaces were not used for cell experiments. Unspecific protein adsorption was determined by direct comparison of adsorption processes on sensors with and without NA-binding sides, e.g., for each measurement, two sensors were functionalized with cFN and two

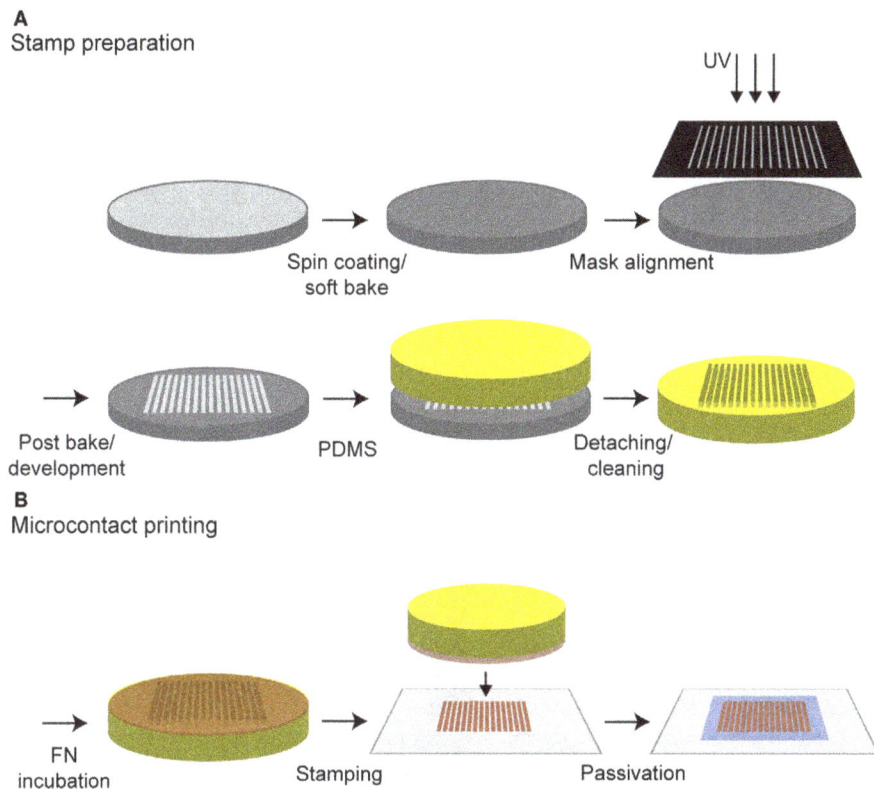

A
Stamp preparation

UV

Spin coating/
soft bake

Mask alignment

Post bake/
development

PDMS

Detaching/
cleaning

B
Microcontact printing

FN
incubation

Stamping

Passivation

FIGURE 1 | Procedure for microcontact printing. (A) A silicon wafer was spin coated with a negative photoresist and treated according the manufacturer's instructions. Contact exposure through a chrome mask with UV light and further processing resulted in the stamp master. PDMS was poured on it, cured in an oven and was ready to use after a cleaning step in *n*-hexane. **(B)** The stamp was incubated with a cFN solution and the protein was adsorbed on the stamp surface. After a washing step, the stamp was dried, inverted, and gently pressed on an oxygen plasma-treated glass substrate whereby the protein structure was transferred to the glass. A final incubation with PLL–PEG passivated the surface in between the protein structure to prevent unspecific cell adhesion.

sensors were coated with cFN-biotin. All samples were measured in real-time under the same conditions. They were incubated simultaneously and under the same conditions in NA and washed before mounting the crystals in the QCM-D machine. The temperature was adjusted to laboratory conditions and the stable oscillation of the sensor was validated. Two-hundred microliters of PBS were added in each chamber. The baseline was detected for a few minutes. Next, the buffer was exchanged by 200 µl of BMP-2-biotin (5 µg/cm^2) for 1 h and afterwards the sensors were washed with PBS until a final plateau was reached.

Enzyme-Linked Immunosorbent Assay

An enzyme-linked immunosorbent assay (ELISA) kit (DuoSet ELISA, R&D Systems) was used to detect the BMP-2-biotin release. Homogeneously stamped cFN-biotin surfaces were prepared as described in Section "Photolithography and Microcontact Printing," in the presence of cFN-biotin or cFN without biotinylation as negative control. The passivation step was omitted, as in the QCM-D characterization. After incubation with BMP-2-biotin *CHO*, the solutions containing the unbound proteins were collected as well as the two washing solutions and the overnight washing solutions at 4°C. The samples were treated according to the manufacturer's instructions. In brief, the 96-well

microplate was coated with capture antibody (part#840968 of DuoSet ELISA, R&D Systems) and the samples were incubated after a blocking step in reagent diluent (1% BSA in PBS, pH 7.2–7.4, 0.2 µm filtered). The detection antibody system [consisting of biotinylated anti-BMP-2 mouse IgG and streptavidin horseradish peroxidase (HRP)] was replaced with BMP-2 antibody directly coupled to HRP (part#892142 of Quantikine, BMP-2 Immunoassay, R&D Systems) as it would interfere with the detection of BMP-2-biotin. The absorbance was measured at 450 nm with a reference point at 570 using a plate reader (Infinite M200, Tecan, Männedorf, Switzerland). All values were corrected by the zero standard. Plotting the common logarithm of the absorbance of averaged standard samples against the common logarithm of the concentration generates a linear standard curve, which was used for quantification of BMP-2 concentrations in solution.

Cell Culture

Mouse C2C12 myoblasts (ATCC CRL-1772) were cultured as sub-confluent monolayers in Dulbecco's modified Eagle's medium containing 4.5 mg/ml glucose, 4 mM L-glutamine, and 1 mM sodium pyruvate (DMEM, 41966-029, Gibco Life Technologies, Carlsbad, CA, USA) supplemented with 10% (v/v) fetal bovine serum (FBS, S0115m, Biochrom AG, Berlin, Germany) and 1% (v/v) penicillin/streptomycin (15140, Gibco) at 37°C and 5% CO_2.

Indirect Immunofluorescent Staining and Microscopy

The translocation of the Smad complex into the nucleus was analyzed to investigate the short-term effect of BMP-2 *E. coli* on myoblasts. Following serum starvation overnight, C2C12 cells were seeded on homogeneously stamped cFN surfaces at a density of 10,000 cells were seeded on a 20 mm × 20 mm glass coverslip and incubated for 30 min to allow adhesion on the substrates. Thereafter, 0.5 μg of BMP-2 was added to the medium (sBMP-2), which was considered time point 0. All samples were fixed after different time points (t_0, 10, 30, 45, 60, 90 min) with 4% (w/v) paraformaldehyde (PFA) in PBS for 30 min, rinsed with PBS, and permeabilized with 0.1% (v/v) Triton-X-100 in PBS (Sigma-Aldrich) for 5 min. After blocking of unspecific binding sites with 1% (w/v) BSA in PBS (1% BSA) for 30 min, the surfaces were incubated with the primary antibody anti-p-Smad 1/5 rabbit IgG (S463/465, clone 41D10, 9516S, Cell Signaling, Danvers, MA, USA) at a dilution of 1:50 (according to the manufacturer's recommendation) in 1% BSA at RT for 1 h. After washing twice with 1% BSA for 10 min, the samples were incubated with the respective secondary antibody Alexa Fluor 488® goat anti-rabbit IgG (Life technologies, A11034) at a final concentration of 5 μg/ml in 1% BSA as well as with Phalloidin-TRITC (0.2 μg/ml) at RT for 1 h and washed again twice with 1% BSA for 10 min. Finally, the samples were embedded in Mowiol (Sigma-Aldrich) containing 0.1% (v/v) DAPI for an additional staining of the nucleus. Stained samples were imaged with an upright wide field microscope (Leica DM6000B, Leica Microsystems GmbH, Wetzlar, Germany) using a 40× (HCX PL APO 40×/0.85 CORR) objective lens. Image processing was done using ImageJ software (version 1.48c, Rasband, W.S., ImageJ, U.S. National Institutes of Health, Bethesda, MD, USA)[1]. For analysis, a binary image of the nucleus and the cytosol was produced. The obtained masks were used to quantify the pSmad signal in these areas. To calculate the integrated densities, the area was multiplied by the mean gray value. In addition, the integrated density of the cytosol was divided by the integrated density of the nucleus.

Since the presence of BMP-2 suppresses the differentiation of C2C12 cells into myotubes and promotes osteogenic differentiation, the myogenic phenotype was assessed by staining for myosin heavy chain (MHC) in confluent cell monolayers. C2C12 cells were serum-starved overnight and cultured at a density of 5,000 cells/cm² on homogeneous stamped cFN-biotin surfaces under high serum conditions for 6 days at 37°C and 5% CO_2. Afterwards, cells were fixed and stained with anti-MHC mouse IgG (MF20, DSHB, Iowa City, IA, USA) at a concentration of 2.3 μg/ml followed by Alexa Fluor® 488 goat anti-mouse IgG (Life Technologies, A11001) and DAPI.

Western Blot

Short-term response was evaluated by western blot detection of phosphorylated Smad 1/5. C2C12 cells were serum-starved overnight and 10,000 cells for each sample were seeded for 30 min at 37°C and 5% CO_2 at a 1 cm² homogeneously stamped cFN surface with or without BMP-2 *E. coli*, as described in Section "Enzyme-Linked Immunosorbent Assay." After different time points (0, 30, 45, 60 min), cells were lysed in 2× Laemmli Buffer (4% SDS, 20% Glycerol, 120 mM Tris–HCl, pH 6.8, 200 mM DTT, 0.02% Bromphenolblue) at −80°C overnight and boiled at 95°C for 5 min. The total proteins homogenates were loaded onto SDS-PAGE NuPAGE 4–12% Bis–Tris Gel, NuPAGE MES Running Buffer (Novex, Life Technologies, Carlsbad, CA, USA) and blotted into nitrocellulose membrane (GE Healthcare, Little Chalfont, UK) in NuPAGE Transfer Buffer (Novex, Life Technologies, Carlsbad, CA, USA). The blots were blocked with 3% milk (Carl Roth, Karlsruhe, Germany) in Tris-buffered saline with 0.1% Tween-20 (TBST, 50 nM Tris, pH 8.0, 150 mM NaCl, 0.1% Tween-20) at RT for 1 h and incubated at RT overnight in TBST 1% milk 1/1000 rabbit anti pSmad 1/5 (#9516, Cell Signaling, Danvers, MA, USA) or 1 h in TBST 1% milk 1/2000 mouse anti β-actin (A1978, Sigma-Aldrich, St. Louis, MO, USA). Blots were then washed in TBST and incubated for 1 h in TBST 1% milk at RT with HRP-conjugated secondary antibodies 1:5000 goat anti-rabbit or goat anti-mouse (Santa Cruz Biotechnology, Heidelberg, Germany). After washing, the membranes were incubated in ECL prime western blotting detection reagent (GE Healthcare, Little Chalfont, UK) and chemiluminescence detected using a LAS 3000 (Fujifilm, Tokyo, Japan).

Time-Lapse Video Microscopy and Analysis of Cell Migration

Due to the dimension of the stripes, the cells were restricted to only migrate in a linear manner. For migration experiments, C2C12 cells were serum-starved overnight. Ten thousand cells were seeded in 2 ml medium at 37°C and 5% CO_2 on 20 mm × 20 mm glass surfaces with microcontact printed stripes. Using an Olympus IX inverted microscope (Olympus, Hamburg, Germany) with a Delta Vision RT system (Applied Precision Inc., Issaquah, WA, USA), 25 fields of view (603.03 μm × 603.06 μm) were recorded every 10 min for at least 10 h using a 10× air objective lens (EC-PlanNeoFluor 10×/0.3 Ph1, Zeiss, Oberkochen, Germany) and detected with a cooled CCD camera (Photometrics, Kew, Australia). Image acquisition was performed with Resolve 3D (AppliedPrecision Inc.). Cell nuclei were tracked by the ImageJ plugin manual tracking. Thus, the velocity of the cells was analyzed and the net distances per hour were calculated and also summed up to determine the total path lengths of the cells.

Statistic Analysis

All experiments were performed in at least two technical repeats. Plots and histograms were generated with Microsoft Office Excel 2007, while box-plots were created with Prism 6 [version 6.04 (Trial), GraphPad][2]. Values of the standard error of the mean (SEM) were calculated from the raw data and were used for error bars on graphs. Comparison between two sets of measures was performed using Mann–Whitney test (two-tailed, 95% confidence level: ***$P < 0.001$, **$P < 0.01$, *$P < 0.1$).

---

[1]http://imagej.nih.gov/ij/

[2]http://www.graphpad.com/demos/

Results

BMP-2 is Successfully Immobilized on Homogenous cFN-Coated Surfaces and is Not Released After Immobilization

Prior to cell experiments, we characterized the surfaces by two different methods, namely QCM-D and ELISA. To directly monitor the binding of BMP-2 to cFN, we used QCM-D, which detects the subsequent adsorption of mass to a quartz crystal, resulting in a shift in the crystal's resonance frequency. As already described above "BMP-2 is Successfully Immobilized on Homogenous cFN-Coated Surfaces and is Not Released After Immobilization," cFN/cFN-biotin was stamped on the QCM-D crystal. After a washing step with PBS, NA was incubated on the crystal followed by another washing step. Finally, BMP-2-biotin was added to the system. Note the difference in adsorption of BMP-2 in absence and presence of biotinylated cFN (**Figure 2A**). This difference was especially visible during the washing step following the initial adsorption of the protein. Due to its unspecific interactions with materials, BMP-2 easily adsorbs to both surfaces but it is released after washing with PBS if NA is not bound to the biotinylated cFN. However, not all BMP-2 was removed by the washing step, suggesting a persisting interaction of BMP-2 with cFN at $-2\,Hz$. In the presence of biotinylated cFN, a plateau was reached at $-11\,Hz$ after washing for several minutes, indicating the presence of a fraction of BMP-2 stably bound to the surface.

With ELISA, we assessed the amount of iBMP-2 by measuring the amount of the protein released in solution after 60 min of incubation and for each of the three washing steps (**Figure 2B**). Here, cFN/cFN-biotin was homogenously stamped on glass substrates and then incubated with NA and BMP-2-biotin. We derived the amount of surface iBMP-2 by subtracting the amount of protein detected in incubation and washing solutions from the initial

amount of BMP-2 in solution. **Figure 2B** depicts the three conditions, namely cFN-biotin without NA and BMP-2, cFN-biotin with BMP-2 but without NA, and cFN-biotin with BMP-2 and NA. This corresponds to a surface concentration of iBMP-2, which was approximately $520\,ng/cm^2$.

Matrix-Immobilized BMP-2 Induces Smad 1/5 Phosphorylation and Prevents Myotube Formation in C2C12

To investigate the bioactivity of iBMP-2, Smad 1/5 activation was evaluated by western blotting and indirect immunofluorescent staining. Cells were left to adhere on the surfaces for 30 min (indicated as time point 0) and then Smad 1/5 (pSmad 1/5) phosphorylation and nuclear translocation were monitored over time. The initial 30-min incubation time is necessary since addition of sBMP-2 is not sufficient to activate the Smad pathway in spreading cells, because of rapid depletion of the GF from the medium (data not shown). For the assessment of Smad phosphorylation, C2C12 myoblasts were seeded on surfaces coated with cFN in absence of BMP-2 (negative control), whereas cells incubated in presence of sBMP-2 in the media served as positive control. Cells were lysed after 0, 30, 45, and 60 min and the phosphorylation levels and kinetics of Smad 1/5 were determined by western blotting. Smad phosphorylation is detected only in cells exposed to sBMP-2 and iBMP-2 after 30 min, whereas only a faint band is present in the samples without BMP-2 (**Figure 3**). iBMP-2 is able to trigger Smad-dependent signaling and the levels of Smad phosphorylation are comparable to those observed when BMP-2 is added to the media (sBMP-2).

Next, we monitored the shuttling of pSmad 1/5 from the cytoplasm to the nucleus. Upon phosphorylation, Smad 1/5/8 forms the Smad complex, which acts as transcription factor in the nucleus. C2C12 cells were first allowed to adhere to the surface for 30 min and then fixed after additional 10, 30, 45, and 60 min

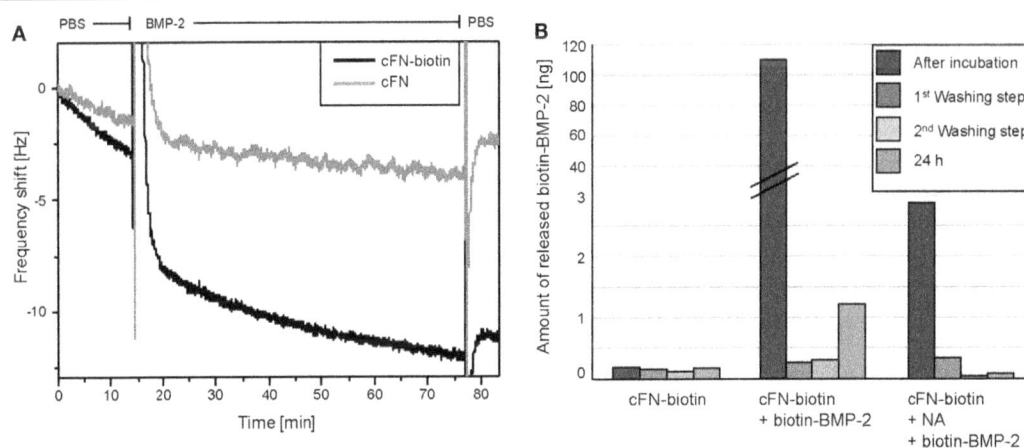

FIGURE 2 | (A) Frequency shifts of F7 measured by QCM-D. Measurements of the adsorption of BMP-2 on QCM-D sensors coated with cFN-biotin (black) and cFN without biotinylation (gray) followed by the binding of NA and BMP-2-biotin. Here, the detail of the exchange from buffer to BMP-2-biotin and the following washing step with PBS is shown in the graph. Note the peaks represent the addition of the appropriate agent and the difference in frequency shift corresponding to a higher mass adsorption on the sensor with biotinylated cFN (black). **(B)** ELISA quantification of the release of BMP-2 from the incubated surfaces. cFN-biotin surfaces in absence of BMP-2 served as negative control. For the other two conditions, surfaces exposed to BMP-2-biotin with and without NA as cross-linker were used. The release was determined in the removed incubation solution as well as in the three washing solutions [first washing step, second washing step, third washing step (24 h)].

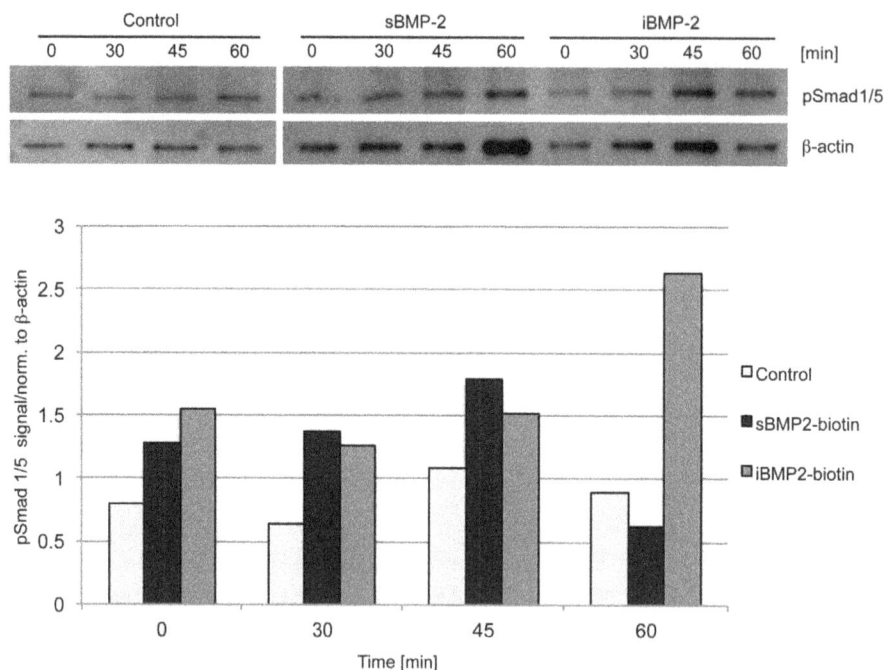

FIGURE 3 | Western blot of Smad 1/5 phosphorylation in C1C12 cells.
Serum-starved cells were seeded on the surfaces for 30 min (indicated as time point 0) and lysed after 30, 45, and 60 min. cFN surfaces serve as control, sBMP-2 indicates cFN surfaces where BMP-2 has been added to the media at the indicated durations. iBMP-2 indicates cFN surfaces with crosslinked biotinylated-BMP-2. Non-stimulated cells adhering to the control surfaces show basal Smad 1/5 phosphorylation signals, which are time-independent, whereas cells stimulated with sBMP-2 and iBMP-2 present pronounced Smad phosphorylation. β-actin served as loading control.

time (**Figure 4**). The quantification of the shuttling of the active Smad complex from the cytoplasm to the nucleus shows a peak at 30 min in cells exposed to sBMP-2 that drops hereafter to control levels (**Figure 5**). The nuclear translocation of pSmad 1/5 in cells on iBMP-2 instead presents a different pattern, with an initial increase above the levels observed for the sBMP-2 at 10 min, followed by a drop at 30 min. It should be noted that cells seeded on iBMP-2 surfaces were exposed to BMP-2 upon surface contact. After 45 min, iBMP-2 leads again to an increased and sustained accumulation of nuclear pSmad in comparison to the control and the sBMP-2 groups. This increase could be explained by the progression of cell-surface interactions, i.e., cells are exposed to additional matrix-bound GFs.

C2C12 cells spontaneously fuse and form contractile multi-inucleated myotubes after few days in culture. In presence of osteoinductive GFs, such as BMP-2, this process is suppressed. Here, we investigated the influence of iBMP-2 on myotube formation in C2C12 cell cultured for 6 days on control surfaces (cFN only, without BMP-2), in presence of BMP-2 added to the culture media (sBMP-2) and on iBMP-2. MHC was stained by indirect immunofluorescence as myotube-specific marker. **Figure 6** clearly depicts myotube formation in cells not exposed to BMP-2 as indicated by the green staining. Both sBMP-2 and iBMP-2 successfully suppress myotube formation, as can be seen in the reduced staining of MHC. Upon conjugation with biotin, we observed a slight decrease in the bioactivity of BMP-2 due to the biotinylation (see Figure S2 in Supplementary Material).

Matrix-Immobilized BMP-2 Affects Cell Migration on Microcontact Printed Structures

For the investigation of cell migration in presence of iBMP-2, cFN was micropatterned in stripes, which served as adhesive and directional guidance. The dimensions of the stripes were chosen in accordance to the cell size and morphology; thus to ensure that only single cells would migrate in a directed fashion and would not bridge over several stripes, the stripes had a width of 20 μm and spacing between the stripes 50 μm. The surface between the cFN stripes was passivated with PLL–PEG to prevent unspecific cell adhesion to the glass. **Figure 7A** shows an example of a micropatterned glass surface. Fluorescently labeled cFN mixed with unconjugated cFN at a ratio of 1:1 is microcontact printed to visualize the integrity of the patterned stripes. The stripes were inspected after each preparation step and remained intact throughout the entire process (Figure S1 in Supplementary Material). C2C12 myoblasts are able to adhere to the cFN pattern and restricted to migrate on the stripes only, as can be seen in **Figure 7B**.

As described in previous sections for the homogenously stamped surfaces, BMP-2-biotin was immobilized on cFN/cFN-biotin micropatterned stripes using NA as cross-linker. The surface in between the cFN stripes was passivated to prevent adhesion. As positive control, sBMP-2 was added to the cell media while as negative control only cFN stripes without addition sBMP-2 were used. **Figure 8A** shows a time course of cell migration along micropatterned stripes in the three different conditions, namely control, sBMP-2, and iBMP-2 (see also Video S1–S3 in

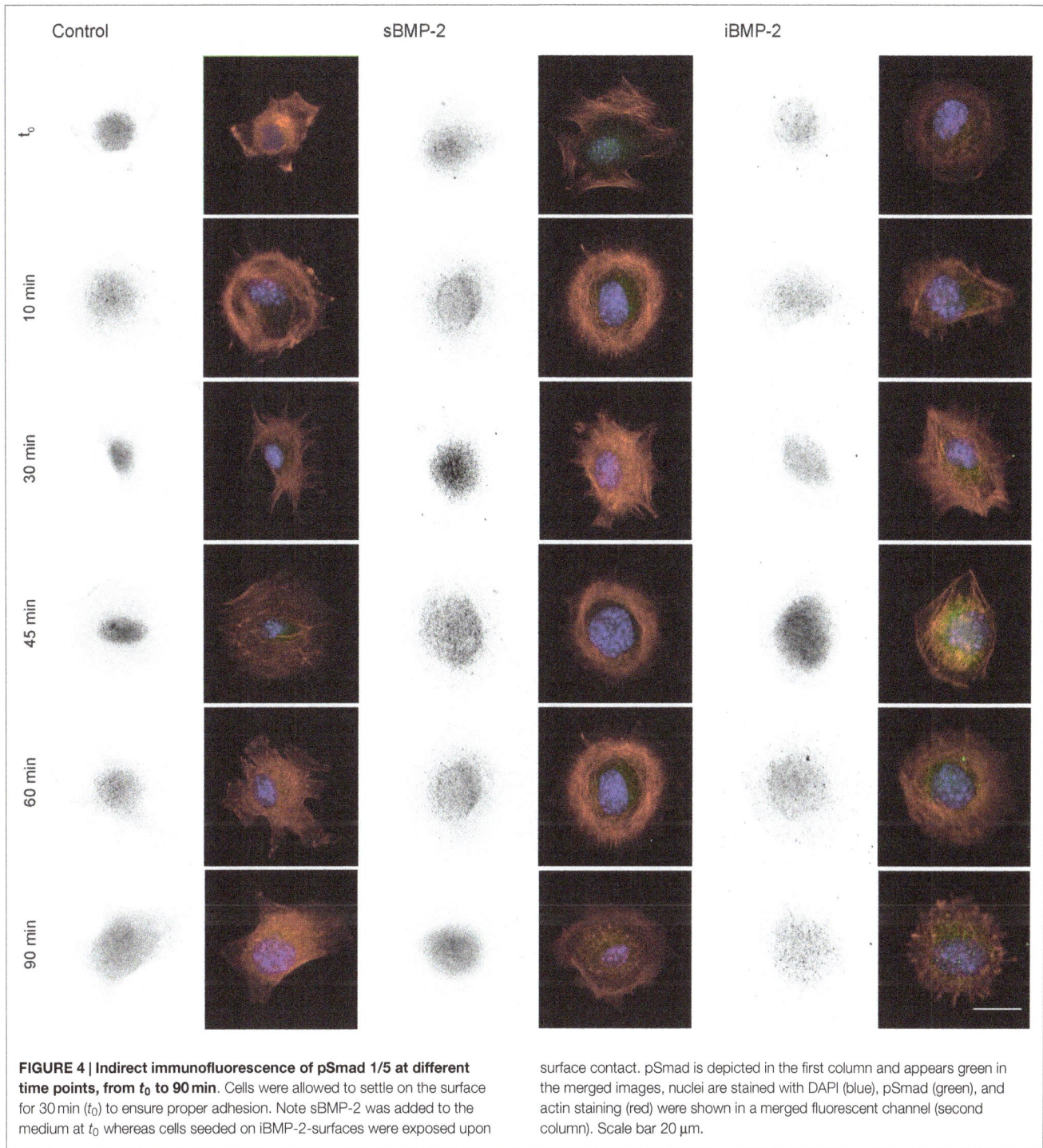

FIGURE 4 | Indirect immunofluorescence of pSmad 1/5 at different time points, from t_0 to 90 min. Cells were allowed to settle on the surface for 30 min (t_0) to ensure proper adhesion. Note sBMP-2 was added to the medium at t_0 whereas cells seeded on iBMP-2-surfaces were exposed upon surface contact. pSmad is depicted in the first column and appears green in the merged images, nuclei are stained with DAPI (blue), pSmad (green), and actin staining (red) were shown in a merged fluorescent channel (second column). Scale bar 20 µm.

Supplementary Material). The arrows indicate the starting point of one cell per condition over time. The velocities of the three conditions are depicted in **Figure 8B** as box-plots, where the median is displayed. Cells on all three conditions feature a similar velocity pattern with only slightly differing median values (control: 0.196 µm/min; sBMP-2: 0.265 µm/min; iBMP-2: 0.227 µm/min). When analyzing the steadiness of cell migration by calculating the net distances per hour, we found differences in the distance pattern covered by the cells on the three conditions. **Figure 8D** shows the migration profile divided into 1 h intervals. Cells on sBMP-2 and iBMP-2 display a similar preference to higher distances, especially at later time points. In contrast, in absence of BMP-2, cells show a rather constant behavior. **Figure 8C** summarizes the total path length of the cells as box-plot taking all net distances into account. Accordingly, cells upon BMP-2 exposure tend to cover larger distances, as can be seen at the varying median values (control: 137 µm; sBMP-2: 245 µm; iBMP-2: 202 µm).

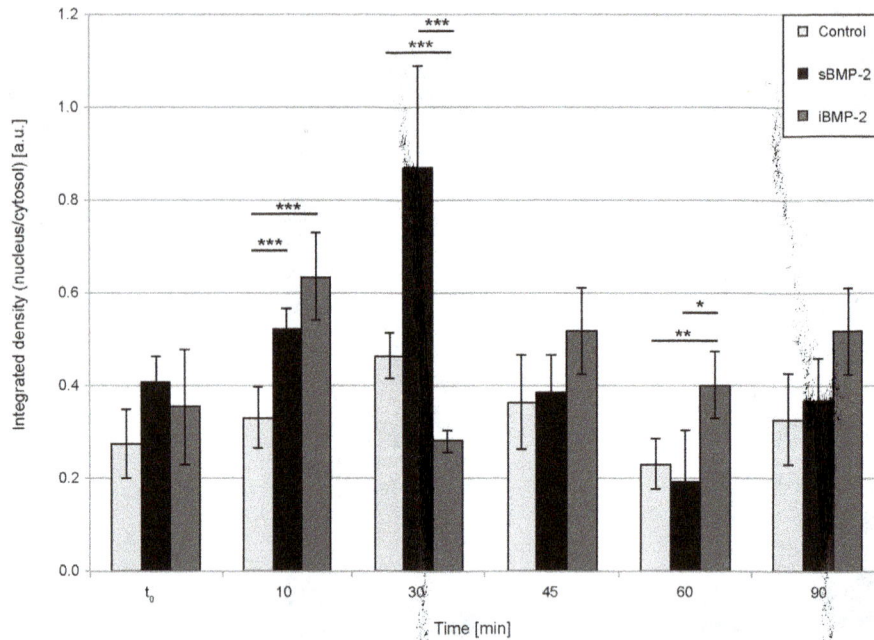

FIGURE 5 | Quantification of pSmad translocation. Ratio of integrated densities for the pSmad signal in the cytosol and nucleus at the indicated time points. ***$P < 0.001$, **$P < 0.01$, *$P < 0.1$.

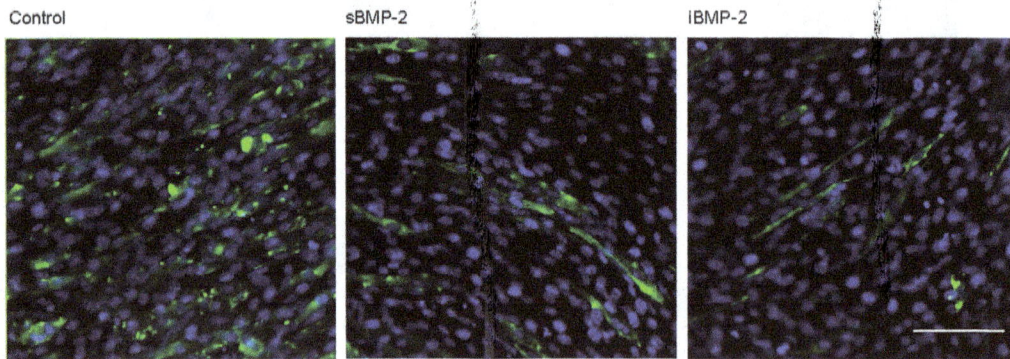

FIGURE 6 | Long-term response of C2C12 cells after 6 days in the presence of BMP-2. Indirect immunofluorescence was employed to stain the myosin heavy subunit expressed in myotubes (green). The cell nuclei were stained with DAPI (blue). Myotube formation was suppressed by sBMP-2 and iBMP-2 but not for cultures of cells adhering to the control samples. Scale bar 100 μm.

Discussion

The study presented here illustrates the immobilization of BMP-2, on cFN by employing the specific interaction between two biotinylated proteins and NA as cross-linker. The immobilized molecule retains its bioactivity since it activates short-term signaling pathways, such as the Smad-dependent pathway as well as long-term signaling pathways, such as suppression of myotube formation. The amount of conjugated linkers per BMP-2 molecule was assumed using structural information of BMP-2 by considering only accessible lysine residues (11 and 15), which do not interfere with receptor binding (Pohl et al., 2012). The less accessible and less favorable lysine residues (73, 76, 97, and 101) might be as well targeted during conjugation, although the orientation

of BMP-2 onto cFN might be not essential for maintaining its activity.

After immobilization of the biotinylated BMP-2 and removal of protein excess, the release from the surface was determined by ELISA during two successive washing steps and after 24 h. The amount of BMP-2 released during the washing steps were below the detection limit. The methods currently used for quantification of GFs in solution allow detection as low as 0.25 ng. Thus, it cannot be excluded that small amounts of BMP-2 might be released but these are below the detection limit of the here employed ELISA.

Surface immobilization of BMP-2 via chemical linkers offers the advantage of having a sustained presentation while reducing the amount of the GF needed to trigger cell responses. Lagunas et al. introduced a system to generate BMP-2 gradients, with

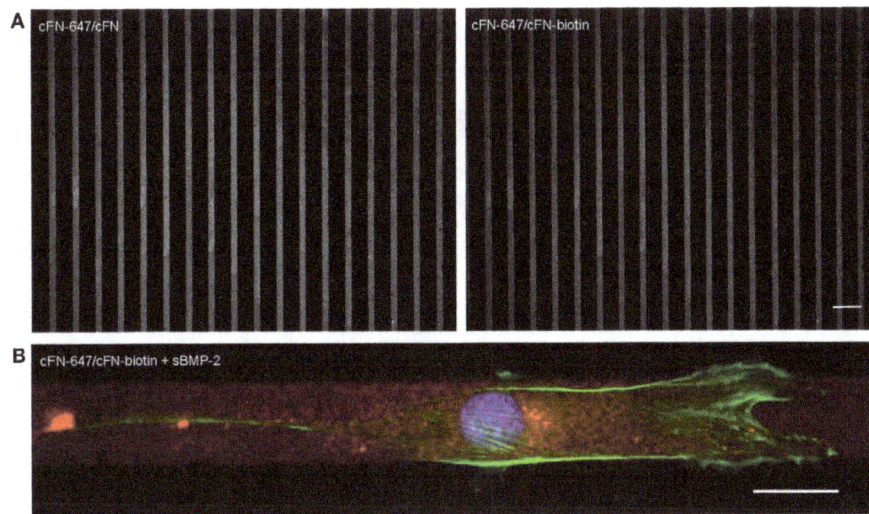

FIGURE 7 | (A) Cell adhesion on microcontact printed stripes of 20 μm width. A mixture of fluorescently labeled cFN-647 and cFN (left), and cFN-647/cFN-biotin (right) was transferred to a glass slide previously activated by oxygen plasma treatment. The spacing between the stripes is 50 μm. Scale bar 100 μm. **(B) Single C2C12 cell migrating on 20 μm cFN-biotin stripes in the presence of sBMP-2**. The actin cytoskeleton was stained with phalloidin-TRITC (green) and the nucleus with DAPI (blue), whereas the cFN-647 stripe is labeled in red. Scale bar 20 μm.

a ligand density ranging from 1.4 to 2.3 pmol/cm^2 (Lagunas et al., 2010, 2013). Chemical surface gradients were established by hydrolysis of PMMA. Due to the strong electrostatic interactions of the BMP-2 molecule with biocompatible materials, other approaches rely on mere physisorption or embedding in films or gels such as PLL–HA as was shown by Crouzier et al. (2011) and Almodóvar et al. (2014). They attached polyelectrolyte multilayer films to substrates by alternating the deposition of PLL and hyaluronan. BMP-2 was loaded and entrapped within these films. The concentration of the entrapped BMP-2 was approximately 700 ng/cm^2, while only superficial molecules of the multilayer are accessible for the cells.

Triggering Smad and non-Smad signaling pathways by iBMP-2 pinpoint that ligand–receptor interaction rather than cellular uptake of the GF is of particular importance. In fact, it has been shown that the initial interactions at the plasma membrane are sufficient for triggering Smad-dependent signaling (Bonor et al., 2012) and that ligand internalization is not necessary for such responses (Pohl et al., 2012). Smad signaling might occur independently of endocytosis involving clathrin-coated pit but rather require caveolin-mediated receptor internalization (Bonor et al., 2012). In the current study, we cannot exclude that the GF alone or the complex of GF–FN molecules are internalized over time. At the same time, it could be possible that activated receptors might traffic upon ligand recognition and binding, even without internalization of the ligand. However, the mode of presentation and delivery in vivo is still a matter of debate. Recently, binding sites for GFs belonging to the TGF-β superfamily were verified in several ECM glycoproteins. Also, other GF binding sites have been found in ECM proteins, such as collagen and FN (Wijelath et al., 2006; Hynes, 2009; Martino and Hubbell, 2010). In vivo, the ECM increases the GFs' bioavailability by serving as a reservoir. GFs can be constitutively available or presented upon exogenous or cellular action. Cryptic binding sites are exposed upon injury

or proteolytic processing leading to a rapid localized availability of GFs. Also, tension forces (Zhu and Clark, 2014) affect GF presentation. The juxtaposition with RGD-motives in the ECM facilitates integrin-mediated cell adhesion and directly links GF signaling to integrin signaling (Lin et al., 2011; Motegi et al., 2011; Fujita et al., 2012).

The mode of GF presentation is essential for medical applications. Amongst other issues, the amount of bioactive factors is a critical subject, since too high dosages bear the risks of side effects and are cost ineffective. To evaluate the minimal amount of BMP-2 necessary to trigger the desired cellular responses, BMP-2 has been immobilized on hexagonally ordered gold nanoparticle arrays with varying interparticle distances (Schwab et al., 2015). In this study, cells were exposed to the GF by sandwiching the BMP-2 bearing surfaces head first on the adherent cells. The cell interacts with the GF at their apical side. In contrast to this approach, we present simultaneously BMP-2 and FN, being both cues at the basal side of the cell. Such mode of presentation effectively triggered the Smad-dependent signaling as shown by Smad phosphorylation and nuclear shuttling of the Smad signaling complex as well as by suppression of myotube formation. The activation of the Smad-dependent signaling pathway as assessed here by Smad translocation into the nucleus depicted a strong peak for sBMP-2 at around 30 min followed by a decrease to control levels. iBMP-2 on the other hand exhibited overall lower values but sustained a higher activity level during the time of observation. This behavior might be explained by considering that sBMP-2 is only available for a short period of time whereas in the case of iBMP-2, the cells are constantly exposed to the GF while interacting with the surface.

Here, we also investigated the non-transcriptional effect of BMP-2 by assessing the influence of matrix-iBMP-2 on cell migration mediated by cytoskeletal rearrangements. We chose micropatterned stripes to restrict cell migration to only two

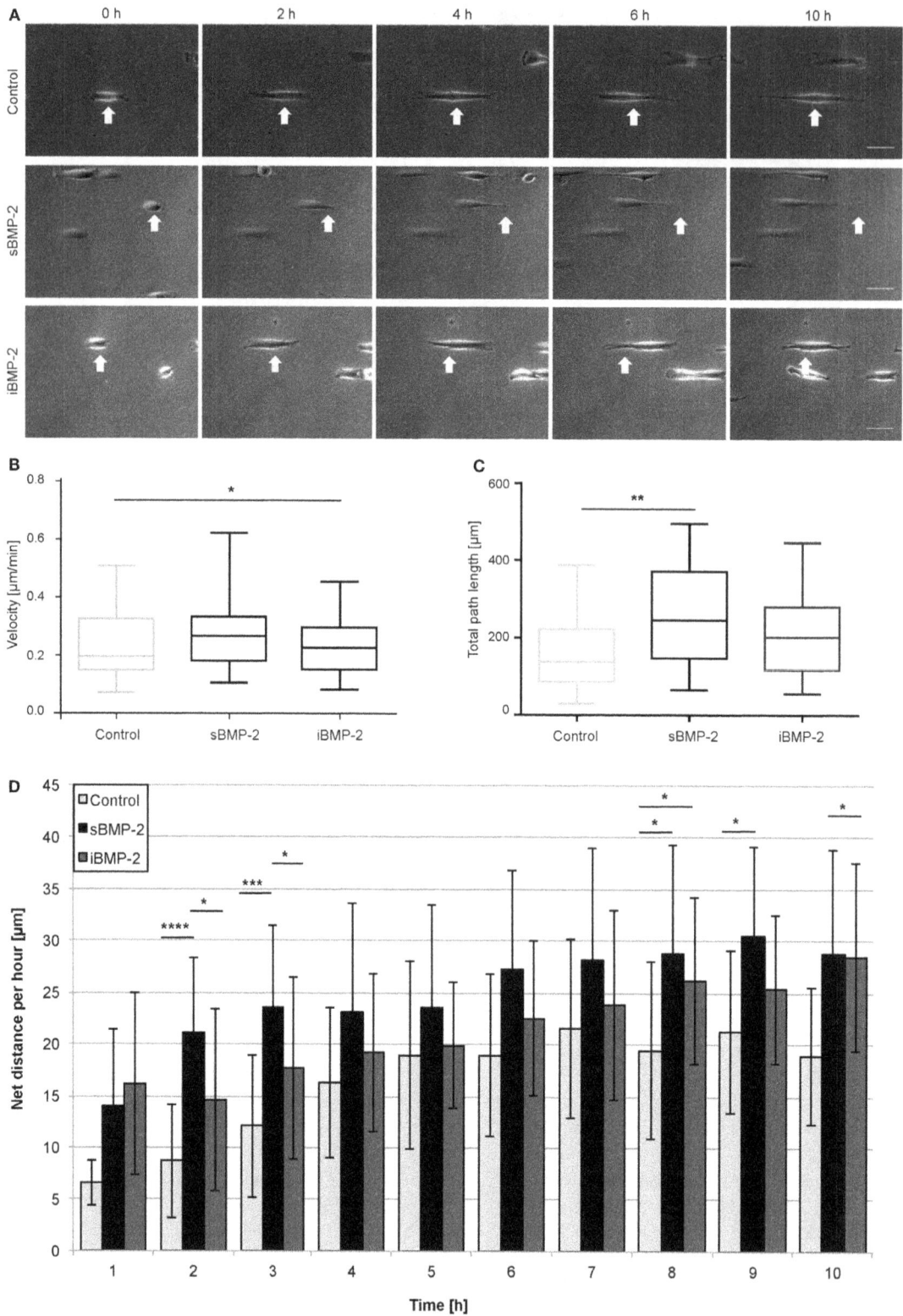

FIGURE 8 | C2C12 migration on microcontact printed stripes. (A) Cells were cultured in serum conditions on 20 μm cFN-biotin stripes. Within the first 10 h, the migration behavior upon sBMP-2, iBMP-2, and no BMP-2 exposure is shown. All experiments were carried out in two technical repeats, with at least 25 cells per condition. Scale bar 50 μm. (B) Cell velocities upon different BMP-2 exposures on cFN-biotin stripes over a period of 10 h. *$P < 0.1$. Horizontal bars represent the median. (C) Averaged total path lengths of cells upon different BMP-2 exposures. **$P < 0.01$. Horizontal bars represent the median. (D) Averaged net distances of cells in 1 h intervals. ****$P < 0.0001$, ***$P < 0.001$, *$P < 0.1$.

directions. Previous studies have indicated that 1D topography can mimic many aspects of fibrillar-oriented 3D cell-derived ECMs. In both 1D and 3D, cell migration is a rapid and uniaxial process, whereby external physical stimuli in the form of linear topographical cues can regulate cell behavior (Doyle et al., 2009). On single 1D micropatterned lines, myoblasts can align, polarize, and migrate directionally (Ghibaudo et al., 2009). Thus, these type of patterned structures provide at the same time a simpler and more representative system than 2D systems for understanding 3D fibrillar matrix regulation of the dynamics of cell adhesion and signaling during cell migration (Cukierman et al., 2002). However, in the system we presented here, the line width of 20 μm is too large to observe quasi-3D migration patterns.

We show that during the first 4 h of observation, BMP-2 affects cell migration regardless of the mode of BMP-2 presentation. In fact, C2C12 cells tend to enhance their migratory behavior as compared to the control. This observation is in agreement with Hiepen et al. (2014), although we did not apply chemotactic gradients.

While guidance cues provided by physical and structural properties of the ECM have emerged as key parameters for directing cell migration, additional signals provided by gradients of soluble chemoattractants are still considered as leading factors for orchestrating cell movements (Tzvetkova-Chevolleau et al., 2008).

Hiepen et al. (2014) demonstrated the importance of BMP-2-induced PI3K signaling for chemotaxis. Thus, the application of a linear BMP-2 gradient resulted in an overall gain in directionality of cell migration toward the source of BMP-2 as well as in an increase of the covered distance. However, the nature of receptor interaction and the mechanism determining polarity at the plasma membrane level still needs to be elucidated. To this end, our approach presented here on the immobilization of GFs to ECM components can be further developed by establishing GF gradients by microfluidics (Almodóvar et al., 2014).

Acknowledgments

We acknowledge the Max Planck Society and the Deutsche Forschungsgemeinschaft (DFG SFB TRR79 project M9) for funding. The authors would like to thank Prof. Dr. J. P. Spatz and Prof. Dr. Ralf Kemkemer for their support. We furthermore thank Jan-Willi Janiesch and Marian Weiss for fruitful discussions on migration analysis and for carefully reading the manuscript.

References

Almodóvar, J., Guillot, R., Monge, C., Vollaire, J., Selimović, S., Coll, J. L., et al. (2014). Spatial patterning of BMP-2 and BMP-7 on biopolymeric films and the guidance of muscle cell fate. *Biomaterials* 35, 3975–3985. doi:10.1016/j.biomaterials.2014.01.012

Bonor, J., Adams, E. L., Bragdon, B., Moseychuk, O., Czymmek, K. J., and Nohe, A. (2012). Initiation of BMP2 signaling in domains on the plasma membrane. *J. Cell Physiol.* 227, 2880–2888. doi:10.1002/jcp.23032

Bragdon, B., Moseychuk, O., Saldanha, S., King, D., Julian, J., and Nohe, A. (2011). Bone morphogenetic proteins: a critical review. *Cell. Signal.* 23, 609–620. doi:10.1016/j.cellsig.2010.10.003

Carragee, E. J., Hurwitz, E. L., and Weiner, B. K. (2011). A critical review of recombinant human bone morphogenetic protein-2 trials in spinal surgery: emerging safety concerns and lessons learned. *Spine J.* 11, 471–491. doi:10.1016/j.spinee.2011.04.023

Cheung, A., and Phillips, A. M. (2006). Bone morphogenetic proteins in orthopaedic surgery. *Curr. Orthop.* 20, 424–429. doi:10.1016/j.cuor.2006.09.003

Crouzier, T., Fourel, L., Boudou, T., Albigès-Rizo, C., and Picart, C. (2011). Presentation of BMP-2 from a soft biopolymeric film unveils its activity on cell adhesion and migration. *Adv. Mater.* 23, H111–H118. doi:10.1002/adma.201004637

Csucs, G., Michel, R., Lussi, J. W., Textor, M., and Danuser, G. (2003). Microcontact printing of novel co-polymers in combination with proteins for cell-biological applications. *Biomaterials* 24, 1713–1720. doi:10.1016/S0142-9612(02)00568-9

Cukierman, E., Pankov, R., and Yamada, K. M. (2002). Cell interactions with three-dimensional matrices. *Curr. Opin. Cell Biol.* 14, 633–639. doi:10.1016/S0955-0674(02)00364-2

Doyle, A. D., Wang, F. W., Matsumoto, K., and Yamada, K. M. (2009). One-dimensional topography underlies three-dimensional fibrillar cell migration. *J. Cell Biol.* 184, 481–490. doi:10.1083/jcb.200810041

Folch, A., and Toner, M. (2000). Microengineering of cellular interactions. *Annu. Rev. Biomed. Eng.* 2, 227–256. doi:10.1146/annurev.bioeng.2.1.227

Folkman, J., Klagsbrun, M., Sasse, J., Wadzinski, M., Ingber, D., and Vlodavsky, I. (1988). A heparin-binding angiogenic protein – basic fibroblast growth-factor – is stored within basement-membrane. *Am. J. Pathol.* 130, 393–400.

Fujita, M., Ieguchi, K., Davari, P., Yamaji, S., Taniguchi, Y., Sekiguchi, K., et al. (2012). Cross-talk between integrin alpha 6 beta 4 and insulin-like growth factor-1 receptor (IGF1R) through direct alpha 6 beta 4 binding to IGF1 and subsequent alpha 6 beta 4-IGF1-IGF1R ternary complex formation in anchorage-independent conditions. *J. Biol. Chem.* 287, 12491–12500. doi:10.1074/jbc.M111.304170

Gamell, C., Osses, N., Bartrons, R., Ruckle, T., Camps, M., Rosa, J. L., et al. (2008). BMP2 induction of actin cytoskeleton reorganization and cell migration requires PI3-kinase and Cdc42 activity. *J. Cell. Sci.* 121, 3960–3970. doi:10.1242/jcs.031286

Ghibaudo, M., Trichet, L., Le Digabel, J., Richert, A., Hersen, P., and Ladoux, B. (2009). Substrate topography induces a crossover from 2d to 3d behavior in fibroblast migration. *Biophys. J.* 97, 357–368. doi:10.1016/j.bpj.2009.04.024

Hartung, A., Bitton-Worms, K., Rechtman, M. M., Wenzel, V., Boergermann, J. H., Hassel, S., et al. (2006). Different routes of bone morphogenic protein (BMP) receptor endocytosis influence bmp signaling. *Mol. Cell. Biol.* 26, 7791–7805. doi:10.1128/MCB.00022-06

Hiepen, C., Benn, A., Denkis, A., Lukonin, I., Weise, C., Boergermann, J. H., et al. (2014). BMP2-induced chemotaxis requires PI3K P55 /P110α-dependent phosphatidylinositol (3,4,5)-triphosphate production and LL5β recruitment at the cytocortex. *BMC Biol.* 12:43. doi:10.1186/1741-7007-12-43

Horiguchi, M., Ota, M., and Rifkin, D. B. (2012). Matrix control of transforming growth factor – function. *J. Biochem.* 152, 321–329. doi:10.1093/jb/mvs089

Hynes, R. O. (2009). The extracellular matrix: not just pretty fibrils. *Science* 326, 1216–1219. doi:10.1126/science.1176009

Igwe, J. C., Mikael, P. E., and Nukavarapu, S. P. (2012). Design, fabrication and in vitro evaluation of a novel polymer-hydrogel hybrid scaffold for bone tissue engineering. *J. Tissue Eng. Regen. Med.* 8, 131–142. doi:10.1002/term.1506

Jackman, R. J., David, C. D., Oksana, C., and George, M. W. (1999). Using elastomeric membranes as dry resists and for dry lift-off. *Langmuir* 15, 2973–2984. doi:10.1021/la981591y

Kang, M. H., Oh, S. C., Lee, H. J., Kang, H. N., Kim, J. L., Kim, J. S., et al. (2011). Metastatic function of BMP-2 in gastric cancer cells: the role of PI3K/AKT, MAPK, the NF- B pathway, and MMP-9 expression. *Exp. Cell Res.* 317, 1746–1762. doi:10.1016/j.yexcr.2011.04.006

Kasten, A., Naser, T., Brüllhoff, K., Fiedler, J., Müller, P., Möller, M., et al. (2014). Guidance of mesenchymal stem cells on fibronectin structured hydrogel films. *PLoS ONE* 9:e109411. doi:10.1371/journal.pone.0109411

Katagiri, T., Yamaguchi, A., Komaki, M., Abe, E., Takahashi, N., Ikeda, T., et al. (1994). Bone morphogenetic protein-2 converts the differentiation pathway of C2C12 myoblasts into the osteoblast lineage. *J. Cell Biol.* 127, 1755–1766. doi:10.1083/jcb.127.6.1755

Lagunas, A., Comelles, J., Martínez, E., and Samitier, J. (2010). Universal chemical gradient platforms using poly(methyl methacrylate) based on the biotin-streptavidin interaction for biological applications. *Langmuir* 26, 14154–14161. doi:10.1021/la102640w

Lagunas, A., Comelles, J., Oberhansl, S., Hortigüela, V., Martínez, E., and Samitier, J. (2013). Continuous bone morphogenetic protein-2 gradients for concentration effect studies on C2C12 osteogenic fate. *Nanomedicine* 9, 694–701. doi:10.1016/j.nano.2012.12.002

Lin, F., Ren, X. D., Pan, Z., Macri, L., Zong, W. X., Tonnesen, M. G., et al. (2011). Fibronectin growth factor-binding domains are required for fibroblast survival. *J. Invest. Dermatol.* 131, 84–98. doi:10.1038/jid.2010.253

Luca, L., Rougemont, A. L., Walpoth, B. H., Gurny, R., and Jordan, O. (2010). The effects of carrier nature and ph on rhbmp-2-induced ectopic bone formation. *J. Control. Release* 147, 38–44. doi:10.1016/j.jconrel.2010.06.011

Martino, M. M., and Hubbell, J. A. (2010). The 12th-14th type III repeats of fibronectin function as a highly promiscuous growth factor-binding domain. *FASEB J.* 24, 4711–4721. doi:10.1096/fj.09-151282

Miyazono, K., Maeda, S., and Imamura, T. (2005). BMP receptor signaling: transcriptional targets, regulation of signals, and signaling cross-talk. *Cytokine Growth Factor Rev.* 16, 251–263. doi:10.1016/j.cytogfr.2005.01.009

Motegi, S., Garfield, S., Feng, X., Sárdy, M., and Udey, M. C. (2011). Potentiation of platelet-derived growth factor receptor-beta signaling mediated by integrin-associated MFG-E8. *Arterioscler. Thromb. Vasc. Biol.* 31, 2653–U2747. doi:10.1161/ATVBAHA.111.233619

Nohe, A. (2001). The mode of bone morphogenetic protein (BMP) receptor oligomerization determines different BMP-2 signaling pathways. *J. Biol. Chem.* 277, 5330–5338. doi:10.1074/jbc.M102750200

Patterson, J., Siew, R., Herring, S. W., Lin, A. S., Guldberg, R., and Stayton, P. S. (2010). Hyaluronic acid hydrogels with controlled degradation properties for oriented bone regeneration. *Biomaterials* 31, 6772–6781. doi:10.1016/j.biomaterials.2010.05.047

Petrie, R. J., Doyle, A. D., and Yamada, K. M. (2009). Random versus directionally persistent cell migration. *Nat. Rev. Mol. Cell Biol.* 10, 538–549. doi:10.1038/nrm2729

Phillippi, J. A., Miller, E., Weiss, L., Huard, J., Waggoner, A., and Campbell, P. (2008). Microenvironments engineered by inkjet bioprinting spatially direct adult stem cells toward muscle- and bone-like subpopulations. *Stem Cells* 26, 127–134. doi:10.1634/stemcells.2007-0520

Pohl, T. L., Boergermann, J. H., Schwaerzer, G. K., Knaus, P., and Cavalcanti-Adam, E. A. (2012). Surface immobilization of bone morphogenetic protein 2 via a self-assembled monolayer formation induces cell differentiation. *Acta Biomater.* 8, 772–780. doi:10.1016/j.actbio.2011.10.019

Rosen, V. (2009). BMP2 signaling in bone development and repair. *Cytokine Growth Factor Rev.* 20, 475–480. doi:10.1016/j.cytogfr.2009.10.018

Schwab, E. H., Pohl, T. L., Haraszti, T., Schwaerzer, G. K., Hiepen, C., Spatz, J. P., et al. (2015). Nanoscale control of surface immobilized BMP-2: toward a quantitative assessment of BMP-mediated signaling events. *Nano Lett.* 15, 1526–1534. doi:10.1021/acs.nanolett.5b00315

Sieber, C., Kopf, J., Hiepen, C., and Knaus, P. (2009). Recent advances in BMP receptor signaling. *Cytokine Growth Factor Rev.* 20, 343–355. doi:10.1016/j.cytogfr.2009.10.007

Sotobori, T., Ueda, T., Myoui, A., Yoshioka, K., Nakasaki, M., Yoshikawa, H., et al. (2006). Bone morphogenetic protein-2 promotes the haptotactic migration of murine osteoblastic and osteosarcoma cells by enhancing incorporation of integrin beta1 into lipid rafts. *Exp. Cell Res.* 312, 3927–3938. doi:10.1016/j.yexcr.2006.08.024

Taipale, J., and Keski-Oja, J. (1997). Growth factors in the extracellular matrix. *FASEB J.* 11, 51–59.

Tzvetkova-Chevolleau, T., Stéphanou, A., Fuard, D., Ohayon, J., Schiavone, P., and Tracqui, P. (2008). The motility of normal and cancer cells in response to the combined influence of the substrate rigidity and anisotropic microstructure. *Biomaterials* 29, 1541–1551. doi:10.1016/j.biomaterials.2007.12.016

Vedula, S. R., Leong, M. C., Lai, T. L., Hersen, P., Kabla, A. J., Lim, C. T., et al. (2012). Emerging modes of collective cell migration induced by geometrical constraints. *Proc. Natl. Acad. Sci. U.S.A* 109, 12974–12979. doi:10.1073/pnas.1119313109

Whitesides, G. M., Ostuni, E., Takayama, S., Jiang, X. Y., and Ingber, D. E. (2001). Soft lithography in biology and biochemistry. *Annu. Rev. Biomed. Eng.* 3, 335–373. doi:10.1146/annurev.bioeng.3.1.335

Wijelath, E. S., Rahman, S., Namekata, M., Murray, J., Nishimura, T., Mostafavi-Pour, Z., et al. (2006). Heparin-II domain of fibronectin is a vascular endothelial growth factor-binding domain – enhancement of VEGF biological activity by a singular growth factor/matrix protein synergism. *Circ. Res.* 99, 853–860. doi:10.1161/01.RES.0000246849.17887.66

Xu, Q. J., Yan, B., Li, S. H., and Duan, C. M. (2004). Fibronectin binds insulin-like growth factor-binding protein 5 and abolishes its ligand-dependent action on cell migration. *J. Biol. Chem.* 279, 4269–4277. doi:10.1074/jbc.M311586200

Yamaguchi, H., Wyckoff, J., and Condeelis, J. (2005). Cell migration in tumors. *Curr. Opin. Cell Biol.* 17, 559–564. doi:10.1016/j.ceb.2005.08.002

Zheng, W., Zhang, W., and Jiang, X. (2012). Precise control of cell adhesion by combination of surface chemistry and soft lithography. *Adv. Healthc. Mater.* 2, 95–108. doi:10.1002/adhm.201200104

Zhu, J., and Clark, R. A. (2014). Fibronectin at select sites binds multiple growth factors and enhances their activity: expansion of the collaborative ECM-GF paradigm. *J. Invest. Dermatol.* 134, 895–901. doi:10.1038/jid.2013.484

Conflict of Interest Statement: The authors declare that the research was conducted in the absence of any commercial or financial relationships that could be construed as a potential conflict of interest.

17

3D printing of octacalcium phosphate bone substitutes

Vladimir S. Komlev[1]*, Vladimir K. Popov[2], Anton V. Mironov[2], Alexander Yu. Fedotov[1], Anastasia Yu. Teterina[1], Igor V. Smirnov[1], Ilya Y. Bozo[3,4,5], Vera A. Rybko[6] and Roman V. Deev[3,7]

[1] A.A. Baikov Institute of Metallurgy and Materials Science, Russian Academy of Sciences, Moscow, Russia, [2] Institute of Laser and Information Technologies, Russian Academy of Sciences, Moscow, Russia, [3] Human Stem Cells Institute, Moscow, Russia, [4] A.I. Evdokimov Moscow State University of Medicine and Dentistry, Moscow, Russia, [5] A.I. Burnazyan Federal Medical Biophysical Center of FMBA of Russia, Moscow, Russia, [6] Institute of Carcinogenesis, N.N. Blokhin Russian Cancer Research Center, Moscow, Russia, [7] Kazan Federal University, Kazan, Russia

Edited by:
Janina Burk,
University of Leipzig, Germany

Reviewed by:
Simona Casarosa,
University of Trento, Italy
Sourabh Ghosh,
Indian Institute of Technology Delhi,
India

*Correspondence:
Vladimir S. Komlev,
A.A. Baikov Institute of Metallurgy and
Materials Science, Russian Academy
of Sciences, Leninsky Prospect 49,
Moscow 119991, Russia
komlev@mail.ru

Biocompatible calcium phosphate ceramic grafts are able of supporting new bone formation in appropriate environment. The major limitation of these materials usage for medical implants is the absence of accessible methods for their patient-specific fabrication. 3D printing methodology is an excellent approach to overcome the limitation supporting effective and fast fabrication of individual complex bone substitutes. Here, we proposed a relatively simple route for 3D printing of octacalcium phosphates (OCP) in complexly shaped structures by the combination of inkjet printing with post-treatment methodology. The printed OCP blocks were further implanted in the developed cranial bone defect followed by histological evaluation. The obtained result confirmed the potential of the developed OCP bone substitutes, which allowed 2.5-time reducing of defect's diameter at 6.5 months in a region where native bone repair is extremely inefficient.

Keywords: 3D printing, tricalcium phosphate, octacalcium phosphate, ceramics, bone graft, *in vivo* test, osteoconductivity

Introduction

Biocompatible synthetic grafts and/or tissue engineering constructions prevail over conventional approaches based on autologous, allogenous, or xenogenous bone tissue. However, complex structure and properties of natural bone limit the spectrum of synthetic materials and fabrication techniques that could be used as custom-designed implants or scaffolds for bone defects replacement or guided bone regeneration. Currently, this problem might be solved via a 3D printing technique (Bergmann et al., 2010; Bose et al., 2013; Popov et al., 2014).

Synthetic calcium phosphates' (CP) chemical similarity to the natural bone mineral content allows to apply it successfully as bone substitutes among a variety of other materials (ceramics, bioglasses, polymers, and their combinations). A number of CP biomaterials with different phase compositions [hydroxyapatite (HA), tricalcium phosphate (TCP), ion-substituted CP, etc.] and several formulations have been developed over the last few decades (Bohner, 2010; Dorozhkin, 2011). Most of these biomaterials are used in clinical practice as granules, cements, or porous blocks (Bohner, 2010). TCP ceramics are a reliable, osteoconductive, and biodegradable material, and it is already commercially available (Suba et al., 2006; Horowitz et al., 2009; Stavropoulos et al., 2010). However, it has recently been demonstrated that octacalcium phosphate (OCP) spherical microporous ceramic granules are three times more effective than TCP for bone marrow mesenchymal stromal cells differentiation *in vivo* (Zorin et al., 2014). Additionally, OCP ceramics possess osteogenic features of interest, e.g., stimulate lamellar bone formation for 2 months after *in vivo* implantation. About 4–5 months after OCP ceramics implantation in clinical trials computer tomography (CT) and histological examinations of patient' biopsies of the bone defect revealed new bone formation (Komlev et al., 2014). Thus, OCP-based implants are the most promising for 3D printing.

There are two major techniques currently available for ceramics 3D printing. The first one is mixing of CP powders or agglomerates with polymers, e.g., collagen, followed by their chemical solidification, and finally high-temperature processing (Detsch et al., 2011; Rath et al., 2012). Another technique comprises sacrificial inverse matrix printing, its infiltration with ceramic slurry, and burning out the negative (Guo et al., 2009; Schumacher et al., 2010).

The main concept of our work is based on an approach, which involved chemical interaction between initial CP powder, such as TCP, and binder liquid ("ink"), such as diluted phosphoric acid, followed by chemical treatment of the printed dicalcium phosphate dihydrate (DCPD) structures in solutions. Therefore, a support material burning out was not necessary that prevented undesirable contamination and risk of OCP decomposition.

Materials and Methods

Chemicals and Reagents

All reagents were purchased from Sigma-Aldrich: high-purity-grade calcium nitrate (Cat. No: 13477-34-4), ammonium carbonates (Cat. No: 506-87-6), ammonium phosphate monobasic (Cat. No: 7722-76-1), potassium carbonate-sodium carbonate mixture (Cat. No: 10424-09-6), and sodium acetate (Cat. No: 127-09-3).

Tricalcium phosphate powder was synthesized in an aqueous medium by slow addition of diammonium phosphate $[(NH_4)_2HPO_4]$ solution into calcium nitrate $[Ca(NO_3)_2 4H_2O]$ solution, containing NH_4OH, under constant stirring. The pH of the mixture was about 7 with Ca/P molar ration of 1.5/1. After total addition of the reactants, the suspension was filtered, dried at 80°C and sintered at 700°C for 2 h. TCP agglomerates with mean size 40–80 μm were used for printing. TCP crystal aggregates were prepared by light grinding using a pestle and then passing through a standard testing sieve.

1.0% aqueous solution of salts of phosphoric acid (pH 4.75) was used as "ink" for the 3D printer. The buffer solution was prepared by dissolving in water of 1.5 ± 0.1M sodium acetate, 1.0 ± 0.1M phosphoric acid, and 0.15 ± 0.01M glutamic acid.

Printing Process

To develop the process of layer-by-layer 3D printing of OCP bone substitutes, we used our custom-designed 3D printer (shown in **Figure 1**). Briefly, it consists of a ceramic powder stuffer with a spreader (3) and Z-piston (4) inside a building box (5), providing TCP powder layer up and down movement according to computer-controlled algorithm. Bidirectional (X–Y) positioning system with a printing head (2) made from modified cartridges for standard inkjet printer (HP C6602A, Hewlett-Packard, USA). Both Z-piston and X–Y movement of printing head ("ink" container with nozzles producing droplet size ca. 40 pL) are driven with stepper motors (6) with X–Y–Z accuracy of ca. 40 μm.

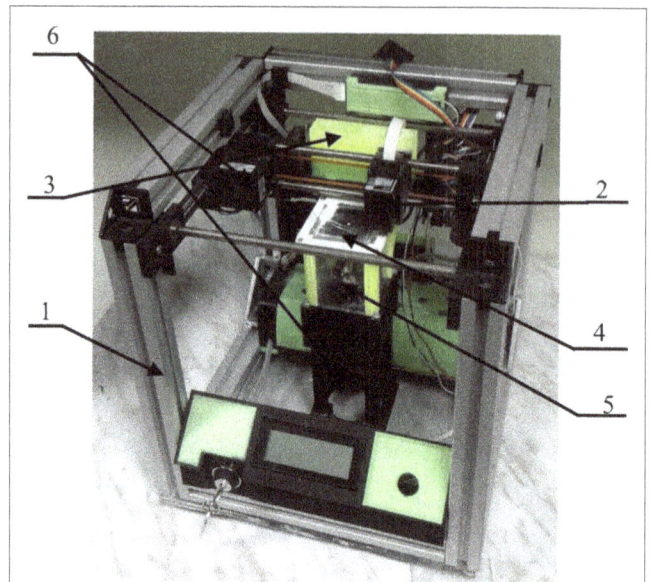

FIGURE 1 | Custom-designed 3D printer. 1, 3D printer frame; 2, printing head; 3, stuffer with spreader; 4, Z-piston; 5, building box; 6, stepper motors.

Flexibility of our 3D printer design comprising relatively small building envelope (60 mm × 60 mm × 60 mm) permits testing of small amounts of powder materials. It makes possible fast and inexpensive study of both new process techniques and new material combinations.

Initially, a 3D dataset of desired ceramic model (a bulging disk with a diameter 20 mm and 16 perforations of 1 mm in diameter) in the STL format is uploaded to the system. The recoating mechanism (3) carries an amount of fine (40–80 μm) TCP powder to the building box, creating a thin (ca./200 μm) layer of powder on the top of the Z-piston plane (4) inside the building box (5) at room temperature. The liquid binder (200 pL/point) is ejected from the printing head onto the powder layer with linear speed up to 10 mm/s, wetting individual cross-section. When the layer is completed, Z-piston moves down by the thickness of a layer (ca./200 μm) and a new layer of powder is deposited on the printed one. These process steps are repeated until the whole sample is formed within the powder bed. The surrounding powder material supports the ceramic model during the printing process. Thus, there is no necessity for further maintenance structures for such features as overhangs and undercuts. Upon completion, the sample is removed from the building box, cleaned using an air blower, and air dried at room temperature for further chemical treatment.

Post-Treatment of Printed Structures

After printing, the samples were placed in aqueous solution, which was prepared by dissolving of 115 g of $NH_4H_2PO_4$ in 500 mL of distilled water at room temperature. The pH of the solution was 4.1 ± 0.1. The samples were kept for 168 h at 40°C. After incubation, the samples were thoroughly washed in distilled water at least 10 times, dried at 37°C and placed in a second solution, which was prepared by dissolving 95.2 g of CH_3COONa in 700 mL of distilled water at 40°C and pH 8.2 ± 0.2. The samples were again kept for 168 h at 40°C, thoroughly washed in distilled water at least five times and dried overnight at 37°C (Komlev et al., 2014).

Material Characterization

Phase composition was analyzed by conventional X-ray diffraction (XRD) technique [Shimadzu XRD-6000 (Japan), Ni-filtered CuKα_1 target, $\lambda = 1.54183$ Å]. The samples were scanned from $2\theta = 3°$–$60°$ with a 0.02° step a preset time of 5 s.

Scanning electron microscopy (SEM) apparatus (Tescan Vega II, Czech Republic), working in secondary and backscattered electron modes, was used for microstructure studies. The samples were sputter-coated with a 25 nm-thick gold layer prior imaging to impart electrical conductivity to the surfaces.

The compressive strength of samples was evaluated in accordance with the ISO standard 9917E. The 3D printed cylindrical samples were about 12 mm in height and 6 mm in diameter. Five samples for each point were used. Compression testing was carried out using an Instron 4082 (Bucks, UK) testing machine operating at a crosshead speed of 1 mm × min^{-1}. Statistical analysis was performed using SPSS software, version 17.0 (Statistical Package for Social Sciences, SPSS Inc., USA). The means and SD of compressive strength were calculated.

In vivo Test: Cranial Model

All manipulations with rabbits ($n = 5$) were carried out in accordance with Animal Welfare Act in the vivarium of the A.I. Burnazyan Federal Medical Biophysical Center. The experimental study protocol was approved by the Moscow Interuniversity Ethics Committee (protocol No. 12–13 from December 12, 2013).

Implantation of the 3D Printed Bone Graft

The animals underwent intramuscular premedication (Sol. Atropini sulfatis 0.1% – 0.04 mg/kg; Sol. Cefazolini 1.0 – 25 mg/kg) and sedation (Sol. Zoletili 100 – 15 mg/kg) before positioning on the operating table special for rabbits and fixation: lying on an abdomen with the paws extended and attached. A linear 3 cm skin incision was performed to a periosteum over sagittal suture from occipital protuberance to the frontal area under local anesthesia (Sol. Ultracaini 1.7 mL). Local anesthetic was applied into the skin and underlying tissues infiltrating periosteum. Soft tissues were lateralized, and the cranial bones surface was exposed. Previously prepared sterile template (disk 20 mm in diameter) was positioned in the center of calvaria from occipital to frontal bone and was used for marking of the defect edges. After that, a template was removed, and osteotomy was made with a bur to form the full-thickness defect (diameter 20 mm) keeping a dura mater uninjured and preserving the small fragments of inner cortical bone (1 mm × 1 mm) in the 1, 5, 7, and 11 o'clock positions as the points of support. Bleeding from the damaged sagittal sinus was stopped by coagulation. 3D printed block exactly corresponding to the defect form was implanted on the retained cortical bone fragments. Surgical wound was closed on multiple tissue levels with interrupted sutures (MonoSyn 4/0). No pain management was required postoperatively. The rabbits were deceased at 6.5 months after surgery. Each calvaria with the bone defect region was removed, fixed in 4% neutral formalin, and subjected to further studies.

Computer Tomography

Explanted material underwent a CT after 3 days of fixation. Scanning parameters were as follows: voxel size 8 μm, 80 kV, and 2 mA.

The tomograms were analyzed with Planmeca Romexis viewer (Planmeca Oy, Finland). Additionally, we carried out a manual segmentation of the area with implanted 3D printed samples and calculated a density (HU) of selected zone in a standard module of 3D-Slicer (NHI, USA).

Histological Examination

Histological slices were made according to the standard procedure after decalcification of the explanted calvaria in the "Biodek-R" solution (Bio-Optica, Italy). All sections were made strictly in the frontal plane through the center of the implant with preservation of parietal bones fragments attached to each side of the 3D printed block (length of the sample was about 25 mm). Histological sections were stained with hematoxylin and eosin and subjected to scanning (Mirax scanner, Carl Zeiss, Germany). Digital images of the histotopograms were analyzed at various magnifications.

Results and Discussion

3D printing technique based on cement powders is an effective and inexpensive method for individual and complex bone substitute's fabrication since there is neither support materials burning out nor organic solvent required (Castilho et al., 2014). Setting and hardening processes during 3D printing are based on two types of interaction, which depend on the raw materials used. The first is an acid–base reaction with the formation of a neutral compound. The second one is the hydrolysis reaction of the metastable CP. Both resulted in an adhesive effect between the particles. The final phases of the cement product are apatite or DCPD (Khalyfa et al., 2007; Gbureck et al., 2008; Klammert et al., 2010). An approach was reported utilizing further cement matrix formation consisting of a mixture of HA/TCP by following heat treatment (Castilho et al., 2014). CP materials printed with these techniques are biocompatible and possess certain osteoconductive properties.

Our work is a combination and further development of the processes involving chemical interaction between initial CP powder, such as TCP and binder liquid ("ink") such as diluted phosphoric acid (Popov et al., 2014), followed by chemical treatment of the printed DCPD structure with chemical solutions at physiological temperatures. It is known that TCP upon treatment with phosphoric can be used as bone cement forming DCPD, which further can be transformed into OCP (Heughebaert et al., 1983). The 3D printing process of TCP powders with phosphoric acid is based on a hydraulic setting reaction leading to DCPD crystallization, and thus to layer-crossing bonding of the powder finally resulting in the formation of a 3D structure. The printed samples consist of unreacted TCP and certain amounts of DCPD (**Figure 2A**). SEM photomicrographs of both TCP and DCPD phases are presented in **Figures 2B1,B2**. Size of the unreacted TCP particles was 5–15 μm (**Figure 2B1**). The DCPD crystals had a flower-like morphology. The width of the DCPD crystals was in range from 1 to 50 μm, and their thickness ranged from a fraction of few microns (**Figure 2B2**). Compressive strength of the 3D printed samples is shown in **Figure 3** and was only about 2.5 MPa.

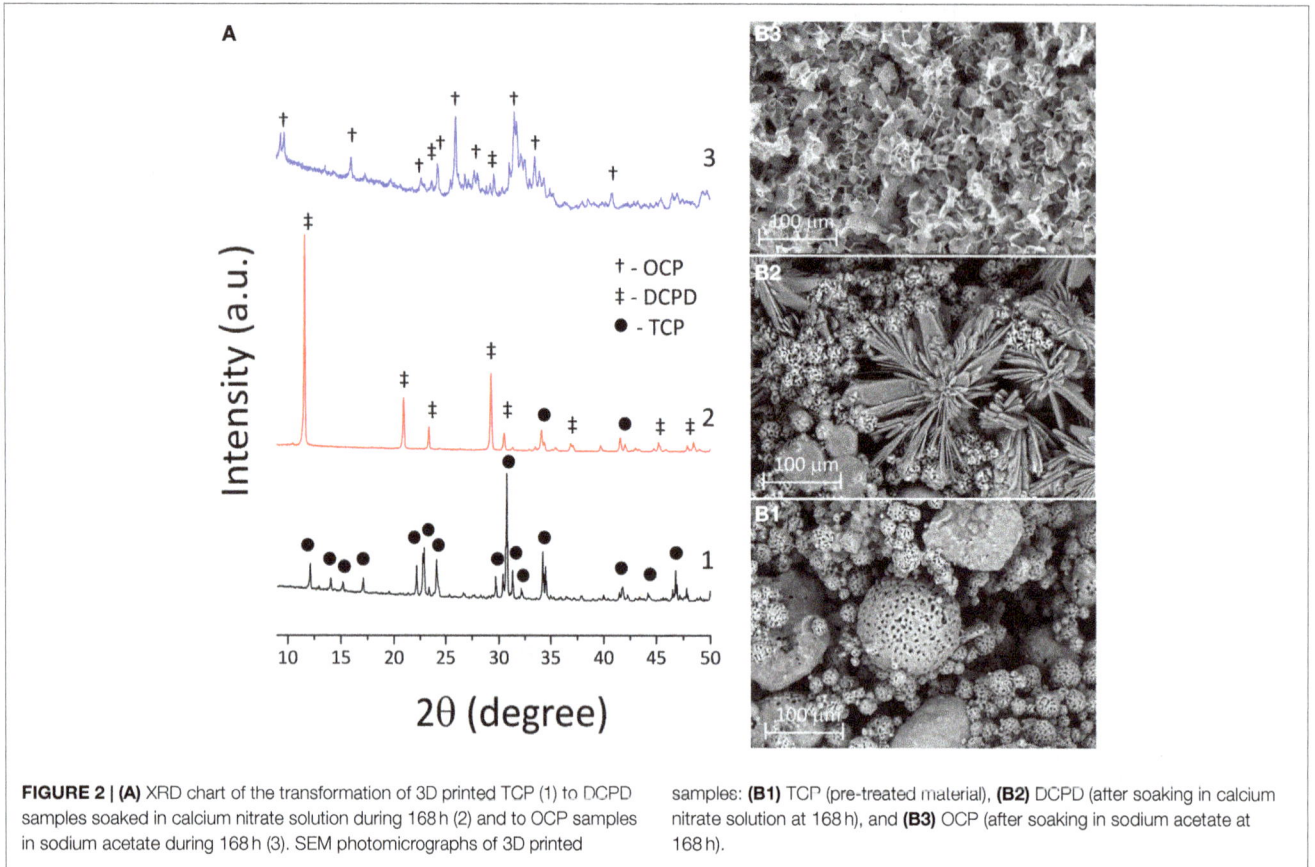

FIGURE 2 | (A) XRD chart of the transformation of 3D printed TCP (1) to DCPD samples soaked in calcium nitrate solution during 168 h (2) and to OCP samples in sodium acetate during 168 h (3). SEM photomicrographs of 3D printed samples: (B1) TCP (pre-treated material), (B2) DCPD (after soaking in calcium nitrate solution at 168 h), and (B3) OCP (after soaking in sodium acetate at 168 h).

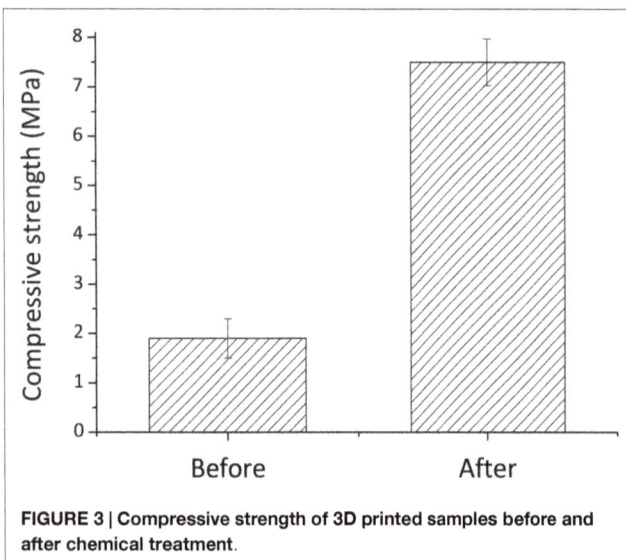

FIGURE 3 | Compressive strength of 3D printed samples before and after chemical treatment.

To this end, the chemical and phase composition of the 3D printed samples is to be fixed by completing acid–base reaction with DCPD compound formation. Further hydrolysis reaction of the metastable CP results in the formation of OCP phase and an adhesive effect between particles. This process is represented in **Figure 2A**, where the transformation from TCP to DCPD was completed after 168 h of soaking in the solution. The obtained 3D printed samples with DCPD phase composition were transformed into OCP of soaking in sodium acetate, according to XRD (**Figure 2A**). XRD of the OCP samples devoted predominant OCP phase with (100) reflection at $2\theta = 4.9°$. However, the modified samples contained small amounts of unreacted DCPD, as well as new nucleated HA phase (after 168 h of soaking in sodium acetate). High intensity of diffraction peaks indicate high crystallinity of OCP materials (**Figure 2A**). OCP plates were needle-like 2–5 µm long and 1–2 µm wide (**Figure 2B3**).

From the data that were presented in **Figure 2**, the following mechanism can be established: in the initial stage, the pH was low due to the presence of phosphoric acid, and the reaction between $Ca_3(PO_4)_2$ and H_3O^+ yielded Ca^{2+} ions. The Ca^{2+} ions reacted with HPO_4^{2-} ions, which formed $CaHPO_4 \cdot 2H_2O$. The further increase of the values of pH of the solution during the post-treatment leads to OCP nucleation and growth.

Compressive strength of 3D printed samples and post treated structures is shown in **Figure 3**. The compressive strength of the post treated material increased with time from 2.5 MPa up to about 7.5 MPa at $P \leq 0.005$. The increase in the compressive strength after treatment can be explained by the formation of new OCP crystals within 3D printed samples, which improve the bonding between particles. These OCP samples were used for *in vivo* experiments.

An adequate *in vivo* model for objective evaluation of qualitative and quantitative parameters of substitute's biological action is utterly important for successful development of 3D printed bone grafts. There are numerous orthotropic animal models: various defects of long bones, mandible, parietal, and frontal bones. However, the majority of bone defects in these models is not large enough or require complex fixation. By choosing an appropriate model for our study, we considered the following criteria: bone defect should be the "maximum-sized" but should not require additional methods of fixation, e.g., osteosynthesis with miniplates, screws, etc., affecting bone regeneration process and, in general, the study results. For this purpose, we developed the original experimental model of a cranial bone defect characterized

by large diameter (20 mm) and preservation of four fragments of inner cortical bone in special positions (1, 5, 7, and 11 o'clock) as points for implant support. This model allowed 3D printed block to be optimally immobilized into the bone defects without additional fixation methods (**Figures 4A,B**).

Postoperatively, there were no signs of acute inflammation, edema, and other adverse events; wound healed by primary intention. According to CT, the peripheral sides of implanted material were fully integrated with surrounding bone tissue (**Figure 4**). Moreover, there were sites of newly formed tissue, apparently

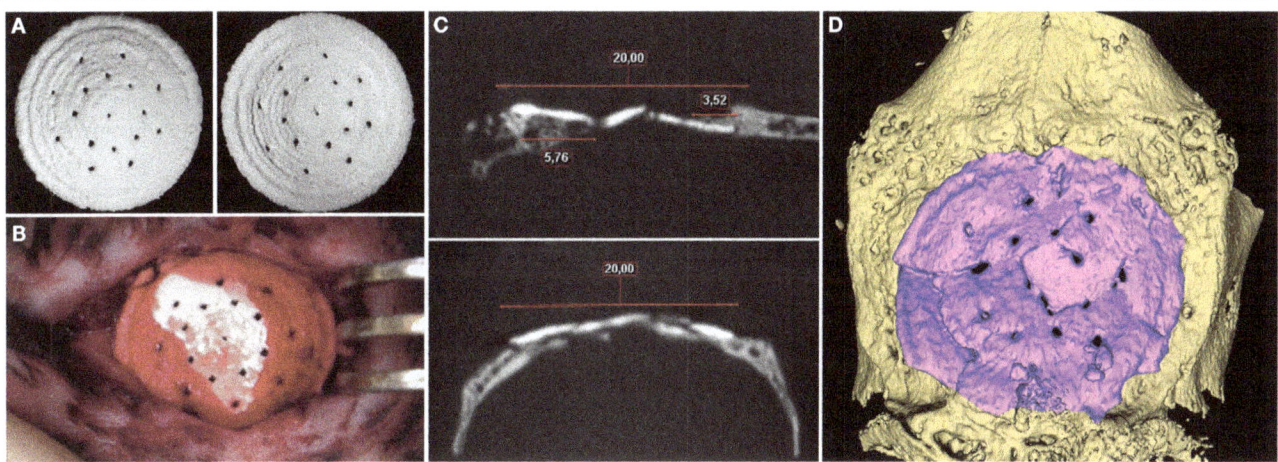

FIGURE 4 | (A) General view of 3D printed samples to be implanted. **(B)** Photomicrograph of the cranial defect produced. **(C)** 2D slices in different areas. **(D)** 3D CT reconstruction for 3D printed block at 6.5 months after implantation.

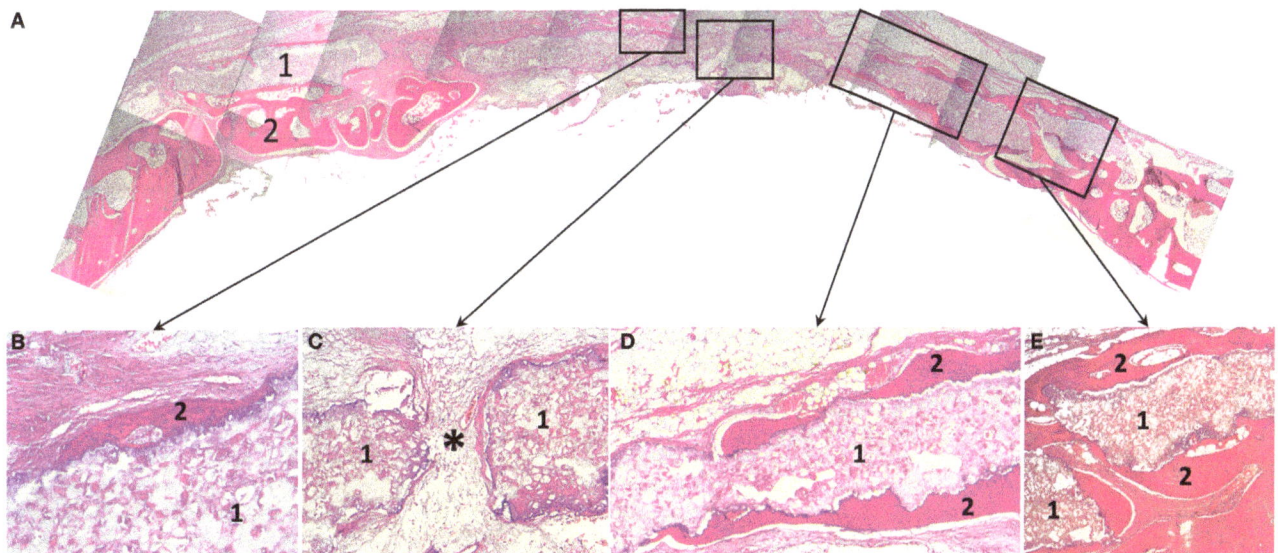

FIGURE 5 | Histological slides of the rabbit's calvaria bones, slice made in the coronal plane: (A) Histotopogram, including two regions of newly formed bone tissue growing toward each other; (B) the central area, where a fragment of the woven bone tissue formed on the implant surface without fibrous tissue interlayer; (C) the central area with pore in the 3D printed implant a fibrous tissue with single vascular vessels grow out through (*); (D) a fragment of the marginal part of the regenerate where newly formed bone tissue grew directly on the 3D printed block surface; **(E) the marginal part of the regenerate having pronounced newly formed bone trabecule retaining the implant**. 1, 3D printed block made of octacalcium phosphate; 2, newly formed bone tissue; *vascular vessel. Staining: hematoxylin and eosin, paraffin sections. Magnification: **(A)** ×4, **(C–E)** ×100, **(B)** ×200.

consisting of bone (767.56 ± 145.81 HU), grown centripetally from the temporal edges and tightly adjacent to the inner and external surfaces of the 3D printed block as though enfolding its peripheral parts. A bone regenerate proceeded from occipital bone had the most length that was defined, apparently, by its greater thickness. The average density of the material was 1851.29 ± 58.26 HU 6.5 months after implantation that impeded evaluation of tissue ingrowths into the 3D printed sample. Indirectly, the presence of gaps and sites of superposed edges of the material fragments in the block could identify this process. However, the fragmentation could be related to a mechanical impact of a rabbit's activity.

Histological study revealed that 3D printed block was biocompatible: in spite of the large dimensions and the absence of a firm fixation to surrounding structures, material directly contacted with newly formed bone without fibrous encapsulation or even slight connective tissue areas making them apart (**Figure 5**). In the central part of the defect, no signs of osteogenesis were observed; material here was surrounded by fibrous tissue grown into the block's pores.

A cross-section shows that a "material–bone tissue" interaction could occur by two ways. First, the bone tissue grows over external and under internal surfaces of the OCP block, but does not penetrate it as the structure was not porous that preserved mechanical qualities of the material. Second, regenerating calvarial bones can grow under the block using it as a conductor. The second way is probably associated with surgical implantation technique.

General feature of this 3D printed block is blood vessels, cells of granulation tissue, as well as osteogenic cells permeability. Bone formation occurred in the sites of close contact with the material that could also be found in the central part of the defect, without any apparent connection with regenerate grown from the edges. In crack sites, the material fragments injured regenerating tissues that led to local giant cell reaction. This finding together with abovementioned confirmed that the gaps were caused by animal activity rather than tissues ingrowths.

The printed implants supported bone regeneration that allowed 2.5-time reducing of defect's diameter at 6.5 months in a region where native bone repair is extremely inefficient.

Conclusion

The results of our study demonstrate that combination of 3D inkjet printing with post-treatment methodology is a promising approach to overcome current limitations in effective and fast fabrication of individual constructions for guided bone regeneration. We proposed and developed a relatively simple route and materials for 3D printing process, targeted to production of complexly shaped and structured OCP bone substitutes. We showed experimentally that 3D inkjet powder printing is a suitable technique for custom-designed critical size OCP bone grafts production.

Acknowledgments

This work was supported by the Russian Foundation for Basic Research (grant No. 13-03-12021 and 13-02-12041) in the parts of initial materials and 3D printing process development, the Russian Science Foundation (grant No. 14-25-00055), and Government of the Russian Federation (contract No. 14.B25.31.0019) in the part of OCP grafts physical–chemical analysis. The authors would like to thank V. Grachev (3D-lab) for CT scanning.

References

Bergmann, C., Lindner, M., Zhang, W., Koczur, K., Kirsten, A., Telle, R., et al. (2010). 3D printing of bone substitute implants using calcium phosphate and bioactive glasses. *J. Eur. Ceram. Soc.* 12, 2563–2567. doi:10.1016/j.jeurceramsoc.2010.04.037

Bohner, M. (2010). Resorbable biomaterials as bone graft substitutes. *Mater. Today* 13, 24–30. doi:10.1016/S1369-7021(10)70014-6

Bose, S., Vahabzadeh, S., and Bandyopadhyay, A. (2013). Bone tissue engineering using 3D printing. *Mater. Today* 12, 496–504. doi:10.1016/j.mattod.2013.11.017

Castilho, M., Moseke, C., Ewald, A., Gbureck, U., Groll, J., Pires, I., et al. (2014). Direct 3D powder printing of biphasic calcium phosphate scaffolds for substitution of complex bone defects. *Biofabrication* 6, 015006. doi:10.1088/1758-5082/6/1/015006

Detsch, R., Schaefer, S., Deisinger, U., Ziegler, G., Seitz, H., and Leukers, B. (2011). In vitro-osteoclastic activity studies on surfaces of 3D printed calcium phosphate scaffolds. *J. Biomater. Appl.* 26, 359–380. doi:10.1177/0885328210373285

Dorozhkin, S. (2011). Calcium orthophosphates: occurrence, properties, biomineralization, pathological calcification and biomimetic applications. *Biomatter* 1, 121–164. doi:10.4161/biom.18790

Gbureck, U., Hölzel, T., Biermann, I., Barralet, J. E., and Grover, L. M. (2008). Preparation of tricalcium phosphate/calcium pyrophosphate structures via rapid prototyping. *J. Mater. Sci. Mater. Med.* 19, 1559–1563. doi:10.1007/s10856-008-3373-x

Guo, D., Xu, K., and Han, Y. (2009). The in situ synthesis of biphasic calcium phosphate scaffolds with controllable compositions, structures, and adjustable properties. *J. Biomed. Mater. Res.* 88, 43–52. doi:10.1002/jbm.a.31844

Heughebaert, J. C., Zawacki, S. J., and Nancollas, G. H. (1983). The growth of octacalcium phosphate on beta tricalcium phosphate. *J. Cryst. Growth* 63, 83–90. doi:10.1016/0022-0248(83)90431-1

Horowitz, R. A., Mazor, Z., Miller, R. J., Krauser, J., Prasad, H. S., and Rohrer, M. D. (2009). Clinical evaluation alveolar ridge preservation with a beta-tricalcium phosphate socket graft. *Compend. Contin. Educ. Dent.* 30, 588–590.

Khalyfa, A., Vogt, S., Weisser, J., Grimm, G., Rechtenbach, A., Meyer, W., et al. (2007). Development of a new calcium phosphate powder-binder system for the 3D printing of patient specific implants. *J. Mater. Sci. Mater. Med.* 18, 909–916. doi:10.1007/s10856-006-0073-2

Klammert, U., Gbureck, U., Vorndran, E., Rödiger, J., Meyer-Marcotty, P. H., and Kübler, A. C. (2010). 3D powder printed calcium phosphate implants for reconstruction of cranial and maxillofacial defects. *J. Craniomaxillofac. Sur.* 8, 565–570. doi:10.1016/j.jcms.2010.01.009

Komlev, V. S., Barinov, S. M., Bozo, I. I., Deev, R. V., Eremin, I. I., Fedotov, A. Y., et al. (2014). Bioceramics composed of octacalcium phosphate demonstrate enhanced biological behavior. *ACS Appl. Mater. Interfaces* 6, 16610–16620. doi:10.1021/am502583p

Popov, V. K., Komlev, V. S., and Chichkov, B. N. (2014). Calcium phosphate blossom for bone tissue engineering. *Mater. Today* 2, 96–97. doi:10.1016/j.mattod.2014.01.015

Rath, S. N., Strobel, L. A., Arkudas, A., Beier, J. P., Maier, A. K., Greil, P., et al. (2012). Osteoinduction and survival of osteoblasts and bone-marrow stromal cells in 3D biphasic calcium phosphate scaffolds under static and dynamic culture conditions. *J. Cell. Mol. Med.* 16, 2350–2361. doi:10.1111/j.1582-4934.2012.01545.x

Schumacher, M., Deisinger, U., Detsch, R., and Ziegler, G. (2010). Indirect rapid prototyping of biphasic calcium phosphate scaffolds as bone substitudes: influence of phase composition, macroporosity and pore geometry on mechanical properties. *J. Mater. Sci. Mater. Med.* 21, 3119–3127. doi:10.1007/s10856-010-4166-6

Stavropoulos, A., Windisch, P., Szendröi-Kiss, D., Peter, R., Gera, I., and Sculean, A. (2010). Clinical and histologic evaluation of granular beta-tricalcium phosphate for the treatment of human intrabony periodontal defects: a report on five cases. *J. Periodontol.* 81, 325–334. doi:10.1902/jop.2009.090386

Suba, Z., Takács, D., Matusovits, D., Barabás, J., Fazekas, A., and Szabó, G. (2006). Maxillary sinus floor grafting with β-tricalcium phosphate in humans: density and microarchitecture of the newly formed bone. *Clin. Oral Implants Res.* 17, 102–108. doi:10.1111/j.1600-0501.2005.01166.x

Zorin, V. L., Komlev, V. S., Zorina, A. I., Khromova, N. V., Solovieva, E. V., Fedotov, A. Y., et al. (2014). Octacalcium phosphate ceramics combined with gingiva-derived stromal cells for engineered functional bone grafts. *Biomed. Mater.* 9, 055005. doi:10.1088/1748-6041/9/5/055005

Conflict of Interest Statement: The authors declare that the research was conducted in the absence of any commercial or financial relationships that could be construed as a potential conflict of interest.

18

Tissue engineering of ureteral grafts: preparation of biocompatible crosslinked ureteral scaffolds of porcine origin

Holger Koch[1]*, Niels Hammer[2], Susann Ossmann[3], Katrin Schierle[4], Ulrich Sack[1,5], Jörg Hofmann[6], Mike Wecks[6] and Andreas Boldt[1,5]

[1] Translational Centre for Regenerative Medicine (TRM), University of Leipzig, Leipzig, Germany, [2] Institute of Anatomy, Faculty of Medicine, University of Leipzig, Leipzig, Germany, [3] Heart Center, Clinic for Cardiac Surgery, University of Leipzig, Leipzig, Germany, [4] Institute of Pathology, University of Leipzig, Leipzig, Germany, [5] Institute for Clinical Immunology, Faculty of Medicine, University of Leipzig, Leipzig, Germany, [6] Institut für Nichtklassische Chemie e. V., Leipzig, Germany

Edited by:
Verena Charwat,
University of Natural Resources and
Life Sciences Vienna, Austria

Reviewed by:
Martin Kaefer,
Indiana University School of
Medicine, USA
Trinity Jude Bivalacqua,
Johns Hopkins Hospital, USA
Giuseppe Orlando,
Wake Forest University Health
Sciences, USA

*Correspondence:
Holger Koch,
Translational Centre for Regenerative
Medicine (TRM), University of Leipzig,
Philipp-Rosenthal-Street 55, Leipzig
D-04103, Germany
holger.koch@trm.uni-leipzig.de

The surgical reconstruction of ureteric defects is often associated with post-operative complications and requires additional medical care. Decellularized ureters originating from porcine donors could represent an alternative therapy. Our aim was to investigate the possibility of manufacturing decellularized ureters, the characteristics of the extracellular matrix (ECM) and the biocompatibility of these grafts *in vitro/in vivo* after treatment with different crosslinking agents. To achieve these goals, native ureters were obtained from pigs and were decellularized. The success of decellularization and the ECM composition were characterized by (immuno)histological staining methods and a DNA-assay. *In vitro*: scaffolds were crosslinked either with carbodiimide (CDI), genipin (GP), glutaraldehyde, left chemically untreated or were lyophilized. Scaffolds in each group were reseeded with Caco2, LS48, 3T3 cells, or native rat smooth muscle cells (SMC). After 2 weeks, the number of ingrown cells was quantified. *In vivo*: crosslinked scaffolds were implanted subcutaneously into rats and the type of infiltrating cells were determined after 1, 9, and 30 days. After decellularization, scaffold morphology and composition of ECM were maintained, all cellular components were removed, DNA destroyed and strongly reduced. *In vitro*: GP and CDI scaffolds revealed a higher number of ingrown 3T3 and SMC cells as compared to untreated scaffolds. *In vivo*: at day 30, implants were predominantly infiltrated by fibroblasts and M2 anti-inflammatory macrophages. A maximum of MMP3 was observed in the CDI group at day 30. TIMP1 was below the detection limit. In this study, we demonstrated the potential of decellularization to create biocompatible porcine ureteric grafts, whereas a CDI-crosslink may facilitate the remodeling process. The use of decellularized ureteric grafts may represent a novel therapeutic method in reconstruction of ureteric defects.

Keywords: ureter, scaffold, decellualrization, tissue engineering, crosslinking

Introduction

The surgical removal of tissues or organs is an aggressive therapeutic strategy to treat innate or acquired pathologies of the urinary tract. Surgical removal will present the patient and surgeon with challenges in the reconstruction of the excretory function of the urinary tract. In the case of extensive ureteral resection, surgical reconstruction by means of end-to-end anastomoses remains a major issue. Various surgical techniques were employed such as the psoas hitch (Warwick and Worth, 1969), the Boari flap (Boari, 1894) and the downward mobilization of the respective kidney (Sullivan et al., 1982), as well as the replacement of the ureters with ileal or bladder tissue or even nephrectomy (del Pizzo et al., 1998; Corvin et al., 2004; Schlote et al., 2004; Wolff et al., 2011; Takeuchi et al., 2014). These surgical techniques were frequently accompanied by serious complications, ranging from mucus formation, stenosis, and infection to renal failure (Corvin et al., 2004; Schlote et al., 2004; Wolff et al., 2011). To circumvent these complications, tissue-engineered scaffolds may be an alternative in the surgical reconstruction of the urinary tract.

Recently, various types of synthetic or biologic scaffolds (Ulm and Krauss, 1960; Block et al., 1977) and hydrogels (Dahms et al., 1997) were introduced in ureteral reconstruction, including decellular scaffolds. Synthetic scaffolds often have a lack in biocompatibility, peristaltic motion, and incrustation. Decellular scaffolds have several advantages over other implants. They can be obtained easily from various species. The cellular components can be removed from the tissues using a broad range of methods (Gilbert et al., 2006; Koch et al., 2012), resulting in decellular extracellular matrix (ECM). Mostly, the structural ECM proteins remain intact three dimensionally, facilitating host cell ingrowth (Badylak, 2004; Koch et al., 2012). Furthermore, antigenic binding sites were strongly reduced due to the removal of DNA and other cellular components. On the other hand, inflammatory reactions within the tissue and degradation cannot entirely be excluded. Inflammatory reactions are likely to be caused by the ECM proteins, providing co-stimulatory signals to immune cells (Lider et al., 1995; Tanemura et al., 2000; Allman et al., 2001, 2002; Badylak, 2004; Konakci et al., 2005; Morwood and Nicholson, 2006; Adair-Kirk and Senior, 2008; Badylak and Gilbert, 2008; Koch et al., 2012). The intensity of the inflammatory reaction and the subsequent degradation and remodeling of decellular scaffolds is strongly tissue dependent and also influenced by the chemical treatment (Badylak, 2004; Gilbert et al., 2006; Valentin et al., 2006; Badylak and Gilbert, 2008; Koch et al., 2012). Though preliminary results with decellular matrices yielded promising results concerning the ingrowth of urothelium, of smooth muscle cells (SMC) and nerve fibers (Dahms et al., 1997). Therefore, decellular scaffolds have to meet two goals. First, ECM scaffolds should maintain their mechanical properties, providing an adequate matrix that allows the cell ingrowth *in vivo*. Second, moderate scaffold degradation is necessary to allow for tissue remodeling. To meet these goals, chemical crosslinking agents are applied (Koch et al., 2012).

The goals of the given study were as follows: (A) to characterize tissue-engineered decellular porcine ureteral scaffolds and (B) to determine the influence of crosslinking agents on the morphological matrix properties and cell ingrowth *in vitro*. Furthermore, we aimed (C) to investigate whether decellular ureters might provoke inflammatory responses or rejection reactions. Another goal of the given study was to evaluate a method to manufacture scaffolds suitable for storage by means of lyophilization.

We addressed the following hypotheses:

1. Porcine ureters can be decellularized successfully, thus preserving ECM composition.
2. Tissue-engineered decellular ureteral scaffolds can be reseeded with different cells *in vitro* and do not provoke rejection reactions *in vivo*.
3. Inflammatory reactions and degradation rate might be influenced by different crosslinking agents *in vivo*.

Materials and Methods

Porcine Ureteral Scaffolds

All experiments were performed with ureters from pigs (*Deutsche Landrasse*, 25–65 kg). The methods used in the present study were similar in some aspects to those of earlier published work (Koch et al., 2012) and complemented by DNA- (2.2), SDS- (2.3), and reseeding-assays (2.6). The organs were obtained under sterile conditions and were stored at 4°C in a 0.9% NaCl solution. For decellularization, ureters were cut into pieces of 8 cm length. The tunica adventitia was removed mechanically. Ureters were then placed in a 1% sodium dodecyl sulfate solution (SDS; Roth, Karlsruhe, Germany) for 7 days. Afterwards, the scaffolds were washed in distilled water for 7 days, sterilized by gamma radiation (25 kGy from a ^{60}Co source) and stored in PBS at 4°C for a maximum of 4 weeks. SDS solution and distilled water were changed daily.

DNA Quantification and Qualitative Fragment Analysis

The isolation and quantification of DNA in the decellular tissue scaffolds was performed using the protocol of Qiagen (DNeasy™, Hilden, Germany) and as previously described (Koch et al., 2012). In brief, decellular ureteral scaffolds were cut into small cross-sectional pieces of 25 mg each and proteinase K (Qiagen, in lysis buffer) was added. Following incubation for 12 h in a shaking water bath (56°C), the DNA was purified and measured spectrophotometrically using a Nanodrop Spectrophotometer (Peqlab, Erlangen, Germany). The DNA content of matrix scaffolds undergoing enzymatic digestion with DNase (200 µg/ml; Sigma, Deisenhofen, Germany; 12 h at 37°C) was compared to the scaffolds without enzymatic digestion (both $n = 9$). Native ureters with the same origin served as positive control ($n = 9$). For qualitative fragment length analysis, 5–12 µg of total DNA was electrophoretically separated in a 1.5% agarose gel (50 min, 120 V). After the run, the gel was documented by light exposure in the FastGeneGelPic LED Bos (Nippon Genetics Europe, Dueren, Germany).

SDS Assay

The determination of residual SDS was performed using an anionic surfactants test kit (Nanocolor®, Macherey-Nagel GmbH & Co. KG, Düren, Germany). Dried decellular ureteral scaffolds were cut into small cross-sectional pieces of 100 mg and were homogenized using liquid nitrogen. In addition, scaffold powder was dissolved in distilled water (4 ml) and added to test tubes containing 4 ml chloroform and 2 ml methanol (5%). Furthermore, 0.5 ml of a methylene blue solution (1%) was added and mixed intensively for 1 min. After incubation time of 10 min, the absorption of the chloroform-containing phase was measured spectrophotometrically at the absorption maximum of 660 nm. For the calculation of residual SDS concentrations within scaffold pieces before and after washing ($n = 12$), a calibration curve was prepared.

Lyophilization of Ureteral Scaffolds

For lyophilization, the sterilized scaffolds were placed in a plastic bowl filled with distilled water at room temperature. The bowls were immersed in a vessel filled with liquid nitrogen until distilled water containing the scaffolds was frozen. The frozen scaffolds were then placed in a freeze-dryer (Alpha 1–4 LDC-1, Martin Christ Gefriertrocknungsanlagen GmbH, Osterode, Germany) and scaffolds were lyophilized applying a constant vacuum (0.05 mbar, RZ-5, Vacuubrand, Wertheim, Germany) in a range from −40 to 0°C.

Crosslinking of Ureteral Scaffolds

Scaffold-crosslinking with different agents was performed as previously described (Koch et al., 2012). In brief, for genipin (GP) crosslinking, the scaffolds were incubated in a 0.33% GP/ethanol solution (Alexis, Lausen, Switzerland) for 3 days at 37°C. Then the scaffolds were removed and rinsed in 75% ethanol for 2 h and in PBS for 3 days (Sung et al., 1999b; Liang et al., 2004; Mantovani et al., 2005; Koch et al., 2012). For carbodiimide (CDI) crosslinking circular pieces of ureter scaffolds (3 mm thickness) were immersed in 2-(N-morpholino) ethanesulfonic acid buffer (MES buffer; 0.2 M, pH 5.0; Sigma, Munich, Germany). After 1 h, the MES buffer was discarded and the scaffolds were incubated in a solution consisting of MES buffer (0.2 M, pH 5.0), N-hydroxysuccinimide (NHS; 0.12 M), and N-(3-dimethylaminopropyl)-N-ethylcarbodiimide (EDC; 0.3 M). After 16 h, the scaffolds were removed and rinsed in MES buffer for 24 h and in PBS for at least 24 h (Cao and Xu, 2008; Everaerts et al., 2008; Koch et al., 2012). For glutaraldehyde (GA) crosslinking, the scaffolds were immersed in 0.625% glutaraldehyde/distilled water (Sigma) for 3 days at 37°C. Subsequently, the scaffolds were removed and washed in PBS for 3 days (Chang et al., 2005; Koch et al., 2012).

Reseeding Decellular Ureteral Scaffolds

Sterilized decellular scaffold pieces of 1 cm, which were either crosslinked, chemically untreated or lyophilized were placed in tubes (15 ml, BD Falcon®, Becton, Dickinson and Company, Heidelberg, Germany) containing different cell lines (Caco2, LS48, 3T3) or native rat SMC. Scaffolds and cells were incubated (each 1.5–2.0×10^6 cells/tube) on a rotator (Multi-RS 60, Biosan, Riga, Latvia) at room temperature for 4 h. Afterwards, scaffolds were placed in well plates and incubated under constant conditions (37°C, 5% CO_2) for 2 weeks ($n = 7$–9). After incubation, scaffold pieces were fixed in 4% paraformaldehyde solution and embedded in paraffin for further histological investigations.

Subcutaneous Rat Model

110 Sprague-Dawley rats were grouped according to scaffold crosslinking: GA, GP, CDI, BP, untreated group, and sham

group (each treatment group: $n = 18$; sham group: $n = 20$; for more details please refer to **Table 1**). One scaffold was implanted subcutaneously into each of the individuals of the respective groups. Animals of the sham group underwent the same surgical procedure but received no implant. The subcutaneous implantation of scaffold pieces was performed as previously described (Koch et al., 2012). In brief, animals were anesthetized with 5% isoflurane (Baxter Deutschland GmbH, Unterschleissheim, Germany) in a N_2/O_2 gas mixture. After anesthetization, the concentration of isoflurane was reduced to 2% isoflurane in a N_2/O_2 gas mixture to maintain anesthesia. Circular pieces of ureteral scaffolds (3 mm thickness, 1 cm diameter) were implanted into one of the subcutaneous back pockets of rats (1 cm length). The wound was sewn with two stitches. Finally, the concentration of isoflurane was reduced to allow rats to recover from anesthesia. All surgical interventions were performed under sterile conditions. Postoperatively, rats were given carprofen (5 mg/kg s.c., Pfizer, Berlin, Germany) for 3 days. After a follow-up of one, nine, or 30 days, the animals were again narcotized, euthanized, and the scaffolds were explanted for further histological investigation. Therefore, the scaffolds were immersed in 4% paraformaldehyde solution and embedded in paraffin. All procedures were approved by the committee of Animal Care and Use of the relevant local governmental body (TVV15/10) in accordance with the Animal Welfare Act. Every effort was made to minimize the number of animals used.

Histology

Following decellularization and explantation at days 1, 9, and 30 post implantation, the scaffolds were fixed in paraformaldehyde solution. Representative areas were embedded in paraffin wax, cut into slices (5 μm thickness), and routinely stained with Hematoxylin–Eosin and Azan (Boldt et al., 2006; Koch et al., 2012). Using these slices, matrix morphology of decellular porcine scaffolds was compared to that of native ureters using light microscopy. Furthermore, the degree of scaffold infiltration by giant cells, granulocytes, capillaries, collagen fibers, lymphocytes, and fibroblasts at days 1, 9, and 30 post implantation was analyzed using these slices.

TABLE 1 | Group composition with type and crosslinking of scaffolds.

Group	n	Type of scaffold	Scaffold crosslinking
Untreated	18	Decellularized, sterilized ureter scaffold	Untreated
GA	18	Decellularized, sterilized ureter scaffold	Glutaraldehyde
GP	18	Decellularized, sterilized ureter scaffold	Geripin
CDI	18	Decellularized, sterilized ureter scaffold	Carbodiimide
BP (control)	18	Decellularized, sterilized bovine pericard scaffold	Glutaraldehyde (bovine pericardium; St. Jude, USA)
Sham (negative control)	20	–	–

Immunohistochemistry

Immunohistochemical analysis of decellular ureters was performed as previously described (Koch et al., 2012). Briefly, formalin-fixed, paraffin-embedded ureteral tissue sections of 5 μm thickness were deparaffinized. Subsequently, the slices were heated in 50 mM Tris buffered saline solution at 95°C for 15 min. After cooling, the slides were incubated with protein-ase K (250 μg/ml) for 10 min and washed in distilled water. Endogenous enzyme activity was blocked (10 min, DAKO staining kit; DAKO Deutschland GmbH, Hamburg, Germany) and the tissue slides were incubated with primary antibodies. The staining steps with anti-collagen I (Acris Antibodies, Herford, Germany), anti-collagen III (Acris Antibodies), anti-collagen IV (Acris Antibodies), anti-elastin (Acris Antibodies), and anti-fibronectin (Dianova, Berlin, Germany) were performed following the manufacturer's instruction (Envision DAB Staining Kit, DAKO). Control experiments were carried out without primary antibodies. All antibodies were diluted 1:100 in PBS. In the stained slices, the ECM composition of decellular and native scaffolds was investigated under light microscopy. To investigate cellular infiltration in explanted scaffolds of the rat model, anti-CD68 and anti-CD163 (all Serotec, Oxford, UK) antibodies were used. All antibodies were diluted 1:50 in PBS. Control experiments were carried out without primary antibodies. To visualize the nuclei, all slices were counterstained with Mayer's hemalaun solution. In stained slices, from each section the CD68 and CD163 positive cells as well as their nuclei were counted from each section in 5 × 6 random microscopic fields by two observers, blinded to the origin of the tissue and each other's ratings (magnification × 1000). The data are represented as a ratio of CD-positive cells/nuclei [mean value ± (SEM)]. To investigate the degradation of the collagen in the scaffolds, metallopeptidase 3 (MMP3) and the metallopeptidase inhibitor 1 (TIMP1) levels were analyzed, using the respective antibodies: anti-MMP3 and anti-TIMP1 (Bioss Inc., Woburn, MA, USA). All antibodies were diluted 1:100 in PBS. Control experiments were carried out without primary antibodies.

Statistics

The Shapiro–Wilk test was used to determine normal distribution of the data, except immunohistochemistry data. The statistical evaluation of the immunohistochemistry including CD68 + or CD163 + cells was performed using Kruskal–Wallis one-way analysis of variance (ANOVA) on ranks with *post hoc* Tukey test. Statistical evaluation of the reseeding procedure, the effectiveness of the washing of the decellular scaffolds on residual SDS and the respective DNA concentration was performed with the one-way repeated measures (RM) ANOVA on ranks with *post hoc* Tukey test. *P*-values of $P < 0.05$ were considered statistically significant.

Results

Porcine Ureteral Scaffolds

After decellularization, the ECM composition is similar to native ureteral tissue. Azan staining of natural (**Figure 1A**) and decellular ureteral scaffolds (**Figure 1B**) revealed morphologically

intact structures, ideal matrix geometry, and no remaining cellular structures. Histological analysis after lyophilization also showed preserved morphological structures and matrix geometry (**Figure 1C**) similar to the native and decellular conditions. After decellularization, collagen I (**Figure 2A**), collagen III (**Figure 2B**), and fibronectin (**Figure 2C**) could be observed in large amounts in all tissue areas similar to native conditions (small pictures, **Figures 2A–C**). The vessels expressed collagen IV (**Figure 2D**) and elastin, which are also located in tunica muscularis (**Figure 2E**).

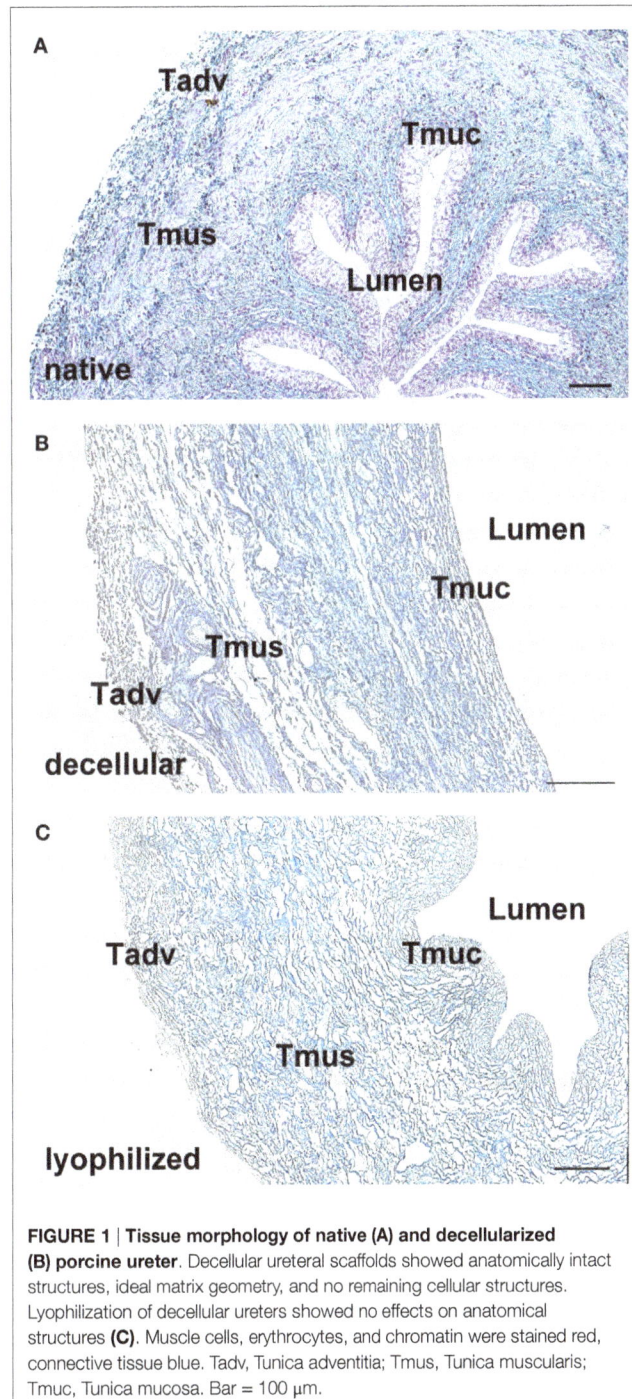

FIGURE 1 | Tissue morphology of native (A) and decellularized (B) porcine ureter. Decellular ureteral scaffolds showed anatomically intact structures, ideal matrix geometry, and no remaining cellular structures. Lyophilization of decellular ureters showed no effects on anatomical structures **(C)**. Muscle cells, erythrocytes, and chromatin were stained red, connective tissue blue. Tadv, Tunica adventitia; Tmus, Tunica muscularis; Tmuc, Tunica mucosa. Bar = 100 μm.

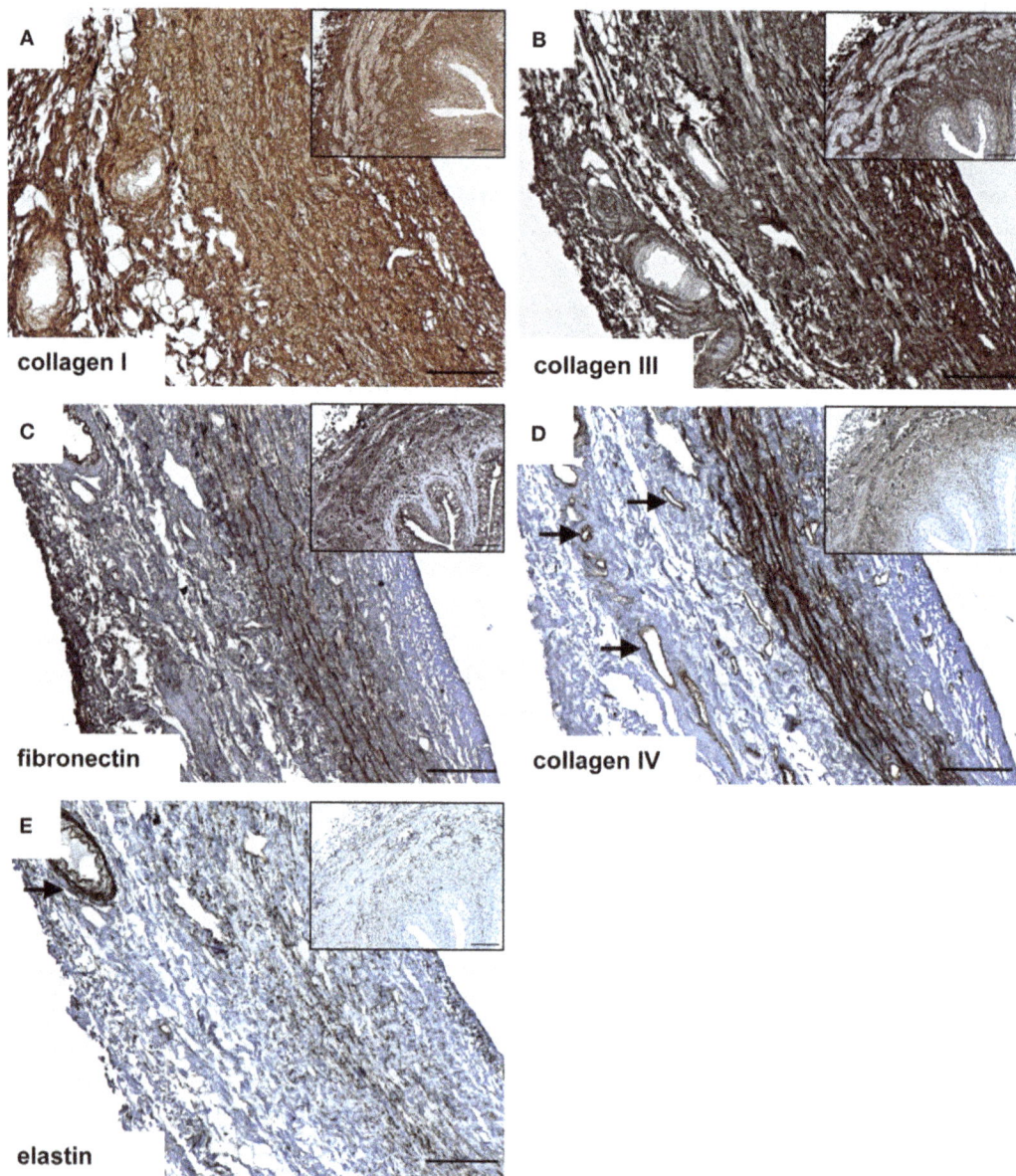

FIGURE 2 | Immunohistochemical DAB-staining of decellular porcine ureteral scaffolds for collagen I (A), collagen III (B), fibronectin (C), collagen IV (D), and elastin (E) in comparison to natural tissue (small pictures). Decellular ureteral scaffolds were shown to maintain native extracellular matrix composition. The arrows mark vessels. Bar = 100 μm.

DNA Quantification

The analysis of the DNA content revealed significant differences among native ureters, decellular ureters, and decellular ureters + DNA digestion [$P < 0.001$; each $n = 9$]. The DNA content in decellular scaffolds was significantly lower ($85.01 \pm 3.1\% = 966.1 \pm 188.2$ ng/mg tissue; $P < 0.001$) compared to that in native ureter samples ($100\% = 6,468.11 \pm 646.9$ ng/mg tissue). An additional DNA digestion further reduced the amount of the DNA to $97.32 \pm 0.7\%$ (173.28 ± 36.6 ng/mg tissue) compared to native ureter samples ($P < 0.001$; **Figure 3A**. Differences between decellular scaffolds and decellular scaffolds+ DNA digestion did not reach a level of significance ($P = 0.31$).

The percentage of remaining DNA after both procedures was decreased by about 91.2% compared with native ureteral tissue ($P < 0.001$). Qualitative analysis by gel electrophoresis showed intact DNA bands in the native samples with a size larger than 3,000 base pairs. Decellularization caused a gross but incomplete removal of this band, accompanied by a visible DNA-smear. When treating the decellular scaffolds with DNase, the smear was grossly removed (**Figure 3B**).

Residual SDS

A significant effect of the washing duration on the SDS-concentration was observed, resulting in a 99.93% decrease,

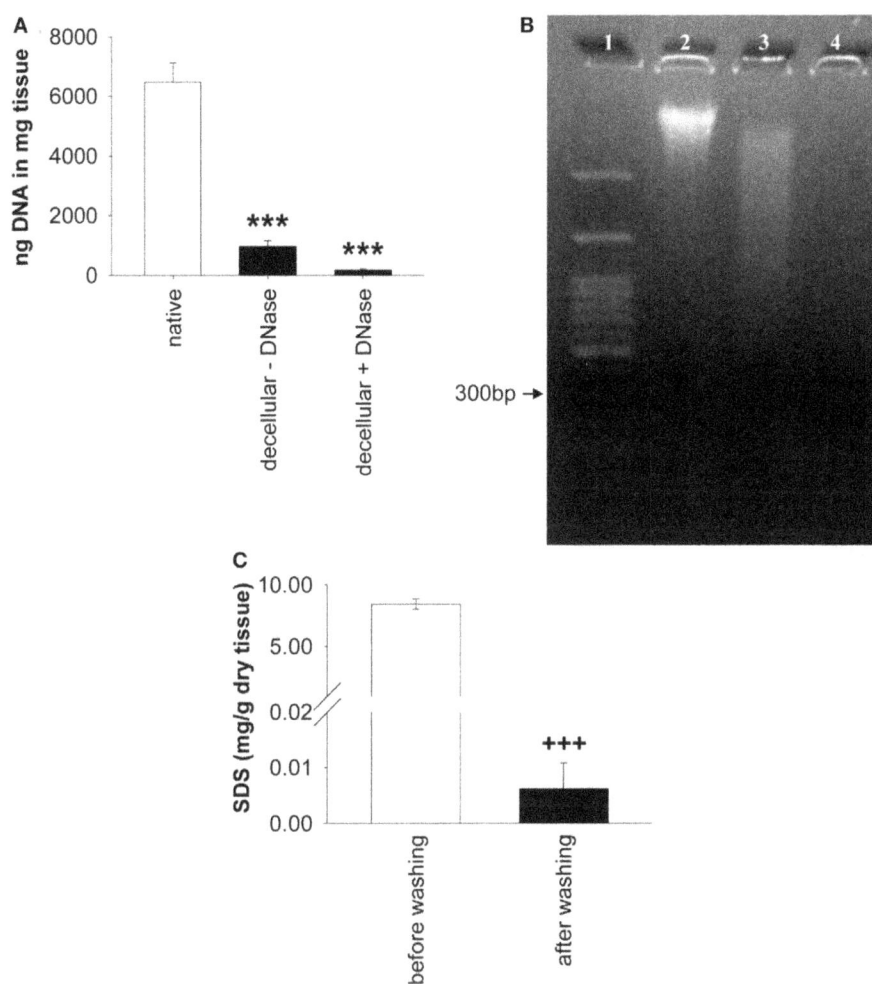

FIGURE 3 | (A) Shows the comparison of remnant DNA in decellular ureteral tissue with and without DNA digestion (both $n = 9$). Significant differences between both groups were not found. Native, untreated ureteral tissue served as control ($n = 9$). In **(B)**, gel electrophoresis of native ureter sample (2) and corresponding decellular scaffold without (3) and with DNase (4) is shown. Lane numbers indicate the respective sample. **(C)** shows the analysis of residual SDS before and after washing in distilled water ($n = 12$). Decellular ureteral scaffolds showed high SDS-concentrations (8.45 ± 0.43 mg/g dry tissue) before washing compared to non-toxic SDS-concentration after washing with distilled water (0.01 ± 0.01 mg/g dry tissue). Washed scaffold pieces show residual SDS-concentrations of $0.07 \pm 0.05\%$ compared to scaffolds before washing ($P < 0.001$; not shown). ***$P < 0.001$ vs. native group. +++$P < 0.001$ vs. decellular ureteral scaffolds before washing.

compared to residual SDS before washing. The concentration of SDS within the scaffolds after washing in distilled water was 0.006 ± 0.01 mg/g dry tissue vs. 8.449 ± 0.43 mg/g dry tissue in scaffolds before washing ($[F_{(1,11)} = 391.89, P < 0.001]$, each $n = 12$, **Figure 3C**).

Reseeding Decellular Ureteral Scaffolds

After incubation for 2 weeks, the ureteral scaffolds were increasingly infiltrated by tested cell lines (**Figures 4** and **5**). LS48 cells were uniformly distributed at the scaffold surface (**Figures 5A–D**). No significant effects of crosslinking were observed on cell growth (**Figure 4A**). 3T3 cells showed a higher infiltration after crosslinking with CDI or GP ($[F_{(3,24)} = 6.84, P = 0.002]$; CDI: $P < 0.05$, GP: $P = 0.001$; **Figure 4B**). Furthermore, multilayer formation (GA, CDI, GP) and moderate scaffold infiltration (CDI, GP) were detected in crosslinked scaffolds, whereas only sporadic cells could

be detected in the untreated scaffold group (**Figures 5E–H**). After incubation with Caco2 cells, the relative amount of cells did not differ between any of the groups (**Figure 4C**). However, scaffold infiltration and multilayer formation were predominant after crosslinking with GP or CDI (**Figures 6A–D**). Furthermore, SMC showed a preference for crosslinked scaffolds (**Figures 6E–H**), whereas the highest infiltration was observed after crosslinking with GP ($[F_{(3,18)} = 5.32, P < 0.008]$; $P < 0.01$; **Figure 4D**). However, reseeding of lyophilized scaffolds failed; neither cell lines nor native cells were grown on dried scaffolds (data not shown). Interestingly, lyophilized implants were degraded by cell lines within 2 weeks.

Response to Implanted Decellular Ureteral Scaffolds

The cell infiltration in untreated (**Figures 7A,C,E**) and crosslinked scaffolds (**Figures 7B,D,F**) was analyzed histologically after

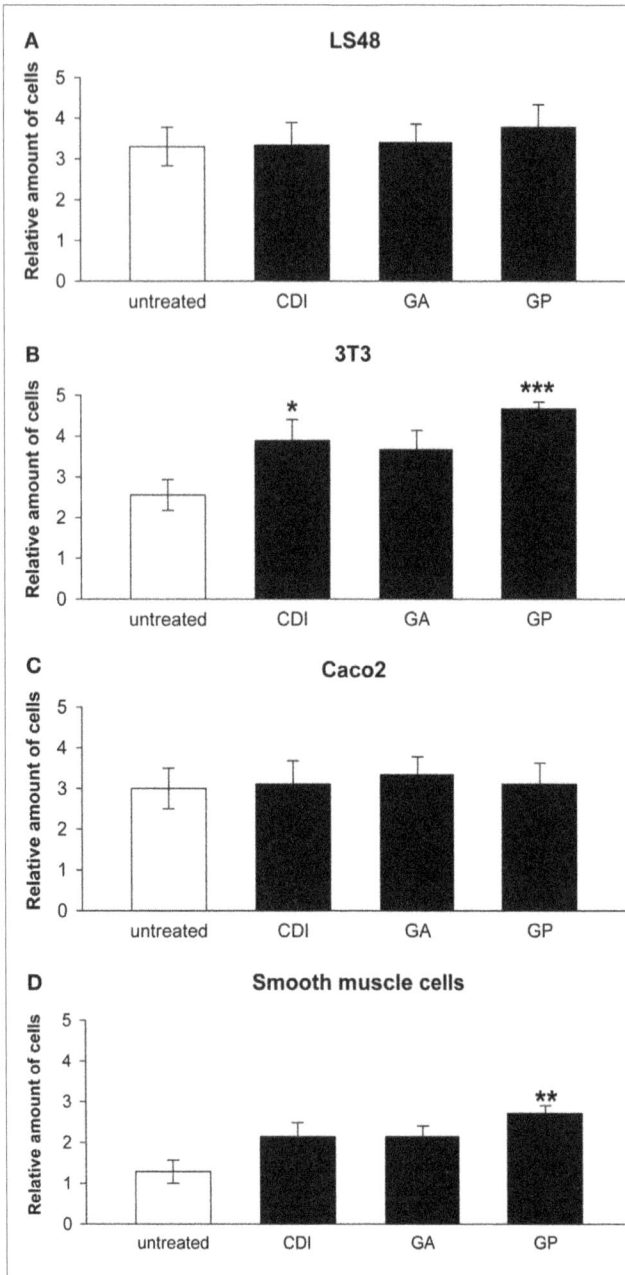

FIGURE 4 | Reseeding of crosslinked or chemical untreated ureteral scaffolds with LS48 (A), 3T3 (B), aco2 (C), and smooth muscle cells (D). Cells are able to grow on chemically untreated and crosslinked scaffolds after incubation for 2 weeks. Effects of crosslinking on relative amount of cells could not be detected under seeding with LS48 [(A), $n = 9$] and Caco2 [(C), $n = 9$] cells. However, 3T3 cells show an increased infiltrating rate into CDI and GP crosslinked scaffolds, compared to the untreated group [(B), $n = 9$]. Furthermore, crosslinking with GP caused an increase of smooth muscle cells, grown on surface and infiltrate scaffolds [(D), $n = 7$]. Data were calculated based on the scoring by two blinded observers: 1 = no cells; 2 = in total <20 cells; 3 = partially 1 cell layer, in total <50 cells, 4 = 1 cell layer around the scaffold; 5 = cells are arranged in multilayer, with matrix-infiltration. Untreated, untreated decellular ureteral tissue; GP, genipin; GA, glutaraldehyde; CDI, carbodiimide. $^*P < 0.05$, $^{**}P < 0.01$, $^{***}P < 0.001$ vs. decellular ureteral scaffolds.

explantation at days 1, 9, and 30 post implantation. At day 1 after implantation, a cellular infiltration directed from the periphery to the center of the respective tissue was observed in untreated scaffolds (**Figure 7A**). After crosslinking with CDI (**Figure 7B**), a cellular layer was detectable at the periphery and only a few number of cells infiltrated the central parts of the scaffolds. At day 9 post implantation, a decrease of cell infiltration was observed in crosslinked scaffolds (**Figure 7D**) compared to that in untreated scaffolds (**Figure 7C**). At day 30 post implantation, the untreated implants were largely degraded and completely infiltrated with cells (**Figure 7E**). In the CDI crosslinked group only an immaterial cellular infiltration could be detected (**Figure 7F**). In all crosslinked groups (GP, GA, CDI, BP), the cell infiltration was lower compared to the untreated scaffold group but without significant differences among the groups.

Only the GA crosslinked group showed a significant increase of giant cells compared to untreated group at day 9 post implantation (**Figure 8A**, $P < 0.01$). At day 1 post implantation, granulocytes were present in each group. Their number decreased and diminished toward day 30 post implantation in most groups, excepting the untreated and BP group (**Figure 8B**). Neovascularization (**Figure 8C**), new collagen fibers (**Figure 8D**), and fibroblasts (**Figure 8F**) were present in all groups without significant differences. At day 1 after implantation, lymphocytes were present in each group and did not differ to day 9 or 30 post-operative (**Figure 8E**).

At day 1 after implantation, MMP3 was activated in all groups (untreated: **Figure 9A**, crosslinked: **Figure 9B**) and increased to day 9 (untreated: **Figure 10A**, crosslinked: **Figure 10B**), whereas the reactivity was weaker in crosslinked than in untreated scaffolds. At day 30, MMP3 was detectable in both untreated (**Figure 11A**) and crosslinked (**Figure 11B**) scaffolds with same intensity. Scaffolds of all groups were negative for TIMP1 at all time-points (**Figures 9C,D**; **Figures 10C,D**; **Figures 11C,D**).

A detailed macrophage analysis showed only a few number of CD163 positive cells at the periphery of BP and CDI crosslinked samples at day 1 after implantation. Furthermore, the number of CD68 positive cells was higher in the BP group compared to that in untreated scaffolds ([$F_{(4,25)} = 9.80$, $P < 0.001$]; $P < 0.001$, **Figure 12A**). Scaffold analysis at day 9 after implantation revealed a significant increase of CD68 positive macrophages after crosslinking with GA compared to the untreated group ([$F_{(4,25)} = 4.40$, $P = 0.008$]; $P < 0.05$). At day 30 post-operative, there were no significant effects of crosslinking on the number of CD68 and CD163 positive cells (**Figure 12B**). Additionally, in most groups, the amount of the anti-inflammatory, pro-remodeling macrophage M2 phenotype increased from day 9 to day 30, indicated by a positive CD163/CD68 ratio (untreated: +10.05%; BP: +65.37%; CDI + 114.03%), whereas it decreased in the GP (−28.31%) and GA (−58.48%) groups (**Figure 12C**).

Discussion

Different surgical techniques were employed for ureter reconstruction such as Boari flap, psoas hitch, downward mobilization of the kidney, and replacement with ileal or bladder tissue. These

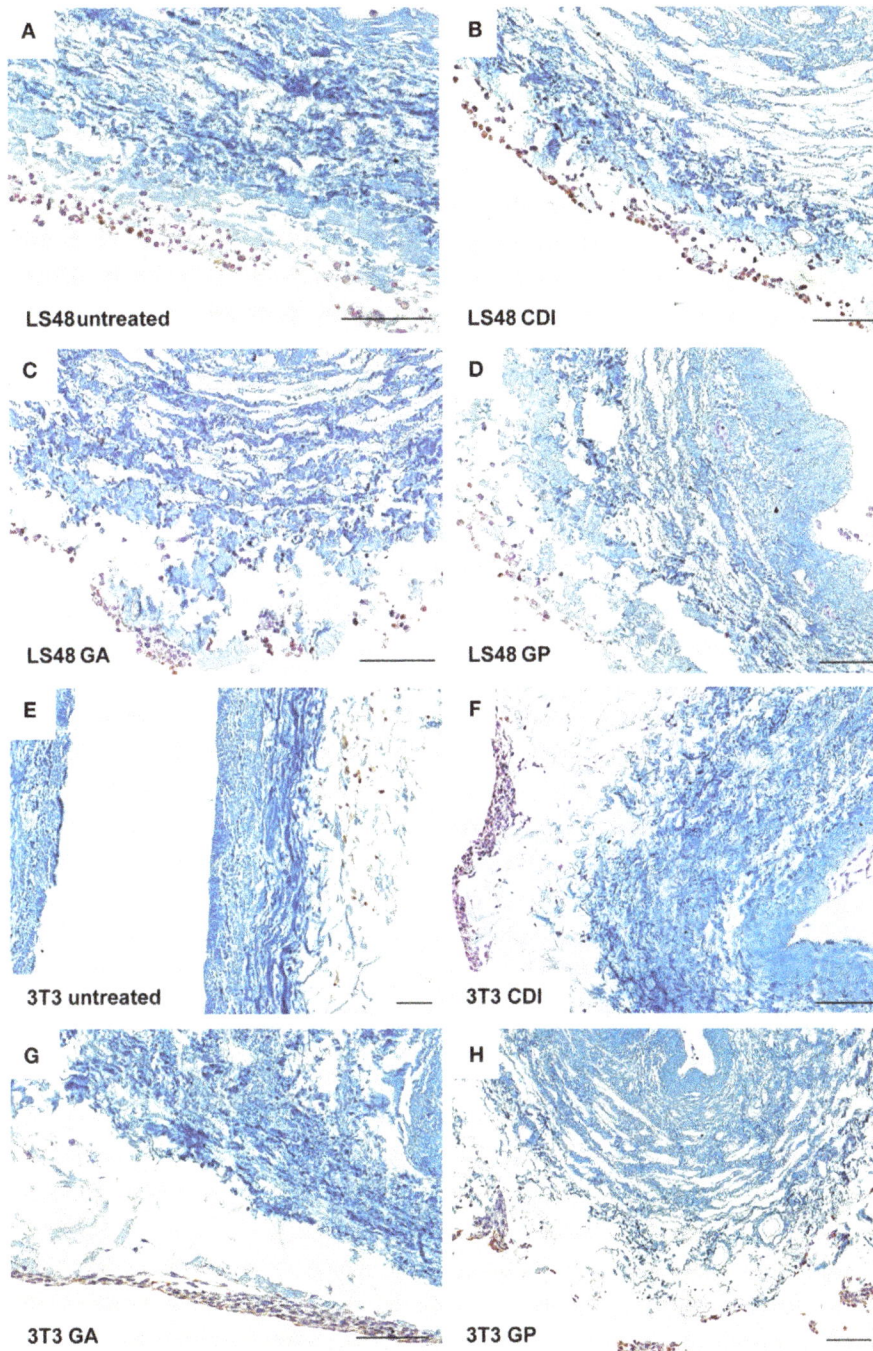

FIGURE 5 | Reseeding of crosslinked or chemical untreated ureteral scaffolds with LS48 and 3T3 cells. LS48 cells grew sporadically on scaffolds and showed small clusters. However, crosslinking showed no effect on capability of cells to grow on scaffolds **(A–D)**. Furthermore, 3T3 cells prefer crosslinked scaffolds **(E–H)**. Multilayer formations and infiltration was predominant in CDI **(F)** and GP **(H)** crosslinked scaffolds, whereas only few cells were detectable in untreated scaffold group.

reconstructing techniques are accompanied by several complications (i.e., excessive formation of mucus, ureteral stenosis, infection, renal, chronic renal failure, and metabolic disturbances or urolithiasis) (Corvin et al., 2004; Schlote et al., 2004; Wolff et al., 2011). Therefore, the development of a biocompatible ureteral implant would be of high clinical interest. Different types of scaffold materials such as hydrogels, synthetic, or natural scaffolds have already been studied in tissue engineering (Dahms et al., 1997). Partial or total ureteral replacement by synthetic materials such as teflon (Ulm and Krauss, 1960) or dacron (Block et al., 1977)

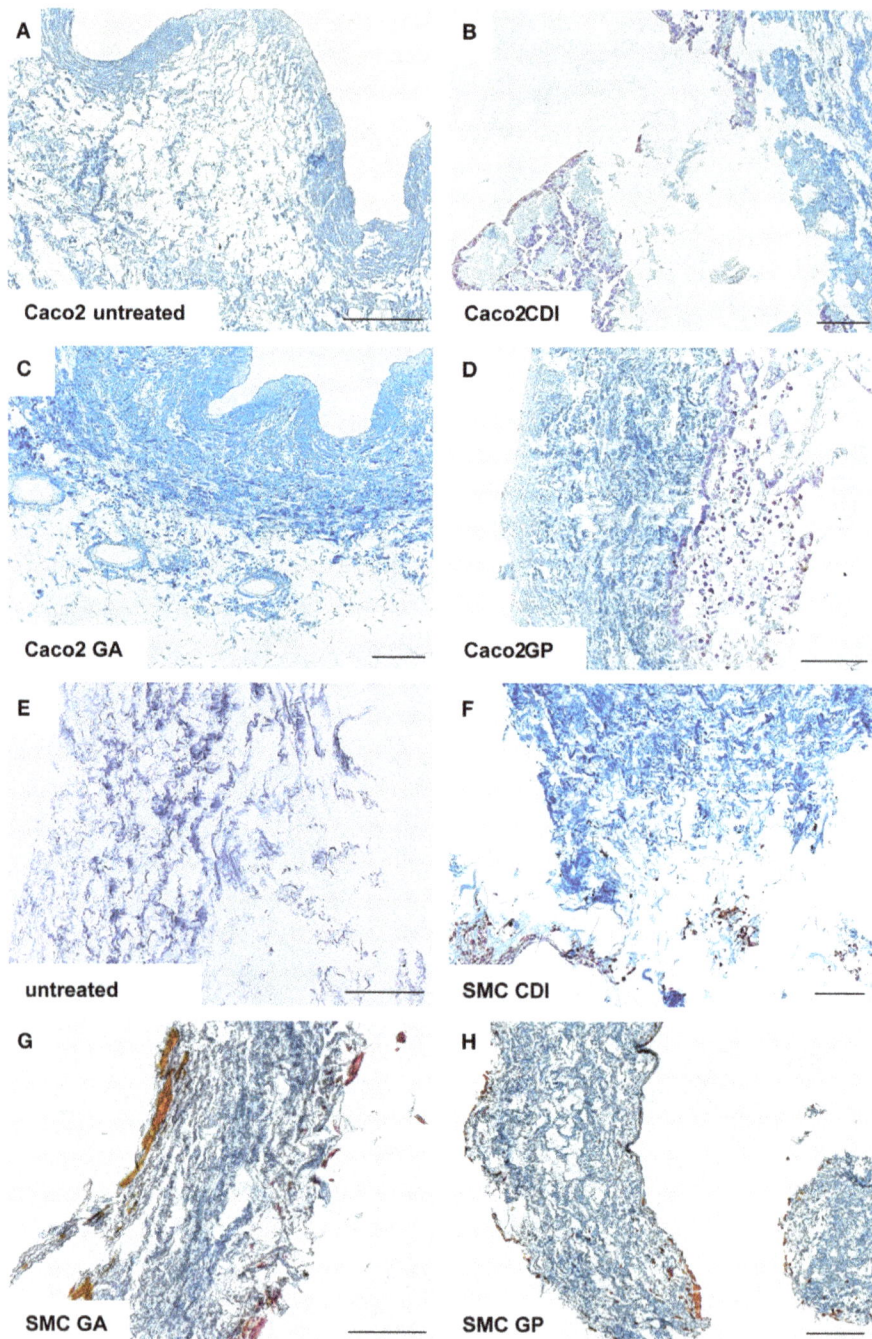

FIGURE 6 | Reseeding of crosslinked or chemically untreated ureteral scaffolds with Caco2 and rat smooth muscle cells. Only a low rate of Caco2 cells was detectable in untreated **(A)** and GA crosslinked **(C)** scaffolds. After CDI **(B)** and GP **(D)** crosslinking, Caco2 cells showed multilayer formation and scaffold infiltration. Smooth muscle cells also preferred crosslinked scaffolds **(E–H)**, whereas cell-cluster and infiltration were observed. Untreated, untreated decellular ureteral tissue; GP, genipin; GA, glutaraldehyde; CDI, carbodiimide. Bar = 100 μm.

was examined. Unfortunately, these materials showed a lack of biocompatibility, peristalsis, and moderate incrustation. Biological ECM scaffolds possess intact structural proteins and growth factors that reduce inflammatory responses (Badylak, 2004; Chang et al., 2005; Badylak and Gilbert, 2008). Nevertheless, decellular scaffolds have several advantages over synthetic implants. The scaffold materials can be easily obtained from different species. The cellular components can be removed from the tissue/organ by a broad range of various methods (Gilbert et al., 2006; Koch et al., 2012), resulting in decellular ECM. Structural proteins of the ECM remain intact and ECM scaffolds have a three-dimensional structure that facilitates host cell ingrowth (Badylak, 2004; Koch et al., 2012).

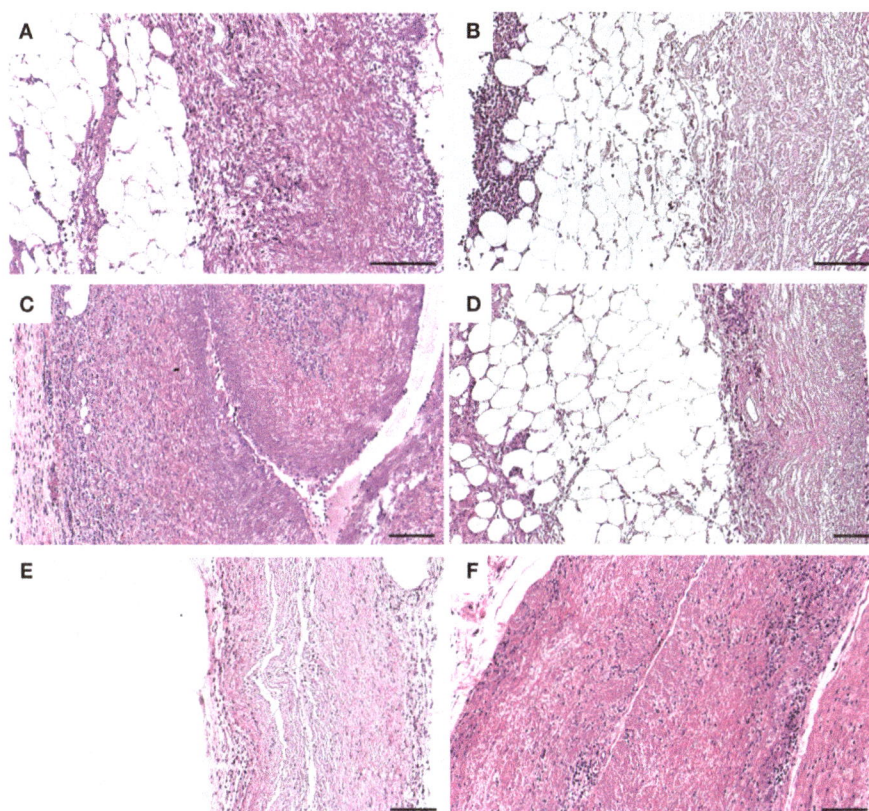

FIGURE 7 | Histological analysis of HE-stained subcutaneous implanted untreated (A,C,E) and CDI crosslinked scaffolds (B,D,F) explanted at days 1, 9, and 30 post-operative. At day 1 post implantation, cellular infiltration with granulocytes, fibroblasts, and macrophages could be observed in untreated scaffolds **(A)**, whereas in CDI crosslinked scaffolds **(B)** only a cellular layer was detectable at the periphery. At day 9 post implantation, a notable increase of infiltrating cells into untreated scaffolds **(C)** was detected as a sign of encapsulation. CDI crosslinked **(D)** scaffolds showed a mild cellular infiltration with granulocytes, fibroblasts, and macrophages. At day 30 post implantation, in contrast to the untreated scaffold group **(E)**, CDI crosslinked scaffolds **(F)** showed only a marginal cellular infiltration by granulocytes, fibroblasts, and macrophages. Untreated scaffolds were completely infiltrated by cells and largely degraded. Detailed cellular analysis is displayed in **Figure 8**. Bar = 100 μm.

Due to removing the DNA and cellular components, the antigenic binding sites were strongly reduced. Therefore, one might assume that decellular scaffolds do not provoke a chronic rejection reaction after implantation, even if originating from another species. In 1997, first preliminary experiments with decellular matrixes showed promising results concerning the ingrowth of urothelium, SMC and nerve cells (Dahms et al., 1997). However, complications such as ureteral occlusion and finally hydronephrosis were also described (Sofer et al., 2002). In addition, previously published data suggest that the host response to the ECM scaffolds was strongly dependent on the species and chemical pre-treatment (Sung et al., 1999a,b; Chang et al., 2002, 2005; Liang et al., 2004; Badylak and Gilbert, 2008; Cao and Xu, 2008; Everaerts et al., 2008; Koch et al., 2012). Therefore, currently published data are not universally consistent. Thus, it was first essential to test the morphological characteristics and the biocompatibility of the ureteral scaffolds.

To the best of our knowledge, we are the first to describe the decellularization of porcine ureters and investigated the influence of different crosslinking agents on cellular reseeding *in vitro* and on the inflammatory response *in vivo* in one study.

Ureter Decellularization and Matrix Composition

According to our hypothesis, porcine ureters can be easily decellularized. After decellularization, histological analysis revealed morphological intact structures, optimal matrix geometry and no remaining cellular structures. Lyophilized ureters showed intact morphological structures, whereas collagen I, III, IV, fibronectin, and elastin could be observed in amounts similar to natural or decellular ureters.

Success of *In Vitro* Reseeding Depends on Crosslinker

In vitro data showed a considerable ingrowth of different cell lines (LS48, 3T3, Caco2) and SMC), depending on crosslinking. Highest infiltration was offered by the crosslinkers CDI and GP compared to other crosslinkers and chemically untreated scaffolds. These findings reflect not only the positive effects of crosslinking but also the effectiveness of washing out residual cytotoxic SDS concentrations (remove of 99.93% SDS). In contrast to crosslinking with GP or CDI, the infiltration of cells into GA crosslinked scaffolds was comparable to untreated scaffolds *in vitro* as a sign of non-optimal

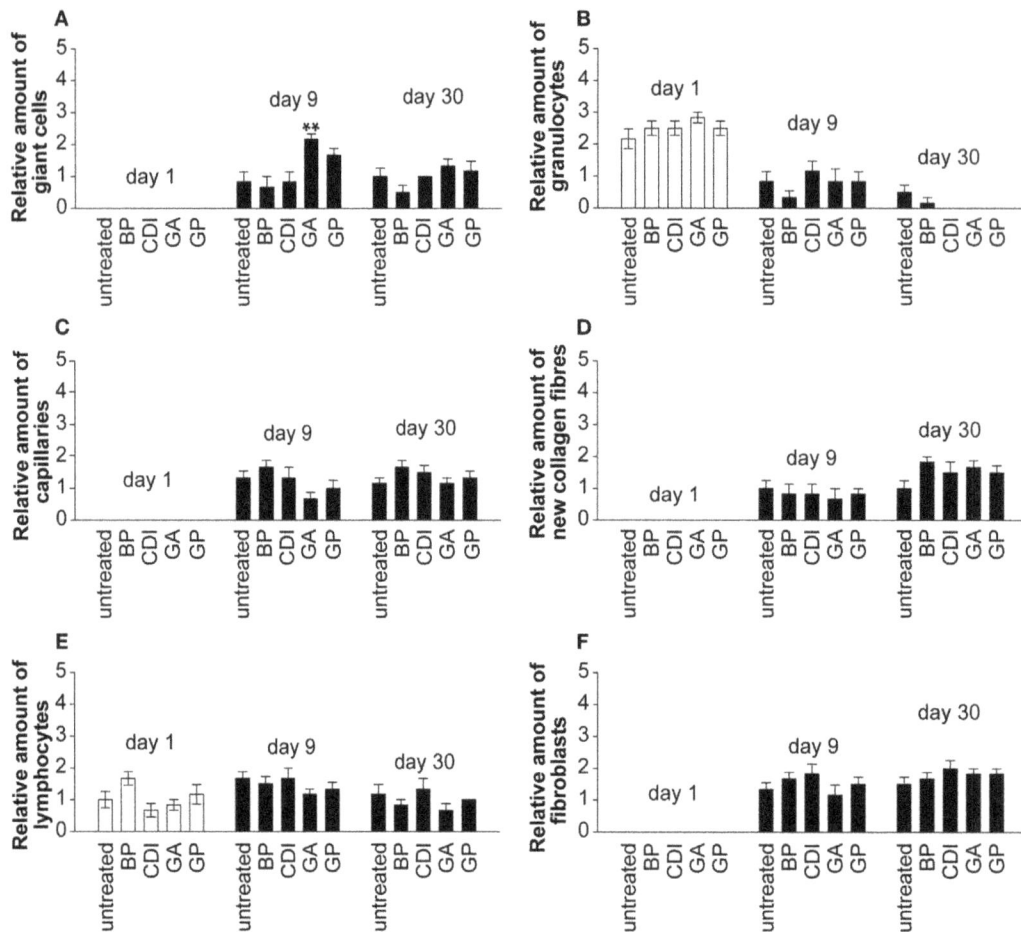

FIGURE 8 | Histological analysis of the degree of scaffold infiltration by giant cells (A), granulocytes (B), capillaries (C), collagen fibers (D), lymphocytes (E), and fibroblasts (F) at days 1, 9, and 30 post implantation. In all implants, an increase of infiltrating giant cells, lymphocytes, fibroblasts, capillaries, and collagen fibers could be detected over time. Furthermore, a decrease of infiltration by granulocytes could be observed in all implants at day 30 compared to day 1 post implantation. A blinded pathologist evaluated the presence of cells (granulocytes, lymphocytes, giant cells, and fibroblasts), capillaries and new collagen fibers and generated a semiquantitative score in repeat determination (0 = negative, 1 = mild, 2 = moderate, 3 = serve; n = 6/group and day; five microscopic fields per slide and rat; each 5 mm²). Untreated, untreated decellular ureteral tissue; BP, bovine pericardium (St. Jude, USA); GP, genipin; GA, glutaraldehyde; CDI, carbodiimide. **P < 0.01 vs. untreated decellular ureteral tissue.

growth conditions. After GP crosslink, an increase of ingrown cells was described compared to GA crosslink (Sung et al., 1999b; Koch et al., 2012), whereas signs of calcification were not detected in GP fixed tissue (Sung et al., 1999a). In the present study, we found a significantly increased ingrowth and multilayer formation of 3T3 and SMC after GP crosslinking compared to that in untreated scaffolds *in vitro*. In comparison to untreated scaffolds, CDI crosslinked scaffolds showed an increase of infiltrating 3T3-cells and multilayer formation as a sign of optimal environment comparable to GP-treated group. In contrast to recent studies, cells did not grow on lyophilized ureters (Kim et al., 2012; Woon et al., 2012); this might indicate that molecular characteristics were changed during lyophilization. On the basis of the facts, lyophilization could not be an optimal alternative to store ureteral scaffolds at this time. However, it would be relevant to analyze molecular changes after lyophilization of crosslinked scaffolds in further studies.

Inflammation, Tissue Resorption and Remodeling Processes Depend on Crosslinker *In Vivo*

In addition, it is fundamental to determine the host response after subcutaneous implantation of different crosslinked ureteral scaffolds. Since the scaffolds were decellular and morphologically intact, we could show in a subcutaneous rat model with decellular esophagus scaffolds that chronic rejection will not occur and implants are well tolerated (Koch et al., 2012). The present work supplements the biocompatible characteristics of acellular scaffolds by reseeding experiments, DNA analysis, and an SDS assay. At days 9 and 30 post implantation, signs of inflammation such as encapsulation and scaffold infiltration by macrophages and fibroblasts were observed and consistent with our expectations. We do not assume that DNA remnants of the scaffolds were the cause of inflammatory reactions in our experiments.

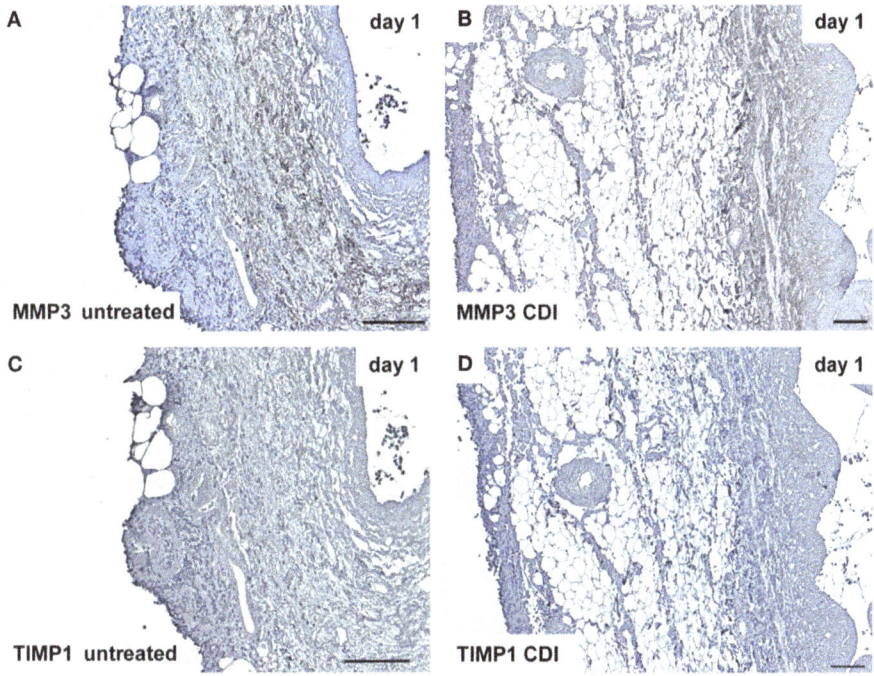

FIGURE 9 | Immunohistochemical DAB-staining of decellular CDI crosslinked implants for MMP3 and TIMP1 in comparison to chemical untreated scaffolds after 1, 9, and 30 days *in vivo* (*n* = 6/ day/group). One day post implantation, MMP3 were detectable in both untreated **(A)** and CDI crosslinked **(B)** scaffolds, whereas CDI crosslinked scaffolds showed a weaker intensity. However, scaffolds of both groups were negative for TIMP1 [untreated: **(C)**, CDI: **(D)**].

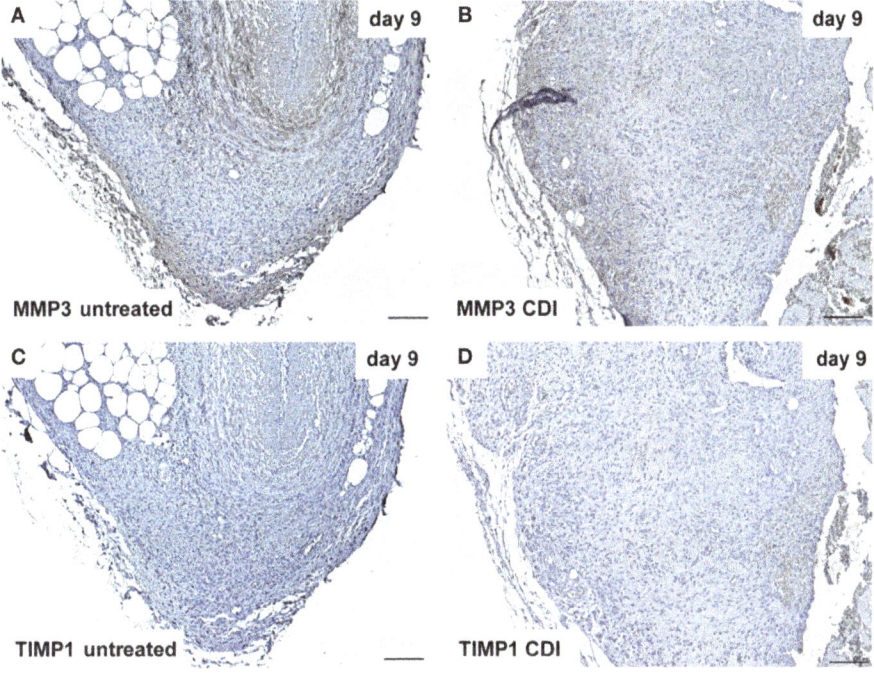

FIGURE 10 | Immunohistochemical DAB-staining of decellular CDI crosslinked implants for MMP3 and TIMP1 in comparison to chemical untreated scaffolds after 1, 9, and 30 days *in vivo* (*n* = 6/day/group). Nine days post-implantation, the rate of MMP3 [untreated: **(A)**, CDI: **(B)**] reactivity increased compared to post-operative day 1. TIMP1 reactivity could not be detected in both untreated **(C)** and crosslinked **(D)** scaffolds.

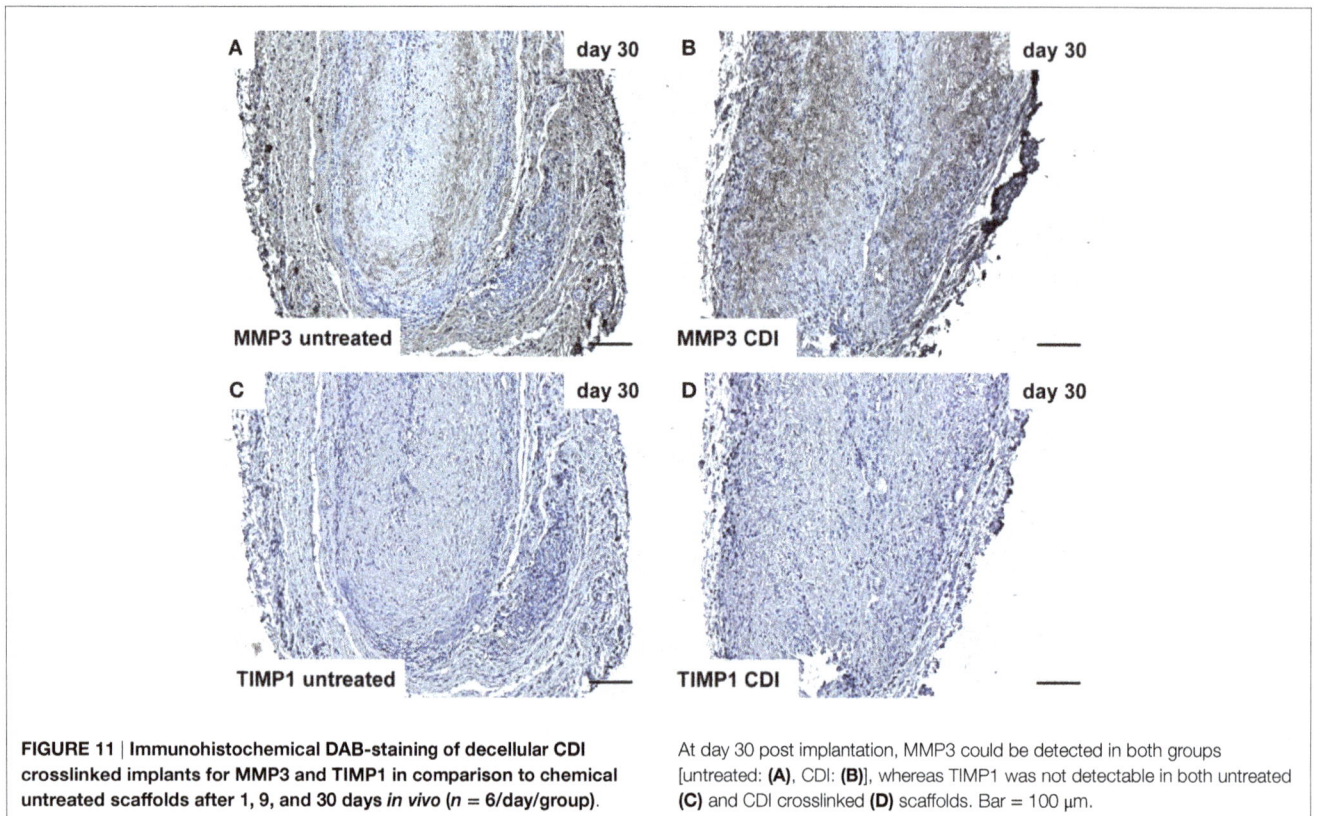

FIGURE 11 | **Immunohistochemical DAB-staining of decellular CDI crosslinked implants for MMP3 and TIMP1 in comparison to chemical untreated scaffolds after 1, 9, and 30 days *in vivo* (*n* = 6/day/group).** At day 30 post implantation, MMP3 could be detected in both groups [untreated: **(A)**, CDI: **(B)**], whereas TIMP1 was not detectable in both untreated **(C)** and CDI crosslinked **(D)** scaffolds. Bar = 100 µm.

After DNA extraction, we could not detect large remnant DNA fragments. Furthermore, we could show a reduction in remnant DNA of 91.2% compared to that of native ureters. In most biological material, remaining DNA consisted of fragments <300 bp, whereas DNA in our experiments almost disappeared. The small amount of remnant DNA is subject to fast enzymatic degradation *in vivo* (Badylak and Gilbert, 2008). It is more plausible, that free amino (–NH₂), carboxyl (–COOH) and hydroxyl (–OH) groups of collagen may be responsible for the immunological reactions (Sung et al., 1999b; Liang et al., 2004; Chang et al., 2005; Cao and Xu, 2008; Koch et al., 2012). These free groups can be bound by chemical crosslinking, which prevents the development of antigenic properties (Ye et al., 1996; Khor, 1997). Another side effect of crosslinking is an increase in mechanical stability. However, some crosslinking agents (e.g., GA) are toxic or promote the calcification of scaffolds *in vivo* (Khor, 1997; Sung et al., 1999a; Chang et al., 2002; Everaerts et al., 2008; Koch et al., 2012). In the present study, the crosslinkers GA, GP, and CDI were selected in accordance with descriptions of the biocompatibility in the recent literature (Khor, 1997; Sung et al., 1999b; Liang et al., 2004; Chang et al., 2005; Cao and Xu, 2008; Koch et al., 2012; Jeong et al., 2013).

Glutaraldehyde is an aggressive, indiscriminant crosslinking reagent that is commonly used in commercially available tissues (Badylak and Gilbert, 2008). GA crosslinked tissue exhibits a stabilized collagen matrix and decreased immunological reaction (Jeong et al., 2013; Awang et al., 2014). However, we observed that the immunological response (giant cells, CD68+ macrophages) in GA crosslinked ureteral scaffolds was higher compared to that

in chemically untreated scaffolds. Furthermore, the polarization of macrophages is important to the remodeling outcome. M1-activated macrophages produce inflammatory cytokines, which promote active inflammation and were associated with rejection reactions. In contrast, M2-activated macrophages (CD163+) are able to facilitate tissue repair and constructive remodeling (Mantovani et al., 2005; Brown et al., 2009; Chin et al., 2011). Macrophages are able to change their polarization in response to local stimuli during the process of wound healing (Mantovani et al., 2004; Stout and Suttles, 2005; Martinez et al., 2008; Kushiyama et al., 2011). The recognition of the predominant phenotype of macrophages provides an indication of scaffold rejection, inflammation, or acceptance after implantation. Interestingly, in contrast to the untreated, BP, and CDI groups, the CD163/CD68 ratio was decreased after GA treatment at day 30 post implantation. This might indicate a switch to a pro-inflammatory and destructive M1 macrophage phenotype after GA treatment. Furthermore, cellular toxicity and cytotoxic T-cell activation have been described after incomplete suppression of immunological actions of GA crosslinked scaffolds (Nishi et al., 1995; Chang et al., 2002; Kim et al., 2014; Manickam et al., 2014). On the other hand, cytotoxic effects of GA crosslinked scaffolds for host cells (fibrocytes, fibroblasts, and macrophages) were described (Huang et al., 1998). We did not observe any cytotoxic effect of GA crosslinked ureteral scaffolds on host fibroblasts or macrophages *in vivo*. In addition, further disadvantages of GA (e.g., scaffold calcification and depolymerization of GA crosslinks) have been reported (Khor, 1997; Schoen and Levy, 2005; Liu et al., 2014). The data suggest that

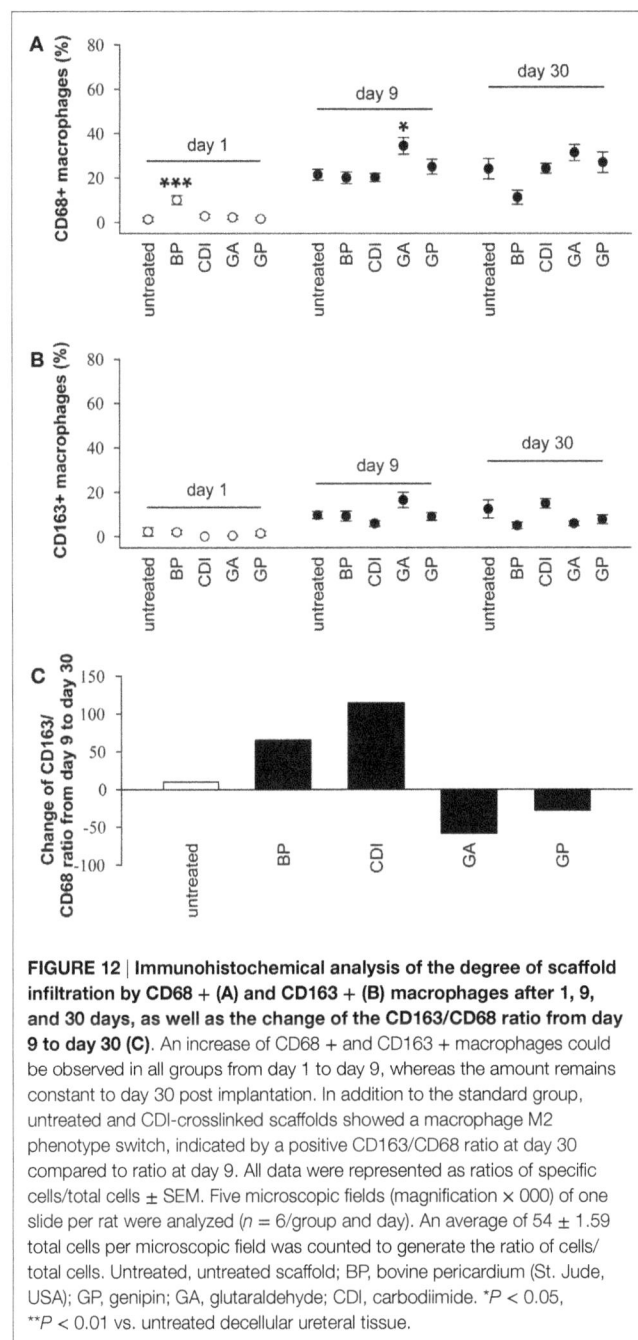

FIGURE 12 | Immunohistochemical analysis of the degree of scaffold infiltration by CD68 + (A) and CD163 + (B) macrophages after 1, 9, and 30 days, as well as the change of the CD163/CD68 ratio from day 9 to day 30 (C). An increase of CD68 + and CD163 + macrophages could be observed in all groups from day 1 to day 9, whereas the amount remains constant to day 30 post implantation. In addition to the standard group, untreated and CDI-crosslinked scaffolds showed a macrophage M2 phenotype switch, indicated by a positive CD163/CD68 ratio at day 30 compared to ratio at day 9. All data were represented as ratios of specific cells/total cells ± SEM. Five microscopic fields (magnification × 000) of one slide per rat were analyzed ($n = 6$/group and day). An average of 54 ± 1.59 total cells per microscopic field was counted to generate the ratio of cells/total cells. Untreated, untreated scaffold; BP, bovine pericardium (St. Jude, USA); GP, genipin; GA, glutaraldehyde; CDI, carbodiimide. $*P < 0.05$, $**P < 0.01$ vs. untreated decellular ureteral tissue.

GA was not an optimal crosslinker for constructive remodeling in the present study (e.g., giant cell and CD68 + macrophage infiltration *in vivo*, poor biocompatibility *in vitro*), which corresponds with other disadvantages described in the literature (Nishi et al., 1995; Huang et al., 1998; Koch et al., 2012).

Genipin has been widely used as a natural crosslinker as a substitute for chemical crosslinkers. It reacts with collagen amino groups and is approximately 10,000 times less cytotoxic than GA (Sung et al., 1999b). The stable GP crosslinked products protect against inflammation, degradation, react antiphlogistically and resulted in faster tissue regeneration compared to GA (Liang et al., 2004; Koo

et al., 2006; Li et al., 2012). Furthermore, a significantly decreased inflammatory response compared to untreated and GA crosslinked scaffolds is described after implantation of GP and GA crosslinked decellular bovine pericardia (Chang et al., 2002). However, in our subcutaneous rat model, we could show that macrophages were present in all scaffolds (untreated and crosslinked) at days 1, 9, and 30 post implantation. In contrast to previous studies (Koch et al., 2012), we also detected a M1 macrophage phenotype switch after GP crosslinking comparable to the GA group, indicating pro-inflammatory and destructive processes. In this way, our data suggest that GP was not the optimal crosslinker for constructive remodeling.

The alternative crosslinker, CDI, activates carboxyl groups for spontaneous reaction with primary amines of aspartic acid and glutamic acid residues of collagen, generating the crosslink (Khor, 1997). Furthermore, recent literature showed that tissue quality was improved, calcification was decreased and tissues offered a good biocompatibility (Khor, 1997). Based on these facts, it is not remarkable that CDI was also used in commercially available tissue products (Badylak and Gilbert, 2008). However, it was reported that CDI crosslinking caused a decrease in elasticity and mechanical toughness (Rafat et al., 2008). In this study, we did not analyze the mechanical properties, but we observed that CDI and GP fixed scaffolds exhibited only a moderate degradation. However, a predominant M1 macrophage phenotype was observed after implantation of CDI crosslinked esophagus scaffolds in a recent study (Koch et al., 2012). Interestingly, we detected a remarkable M2 macrophage phenotype switch after CDI crosslinking *in vivo*, which is known to be associated with constructive remodeling and tissue repair (Khor, 1997; Chang et al., 2002; Koch et al., 2012). Furthermore, the presence of pro-remodeling macrophages and fibroblasts might suggest host repair and constructive remodeling (Chin et al., 2011). Furthermore, the infiltration, survival, and living of the tissue-fibroblasts support the good biocompatibility of CDI scaffolds *in vivo*.

In addition, the activation of MMP3 and the inactivation of TIMP1 indicate remodeling and healthy processes and were also analyzed at each point of time. MMP3 degrades fibronectin, laminin, elastin, collagen (II, IV, IX, X, XI), and activates collagenase1 (Bullard et al., 1999; Shantha Kumara et al., 2014). MMP3 was synthesized by fibroblasts, activated macrophages and keratinocytes adjacent to sites of injury and was found in settings where active ECM remodeling occurs (Bullard et al., 1999). Furthermore, MMP3 can also activate other MMPs such as MMP1, MMP7, and MMP9, rendering MMP3 crucial in connective tissue remodeling (Ye et al., 1996). The enzyme is not only considered to be involved in wound repair but also in progression of atherosclerosis and tumor initiation (Shantha Kumara et al., 2014). In the present study, MMP3 was detectable in each group, whereas reactivity was decreased after crosslinking compared to untreated scaffolds, as a sign of increased stability, required for adequate constructive remodeling processes. The MMP3 reactivity after crosslinking (GA, GP, CDI) reached its maximum in the CDI group, at day 30 post-operative. TIMP1, a tissue inhibitor of metalloproteinases, is a glycoprotein that is expressed from several tissues of organisms, able to promote cell proliferation in a wide range of cell types, and might also have an anti-apoptotic function. In the present study, TIMP1 was not detected at any point in time.

Conclusion

We reported on morphology, *in vitro* biocompatibility, and immune response of tissue-engineered decellular porcine ureteral scaffolds, treated with different crosslinking agents. CDI crosslinked scaffolds exhibited a crucial M2-macrophage phenotype switch, activated MMP3, and inactivated TIMP1 *in vivo*. The results suggested constructive remodeling processes and an improved integration of ureteral scaffolds into their surrounding tissue after implantation. These results were supported by *in vitro* results: a high infiltration of different cells was observed in CDI and GP scaffolds. The sum of the data suggests that CDI offered most benefits for crosslinking ECM scaffolds. The results of the present study help to develop a new biocompatible ureteral xenograft. However, biomechanical data are necessary to investigate a ureteral

scaffold. In the future, we will design experiments to investigate biomechanical characteristics of decellularized tissue compared to native. Furthermore, studies such as large animal models should clarify the functionality of segmental CDI crosslinked ureteral scaffolds in the ureteral location. If this approach is successful, decellular ureteral scaffolds could be an important therapeutic tool for a wide range of applications (e.g., malignant tumor, ureteral stenosis, ureteral atresia, etc.).

Acknowledgments

The work presented in this paper was made possible by funding from the German Federal Ministry of Education and Research (BMBF number 1315883). Special thanks to Bettina Glatte and Ramona Blaschke for excellent laboratory work.

References

Adair-Kirk, T. L., and Senior, R. M. (2008). Fragments of extracellular matrix as mediators of inflammation. Int. J. Biochem. Cell Biol. 40, 1101–1110. doi:10.1016/j.biocel.2007.12.005

Allman, A. J., McPherson, T. B., Badylak, S. F., Merrill, L. C., Kallakury, B., Sheehan, C., et al. (2001). Xenogenic extracellular matrix grafts elicit a TH2-restricted immune response. Transplantation 71, 1631–1640. doi:10.1097/00007890-200106150-00024

Allman, A. J., McPherson, T. B., Merrill, L. C., Badylak, S. F., and Metzger, D. W. (2002). The Th2-restricted immune response to xenogenic small intestinal submucosa does not influence systemic protective immunity to viral and bacterial pathogens. Tissue Eng. 8, 53–62. doi:10.1089/107632702753503054

Awang, M. A., Firdaus, M. A., Busra, M. B., Chowdhury, S. R., Fadilah, N. R., Wan Hamirul, W. K., et al. (2014). Cytotoxic evaluation of biomechanically improved crosslinked ovine collagen on human dermal fibroblasts. Biomed. Mater. Eng. 24, 1715–1724. doi:10.3233/BME-140983

Badylak, S. F. (2004). Xenogenic extracellular matrix as a scaffold for tissue reconstruction. Transpl. Immunol. 12, 367–377. doi:10.1016/j.trim.2003.12.016

Badylak, S. F., and Gilbert, T. W. (2008). Immune response to biologic scaffold materials. Semin. Immunol. 20, 109–116. doi:10.1016/j.smim.2007.11.003

Block, N. L., Stover, E., and Politano, V. A. (1977). A prosthetic ureter in the dog. Trans. Am. Soc. Artif. Intern. Organs 23, 367–370. doi:10.1097/00002480-197700230-00094

Boari, A. (1894). Contribute sperementale alla plastica delle uretere. Atti. Accad. Fisiocrit Siena Med. Fis. 14, 444.

Boldt, A., Scholl, A., Garbade, J., Resetar, M. E., Mohr, F. W., Gummert, J. F., et al. (2006). ACE-inhibitor treatment attenuates atrial structural remodeling in patients with lone chronic atrial fibrillation. Basic Res. Cardiol. 101, 261–267. doi:10.1007/s00395-005-0571-2

Brown, B. N., Valentin, J. E., Stewart-Akers, A. M., McCabe, G.P., and Badylak, S. F. (2009). Macrophage phenotype and remodeling outcomes in response to biologic scaffolds with and without a cellular component. Biomaterials 30, 1482–1491. doi:10.1016/j.biomaterials.2008.11.040

Bullard, K. M., Lund, L., Mudgett, J. S., Mellin, T. N., Hunt, T. K., Murphy, B., et al. (1999). Impaired wound contraction in stromelysin-1 deficient mice. Ann. Surg. 230, 260–265. doi:10.1097/00000658-199908000-00017

Cao, H., and Xu, S. Y. (2008). EDC/NHS-crosslinked type II collagen-chondroitin sulfate scaffold: characterization and in vitro evaluation. J. Mater. Sci. Mater. Med. 19, 567–575. doi:10.1007/s10856-007-3281-5

Chang, Y., Hsu, C. K., Wei, H. J., Chen, S. C., Liang, H. C., Lai P. H., et al. (2005). Cell-free xenogenic vascular grafts fixed with glutaraldehyde or genipin: in vitro and in vivo studies. J. Biotechnol. 120, 207–219. doi:10.1016/j.jbiotec.2005.06.029

Chang, Y., Tsai, C. C., Liang, H. C., and Sung, H. W. (2002). In vivo evaluation of cellular and acellular bovine pericardia fixed with a naturally occurring crosslinking agent (genipin). Biomaterials 23, 2447–2457. doi:10.1016/S0142-9612(01)00379-9

Chin, L., Calabro, A., Rodriguez, E. R., Tan, C. D., Walker, E., and Derwin, K. A. (2011). Characterization of and host response to tyramine substituted-hyaluronan enriched fascia extracellular matrix. J. Mater. Sci. Mater. Med. 22, 1465–1477. doi:10.1007/s10856-011-4325-4

Corvin, S., Feil, G., and Stenzl, A. (2004). Tissue engineering of the urethra and ureter. Urologe A. 43, 1213–1216. doi:10.1007/s00120-004-0689-0

Dahms, S. E., Piechota, H. J., Nunes, L., Dahiya, R., Lue, T. F., and Tanagho, E. A. (1997). Free ureteral replacement in rats: regeneration of ureteral wall components in the acellular matrix graft. Urology 50, 818–825. doi:10.1016/S0090-4295(97)00391-9

del Pizzo, J. J., Jacobs, S. C., Bartlett, S. T., and Sklar, G. N. (1998). The use of bladder for total transplant ureteral reconstruction. J. Urol. 159, 750–752. doi:10.1016/S0022-5347(01)63719-4

Everaerts, F., Torrianni, M., Hendriks, M., and Feijen, J. (2008). Biomechanical properties of carbodiimide crosslinked collagen: influence of the formation of ester crosslinks. J. Biomed. Mater. Res. A 85, 547–555. doi:10.1002/jbm.a.31524

Gilbert, T. W., Sellaro, T. L., and Badylak, S. F. (2006). Decellularization of tissues and organs. Biomaterials 27, 3675–3683. doi:10.1016/j.biomaterials.2006.02.014

Huang, L. L., Sung, H. W., Tsai, C. C., and Huang, D. M. (1998). "Biocompatibility study of a biological tissue fixed with a naturally occurring crosslinking reagent. J. Biomed. Mater. Res. 42, 568–576. doi:10.1002/(SICI)1097-4636(19981215)42:4<568::AID-JBM13>3.0.CO;2-7

Jeong, S., Yoon, E. J., Lim, H. G., Sung, S. C., and Kim, Y. J. (2013). The effect of space fillers in the crosslinking processes of bioprosthesis. Biores. Open Access. 2, 98–106. doi:10.1089/biores.2012.0289

Khor, E. (1997). Methods for the treatment of collagenous tissues for bioprostheses. Biomaterials 18, 95–105. doi:10.1016/S0142-9612(96)00106-8

Kim, B. S., Choi, J. S., Kim, J. D., Choi, Y. C., and Cho, Y. W. (2012). Recellularization of decellularized human adipose-tissue-derived extracellular matrix sheets with other human cell types. Cell Tissue Res. 348, 559–567. doi:10.1007/s00441-012-1391-y

Kim, M., Takaoka, A., Hoang, Q. V., Trokel, S. L., and Paik, D. C. (2014). Pharmacologic alternatives to riboflavin photochemical corneal crosslinking: a comparison study of cell toxicity thresholds. Invest. Ophthalmol. Vis. Sci. 55, 3247–3257. doi:10.1167/iovs.13-13703

Koch, H., Graneist, C., Emmrich, F., Till, H., Metzger, R., Aupperle, H., et al. (2012). Xenogenic esophagus scaffolds fixed with several agents: comparative in vivo study of rejection and inflammation. J. Biomed. Biotechnol. 2012, 948320. doi:10.1155/2012/948320

Konakci, K. Z., Bohle, B., Blumer, R., Hoetzenecker, W., Roth, G., Moser, B., et al. (2005). Alpha-Gal on bioprostheses: xenograft immune response in cardiac surgery. Eur. J. Clin. Invest. 35, 17–23. doi:10.1111/j.1365-2362.2005.01441.x

Koo, H. J., Lim, K. H., Jung, H. J., and Park, E. H. (2006). Anti-inflammatory evaluation of gardenia extract, geniposide and genipin. J. Ethnopharmacol. 103, 496–500. doi:10.1016/j.jep.2005.08.011

Kushiyama, T., Oda, T., Yamada, M., Higashi, K., Yamamoto, K., Sakurai, Y., et al. (2011). Alteration in the phenotype of macrophages in the repair of renal interstitial fibrosis in mice. Nephrology (Carlton) 16, 522–535. doi:10.1111/j.1440-1797.2010.01439.x

Li, C. C., Hsiang, C. Y., Lo, H. Y., Pai, F. T., Wu, S. L., and Ho, T. Y. (2012). Genipin inhibits lipopolysaccharide-induced acute systemic inflammation in mice as evidenced by nuclear factor-κB bioluminescent imaging-guided transcriptomic analysis. Food Chem. Toxicol. 50, 2978–2986. doi:10.1016/j.fct.2012.05.054

Liang, H. C., Chang, Y., Hsu, C. K., Lee, M. H., and Sung, H. W. (2004). Effects of crosslinking degree of an acellular biological tissue on its tissue regeneration pattern. *Biomaterials* 25, 3541–3552. doi:10.1016/j.biomaterials.2003.09.109

Lider, O., Hershkoviz, R., and Kachalsky, S. G. (1995). Interactions of migrating T lymphocytes, inflammatory mediators, and the extracellular matrix. *Crit. Rev. Immunol.* 15, 271–283. doi:10.1615/CritRevImmunol.v15.i3-4.50

Liu, J., Zhong, S., Lan, H., Meng, X., Zhang, H., Fan, Y., et al. (2014). Mapping the calcification of bovine pericardium in rat model by enhanced micro-computed tomography. *Biomaterials* 35, 8305–8311. doi:10.1016/j.biomaterials.2014.06.026

Manickam, B., Sreedharan, R., and Elumalai, M. (2014). 'Genipin' – the natural water soluble crosslinking agent and its importance in the modified drug delivery systems: an overview. *Curr. Drug Deliv.* 11, 139–145. doi:10.2174/15672018113106660059

Mantovani, A., Sica, A., and Locati, M. (2005). Macrophage polarization comes of age. *Immunity* 23, 344–346. doi:10.1016/j.immuni.2005.10.001

Mantovani, A., Sica, A., Sozzani, S., Allavena P., Vecchi, A., and Locati, M. (2004). The chemokine system in diverse forms of macrophage activation and polarization. *Trends Immunol.* 25, 677–686. doi:10.1016/j.it.2004.09.015

Martinez, F. O., Sica, A., Mantovani, A., and Locati, M. (2008). Macrophage activation and polarization. *Front. Biosci.* 13:453–461. doi:10.2741/2692

Morwood, S. R., and Nicholson, L. B. (2006). Modulation of the immune response by extracellular matrix proteins. *Arch. Immunol. Ther. Exp.* (*Warsz*) 54, 367–374. doi:10.1007/s00005-006-0043-x

Nishi, C., Nakajima, N., and Ikada, Y. (1995). In vivo evaluation of cytotoxicity of diepoxy compounds used for biomaterial modification. *J. Biomed. Mater. Res.* 29, 829–834. doi:10.1002/jbm.820290707

Rafat, M., Li, F., Fagerholm P., Lagali, N. S., Watsky, M. A., Munger, R., et al. (2008). PEG-stabilized carbodiimide crosslinked collagen-chitosan hydrogels for corneal tissue engineering. *Biomaterials* 29, 3960–3972. doi:10.1016/j.biomaterials.2008.06.017

Schlote, N., Wefer, J., and Sievert, K. D. (2004). Acellular matrix for functional reconstruction of the urogenital tract. Special form of "tissue engineering"? *Urologe A.* 43, 1209–1212. doi:10.1007/s00120-004-0695-2

Schoen, F. J., and Levy, R. J. (2005). Calcification of tissue heart valve substitutes: progress toward understanding and prevention. *Ann. Thorac. Surg.* 79, 1072–1080. doi:10.1016/j.athoracsur.2004.06.033

Shantha Kumara, H. M., Gaita, D. J., Miyagaki, H., Yan, X., Herath, S. A., Cekic, V., et al. (2014). Minimally invasive colorectal resection is associated with significantly elevated levels of plasma matrix metalloproteinase 3 (MMP-3) during the first month after surgery which may promote the growth of residual metastases. *Surg. Endosc.* 28, 3322–3328. doi:10.1007/s00464-014-3612-9

Sofer, M., Rowe, E., Forder, D. M., and Denstedt, J. D. (2002). Ureteral segmental replacement using multilayer porcine small-intestinal submucosa. *J. Endourol.* 16, 27–31. doi:10.1089/089277902753483682

Stout, R. D., and Suttles, J. (2005). Immunosenescence and macrophage functional plasticity: dysregulation of macrophage function by age-associated microenvironmental changes. *Immunol. Rev.* 205, 60–71. doi:10.1111/j.0105-2896.2005.00260.x

Sullivan, L. D., Masterson, J. S., and Wright, J. E. (1982). Vesicopsoas hitch: a versatile procedure. *Can. J. Surg.* 25, 26–29.

Sung, H. W., Chang, Y., Chiu, C. T., Chen, C. N., and Liang, H. C. (1999a). Crosslinking characteristics and mechanical properties of a bovine pericardium fixed with a naturally occurring crosslinking agent. *J. Biomed. Mater. Res.* 47, 116–126. doi:10.1002/(SICI)1097-4636(199911)47:2<116::AID-JBM2>3.0.CO;2-J

Sung, H. W., Huang, R. N., Huang, L. L., and Tsai, C. C. (1999b). In vitro evaluation of cytotoxicity of a naturally occurring crosslinking reagent for biological tissue fixation. *J. Biomater. Sci. Polym. Ed.* 10, 63–78. doi:10.1163/156856299X00289

Takeuchi, M., Masumori, N., and Tsukamoto, T. (2014). Ureteral reconstruction with bowel segments: experience with eight patients in a single institute. *Korean J. Urol.* 55, 742–749. doi:10.4111/kju.2014.55.11.742

Tanemura, M., Yin, D., Chong, A. S., and Galili, U. (2000). Differential immune responses to alpha-gal epitopes on xenografts and allografts: implications for accommodation in xenotransplantation. *J. Clin. Invest.* 105, 301–310. doi:10.1172/JCI7358

Ulm, A. H., and Krauss, L. (1960). Total unilateral teflon ureteral substitutes in the dog. *J. Urol.* 83, 575–582.

Valentin, J. E., Badylak, J. S., McCabe, G. P., and Badylak, S. F. (2006). Extracellular matrix bioscaffolds for orthopaedic applications. A comparative histologic study. *J. Bone Joint Surg. Am.* 88, 2673–2686. doi:10.2106/JBJS.E.01008

Warwick, R. T., and Worth P. H. (1969). The psoas bladder-hitch procedure for the replacement of the lower third of the ureter. *Br. J. Urol.* 41, 701–709. doi:10.1111/j.1464-410X.1969.tb09981.x

Wolff, B., Chartier-Kastler, E., Mozer P., Haertig, A., Bitker, M. O., and Rouprêt, M. (2011). Long-term functional outcomes after ileal ureter substitution: a single-center experience. *Urology* 78, 692–695. doi:10.1016/j.urology.2011.04.054

Woon, C. Y., Farnebo, S., Schmitt, T., Kraus, A., Megerle, K., Pham, H., et al. (2012). Human flexor tendon tissue engineering: revitalization of biostatic allograft scaffolds. *Tissue Eng. Part A* 18, 2406–2417. doi:10.1089/ten.TEA.2012.0152

Ye, S., Eriksson P., Hamsten, A., Kurkinen, M., Humphries, S. E., and Henney, A. M. (1996). Progression of coronary atherosclerosis is associated with a common genetic variant of the human stromelysin-1 promoter which results in reduced gene expression. *J. Biol. Chem.* 1, 13055–13060.

Conflict of Interest Statement: The authors declare that the research was conducted in the absence of any commercial or financial relationships that could be construed as a potential conflict of interest.

19

High-resolution X-ray techniques as new tool to investigate the 3D vascularization of engineered-bone tissue

Inna Bukreeva[1], Michela Fratini[1,2], Gaetano Campi[3], Daniele Pelliccia[4,5,6], Raffaele Spanò[7], Giuliana Tromba[8], Francesco Brun[8,9], Manfred Burghammer[10,11], Marco Grilli[12,13], Ranieri Cancedda[7], Alessia Cedola[1] and Maddalena Mastrogiacomo[7]*

[1] Consiglio Nazionale delle Ricerche – Istituto NANOTEC, c/o Dipartimento di Fisica, Università Sapienza, Rome, Italy, [2] Department of Science, Roma Tre University, Rome, Italy, [3] Istituto di Cristallografia, Consiglio Nazionale delle Ricerche, Rome, Italy, [4] School of Applied Sciences, RMIT University, Melbourne, VIC, Australia, [5] Australian Synchrotron, Clayton, VIC, Australia, [6] School of Physics and Astronomy, Monash University, Clayton, VIC, Australia, [7] Dipartimento di Medicina Sperimentale dell'Università di Genova, AOU San Martino-IST, Genova, Italy, [8] Elettra – Synchrotron Radiation Trieste S.C.p.A, Trieste, Italy, [9] Dipartimento di Ingegneria e Architettura, Università di Trieste, Trieste, Italy, [10] European Synchrotron Radiation Facility, Grenoble, France, [11] Department of Analytical Chemistry, Ghent University, Ghent, Belgium, [12] Dipartimento di Fisica, Università Sapienza, Rome, Italy, [13] Consiglio Nazionale delle Ricerche – Istituto dei Sistemi Complessi, c/o Dipartimento di Fisica, Università Sapienza, Rome, Italy

Edited by:
Mauro Alini,
AO Foundation, Switzerland

Reviewed by:
Arnaud Scherberich,
University Hospital Basel, Switzerland
Marietta Herrmann,
AO Foundation, Switzerland
Vincent A. Stadelmann,
AO Foundation, Switzerland

*Correspondence:
Maddalena Mastrogiacomo,
Largo Rosanna Benzi,
10 16132 Genova, Italy
maddalena.mastrogiacomo@.unige.it

The understanding of structure–function relationships in normal and pathologic mammalian tissues is at the basis of a tissue engineering (TE) approach for the development of biological substitutes to restore or improve tissue function. In this framework, it is interesting to investigate engineered bone tissue, formed when porous ceramic constructs are loaded with bone marrow stromal cells (BMSC) and implanted *in vivo*. To monitor the relation between bone formation and vascularization, it is important to achieve a detailed imaging and a quantitative description of the complete three-dimensional vascular network in such constructs. Here, we used synchrotron X-ray phase-contrast micro-tomography to visualize and analyze the three-dimensional micro-vascular networks in bone-engineered constructs, in an ectopic bone formation mouse-model. We compared samples seeded and not seeded with BMSC, as well as samples differently stained or unstained. Thanks to the high quality of the images, we investigated the 3D distribution of both vessels and collagen matrix and we obtained quantitative information for all different samples. We propose our approach as a tool for quantitative studies of angiogenesis in TE and for any pre-clinical investigation where a quantitative analysis of the vascular network is required.

Keywords: X-ray phase-contrast tomography, tissue engineering, vascularization, X-ray micro-diffraction, bone tissue

Introduction

Tissue Engineering (TE) is the biotechnology that combines aspects of medicine, biology, and engineering to generate, repair, or replace human tissues. In particular, the TE approach may be used to regenerate bone by implanting a porous ceramic scaffold combined with bone marrow stromal cells (BMSC) *in vivo*. The scaffold plays a fundamental role since it acts as a guide and it stimulates the growth thus creating TE constructs or living bio-composites (Hench and Polak, 2002; Cancedda et al., 2003). An ideal scaffold should present high porosity, maximum surface area for bone growth, and an interconnected pore space with pores having a sufficiently large size to allow the penetration and diffusion of the blood vessels (Quarto et al., 2001). Indeed, the efficiency of an artificially implanted construct depends on the timely delivery and exchange of nutrients (oxygen, glucose, amino acids, etc.) from surrounding blood vessels to the BMSC, and the contemporary removal of the metabolism waste products (CO_2, lactate, and urea) (Carano and Filvaroff, 2003; Jain, 2003). Therefore, the control of the angiogenesis of the microvascular network with proper spatial organization is a key step to obtain tissue regeneration and repair (Carano and Filvaroff, 2003). Furthermore, a deeper understanding of the developmental neo-vascularization is necessary for a better treatment of many pathological conditions, including cancer, diabetes, psoriasis, and articular degeneration.

In this framework, the need to detect subtle changes in tissue microvasculature requires the use of minimally invasive and bulk-sensitive experimental techniques. Currently, conventional characterization techniques have limitations: 2D imaging, such as histology, yields incomplete spatial coverage with possible data misinterpretation, whereas conventional micro-computed tomography (micro-CT) does not achieve sufficient resolution and contrast. In particular, it is virtually impossible to observe blood vessels by conventional X-ray imaging techniques without using contrast agents (Plouraboue et al., 2004; Risser et al., 2007). Recently, new contrast agent method for the synchrotrons radiation X-ray imaging of organisms was developed. As example, the micro-bubble was applied as a phase-contrast agent for angiography applications (Tang et al., 2011). Thus, a 3D imaging spanning from a few millimeters to hundreds of nanometers, able to discriminate the smallest micro-capillaries and the volume of the scaffold with and without invasive contrast agent and without aggressive sample preparation, is extremely desirable.

Conventional X-ray radiography and tomography are well established tool for imaging the internal structure of thick objects, based on absorption properties of the sample. The average thickness and 3D distribution of newly formed bone, at different implantation times, as well as scaffold modifications occurring after implantation, have been largely investigated by synchrotron radiation techniques (Komlev et al., 2006; Mastrogiacomo et al., 2007). Other authors reported *in vivo* quantification of blood vessels in mice, ranging from largest to smallest structures using contrast-enhanced micro-CT for studying the physiological and pathological processes (Nebuloni et al., 2014).

Nevertheless, for weakly absorbing materials (like biological materials), the X-ray attenuation due to the sample becomes often too small to give detectable contrasts. A better contrast can be obtained by imaging the phase modulation induced by the sample in a coherent or partial coherent beam (Cloetens et al., 1996; Di Fonzo et al., 1998). In this case, the phase contrast can be up to 1000 times higher than the absorption contrast (Bravin et al., 2013). The tomography provides the additional benefit to discriminate the different depths inside the sample and to provide a map of the different layers.

In addition, the combination of different investigation techniques (Cedola et al., 2014) on the same sample provides a deeper understanding. In particular, the combination of X-ray micro-diffraction (XRμD) (Cedola et al., 2006) and synchrotron X-ray phase-contrast micro-tomography (Bravin et al., 2013) (XRPCμT) allows to combine the structural information of the regenerated bone system, obtained by XRμD, with the micrometer morphological information obtained by XRPCμT.

The X-ray diffraction is the main technique suitable for studying the atomic order in the matter. It is based on the constructive interference of hard X-ray scattered by the atomic distribution of the sample (Giacovazzo et al., 1993).

In this work, we use high-resolution in-line propagation XRPCμT for imaging the 3D vascular network in bone-engineered constructs, in an ectopic bone formation mouse-model using different staining preparation: (i) with MICROFIL® (Flowtech, Inc., Carver, Massachusetts) (Zagorchev et al., 2010; Ehling et al., 2014); (ii) with phosphotungstic acid (PTA) (Descamps et al., 2014); (iii) without staining. The synchrotron XRPCμT was able to visualize the 3D vascularization network inside the scaffold, without any sample sectioning.

With the aim to provide additional structural information (Campi et al., 2012, 2013), and in order to characterize the well-packed collagen fibers inside the scaffold pores, the X-ray tomographic study was complemented with scanning XRμD. To show the applicability of the technique in different experimental conditions, this combined technique was applied to samples that underwent different staining procedures.

The high quality of the images enabled the extraction of a quantitative information for all the different sample preparations.

In this study, our goal was mainly methodological and we investigated by the combined technique only one sample for each experimental group. However, in addition to show the validity of the method, we were able to obtain also some biological information. Although a statistically significant biological study was far from the scope of the work, we were able to successfully demonstrate the effectiveness of the XRPCμT approach to understand angiogenesis in the engineered bone tissues representative of all experimental groups.

Materials and Methods

Sample Preparation

All experimental animal procedures were carried out in the IRCCS AOU San Martino – IST Animal Facility (Genoa, Italy), in the respect of the national current regulations regarding the protection of animals used for scientific purpose (D.lgsvo 27/01/1992, n. 116). Research protocols have been evaluated and approved by the IRCCS AOU San Martino – IST *Ethical Committee for animal experimentation (CSEA)* as Animal use project n. 336 communicated to The Italian Ministry of Health, having regard to the article 7 of the D.lgs 116/92.

The studied scaffold was Skelite™ (Millenium Biologix Corp., Kingston, Canada), which is a bone graft substitute containing silicon in the form of Si-TCP, and consisting of approximately 67% Si-TCP and 33% HA/B-TCP. The scaffolds were seeded with *ex vivo* expanded sheep BMSC and implanted subcutaneously on the back of immuno-compromised mice (CD-1 nu/nu mice, females, Charles River) according to the methods previously described by Martin[14].

Cell Isolation

Bone marrow aspirates were harvested from the posterior iliac crest of each animal (female sheep of Italian Biellese strain) under approval of the competent ethical committee and legal authorities. Bone marrow samples were washed twice with PBS (phosphate buffered saline). Marrow specimens were stained with a nuclear stain (0.1% methyl violet in 0.1 M citric acid) and the nucleated fraction was counted. Cells were suspended in Coon's modified Ham's F12 medium supplemented with 10% FCS, 100 IU/ml penicillin, and 100 mg/ml streptomycin and plated at a density of 1×10^6 cells/cm^2. Human recombinant fibroblast growth factor 2 (FGF2) (1 ng/ml) was added since the beginning of the culture. Medium was changed 2 days after the original plating and then twice a week. When cells in the culture dishes were nearly confluent (passage 0), BMSC were detached with 0.05% trypsin–0.01% EDTA and 5×10^5 cells were replated in 100-mm dishes (passage 1). At the next confluence, BMSC were detached and used for implants in immuno-deficient (ID) (CD-1 nu/nu) mice.

Cell Seeding

After 3–4 weeks of *in vitro* expansion, sheep BMSC were detached from the Petri dishes with 0.05% trypsin and 0.01% EDTA, washed in serum-free medium, and resuspended at 2.5×10^6 cells/20 μl of fibrinogen solution. The cell suspension was seeded onto each cube of biomaterial (3 mm × 3 mm × 3 mm) and 20 μl of thrombin were added (Tissucol, Baxter, Vienna, Austria). The polymerization reaction was allowed to proceed at 37°C for 10 min, then bioceramic/BMSC composites were subcutaneously implanted in ID mice.

Animal Surgery

Mice were cared and treated according to institutional guidelines approved by the IRCCS AOU San Martino – IST Ethical Committee for animal experimentation (CSEA), in the respect of the national current regulations regarding the protection of animals used for scientific purpose (D.lgs 27/01/1992, n. 116) and communicated to the Italian Ministry of Health, having regard to the article 7 of the D.lgs 116/92. Animals were anesthetized by intraperitoneal injection of ketamine (80–100 mg/kg) and xilazine (5–10 mg/kg). At the end of *the selected implantation time* scaffolds were removed from the host animals for analysis.

All *in vivo* experiments were performed in triplicate, but only one sample for each group was XRPCµT analyzed. As control, one group of scaffolds was implanted without sheep BMSC pre-seeding. Four groups of mice were analyzed as reported in Table I in **Figure 1B**: (A) no BMSC pre-seeding and perfusion with MICROFIL®; (B) BMSC pre-seeding and perfusion with MICROFIL®, a low-viscosity radio opaque polymer (Flowtech, Inc., Carver, Massachusetts) well suited for vascularization studies; (C) BMSC pre-seeding and staining with PTA (PTA solution, Sigma-Aldrich Corp., St. Louis, MO, USA); (D) BMSC pre-seeding and perfusion with saline.

The animals perfused by MICROFIL® at 4 weeks received an intraperitoneal injection of anesthetics (ketamine 80–100 mg/kg and xilazine 5–10 mg/kg) before the treatment. First, to eliminate the blood from the vessels, a solution of heparin 50 U/ml in 0.9% sodium chloride solution was perfused from the left ventricle until the outgoing liquid from the right atrium became clear. Then, a solution of MICROFIL® was injected in the same way with a combination of MV compounds: MV diluent was mixed to MV-130 Red (4:5), with the final addiction of 1/20 of MV curing agent. At the end of perfusion, animals were sacrificed and transferred overnight at 4°C to allow the solidification of the MICROFIL® agent. One day after the perfusion, the scaffolds were recovered from the animal, fixed with a solution of 4% paraformaldehyde for 2 days and maintained in 70% alcohol. For the saline perfusion, the same procedure was followed but the mice were perfused with 0.9% NaCl solution instead of the MICROFIL® agent. For the PTA staining, the scaffolds recovered from the mice were directly placed in a solution containing 0.7% PTA diluted in 70% ethanol for 12 h and kept under slow rotation (Martin et al., 1997). The samples were then transferred to fresh 70% ethanol. For each experimental condition, after the XRPCµT analysis, a chosen sample was dehydrated in ethanol at increasing concentration, embedded in methylmethacrylate and transversally cut using a diamond saw (Gillings–Hamco, Hamco

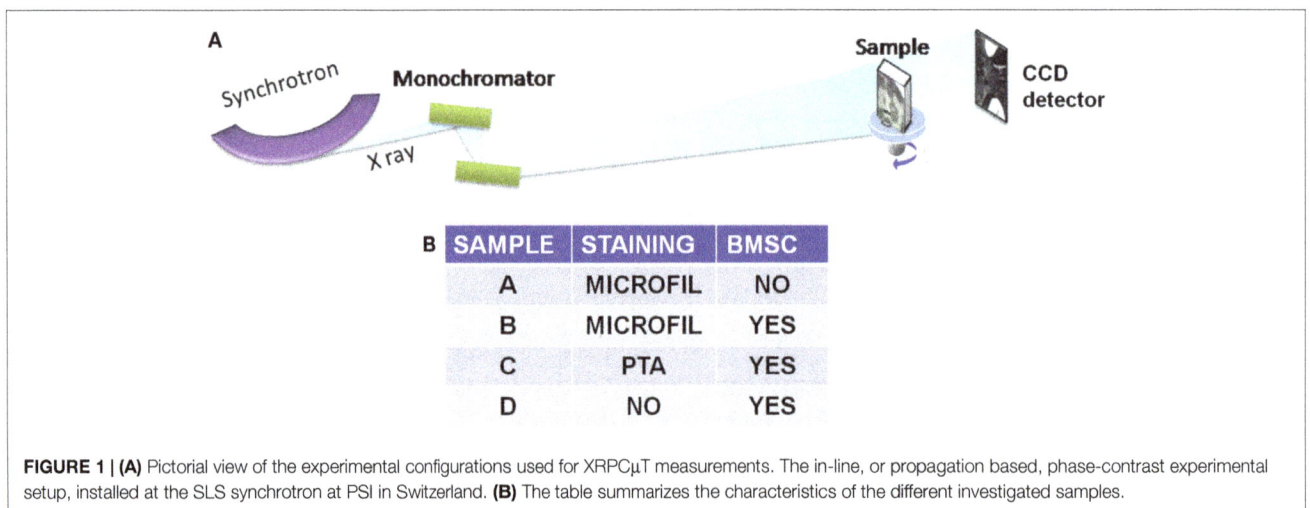

	SAMPLE	STAINING	BMSC
	A	MICROFIL	NO
	B	MICROFIL	YES
	C	PTA	YES
	D	NO	YES

FIGURE 1 | (A) Pictorial view of the experimental configurations used for XRPCµT measurements. The in-line, or propagation based, phase-contrast experimental setup, installed at the SLS synchrotron at PSI in Switzerland. **(B)** The table summarizes the characteristics of the different investigated samples.

Machines, Inc., Rochester, NY, USA) in serial sections ($\approx 150\,\mu m$ thick) for the SXRμD measurements.

X-Ray Phase-Contrast Tomography Measurements

Among the different approaches for XRPCμT (Diemoz et al., 2012), in this work we used in-line free space propagation to reach high spatial resolution for the detection of micro-vessels. This technique is based on the interference fringes produced by the differently refracted beams crossing the sample. Therefore, this technique transforms the phase variation due to the object refraction index in intensity modulation directly detectable by a CCD camera. Suitable algorithms of phase retrieval allow to recover the object refraction index starting from the interference fringes produced by the object itself.

The experiment was carried out at TOMCAT beamline at the Swiss Light Source (SLS) in Villigen (Switzerland). The monochromatic incident X-ray energy was 24 keV and a CCD camera with a pixel size of about 0.64 microns was set at a distance of 5 cm from the sample. The tomography has been acquired with 1601 projections covering a total angle range of 360°. The setup does not comprise optical X-ray elements. For this reason, the spatial resolution is only limited by the detector resolution.

On the other hand, the image captured by in-line propagation always contains mixed absorption and phase-contrast effects. Therefore, specific algorithm must be used to decouple (at least in part) absorption from phase information (Paganin et al., 2002). The phase retrieval algorithm proposed by Paganin et al. (2002) was applied to all projections of the tomographic measurements prior to the slices reconstruction.

Quantitative Analysis of X-Ray Phase-Contrast Tomography

Once the sample volume was reconstructed from the acquired projections, a stack of reconstructed slices of the sample was obtained. The quantitative analysis of the tomographic volumes, to obtain the number and section of the vessels as a function of the depth inside the sample (Plot 1 and Plot 2), was performed exploiting the software *ImageJ*. This software, developed for the image treatment, allows for the visualization and analysis of each reconstructed slice of the stack. The number of branches was calculated exploiting *Skeleton*, a plugin of *ImageJ*. Before applying *Skeleton*, a proper segmentation of the vessels (performed with the software *Volview*) was necessary.

Since within each group, preliminary analyses by histology had shown a high consistency in the data for all scaffolds, the XRPCμT analysis was performed on one selected scaffold for each of the four mice groups. In all cases, data obtained from the XRPCμT analysis of the selected scaffold were comparable to the data derived from the histology analysis of the other scaffolds of the group.

Scanning X-Ray Micro-Diffraction Measurements

We used scanning XRμD for the investigation of the periodical assembly of collagen fibrils in the implanted constructs. Scaffold sections with a thickness of about 100 μm were measured on the ID13 beamline of the European Synchrotron Radiation Facility, ESRF, France. The scanning micro-diffraction setup was constituted by a double-crystal monochromator and a Kirkpatrick–Baez mirror as focusing system, producing a beam size of $1\mu m \times 1\,\mu m$ with a wavelength of 0.976 Å. 2D diffraction patterns were recorded in transmission by a FreLon CCD detector (2048×2048 pixels with size $50\,\mu m^2$) placed at a distance of 110 cm from the sample with an acquisition time of 5s. In this way, we achieved a q range of $[0.5–30]$ nm^{-1} to measure simultaneously the small-angle X-ray scattering and the wide angle X-ray scattering. 2D diffraction patterns have been radially and azimuthally integrated to provide 1D profiles of intensity, I(q), vs. transfer moment, $q = 4\pi \sin(\theta)/\lambda$, and angular intensity distribution I(Φ). We focused on the collagen signal collected at medium angle scattering around $q = 5.6$ nm^{-1}. The samples were scanned by piezo-scanning stage with 0.1 micron repeatability.

The collagen equatorial reflection was modeled with a Gaussian added to second-order polynomial background. The peak position q_C gives the lateral spacing, $D = 2\pi/q_C$, while the area under the peak accounts the total collagen mass. The orientation degree of the collagen molecules are given by the area under the peaks of the azimuthal profiles I(Φ). The total area under the I(Φ) curve is the sum of the area under the peaks, A_Φ, which is proportional to the fraction of aligned molecules, and the area under the constant background (dotted line), A_{BKG}, which is proportional to the fraction of randomly oriented molecules. The orientation degree, corresponding to the fraction of the aligned molecules can be defined as the ratio A_Φ/A_{BKG}.

Results

XRPCμCT Analysis

In order to investigate by XRPCμT the 3D micro-vessels distribution inside the scaffold, a high spatial resolution is required. For this reason, we used the in-line propagation setup of the TOMCAT beamline at SLS, sketched in **Figure 1**, able to achieve a spatial resolution of 0.64 μm. In the table shown in **Figure 1B**, we reported the characteristics of the different investigated sample groups. **Figure 2** shows details of the vessels distribution inside representative samples from the four different groups implanted for 4 weeks in the mice. The first two samples (A and B) were both stained with MICROFIL®, a compound that fills and enhances the opacity of the micro-vascular network. In sample A, no BMSC were seeded on the scaffold, whereas the scaffold of sample B was seeded with BMSC. Sample C was also seeded with BMSC, but, after its recovery from the animal, it was stained with PTA. PTA enhances the soft tissue (ST) signal and thus it was expected to improve the visualization of both the vessels entering the scaffold pores and the collagenous matrix (Campi et al., 2013). **Figure 2D** displays the tomographic image of the sample D, which was seeded with BMSC (like B and C samples), but neither it was prepared with MICROFIL®, nor it underwent staining treatment.

In **Figure 2A**, the vessels in the sample A are rendered in red, the scaffold in blue, and the ST in yellow and green. The inset of **Figure 2A** shows a close-up of a vessel filled with MICROFIL® where bone is not formed. Vessels penetrate the scaffold pores, but at first sight a poor branching is already evident. **Figure 2B** shows the 3D volume of the sample B. The inset of the figure highlights a

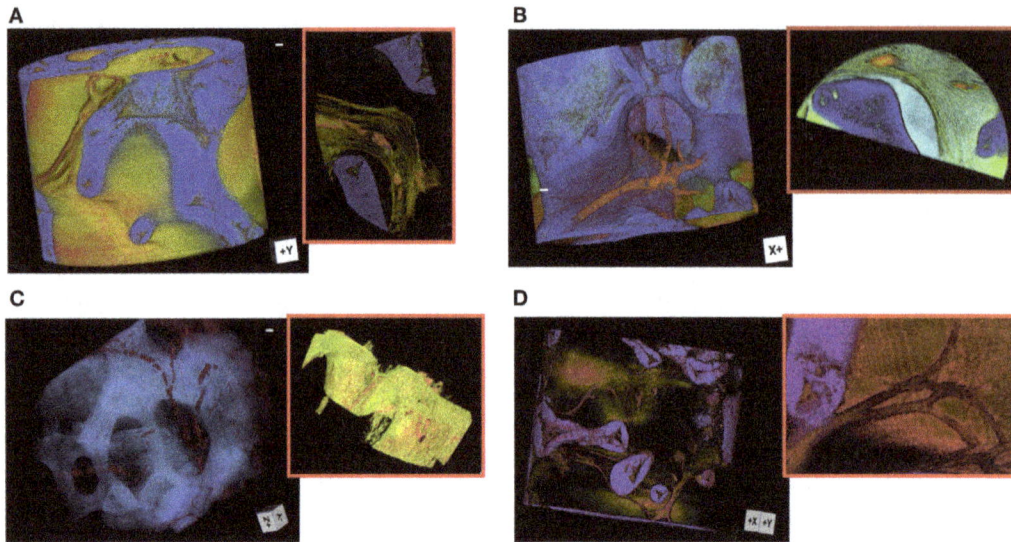

FIGURE 2 | Vessels distributions inside four different samples implanted for 4 weeks in the mice. The size-bar corresponds to 30 μm. The first two samples, A and B, were both prepared with MICROFILL® but, while the sample A was not pre-seeded with BMSCs before implantation, the sample B was pre-seeded with BMSCs. The sample C was also pre-seeded with BMSCs, but after the recovery of the scaffold from the animal it was stained with PTA. The sample D was a BMSC seeded not stained sample. **(A)** The vessels in the sample A are rendered in red, the scaffold in blue, and the soft tissue in yellow and green. The inset shows the main vessel partially filled with MICROFIL®. **(B)** The 3D volume of the sample B was reported. The inset shows a very intricate collagen matrix (rendered in yellow) coexists with the vessels (light green). The newly formed bone is rendered in light blue. **(C)** The 3D volume of sample C is reported. The segmentation renders the vessels in red and the scaffold in blue. The soft tissues were computationally removed from the 3D rendering to highlight the vessels distribution inside the scaffold. The inset shows in red the numerous vessels crossing the soft tissue (segmented in green). **(D)** The sample D was BMSC seeded but not stained. The vessels are rendered in red, the soft tissue in yellow and green. The inset shows one of the ramified vessels in red.

very intricate matrix (rendered in green) which coexists with the vessels (red) and the newly formed bone (segmented in light blue). **Figure 2C** shows the 3D volume of sample C. The segmentation renders the vessels in red and the scaffold in blue. Since the PTA enhances the contrast of both vessels and STs, we highlighted the vessels distribution inside the scaffold, by computationally removing the STs from the 3D rendering. The inset shows, in a portion of the volume, the numerous vessels, segmented in red, crossing the ST, which is segmented in green and yellow. Finally, we report in **Figure 2D** images of sample D. Although the lack of staining makes the visualization of vessels more cumbersome, **Figure 2D** clearly demonstrates that the imaging of the vascular network without invasive treatments is doable. The vessels are rendered in red, the scaffold in blue, and the ST in yellow and green. The inset shows one of the ramified vessels. We report the 3D rendering of sample B in Video S1 in Supplementary Material.

Quantitative Analysis of Tomography Images

While **Figure 2** provides an imaging survey, **Figure 3** contains the results of the quantitative analyses. In this figure, we considered the samples A, B, C, and D. We explored a central cube volume of 1.4 mm side, for all the samples. The precision of the selected volume was assured by the precision of the experimental setup, which allowed one to always illuminate equal portions of the samples. Exploiting the 3D character of the tomographic approach, we systematically analyzed the computed sections (each 640 nm thick) of the samples, perpendicular to any chosen direction, studying the number, section, and distribution of the vessels crossing each

section. To get insights on the structure of the vascular trees in the recovered implants, we first plotted the number of vessels of the vascular network reaching the system at different depths (**Figure 3**, plot 1) and then we investigated the depth distribution of vessels with different size (**Figure 3**, plot 2).

In **Figure 3A** (sample A), we choose the direction of the large vessel entering the scaffold (appearing from zero in plot 1) and we considered the sections perpendicular to this direction. We could not follow the same approach for the B and C samples since no clear directionality was found in the networks, which seemed more isotropically distributed with high connectivity between the pores in the various directions. The plot 1 reports the total number of vessels (i.e., irrespective from their size) upon varying the depth along the chosen direction. A major difference is visible between the sample A and the other three. In the absence of mesenchymal progenitor cells (sample A), the vascular tree has a poor development and is composed of a single large vessel, which only ramifies from 400 to 800 μm in a few small vessels, before they all disappear in the sample at about 1000 μm. On the contrary, the B, C, and D samples display a wide tree of vessels with several branches covering the whole depth of about 1400 μm in **Figure 3B** and 1300 μm in **Figures 3C,D**. The broad distributions of the B, C, and D samples have similar extensions and comparable average values of vessel number.

To get higher level of detail on how vessels of different size are spatially distributed, we divided the vessels into two categories: small vessels with a diameter between 10 and 15 μm and large vessels with a diameter between 15 and 20 μm. Plot 2 reports

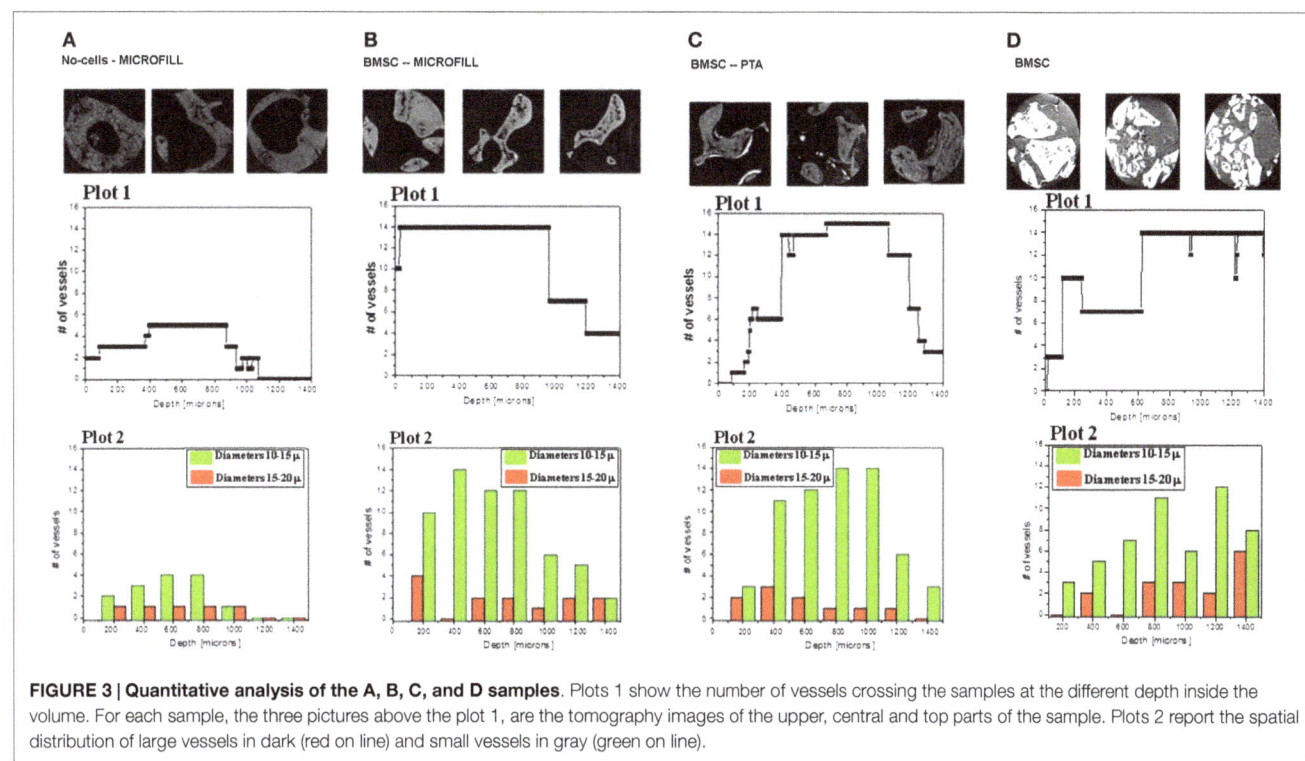

FIGURE 3 | Quantitative analysis of the A, B, C, and D samples. Plots 1 show the number of vessels crossing the samples at the different depth inside the volume. For each sample, the three pictures above the plot 1, are the tomography images of the upper, central and top parts of the sample. Plots 2 report the spatial distribution of large vessels in dark (red on line) and small vessels in gray (green on line).

the number V_m of small vessels (represented in gray) and the number V_M of large vessels (represented in black) at different depths inside the samples. Clearly, in the whole space occupied by the vascular trees of B, C, and D samples, small vessels were by far more numerous and a significant branching occurred. This analysis emphasizes even more strikingly the difference with respect to the A sample, where only one large vessel was present, which intersected the sample, crossing it for about 1 mm, and abruptly disappearing. Few small vessels occupied the first part of the sample, from 400 to 800 μm depth, and then disappeared outside this interval. The table shown in **Figure 4A** extends and summarizes the quantitative comparison of vessels in the four samples. The individual structure of the vessels was similar in the three samples because the maximal sections and the minimal diameters were comparable. Again the major difference laid in the average number of branches forming the vascular trees. The A sample was poorly ramified, while B, C, and D samples displayed thriving trees with many branches. Finally the overall flow rate of the vascular networks for the four samples, represented by the vascularization factor (VF) reported in the last line of the Table in **Figure 4A** and visualized in **Figure 4B**, showed a major difference between sample A and the other three samples. Assuming that for each vessel the blood flow is proportional to its section, this quantity is calculated as the integral of small vessels weighted by their average section ($\sim$123 μm^2) plus the integral of large vessels weighted by their average section ($\sim$240 μm^2) (the sum is then normalized by the total depth of 1400 μm).

Diffraction Analysis

Despite the high resolution of the tomographic images, some ambiguity may still be present, like in the insets of **Figure 2C** where the "hairy" region near the bone might be due to capillaries

or to collagenous bundles. To discriminate in the intricate network of "hairy" structures (in green **Figure 2**) between a capillary network and collagenous oriented fibers, XRµD scanning was already used to explore the time evolution of collagen matrix and structure during the bone mineralization process (Cedola et al., 2006). Here, we used the same technique to confirm that the intricate network was due to collagen fibers matrix. Collagen diffraction gives a broad peak around $q = 5.6$ nm^{-1}, due to the molecular lateral packing. In **Figure 5A**, we show the typical diffraction radial profiles, I(q), measured in the ST, at the ST/Bone (B) interface and in the scaffold. We could clearly observe how the collagen peak becomes more pronounced as the mineralization arises, i.e., at the ST/B interface. The orientation degree of the collagen molecules is given by the area under the peaks of the azimuthal profiles I(Φ). Typical azimuthal profiles measured in ST and at the ST/B interface, are reported in **Figure 5B**. **Figure 5C** shows a typical XRPCµCT image of the ST/B interface, while the spatial distribution of collagen amount and alignment at this interface is reported in **Figure 5D**. Specifically, the collagen amount, corresponding to the collagen peak area on each measured point, is given by the map intensity; at the same time, the collagen molecules orientation angle and orientation degree are represented by the directions and amplitudes of the black arrows, as in a vector plot. These scanning XRµD results identify the packing and alignment of the collagen molecules close to the newly formed bone far from the scaffold, well distinguished from the (micro)vessels network in the XRPCµT imaging.

Discussion

The aim of this study was to assess the effectiveness of our XRPCµT approach, combined with XRµD, to study the

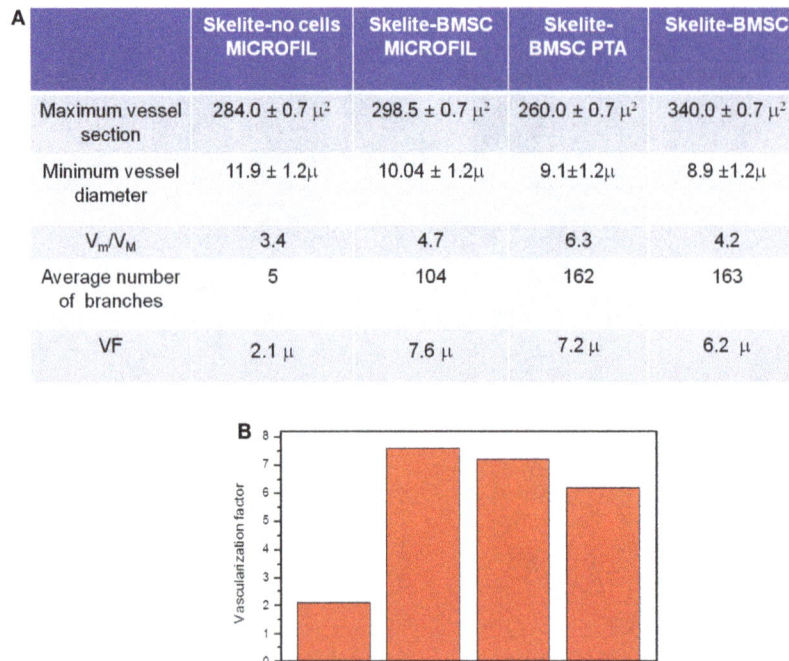

A	Skelite-no cells MICROFIL	Skelite-BMSC MICROFIL	Skelite-BMSC PTA	Skelite-BMSC
Maximum vessel section	$284.0 \pm 0.7\ \mu^2$	$298.5 \pm 0.7\ \mu^2$	$260.0 \pm 0.7\ \mu^2$	$340.0 \pm 0.7\ \mu^2$
Minimum vessel diameter	$11.9 \pm 1.2\mu$	$10.04 \pm 1.2\mu$	$9.1 \pm 1.2\mu$	$8.9 \pm 1.2\mu$
V_m/V_M	3.4	4.7	6.3	4.2
Average number of branches	5	104	162	163
VF	$2.1\ \mu$	$7.6\ \mu$	$7.2\ \mu$	$6.2\ \mu$

FIGURE 4 | (A) Table of quantitative information obtained for the A, B, C, and D samples. V_m and V_M are the total numbers of small and large vessels, respectively (see text). **(B)** Vascularization factor (see text) for the four samples.

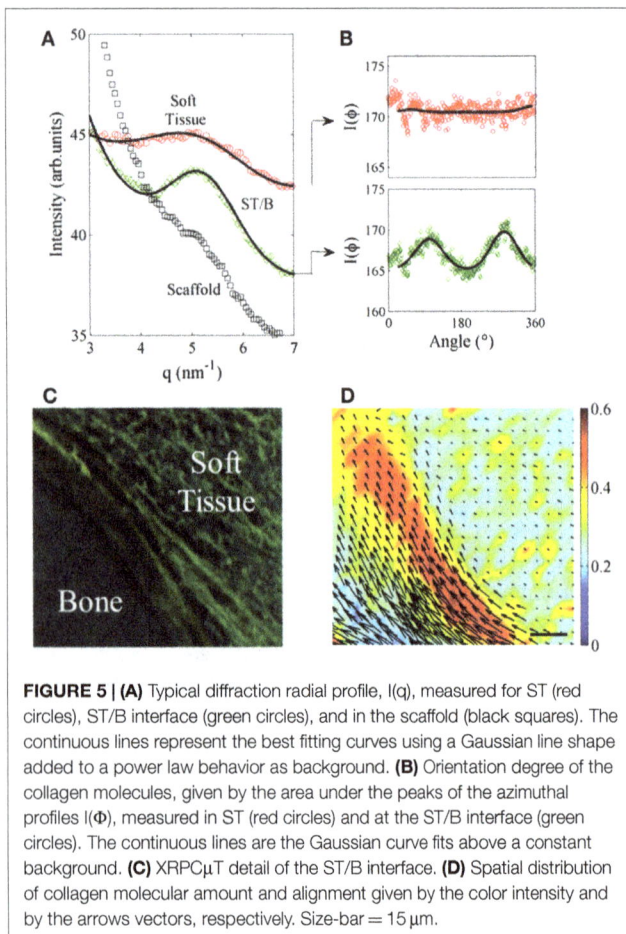

FIGURE 5 | (A) Typical diffraction radial profile, I(q), measured for ST (red circles), ST/B interface (green circles), and in the scaffold (black squares). The continuous lines represent the best fitting curves using a Gaussian line shape added to a power law behavior as background. **(B)** Orientation degree of the collagen molecules, given by the area under the peaks of the azimuthal profiles I(Φ), measured in ST (red circles) and at the ST/B interface (green circles). The continuous lines are the Gaussian curve fits above a constant background. **(C)** XRPCμT detail of the ST/B interface. **(D)** Spatial distribution of collagen molecular amount and alignment given by the color intensity and by the arrows vectors, respectively. Size-bar = 15 μm.

angiogenesis in engineered bone constructs. The understanding of the angiogenesis in bone-engineered scaffolds still remains an important goal for the regenerative medicine and to allow for the clinical application of this approach. The identification of the most appropriate scaffold for bone tissue regeneration is directly related to the ability of the scaffold to recruit osteoprogenitor cells and endothelial progenitors. On the other hand, new technologies should provide the tools for monitoring angiogenesis in the engineered scaffolds. While traditional histology provides unique insight into tissue morphology, it fails to reveal the spatial organization of the microscopic structures, unless a tedious and time-, resource-, and energy-consuming sectioning s of the whole sample – followed by histological analysis – is performed. In addition, histology and image processing inherently result in small, local tissue artifacts that can introduce errors in the determination of the microscopic tissue structure (Martin et al., 2002). Recently, some authors have demonstrated the possibility to perform an *in vivo* quantification of the vascular network in mice using contrast-enhanced micro-CT (Nebuloni et al., 2014). Although a new phase-contrast medium – the micro-bubble – was recently developed and applied to angiography applications (Tang et al., 2011), different papers have shown that XRPCT is able to perform a 3D visualization of the smallest capillaries (Momose et al., 2000; Fratini et al., 2015) in mice, without the use of any contrast agent.

Within this context, we investigated by synchrotron XRPCμT and XRμD samples that underwent different staining procedures. The first two sets were perfused by the radiopaque medium MICROFIL® (Zagorchev et al., 2010), but only one of these two sets was also seeded with BMSC. The third set was stained with PTA immediately after its explantation from the animal, while the fourth set of samples was left unstained in order to obtain evidence that the imaging of the vascular network was also possible without any previous staining treatment. We used XRPCT because the low-density soft matter making up the collagen fibrils (Campi et al., 2012) and the vessels is not visible via conventional micro-CT based on absorption (Gao et al., 1998; Momose et al., 2000). The high quality achieved for the 3D images enabled the extraction of quantitative pieces of information (number, section, and distribution of the vessels crossing each section) for all the different sample preparations.

The main goal of our work was the technical achievement of 3D imaging of a vascular network. This clearly demonstrated and quantitatively analyzed in the samples where this vascularization was present. Moreover, our data also suggest that seeding the scaffolds with BMSC enforces the vascularization. The major difference lies in the average number of branches forming the vascular trees. The sample not seeded with BMSC was poorly ramified, while the other three samples displayed thriving trees with many branches. It is important to emphasize that the histological studies performed on samples unseeded with cells, show a poor vascularization (Figure S1 in Supplementary Material).

Even though XRPCT was able to visualize the 3D vascularization network inside the scaffold without any sample sectioning and preparation, in order to achieve a higher image quality with sub-micrometer spatial resolution, the use of a coherent, highly brilliant X-ray Synchrotron source was mandatory. This could certainly limit a possible future use of this technique in the clinical routine, but remains a highly valuable experimental approach in pre-clinical researches such as those involving investigation of different scaffold vascularization.

Once the capability of this technique has been established, the way is paved for a wealth of further investigations and more firm biological conclusions can be drawn with more extensive analyses and statistics. In this regard, an obvious future work will be the comparative analysis of different types of scaffolds with different implantation times. We therefore propose our approach as a tool for angiogenesis studies in TE and for any other pre-clinical investigations where the quantitative analysis of the vascular network is required.

Acknowledgments

We are grateful to Peter Modregger from the staff of SLS-PSI, Villigen, Switzerland for experimental help. MG acknowledges financial support from "AWARDS Projects" of the University of Rome Sapienza, n. C26H13KZS9.

References

Bravin, A., Coan, P., and Suortti, P. (2013). X-ray phase-contrast imaging: from pre-clinical applications towards clinics. *Phys. Med. Biol.* 58, R1–R35. doi:10.1088/0031-9155/58/1/R1

Campi, G., Pezzotti, G., Fratini, M., Ricci, A., Burghammer, M., Cancedda, R., et al. (2013). Imaging regenerating bone tissue based on neural networks applied to micro-diffraction measurements. *Appl. Phys. Lett.* 103, 253703. doi:10.1063/1.4852056

Campi, G., Ricci, A., Guagliardi, A., Giannini, C., Lagomarsino, S., Cancedda, R., et al. (2012). Early stage mineralization in tissue engineering mapped by high resolution X-ray microdiffraction. *Acta Biomater.* 8, 3411–3418. doi:10.1016/j.actbio.2012.05.034

Cancedda, R., Dozin, B., Giannoni, P., and Quarto, R. (2003). Tissue engineering and cell therapy of cartilage and bone. *Matrix Biol.* 22, 81–91. doi:10.1016/S0945-053X(03)00012-X

Carano, R. A. D., and Filvaroff, E. H. (2003). Angiogenesis and bone repair. *Drug Discov. Today* 8, 980–989. doi:10.1016/S1359-6446(03)02866-6

Cedola, A., Campi, G., Pelliccia, D., Bukreeva, I., Fratini, M., Burghammer, M., et al. (2014). Three dimensional visualization of engineered bone and soft tissue by combined x-ray micro-diffraction and phase contrast tomography. *Phys. Med. Biol.* 59, 189–201. doi:10.1088/0031-9155/59/1/189

Cedola, A., Mastrogiacomo, M., Burghammer, M., Komlev, V., Giannoni, P., Favia, A., et al. (2006). Engineered bone from bone marrow stromal cells: a structural study by an advanced x-ray microdiffraction technique. *Phys. Med. Biol.* 51, N109–N116. doi:10.1088/0031-9155/51/6/N02

Cloetens, P., Barrett, R., Baruchel, J., Guigay, J.-P., and Schlenker, M. (1996). Phase objects in synchrotron radiation hard x-ray imaging. *J. Phys. D Appl. Phys.* 29, 133–146. doi:10.1088/0022-3727/29/1/023

Descamps, E., Sochacka, A., De Kegel, B., Van Loo, D., Van Hoorebeke, L., and Adriaens, D. (2014). Soft tissue discrimination with contrast agents using micro-CT scanning. *Belg. J. Zool.* 144, 20–40.

Di Fonzo, S., Jark, W., Soullié, G., Cedola, A., Lagomarsino, S., Cloetens, P., et al. (1998). Submicrometre resolution phase-contrast radiography with the beam from an X-ray waveguide. *J. Synchrotron Radiat.* 5, 376–378. doi:10.1107/S0909049597019250

Diemoz, P. C., Bravin, A., Langer, M., and Coan, P. (2012). Analytical and experimental determination of signal-to-noise ratio and figure of merit in three phase-contrast imaging techniques. *Opt. Express* 20, 27670–27690. doi:10.1364/OE.20.027670

Ehling, J., Theek, B., Gremse, F., Baetke, S., Möckel, D., Maynard, J., et al. (2014). Micro-CT imaging of tumor angiogenesis: quantitative measures describing micromorphology and vascularization. *Am. J. Pathol.* 184, 431–441. doi:10.1016/j.ajpath.2013.10.014

Fratini, M., Bukreeva, I., Campi, G., Brun, F., Tromba, G., Modregger, P., et al. (2015). Simultaneous submicrometric 3D imaging of the micro-vascular network and the neuronal system in a mouse spinal cord. *Sci. Rep.* 5, 8514. doi:10.1038/srep08514

Gao, D., Pogany, A., Stevenson, A. W., and Wilkins, S. W. (1998). Phase-contrast radiography. *Radiographics* 18, 1257–1267. doi:10.1148/radiographics.18.5.9747618

Giacovazzo, C., Monaco, H. L., Viterbo, F., Scordari, G., Gilli, G., Zanotti, G., et al. (1993). Fundamentals of crystallography. IUCr texts on crystallography no. 2. *Acta Crystallogr. A Found. Crystallogr.* 49, 373–374. doi:10.1107/S0108767392012285

Hench, L. L., and Polak, J. M. (2002). Third-generation biomedical materials. *Science* 295, 1014–1017. doi:10.1126/science.1067404

Jain, R. K. (2003). Molecular regulation of vessel maturation. *Nat. Med.* 9, 685–693. doi:10.1038/nm0603-685

Komlev, V. S., Peyrin, F., Mastrogiacomo, M., Cedola, A., Papadimitropoulos, A., Rustichelli, F., et al. (2006). Kinetics of in vivo bone deposition by bone marrow stromal cells into porous calcium phosphate scaffolds: an X-ray computed microtomography study. *Tissue Eng.* 12, 3449–3458. doi:10.1089/ten.2006.12.3449

Martin, I., Mastrogiacomo, M., De Leo, G., Muraglia, A., Beltrame, F., Cancedda, R., et al. (2002). Fluorescence microscopy imaging of bone for automated histomorphometry. *Tissue Eng.* 8, 847–852. doi:10.1089/10763270260424204

Martin, I., Muraglia, A., Campanile, G., Cancedda, R., and Quarto, R. (1997). Fibroblast growth factor-2 supports ex vivo expansion and maintenance of osteogenic precursors from human bone marrow. *Endocrinology* 138, 4456–4462. doi:10.1210/en.138.10.4456

Mastrogiacomo, M., Papadimitropoulos, A., Cedola, A., Peyrin, F., Giannoni, P., Pearce, S. G., et al. (2007). Engineering of bone using bone marrow stromal cells and a silicon-stabilized tricalcium phosphate bioceramic: evidence for a coupling between bone formation and scaffold resorption. *Biomaterials* 28, 1376–1384. doi:10.1016/j.biomaterials.2006.10.001

Momose, A., Takeda, T., and Itai, Y. (2000). Blood vessels: depiction at phase-contrast X-ray imaging without contrast agents in the mouse and rat-feasibility study. *Radiology* 217, 593–596. doi:10.1148/radiology.217.2.r00oc14593

Nebuloni, L., Kuhn, G. A., Vogel, J., and Müller, R. (2014). A novel in vivo vascular imaging approach for hierarchical quantification of vasculature using contrast enhanced micro-computed tomography. *PLoS ONE* 9:e86562. doi:10.1371/journal.pone.0086562

Paganin, D., Mayo, S. C., Gureyev, T. E., Miller, P. R., and Wilkins, S. W. (2002). Simultaneous phase and amplitude extraction from a single defocused image of a homogeneous object. *J. Microsc.* 206, 33–40. doi:10.1046/j.1365-2818.2002.01010.x

Plouraboue, F., Cloetens, P., Fonta, C., Steyer, A., Lauwers, F., and Marc-Vergnes, J.-P. (2004). X-ray high-resolution vascular network imaging. *J. Microsc.* 215, 139–148. doi:10.1111/j.0022-2720.2004.01362.x

Quarto, R., Mastrogiacomo, M., Cancedda, R., Kutepov, S. M., Mukhachev, V., Lavroukov, A., et al. (2001). Repair of large bone defects with the use of autologous bone marrow stromal cells. *N. Engl. J. Med.* 344, 385–386. doi:10.1056/NEJM200102013440516

Risser, L., Plouraboué, F., Steyer, A., Cloetens, P., Le Duc, G., and Fonta, C. (2007). From homogeneous to fractal normal and tumorous microvascular networks in the brain. *J. Cereb. Blood Flow Metab.* 27, 293–303. doi:10.1038/sj.jcbfm.9600332

Tang, R., Xi, Y., Chai, W.-M., Wang, Y., Guan, Y., Yang, G.-Y., et al. (2011). Microbubble-based synchrotron radiation phase contrast imaging: basic study and angiography applications. *Phys. Med. Biol.* 56, 3503–3512. doi:10.1088/0031-9155/56/12/004

Zagorchev, L., Oses, P., Zhuang, Z. W., Moodie, K., Mulligan-Kehoe, M. J., Simons, M., et al. (2010). Micro computed tomography for vascular exploration. *J. Angiogenes. Res.* 2, 7. doi:10.1186/2040-2384-2-7

Conflict of Interest Statement: The authors declare that the research was conducted in the absence of any commercial or financial relationships that could be construed as a potential conflict of interest.

Permissions

All chapters in this book were first published in FBIOE, by Frontiers; hereby published with permission under the Creative Commons Attribution License or equivalent. Every chapter published in this book has been scrutinized by our experts. Their significance has been extensively debated. The topics covered herein carry significant findings which will fuel the growth of the discipline. They may even be implemented as practical applications or may be referred to as a beginning point for another development.

The contributors of this book come from diverse backgrounds, making this book a truly international effort. This book will bring forth new frontiers with its revolutionizing research information and detailed analysis of the nascent developments around the world.

We would like to thank all the contributing authors for lending their expertise to make the book truly unique. They have played a crucial role in the development of this book. Without their invaluable contributions this book wouldn't have been possible. They have made vital efforts to compile up to date information on the varied aspects of this subject to make this book a valuable addition to the collection of many professionals and students.

This book was conceptualized with the vision of imparting up-to-date information and advanced data in this field. To ensure the same, a matchless editorial board was set up. Every individual on the board went through rigorous rounds of assessment to prove their worth. After which they invested a large part of their time researching and compiling the most relevant data for our readers.

The editorial board has been involved in producing this book since its inception. They have spent rigorous hours researching and exploring the diverse topics which have resulted in the successful publishing of this book. They have passed on their knowledge of decades through this book. To expedite this challenging task, the publisher supported the team at every step. A small team of assistant editors was also appointed to further simplify the editing procedure and attain best results for the readers.

Apart from the editorial board, the designing team has also invested a significant amount of their time in understanding the subject and creating the most relevant covers. They scrutinized every image to scout for the most suitable representation of the subject and create an appropriate cover for the book.

The publishing team has been an ardent support to the editorial, designing and production team. Their endless efforts to recruit the best for this project, has resulted in the accomplishment of this book. They are a veteran in the field of academics and their pool of knowledge is as vast as their experience in printing. Their expertise and guidance has proved useful at every step. Their uncompromising quality standards have made this book an exceptional effort. Their encouragement from time to time has been an inspiration for everyone.

The publisher and the editorial board hope that this book will prove to be a valuable piece of knowledge for researchers, students, practitioners and scholars across the globe.

List of Contributors

T. S. Sampath Kumar and K. Madhumathi
Medical Materials Laboratory, Department of Metallurgical and Materials Engineering, Indian Institute of Technology Madras, Chennai, India

Y. Rubaiya and Mukesh Doble
Department of Biotechnology, Indian Institute of Technology Madras, Chennai, India

Marietta Herrmann, Sophie Verrier and Mauro Alini
AO Research Institute Davos, Davos, Switzerland

Amy H. Van Hove
Department of Biomedical Engineering, University of Rochester, Rochester, NY, USA

Danielle S. W. Benoit
Department of Biomedical Engineering, University of Rochester, Rochester, NY, USA
Department of Chemical Engineering, University of Rochester, Rochester, NY, USA
Department of Biomedical Genetics, University of Rochester Medical Center, Rochester, NY, USA
Department of Orthopaedics, Center for Musculoskeletal Research, University of Rochester Medical Center, Rochester, NY, USA

Shane Browne and Abhay Pandit
Network of Excellence for Functional Biomaterials (NFB), National University of Ireland, Galway, Ireland

Elena Boccardi, Anahí Philippart, Judith A. Juhasz-Bortuzzo and Aldo R. Boccaccini
Institute of Biomaterials, Department of Materials Science and Engineering, Friedrich-Alexander University Erlangen- Nürnberg, Erlangen, Germany

Ana M. Beltrán and Erdmann Spiecker
Center for Nanoanalysis and Electron Microscopy (CENEM), Institute of Micro- and Nanostructure Research, Department of Materials Science and Engineering, Friedrich-Alexander University Erlangen-Nürnberg, Erlangen, Germany

Giorgia Novajra and Chiara Vitale-Brovarone
Institute of Materials Physics and Engineering, Applied Science and Technology Department, Politecnico di Torino, Turin, Italy

Antonietta R. Silini, Anna Cargnoni, Marta Magatti, Stefano Pianta and Ornella Parolini
Centro di Ricerca "E. Menni", Fondazione Poliambulanza Istituto Ospedaliero, Brescia, Italy

Christian Claude Lachaud, Abdelkrim Hmadcha and Bernat Soria
Andalusian Center for Molecular Biology and Regenerative Medicine – Centro Andaluz de Biología Molecular y Medicina Regenerativa (CABIMER), Seville, Spain
Centro de Investigación en Red sobre Diabetes y Enfermedades Metabólicas (CIBERDEM), Madrid, Spain

Berta Rodriguez-Campins
Departamento de I+D, New Biotechnic S.A., Seville, Spain
Fundación Andaluza de Investigación y Desarrollo (FAID), Seville, Spain

Aaron X. Sun
Center for Cellular and Molecular Engineering, Department of Orthopaedic Surgery, University of Pittsburgh School of Medicine, Pittsburgh, PA, USA
Medical Scientist Training Program, University of Pittsburgh School of Medicine, Pittsburgh, PA, USA

Hang Lin
Center for Cellular and Molecular Engineering, Department of Orthopaedic Surgery, University of Pittsburgh School of Medicine, Pittsburgh, PA, USA

Angela M. Beck, Evan J. Kilroy and Rocky S. Tuan
Center for Cellular and Molecular Engineering, Department of Orthopaedic Surgery, University of Pittsburgh School of Medicine, Pittsburgh, PA, USA
Department of Bioengineering, University of Pittsburgh Swanson School of Engineering, Pittsburgh,PA, USA

Vikram Rao, Yu-Ru V. Shih, Harsha Kabra and Shyni Varghese
Department of Bioengineering, University of California San Diego, La Jolla, CA, USA

Heemin Kang
Materials Science and Engineering Program, University of California San Diego, La Jolla, CA, USA

Anne M. Leferink, Clemens A. van Blitterswijk and Lorenzo Moroni
Department of Tissue Regeneration, MIRA Institute, University of Twente, Enschede, Netherlands
Department of Complex Tissue Regeneration, Faculty of Health, Medicine and Life Sciences, Maastricht University, Maastricht, Netherlands

Yhee-Cheng Chng
Quintech Life Sciences Pte Ltd., Singapore, Singapore

Vineet Gupta
Bioengineering Graduate Program, University of Kansas, Lawrence, KS, USA

Neethu Mohan
Division of Tissue Engineering and Regeneration Technologies, Biomedical Technology Wing, Sree Chitra Tirunal Institute for Medical Sciences and Technology, Trivandrum, India

Cory J. Berkland
Bioengineering Graduate Program, University of Kansas, Lawrence, KS, USA
Department of Pharmaceutical Chemistry, University of Kansas, Lawrence, KS, USA

Michael S. Detamore
Bioengineering Graduate Program, University of Kansas, Lawrence, KS, USA
Department of Chemical and Petroleum Engineering, University of Kansas, Lawrence, KS, USA

José Ballester-Beltrán and Manuel Salmerón-Sánchez
Division of Biomedical Engineering, School of Engineering, University of Glasgow, Glasgow, UK

Manus J. P. Biggs and Aldo Leal-Egaña
Network of Excellence for Functional Biomaterials, National University of Ireland, Galway, Ireland

Matthew J. Dalby
Institute of Molecular, Cell and Systems Biology, University of Glasgow, Glasgow, UK

Francesco Baino, Giorgia Novajra and Chiara Vitale-Brovarone
Department of Applied Science and Technology, Institute of Materials Physics and Engineering, Politecnico di Torino, Turin, Italy

Shinya Yamada, Akiko Obata, Hirotaka Maeda and Toshihiro Kasuga
Department of Frontier Materials, Graduate School of Engineering, Nagoya Institute of Technology, Nagoya, Japan

Yoshio Ota
Yabashi Industries Co., Ltd., Ogaki, Japan

Daniele Tartarini
Department of Mechanical Engineering, Insigneo Institute for in silico Medicine, University of Sheffield, Sheffield, UK

Elisa Mele
Department of Materials, Loughborough University, Loughborough, UK

Kristin Hauff
Department of Biophysical Chemistry, Institute of Physical Chemistry, University of Heidelberg, Heidelberg, Germany
Applied Chemistry, University of Reutlingen, Reutlingen, Germany

Chiara Zambarda, Maria Halbig, Rebecca Medda and Elisabetta Ada Cavalcanti-Adam
Department of Biophysical Chemistry, Institute of Physical Chemistry, University of Heidelberg, Heidelberg, Germany
Department of New Materials and Biosystems, Max Planck Institute for Intelligent Systems, Stuttgart, Germany

Miriam Dietrich and Anna Luise Grab
Department of Biophysical Chemistry, Institute of Physical Chemistry, University of Heidelberg, Heidelberg, Germany

Vladimir S. Komlev, Alexander Yu. Fedotov, Anastasia Yu. Teterina and Igor V. Smirnov
A.A. Baikov Institute of Metallurgy and Materials Science, Russian Academy of Sciences, Moscow, Russia

Vladimir K. Popov and Anton V. Mironov
Institute of Laser and Information Technologies, Russian Academy of Sciences, Moscow, Russia

Ilya Y. Bozo
Human Stem Cells Institute, Moscow, Russia
A.I. Evdokimov Moscow State University of Medicine and Dentistry, Moscow, Russia
A.I. Burnazyan Federal Medical Biophysical Center of FMBA of Russia, Moscow, Russia

Vera A. Rybko
Institute of Carcinogenesis, N.N. Blokhin Russian Cancer Research Center, Moscow, Russia

Roman V. Deev
Kazan Federal University, Kazan, Russia

Holger Koch
Translational Centre for Regenerative Medicine (TRM), University of Leipzig, Leipzig, Germany

Niels Hammer
Institute of Anatomy, Faculty of Medicine, University of Leipzig, Leipzig, Germany

Susann Ossmann
Heart Center, Clinic for Cardiac Surgery, University of Leipzig, Leipzig, Germany

Katrin Schierle
Institute of Pathology, University of Leipzig, Leipzig, Germany

Ulrich Sack and Andreas Boldt
Translational Centre for Regenerative Medicine (TRM), University of Leipzig, Leipzig, Germany
Institute for Clinical Immunology, Faculty of Medicine, University of Leipzig, Leipzig, Germany

Jörg Hofmann and Mike Wecks
Institut für Nichtklassische Chemie e. V., Leipzig, Germany

Inna Bukreeva and Alessia Cedola
Consiglio Nazionale delle Ricerche – Istituto NANOTEC, c/o Dipartimento di Fisica, Università Sapienza, Rome, Italy

Michela Fratini
Consiglio Nazionale delle Ricerche – Istituto NANOTEC, c/o Dipartimento di Fisica, Università Sapienza, Rome, Italy
Department of Science, Roma Tre University, Rome, Italy

Gaetano Campi
Istituto di Cristallografia, Consiglio Nazionale delle Ricerche, Rome, Italy

Daniele Pelliccia
School of Applied Sciences, RMIT University, Melbourne, VIC, Australia
Australian Synchrotron, Clayton, VIC, Australia
School of Physics and Astronomy, Monash University, Clayton, VIC, Australia

Raffaele Spanò, Ranieri Cancedda and Maddalena Mastrogiacomo
Dipartimento di Medicina Sperimentale dell'Università di Genova, AOU San Martino-IST, Genova, Italy

Giuliana Tromba
Elettra – Synchrotron Radiation Trieste S.C.p.A, Trieste, Italy

Francesco Brun
Elettra – Synchrotron Radiation Trieste S.C.p.A, Trieste, Italy
Dipartimento di Ingegneria e Architettura, Università di Trieste, Trieste, Italy

Manfred Burghammer
European Synchrotron Radiation Facility, Grenoble, France
Department of Analytical Chemistry, Ghent University, Ghent, Belgium

Marco Grilli
Dipartimento di Fisica, Università Sapienza, Rome, Italy
Consiglio Nazionale delle Ricerche – Istituto dei Sistemi Complessi, c/o Dipartimento di Fisica, Università Sapienza, Rome, Italy

www.ingramcontent.com/pod-product-compliance
Lightning Source LLC
Chambersburg PA
CBHW080515200326
41458CB00012B/4211